Becoming a Nurse

The guidelines and skills required to become a nurse are always changing and it can be difficult to stay up-to-date with the current standards. This book has been specifically designed to address the main skills you need to meet NMC requirements.

Becoming a Nurse will demystify what you need to know, while preparing you to meet NMC standards and become a confident, practising professional. The book introduces the many subjects outside the biological, which are none the less essential for both pre-registration and practising nurses. This new edition has been thoroughly updated throughout, and includes four new chapters on psychological concepts for nursing; sociological concepts for nursing; spiritual care; and preceptorship and transition. Like the previous edition the book also covers:

- law, ethics and policy;
- management and leadership;
- communication, interpersonal skills and interprofessional working;
- evidence-based practice;
- medicines management;
- public health; and
- professional development.

Each chapter is packed full of case studies, discussion questions and further readings to encourage critical thinking and reflection. It is an excellent resource to prepare you for your programme or to refresh your knowledge of NMC standards.

Derek Sellman is Associate Professor, Faculty of Nursing, University of Alberta, Canada. Derek's interests include education for professional practice, health care ethics, and philosophy of nursing. Derek is editor of the journal *Nursing Philosophy*.

Paul Snelling is a Principal Lecturer at the University of Worcester, UK, where he teaches on the BSc Nursing programme. Paul's research interests are in philosophy and ethics of nursing practice and professional regulation.

Becoming a Nurse

Fundamentals of professional practice for nursing

Second edition

Edited by
Derek Sellman and Paul Snelling

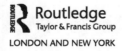

Routledge
Taylor & Francis Group

LONDON AND NEW YORK

Second edition published 2017
by Routledge
2 Park Square, Milton Park, Abingdon, Oxon OX14 4RN

and by Routledge
711 Third Avenue, New York, NY 10017

Routledge is an imprint of the Taylor & Francis Group, an informa business

First edition published by Routledge in 2009

British Library Cataloguing-in-Publication Data
A catalogue record for this book is available from the British Library

Library of Congress Cataloging in Publication Data
Names: Sellman, Derek, editor. | Snelling, Paul, editor. |
Sellman, Derek. Becoming a nurse. Preceded by (work):
Title: Becoming a nurse : fundamentals of professional practice for nursing / edited by Derek Sellman and Paul Snelling.
Other titles: Becoming a nurse (Sellman)
Description: Second edition. | Abingdon, Oxon ; New York, NY : Routledge, 2017. |
Preceded by Becoming a nurse / Derek Sellman and Paul Snelling. 2010.
| Includes bibliographical references and index.
Identifiers: LCCN 2016013293| ISBN 9780415734042 (hardback) |
ISBN 9780273786214 (pbk.) | ISBN 9781315693439 (ebook)
Subjects: | MESH: Nursing | Nurse's Role | Vocational Guidance
Classification: LCC RT42 | NLM WY 16 | DDC 610.73—dc23
LC record available at http://lccn.loc.gov/2016013293

ISBN: 978-0-415-73404-2 (hbk)
ISBN: 978-0-273-78621-4 (pbk)
ISBN: 978-1-315-69343-9 (ebk)

Typeset in Goudy
by Florence Production Ltd, Stoodleigh, Devon, UK

*For Louise and Imogen for their continued
forbearance and love.*

*For Mum with love and thanks,
and in grateful memory of John Snelling.*

CONTENTS

Contents

Contents

Contents

FIGURES

TABLES

CONTRIBUTORS

Mark Broom PhD, RSCN, RGN, Academic Subject Manager – Family Care, Faculty of Life Sciences and Education, University of South Wales. Mark's interests are in promoting high-quality care for acutely ill children, clinical reasoning and the use of IT in nurse education.

Julie Bugler, Lecturer/Clinician, Faculty of Health and Applied Sciences, University of the West of England. Julie has been a registered nurse for people with learning disabilities for almost 30 years and has spent the last 13 years working as a community nurse for children with learning disabilities. Her passion lies in hearing and enabling the 'voice' of service users and has developed an award-winning participation group in the NHS.

Janice Clarke is a Senior Lecturer at the University of Worcester. She is a qualified nurse and her doctoral research about spirituality and nursing has led to publication of a number of papers and conference presentations, which have focused on developing a practical, relational way to improve the overall quality of nursing care by using the principles of spirituality.

Gerard Clinton is a Registered Psychiatric Nurse attached to the School of Nursing and Human Sciences at Dublin City University. He has worked as a researcher and lecturer, and used conversation and discursive analysis strategies in his PhD thesis to study how mental health nurses talk about judgements and decisions.

David Cudlip spent his time prior to being a nurse working as an archaeologist and playing in a number of noisy and inept bands. He didn't find any gold or get on television. Since training as an adult nurse in his late thirties, he has worked in a Minor Injuries Unit and is now a rapid response practitioner in Gloucestershire.

Stephen Evans MA, PGDipOT, BSc (Hons), Associate Head of Department, Radiography and Occupational Therapy, Faculty of Health and Applied Sciences, University of the West of England. Stephen's current interests are in inclusive design in the built environment and the social model of disability.

Daniel Farrelly is a Senior Lecturer in Psychology at the University of Worcester. His research interests include the evolutionary origins of human behaviours such as cooperation, competition (including the role of testosterone) and cognition, as well as emotional intelligence and its links with other psychological traits.

Claire Fullbrook-Scanlon RGN RHV MSc PGCertEd BSc (Hons) is Matron for Stroke and Neurology, lead stroke nurse and non-medical prescribing lead at the Royal United Hospital Foundation Trust, Bath. Claire is also a Senior Lecturer at University of the West of England. Her professional interests include all aspects of the stroke care pathway and stroke care in Ghana, West Africa.

Contributors

Cathryn Havard MSc BA (Hons) RN, FETC is Senior Lecturer in Nursing, Department of Nursing and Midwifery, University of the West of England. Cathryn teaches nursing management and leadership and facilitates other aspects of student learning within the pre-registration curriculum. Her interests and research activities relate to the ongoing professional development of nurses in a range of health care settings and the facilitation of work-based learning projects in her specialist practice area of cancer care.

Sally Hayes, Senior Nurse Lecturer, Faculty of Health and Applied Sciences, University of the West of England. Sally worked in the past as a Heart Failure Specialist Nurse in the Gloucestershire Heart Failure Service, and more recently as a Clinical Nurse Specialist in Palliative Care at Gloucester Royal Hospital, before commencing as senior lecturer focusing on end of life care and non-medical prescribing.

Janet Holt PhD, MPhil, BA (Hons), FHEA, RGN, RM is a Senior Lecturer in the School of Healthcare at the University of Leeds. She is Chair of the Royal College of Nursing Ethics Committee and represents the RCN on the Ethics Committee of the British Medical Association. Janet is also a member of the Editorial Board for the journal *Nursing Philosophy*, a consultant editor for the journal *Nursing Ethics* and is currently Chair of the International Philosophy of Nursing Society.

Clare Hopkinson PhD, MSc, BA (Hons), RN, Senior Lecturer, Adult Nursing, Faculty of Health and Applied Sciences, University of the West of England. Clare has over 20 years' experience of facilitating critically reflexive action inquiry groups working with a variety of professional disciplines predominately in the NHS. Her interests include service improvement through critically reflexive practice, arts and health, collaborative action research, and the emotional cost of caring.

Victoria Lavender, MA (Phil), BA (Hons), RMN, former Senior Lecturer in Mental Health Nursing at the University of the West of England. Victoria has worked as a mental health nurse. Her areas of interest are the mental health of women and the history of mental health care provision.

Pádraig MacNeela is a Lecturer and Director of PhD Studies at the School of Psychology, National University of Ireland, Galway. Pádraig has studied judgement and decision-making with particular reference to psychosocial, informal and organisational dimensions of health care. He also works in the field of youth research, in areas such as sexual health, gender and alcohol use.

Elaine Mahoney MSc, RSCN, RGN, Senior Lecturer, Faculty of Life Sciences and Education, University of South Wales. Elaine's interests are in family-centred care and all aspects of nursing children.

Margaret Miers, PhD, RN, retired from her role as Professor of Nursing and Social Science at the University of the West of England, in 2010. Her research interests include the evaluation of interprofessional learning and she is co-editor of Palgrave's 2010 text *Understanding Interprofessional Working in Health and Social Care: Theory and Practice*.

Katherine Pollard, Senior Research Fellow, Faculty of Health and Applied Sciences, University of the West of England. Katherine worked as a midwife in the NHS before embarking on a research career. Her areas of interest include interprofessional issues, workforce development and service delivery in health and social care.

David Pontin, RN, RSCPHN, PhD, Aneurin Bevan Chair of Community Health. David has worked in a number of senior leadership roles in the NHS in England and Wales, and in the university sector. He is currently a Professor at the School of Care Sciences, Faculty of Life Sciences and Education, University of South Wales.

P. Anne Scott is Professor and Vice President for Equality and Diversity, National University of Ireland, Galway. Anne is a nurse and philosopher. Her main research interests are in the philosophy and ethics of health care and in judgement and decision-making.

Derek Sellman, PhD, RN, Associate Professor, Faculty of Nursing, University of Alberta, Canada. Derek's interests include education for professional practice, health care ethics and philosophy of nursing. Derek is editor of the journal *Nursing Philosophy*.

Iain Snelling is a Senior Fellow at the Health Services Management Centre (HSMC), University of Birmingham. He is a tutor on the Elizabeth Garrett Anderson programme, one of the NHS Leadership Academy's suite of leadership development programmes, and leads HSMC's Leadership for Health Services Improvement programme. For 14 years until 2002 he was a general manager in a number of NHS acute hospitals.

Paul Snelling is a Principal Lecturer at the University of Worcester, where he teaches on the BSc Nursing programme. His research interests are in philosophy and ethics of nursing practice and professional regulation.

Jane Tarr, PhD, formerly Principal Lecturer, School of Education, University of the West of England. She is currently training to be a music therapist working with vulnerable young people who have been traumatised early in their lives. She is leading on a professional development programme for teachers funded through the European Union ERASMUS +. Her work supports collaborative working practice between teachers and therapists to build the well-being of vulnerable young people and support them in their learning.

Jane Thomas, Professor and Director of the Swansea Academy of Learning and Teaching (SALT) and institutional lead on Learning and Teaching at Swansea University. Jane has a working background in primary care and public health and was responsible for establishing postgraduate provision in this area at Swansea. She links with Public Health Wales and is an assessor for the United Kingdom Public Health Register.

Richard Thomas is a Senior Lecturer in the Faculty of Health and Applied Sciences, School of Nursing and Midwifery at the University of the West of England. He is a registered nurse with experience in adult intensive care and teaches Nursing and Healthcare Law at pre- and post-registration levels.

Jackie Younker, RN, MSN, PGCertEd, formerly Senior Lecturer in Adult Nursing at the University of the West of England. She has returned to clinical practice as an advanced nurse practitioner in cardiac surgery. Her areas of interest include advanced practice nursing, critical care and resuscitation education.

1

Introduction

The state of UK nursing

Paul Snelling and Derek Sellman

INTRODUCTION

Keeping abreast of developments in the environment in which nursing has to practise can be very difficult. As editors of a textbook we are acutely aware of how quickly things go out of date, and so how unwise it might seem even to attempt to write an introductory chapter about contemporary nursing practice. Looking back to 2009 when the first edition of this book was published, we can see how much things have changed. The introductory section was finished on New Year's Day in 2009 at a time when the global economic crisis was in full swing, with vast sums of money being printed and given to the banks. But as anyone who gets a loan will tell you, it's only when you have to start paying it back that the consequences become real.

The first edition pre-dated the general election of 2010, which returned, for the first time in many years, no overall majority, and 5 years of Conservative/Liberal Democrat coalition government followed which presided over a strategy to reduce the budgetary deficit prioritising austerity. Even though it was claimed that the health budget would be protected, in reality the spending power of the budget was reduced because costs increase at a higher rate than 'protected' funds. In 2015 the Conservative Party was returned to power and austerity is set to continue for this parliament. Not only does this mean that pay restraint, which has seen the salaries of public servants including most nurses reduce significantly in real terms, seems likely to continue, but the financial climate and changing patterns of disease will continue to pressurise core services of the NHS and other care services. The professional practice of nurses and other health care professionals will inevitably be undertaken in this extremely challenging financial environment for the foreseeable future.

The other major development in the time since the first edition is the publication of the two Francis Reports into the events at Mid-Staffordshire Foundation NHS Trust. (The name of the hospital was Stafford Hospital, and often is abbreviated to 'Mid-Staffs'). These reports investigated a catalogue of poor care, which may have resulted in the deaths of many patients. The alarm bells were rung by statistical data, which showed that more deaths than might have been expected occurred. The inquiry reports were published in 2010 and 2013, and their findings and subsequent responses from a range of bodies continue to have a profound effect on professional practice. This is a common theme running through this book. Politics on a grand scale is important of course, but not everyone is interested in Westminster debates and machinations. However, the results of financial squeezing and the renewed (perhaps rhetorical) emphasis on patient safety constitute a tension between cost and quality, which constrains every nurse's practice. This introductory chapter introduces recent developments in the professional practice of nursing and nursing education.

THE EVENTS AT MID-STAFFORDSHIRE FOUNDATION NHS TRUST

The events at Mid-Staffordshire Foundation NHS Trust were seminal in the development of health care policy and the professional practice of nursing. In 2007, concerns were raised about mortality rates at the Trust when compared with other similar hospitals. Despite the hospital being rated as 'good to fair' in the Healthcare Commission's annual check, the Dr Foster guide showed that the Trust had a higher than average Hospital Standardised Mortality Ratio (HSMR – see Box 1.1). The Healthcare Commission, the regulator at the time, considered the response of the Trust to the high mortality to be inadequate and launched an investigation (Healthcare Commission 2009), which was critical of the Trust.

At about the same time public anger about the care delivered at the hospital grew, co-ordinated by a group called Cure the NHS (Bailey 2012), set up by Julie Bailey, whose mother died in Stafford Hospital. Ms Bailey, who was subsequently awarded a CBE in 2014, and her group became influential and vociferous, and the press maintained a keen interest. Cure the NHS pressed for a full public inquiry into the Trust's failing and the wider NHS. Further reviews were commissioned on specific aspects of the care at Mid-Staffs, but none satisfied public concerns. Still there was to be no full public inquiry, but the Labour Government decided to set up an Independent Inquiry under the chairmanship of Robert Francis QC, as he then was (he became Sir Robert Francis in 2014). The two-volume report was published in February 2010. This report is sometimes referred to as the first Francis Report (Francis 2010) and its findings were wide ranging. The picture painted was of a failing yet complacent organisation, with poor leadership and where the focus of activity was directed at financial control rather than clinical outcomes. Nursing staff were noted to be demoralised and 'many had adopted a survival strategy of going through the motions of doing their job as opposed to pursuing a much valued and necessary vocation' (Francis 2010, p. 412). The letter from Mr Francis to the Secretary of State, which introduced the report, concluded that:

> If there is one lesson to be learnt, I suggest that it is that people must always come before numbers. It is the individual experiences that lie behind statistics and benchmarks and action plans that really matter, and that is what must never be forgotten when policies are being made and implemented.
>
> (Francis 2010, p. 4)

The Inquiry reported 3 months before the general election of 2010, and the incoming coalition Government agreed to hold a full public inquiry. As the name implies evidence

---

BOX 1.1 Hospital Standardised Mortality Ratio (HSMR) and other statistics

The HSMR is a statistical test that is increasingly being used as an indicator of quality in hospitals. It compares actual recorded deaths with the number of deaths that are statistically predicted for the population served, controlled for factors such as deprivation and age. Where the number of deaths are exactly as expected, the ratio is 100. So, under a hundred is better than expected and over 100 is worse. Information about mortality statistics is published in annual guides like the Dr Foster Hospital Guide and also on the NHS Choices website. In 2007 the number was 127 at Stafford Hospital.

There are problems associated with these statistics. They depend on widely available data and the way that this data is coded can affect the results. A review article by Bottle *et al.* (2011) gives further details. The statistics have a role to play in identifying potential issues at hospitals, which can then be investigated further. This is what happened in 2013 when Dr Bruce Keogh investigated patient safety at number of trusts identified by high death rates (Keogh 2013).

Perhaps the biggest problem with these statistics is not how they are calculated but how they are used. The number of 'excess' deaths can be calculated but this is not the same as saying that this number of individuals died as a result of poor care. Sometimes people not schooled in statistical tests can confuse these two things, but there is also a suspicion that the figures are being deliberately misrepresented. For example, in reporting the findings of the Keogh Report the *Daily Telegraph* ran the headline '13,000 died needlessly at 14 worst NHS trusts' (Donnelly and Saweer 2013). The Press Complaints Commission subsequently upheld a complaint about the headlines and the online version of the article carries a clarification at the bottom. But the headline remains the same. Spiegelhalter (2013) explains how the statistics are misrepresented.

More recently, similar arguments about statistics and their misrepresentation have been heard in debates discussing proposed reform to junior doctors' contracts, with claims that there are 6,000–11,000 excess deaths per year at weekends hotly disputed by doctors and academics.

---

given to this inquiry was given in public, and the terms of reference were wider. This time Mr Francis was also asked to consider wider questions of NHS governance, that is how systems failed to notice what was going on and stop it sooner, and so the second Francis Report was more detailed. Mr Francis started his inquiry in November 2010 and published his three-volume report in February 2013 (Francis 2013). A whole chapter, chapter 23 in the third volume, is devoted to nursing containing 29 of the report's 290 recommendations. The introduction to the nursing chapter reported as follows:

23.3 A very significant proportion of the complaints of poor care which the first inquiry and this inquiry have been concerned about have been due to poor nursing and it will be necessary to examine the causes of this. They include:

- inadequate staffing;
- poor leadership;
- poor recruitment;
- deficiencies in initial and continuing training;
- undervaluing the nursing task and those who perform it;
- declining professionalism.

23.4 It is clear that the nursing issues found in Stafford are not confined to the hospital but are found throughout the country. This is not to deny that much high-quality committed and compassionate nursing is carried out day in and day out, often with inadequate recognition. However, all in the profession must surely recognise that the challenges to the maintenance of proper standards and protection of patients have never been greater.

23.5 Until this scandalous decline in standards is reversed, it is likely that unacceptable levels of care will persist and therefore it is an area requiring the highest priority. There is no excuse for not tackling it successfully. Much of what needs to be done does not require additional resources, but changes in attitudes, culture, values and behaviour.

(Francis 2013, pp. 1498–1499)

This is damning criticism indeed, especially perhaps the observation that it was clear that the nursing issues are found throughout the country. The initial chapter of the report discussed the extent to which events described at Mid-Staffs and the explanations for them could be extrapolated more widely. Concerns that the inquiry was making too much of the evidence in a single organisation, which could not be interpreted more widely came from individuals and organisations that were pre-warned via letter that they were facing criticism in the final report. Though some patients asked him to, Mr Francis did not look elsewhere at other trusts because his terms of reference did not allow it, but he made three points to those who claimed too much extrapolation.

First, even if it was the case that there was no other provider as bad as Mid-Staffs, it was of concern that the systems of checks and balances didn't work there. Second, there were a number of other publications at about the same time, for example, the Care Quality Commission (2013), the Alzheimer's Society (2009) and the Patient's Association (2009), which raised general concerns about the state of care in hospitals. Third, he said that the failure to detect the shortcomings of the Trust resulted in it being unlikely that the public had confidence that 'another Stafford' doesn't exist.

It is debateable whether these three points are sufficient to enable the conclusion that the nursing issues highlighted can be 'found throughout the country' or that the recommendations presented in relation to nursing can be derived from the evidence presented in relation to the care at Mid-Staffs. The recommendations concerning nursing cover a good deal of ground and so won't be reproduced here in their entirety. However there were some important themes addressed by further reports and actions, which continue to shape the nursing environment and are worth further consideration.

NURSING EDUCATION

The Willis Commission

In 2012 the Royal College of Nursing (RCN) commissioned Lord Willis to answer this question:

> What essential features of preregistration nursing education in the UK, and what types of support for newly registered practitioners, are needed to create and maintain a workforce of competent, compassionate nurses fit to deliver future health and social care services?
>
> (Willis 2012, p. 4)

Lord Willis sat with a panel of seven senior nurses, managers and academics. It found that:

> The commission found no evidence of any major shortcomings in nursing education that could be held directly responsible for poor practice. It also found it difficult to prove or disprove the perception of a decline in standards of care.
>
> (Willis 2012, p. 43)

The report was supportive of graduate preparation of nurses, which was agreed in 2009 and implemented by 2013, but met with some opposition especially in the national press (Gillette 2012, 2014). Without being overly sceptical, it is worthwhile when reading these reports to bear in mind the function and purpose of the sponsoring organisation, in this case the RCN, which has a mandate to advocate for nurses. Box 1.2 provides details about the types of organisations representing nurses or more concerned with nursing.

Raising the bar: the Shape of Caring Review

A later and more significant review of nurse education was also chaired by Lord Willis. Entitled the Shape of Caring Review, it was commissioned by Health Education England and the Nursing and Midwifery Council. Health Education England is the part of the Department of Health responsible for commissioning education; a review jointly commissioned by government and regulator must be considered a very authoritative source. The report made a number of recommendations, including about the role of health care assistants, building on the earlier Cavendish Review (Cavendish 2013), and the future shape of pre-registration nursing education.

Unregulated 'nursing' roles

There are nearly as many health care assistants as registered nurses working in the National Health Service. Within Europe, the UK, Ireland and Switzerland are the only countries where health care assistants are not regulated (Willis 2015) and currently there is no standardisation of training or titles. Following the Cavendish Review, a care certificate was introduced from April 2015 (NHS Employers 2015). As well as recommending evaluation and making the certificate mandatory, the Shape of Caring Review recommended

---

BOX 1.2 Nursing and other interested organisations

The International Council of Nursing regards nursing organisations as being one of 'three pillars'.

Regulators have a role in protecting the public and deciding matters like Codes of Conduct against which the behaviour of nurses is measured and in approving university courses leading to registration. In the UK, the regulator is the Nursing and Midwifery Council (NMC). Professional bodies promote nursing practice, for example, by promoting evidence-based guidelines, and making library resources available. In the UK the professional body for nursing is the Royal College of Nursing (RCN www.rcn.org.uk/). Trade unions represent the interests of their members, by representing individuals and also by negotiating and campaigning. In the UK, the RCN fulfils this role but other trade unions, like Unison, also represent nurses.

Some organisations fulfil more than one role, and this can be a source of tension. Robert Francis recommended that the RCN consider splitting its dual function of trade union and professional body, but the RCN rejected this (RCN 2013). In other countries, professional bodies also have some regulatory functions and this too can cause some conflict of interests (Duncan *et al.* 2015).

The Government is perhaps the most important influence on nursing practice. With some caveats, like, for example, the extent to which it can command a majority in the House of Commons, it can pass laws and make policy that directly affects nursing and health care. This is why consultations concerning, for example, the establishment of a second level of regulated nurse are undertaken by the Department of Health or its subsidiary organisation Health Education England. The NMC may regulate this new group but can only do so if required by the Government.

Other organisations like the Alzheimer's Society are pressure groups and charities whose function is to promote certain groups of people.

---

that Health Education England should explore the possibility of creating a 'defined care role' (NHS Agenda for Change Band 3) that would act as a bridge between the unregulated care assistant workforce and the registered nursing workforce. As the report noted, assistant practitioners have been around for a number of years, but have never become widespread. As we write this introductory chapter, a consultation exercise is underway and by the time the book appears in print we will know more about the role: its title, level of education, whether it will be regulated, and how it will be incorporated into nursing teams. It is also clear from the review and the consultation exercise that there will be other educational routes, via apprenticeships for example, into the nursing profession. While the qualification for registered nurses will continue as a degree there will be more diverse and flexible methods of obtaining it.

The Shape of Caring Review also made some recommendations about how future pre-registration courses might look. Two possibilities are especially important: the branches, or fields of study, and the actual content of the programmes. Currently there are four branches of nursing: adult is by far the largest, and there are also children's nurses, mental health nurses and learning disability nurses. The report states that discussions with students have identified that there is not 'parity of esteem between physical and mental health' (Willis 2015 p. 42), and this does not support person-centred care. This 'parity of esteem' is of wider concern in the NHS and to address it, the Government has claimed that it is intends to 'revolutionise' mental health care (NHS England 2016; Prime Minister's Office 2016). The report points out that a quarter of people will experience a mental illness at some point of their life, and co-existing mental illness is very common in patients in acute hospital wards as well as people being cared for with physical ailments in the community. In addition, advancements in care and treatment of individuals with learning disabilities have resulted in many more people with learning disabilities living longer, but concerns have been raised that the care that they receive in general acute and community services is not as good as it could be and should be. One reason for this is that general health and care professionals and nursing students (other than in the learning disability field) do not know enough about how to care for individuals with a learning disability (Beacock *et al.* 2015).

The review recommended that to overcome these problems and to increase the ability of nurses to deliver more seamless person-centred care, there should be 2 years' 'whole person core education', which would be studied by all students, in a wide range of acute and community settings. Following completion of this period, students would specialise into their chosen field for their third year. The review also suggested that an additional field of community care be considered. The second Francis Report (2013) had also mooted an additional speciality, that of registered older persons' nurse, but this does not appear part of the current proposal. Following completion of this third specialist year, the review suggests a further year of integrated preceptorship to support transition into full registration status, which would also be aimed at reducing attrition of newly qualified nurses. This model has become known as the 2+1+1 model, and if it is implemented it will be a significant change to current arrangements.

It was also noted that as nursing becomes more established as a wholly graduate profession, more should be expected from nurses. As the title of the review suggested nursing needs to 'raise the bar'. One of the ways that this can be accomplished is by extending the range of the pre-registration curriculum so that it contains some elements of nursing that previously have been considered part of post-registration education. The review gave these examples:

- skills and the underpinning theoretical knowledge to take a structured history and assessment of patients presenting with complex needs, deteriorating condition or psychological crisis;
- diagnostic skills to identify and commence treatment such as venepuncture, cannulation, administration of intravenous additive, diabetes management and chest/lung assessment or utilise psychological solution focused therapies; and
- communication skills for bereavement.

(Willis 2015, p. 46)

The review was clear that its recommendations were suggestions only and that many other options to develop nursing education could also be considered. The actual recommendations are couched in terms of review and consultation rather than firm proposals. For example: 'NMC should gather evidence, explore and consult on the proposed 2+1+1 model, alongside other alternatives to examine whether the existing "four fields" model is fit for the future' (Willis 2015, p. 63).

The nursing workforce has developed through the generations and will continue to do so in order to meet demand and improve performance. Clearly the future nursing workforce is shaped significantly by pre-registration education, and while the *Standards* have been reviewed and amended in the past, most recently in 2004 and 2010 it seems likely that the current review will result in significant change. Consultation is planned for 2016–2017, and should result in new standards being issued by the end of 2017.

Standards for Pre-Registration Nursing Education

Francis made a number of recommendations about nurse education. Most obvious was the recommendation that 'training should be reviewed so that sufficient practical elements are incorporated to ensure that a consistent standard is achieved by all trainees throughout the country. This requires national standards' (Francis 2013, Recommendation 186, p. 1539). In their response the NMC noted that they had already changed the standards in 2010 and these met the recommendations. It's difficult to see exactly what Mr Francis had in mind when he made these recommendations, but it is clearly the case that nurse education will be going through significant change so it's worthwhile reviewing how nurse education is regulated.

As explained in Chapter 2, the Nursing and Midwifery Council is the professional regulator for nursing and midwifery in the UK. This means it maintains a register of nurses and midwives and it also regulates nursing education. It does this in two ways. First it publishes a set of *Standards for Pre-Registration Nursing Education*. This is not a national curriculum but it does maintain some consistency because each university is required to show that its course meets the *Standards* and that its graduates can do everything that they are required to be able to do. This document is supported by the *Essentials Skills Clusters*, which set out in some detail what nurses have to be able to do before they can become registered – for example, there are a number concerned with medicines management as discussed in Chapter 18. Universities are not required to do the same thing, but you will probably be able to see the *Standards* and the *Essential Skills Clusters* referred to in your practice documentation, especially in the sign-off section, so there is some consistency, as the NMC (2013) also pointed out in their response. The second way the NMC regulates education is through regular inspections of universities and the courses they provide. Similar to Ofsted visits to schools and Care Quality Commission visits to hospitals, these visits thoroughly inspect curriculum delivery in theory and practice and the NMC inspectors also talk to mentors and students. The inspections ensure that quality is maintained, and similar to the other sorts of visits, changes can be insisted upon if the course is not up to scratch.

By the time that you read this, the country will have decided whether we are to remain part of the European Union (EU). This organisation has had a major influence on the way that nursing curricula have developed. All programmes in the EU leading to registration are required to follow certain regulations, which can be traced back to 1977. In practice, these regulations stipulate that programmes are to be half theory and half practice, and also must consist of at least 4,600 hours (Salvage and Heijnen 1997). Criticisms that nursing has become too academic, that university-trained nurses are 'too posh to wash' and training should return to its more practice-based roots ignore the fact that the current EU structure has been in place for approaching 40 years, and predates nursing's academic transition. In 1977, training was based in hospitals and students were paid a salary for their work on the wards. The total of 4,600 hours at 37.5 hours per week equates to 40 weeks per year and this explains why you are still studying or in practice while your friends studying history or maths are away on longer summer breaks. Some courses calculate the hours so that there are 45 weeks per year. For the theory half of the course university regulations about teaching and assessment assume rather than measure that students have studied for a certain amount of time (Snelling *et al.* 2010), but practice hours can be and are counted, so that at the end of the course if you have passed everything else but only accumulated 2,250 hours you will have to return to practice to complete the remaining hours in order to reach the required 2,300 hour total.

When the episodes of poor care at Mid-Staffs were occurring, the NMC standards from 2004 were in use and these were detailed in the previous edition of this book. As we write this, courses are using the 2010 standards. As explained in Chapter 19, these standards were additionally rebadged as *Standards for Competence for Registered Nurses* and apply to all nurses so that they now have a dual role – to structure the initial pre-registration course at universities, but also to explain what all nurses are required to be able to do. These standards are now 6 years old and due for review, but potential changes to nursing practice partly in response to the events of Mid-Staffs mean that any resulting change may be more radical than previously anticipated. Whatever happens to the *Standards*, nurses will still need to study law and ethics, communication, and management and leadership and all the other subjects in this book and this is why we haven't mapped the chapters to the *Standards* as we did in the first edition.

Tuition fees

Since tuition fees were introduced in 1999, there have been anomalies in the costs to individuals studying in preparation to enter one of the health professions, with some but not all courses requiring payment. Medical students, for example, pay tuition fees for the first 4 years of their course. Student nurses have been exempt from tuition fees as courses were funded through contracts set by the NHS. These contracts require universities to recruit a fixed number of students set by the contract. Even though bursaries have been low, student nurses have not been required to graduate carrying the burden of large tuition fee debt. However, this is set to change from September 2017, when pre-2017 funding arrangements will no longer apply. Students starting their pre-registration courses from September 2017 will be required to pay tuition fees to universities and for most this will be paid by a student loan repaid over the course of a working life. In the autumn statement, which announced the move, the Chancellor of the Exchequer said that:

> Today there is a cap on student nurses; over half of all applicants are turned away, and it leaves hospitals relying on agencies and overseas staff.
> So we'll replace direct funding with loans for new students – so we can abolish this self-defeating cap and create up to 10,000 new training places in this Parliament.
>
> (Chancellor of the Exchequer 2015)

The justification in the statement was the need to recruit more students, and while it is the case that nursing courses are oversubscribed some of those not recruited will have been deemed unsuitable. It is not known whether numbers applying to nursing courses will be affected, but trade unions have argued that the cost may deter potential applicants (Unison 2015). The cost saving of the measure was not included in the statement but has been estimated at £1.2 billion per year (Nuffield Trust *et al.* 2015) by the end of the parliament. The change in funding arrangements means that the contracts between local education and training boards and universities will no longer be required and universities will be free to recruit more students, constrained only by their ability to find sufficient placements in the NHS and other health care providers to satisfy the NMC's criteria.

Like other university students and following the change scheduled for 2017, most nursing students will graduate with considerable debt. This debt is repaid at the rate of 9 per cent of salary over the £21,000 threshold. For a newly qualified registered nurse earning (from 1 April 2015) £21,692, the monthly repayment would be just £5.25 a month, and thereafter every extra £1,000 of salary will result in an increase of £7.50 per month in repayment. There has been some protest marches and the proposals have so far been opposed by the Labour Party. The RCN have pointed out that the length of the study year for nursing students means that, unlike students on most other university courses, opportunities for student nurses to undertake paid work while studying are limited (RCN 2015). Precise details are yet to be consulted upon and decided, and it remains to be seen what the consequences of this significant change will be. But it is clear that 2 years after preparations for this second edition of the book, the content of pre-registration nursing programmes will be the same as at the time of writing but there will be two different sets of students studying it; some paying and some not, and their experiences may be quite different.

Pre-nursing health care assistant experience

Robert Francis recommended that 'there should be an entry level requirement that student nurses spend a minimum period of time, at least 3 months, working on the direct care of patients under the supervision of a registered nurse' (Francis 2013, p. 1539, Recommendation 187). In its initial response the Government stated that 'every student who seeks NHS funding for nursing degrees should first serve up to a year as a health care assistant to promote frontline caring experience and values as well as academic strength' (DH 2013, p. 67). In its response the NMC pointed out that the structure of its programmes already met this requirement because the programmes are at least 3 years, of which half is undertaken in practice. The recommendation was that completion of this period should be a precondition of continuation in nurse training, but as the NMC pointed out (after noting the concerns that led to the recommendation), the set of standards already in place 'meets the spirit and the letter' (NMC 2013, p. 33) of the recommendation.

Nevertheless a series of pilots were carried out and it was reported that the experience was valued by those undertaking it (Allied Health Solutions 2015). The optimum time was identified as 6 months, as any less than this would impose costs on employing organisations. The recommendations of the pilot refer to the scheme being an 'opportunity' (p. 138) to access pre-registration nursing education, and that it should be 'one of the routes' available (p. 136). It is possible that if the care certificate becomes compulsory, possession of the certificate could be a requirement for starting a pre-registration course, effectively making mandatory the experience necessary to obtain the certificate. However, an evaluation or a pilot scheme cannot answer the question of whether or not this should happen; neither can it hope to shed any light on whether such a scheme will reduce the likelihood of a recurrence of the poor care at Mid-Staffs.

NURSING STRATEGY: COMPASSION IN PRACTICE AND THE 6CS

The Department of Health strategy for nursing is expressed in the 6Cs. The strategy relies on its values being widely shared: 'The greatest impact will come from individuals acting to embed the 6Cs in everything they do, supported . . . by their local organisations and by national bodies' (DH 2012, p. 26). The 6Cs can be seen throughout numerous documents and the language is also embedded within local nursing policies and strategies. The DH recognises that, in themselves, the 6Cs are not new but

> putting them together in this way to define a vision is an opportunity to reinforce the enduring values and beliefs that underpin care wherever it takes place. It gives us an easily understood and consistent way to explain our values as professionals and care staff and to hold ourselves to account for the care and services that we provide.
>
> (DH 2012, p. 13)

The 6Cs are described as values and behaviours comprising care, compassion, competence, communication, courage and commitment. Box 1.3 provides the definitions provided by the Department of Health (2012, p. 13).

The emphasis on values and behaviours rather than on strategic action has been criticised as reductionist, with a suspicion that attempting to address improvements in

---

BOX 1.3 The 6Cs defined

Care is our core business and that of our organisations, and the care we deliver helps the individual person and improves the health of the whole community. Caring defines us and our work. People receiving care expect it to be right for them, consistently, throughout every stage of their life.

Compassion is how care is given through relationships based on empathy, respect and dignity – it can also be described as intelligent kindness, and is central to how people perceive their care.

Competence means all those in caring roles must have the ability to understand an individual's health and social needs and the expertise, clinical and technical knowledge to deliver effective care and treatments based on research and evidence.

Communication is central to successful caring relationships and to effective team working. Listening is as important as what we say and do and essential for 'no decision about me without me'. Communication is the key to a good workplace with benefits for those in our care and staff alike.

Courage enables us to do the right thing for the people we care for, to speak up when we have concerns and to have the personal strength and vision to innovate and to embrace new ways of working.

A Commitment to our patients and populations is a cornerstone of what we do. We need to build on our commitment to improve the care and experience of our patients, to take action to make this vision and strategy a reality for all and meet the health, care and support challenges ahead.

one of the values does not consider the rest or the context in which care takes place (Dewar and Christley 2013). This can result in the 6Cs becomes something of a 'mantra' (Allied Health Solutions 2015) rather than anything more structured and meaningful.

The critique that the 6Cs and other responses to the horrors of Mid-Staffs over-emphasises the role that individual nurses play was developed by John Paley in a well discussed paper published in the journal *Nursing Philosophy* (Paley 2014). Drawing from social psychology, Paley argued that the environment nurses found themselves in had a profound effect on what they noticed or responded to. In simple terms (and as the Francis Report also noted), staffing levels were depleted at Stafford Hospital and this made people so busy that they failed to see that they were not acting compassionately. This is not to excuse the behaviour, but to attempt to explain it. If situationalist factors contributed significantly to the behaviour described in Francis's reports, then directing action at individuals through the 6Cs or addressing nurse education via experience before starting a course will not help remedy the perceived problem or prevent reoccurrence. What is needed is improvement to the environment. Paley's paper provoked a number of responses, which argued that there was indeed a compassion deficit that can be addressed through educational reform (Rolfe and Gardner 2014). This tension between the narratives of personal responsibility for behaviour and outside influences can be seen in a number of situations, from a failure to recycle to a failure to follow health advice. This tension is discussed in Chapter 11.

The response to Francis from Government has been largely to concentrate on individual factors partly via the measures discussed in this chapter: as Traynor *et al.* (2015) call it, concentrating on the 'bad apples'. For example, launching an initiative to introduce patient rounds into the NHS, the Prime Minister was quoted as saying that 'There is a real problem with nursing in our hospitals' (Kirkup and Holehouse 2012). Improvements in staffing, by the introduction of mandatory staffing levels have not been implemented though unsurprisingly there is a wealth of evidence that patient outcomes improve with increased levels of registered nurses (Aiken *et al.* 2014, Griffiths *et al.* 2015). The National Institution for Health and Care Excellence was charged with drawing up guidance on safe staffing levels (NICE 2014) and NHS organisations must now publish staffing information. However, these guidelines are advisory and with the overspend in the NHS budget approaching £2.5 billion in a single year, over half of NHS finance directors who responded to a regular King's Fund survey (King's Fund 2016) believed that the quality of care in their organisations had worsened this year. A recent BBC programme used Freedom of Information requests to report that there were over 20,000 nursing vacancies in England, Wales and Northern Ireland, a rate of 9 per cent with over two thirds of trusts actively recruiting doctors or nurses from abroad (Hughes and Clarke 2016). If these figures are believed, shortages of staff are not improving and if reforms to nurse education do indeed produce more qualified nurses it is difficult to see how trusts will be able to afford to employ them.

The contemporary health care environment is both complex and changeable, and has presented a number of interesting challenges for the development of the profession as highlighted in this introductory chapter. The changes discussed may lead to a greatly different educational and practice environment for nurses who start their courses in 2016 than for their colleagues who start just a year or two later. The themes of change in a complex environment will be revisited throughout the book.

THE STRUCTURE OF THE BOOK

Many nursing textbooks are available, including several large and impressively produced single volumes, which claim to cover what might be regarded as 'the curriculum'. In recommending some of these to our students we have found that the clinical and skills orientation of the texts does not always address the wider aspects of the context of nursing as presented by the NMC *Standards*. Of course, there are many single issue books about, for example, ethics and law, interprofessional working, personal development, and so on, but few that cover the wide range of generic knowledge and skills that pre-registration programmes and professional practice require. This volume has been developed in response to what we perceive as a need for a text that provides the wider range of topics indicated in the NMC *Standards*. We hope that, in this collection, we have brought together valuable contributions from a number of different authors who can offer students of nursing a wide perspective approaching that required by the NMC *Standards*. The discerning reader will notice that we have not covered every topic that appears in the Standards but in introducing the major topic areas we are confident that the majority of the NMC *standards* are addressed. Students looking for a book that discusses, for example, childhood intracranial pressure or diseases of the abdomen are invited to look elsewhere.

Because at the time of writing the NMC is about to consult on new standards for pre-registration education, we have not linked each chapter to existing standards. As discussed, significant change in the standards is likely to come in practical skills, which is not the focus of this book. We believe that while the wording may change, the general thrust of the NMC standards will remain and thus the content of this book will likely remain relevant for some time to come.

Each chapter in the book is presented in three parts:

- In the first part, the chapter topic is outlined and introduced in a broad sense.
- In the second and longest part, the subject matter is explained further.
- In the third part, the subject is explored and in some instances alternative explanations are offered.

While every chapter has its individual style, they all share some common features including:

- Each chapter introduces at least one case to illustrate how the subject matter relates to nursing practice. In some chapters a single case is developed; in other chapters a number of different cases are utilised.
- Each chapter includes activities that aim to assist reflective and active reading. Many of these activities are designed to be undertaken in small groups in order to enhance learning.
- Each chapter offers suggestions for further reading.

A NOTE ON TERMINOLOGY

We acknowledge that nursing is predominantly a female profession and we are keen to avoid promoting stereotypes. We find the constant use of: 'he or she'; 's/he'; or 'his or her' unsatisfactory in this regard: it may avoid promoting stereotypes but it gets in the way of fluid and accessible writing styles. In this volume we have chosen to adopt a convention of using either 'she' or 'he' (or 'hers' or 'his') interchangeably. No gender bias or stereotypical view should be read into the choices made, as these have been purely arbitrary throughout.

REFERENCES

Aiken, L. H., Sloane, D. M., Bruyneel, L., Van den Heede, K., Griffiths, P., Busse, R. *et al.* (2014) Nurse staffing and education and hospital mortality in nine European countries: a retrospective observational study. *Lancet* **383** (9931), 1824–1830.

Allied Health Solutions (2015) *Pre-Nursing Degree Care Experience Pilot: End of evaluation report.* London: Health Education England. www.hee.nhs.uk/sites/default/files/documents/Pre-nursing%20degree%20evalutaion.pdf (accessed 3 January 2016).

Alzheimer's Society (2009) *Counting the Cost: Caring for people with dementia on hospital wards.* London: Alzheimer's Society. www.alzheimers.org.uk/site/scripts/download_info.php?download ID=356 (accessed 3 January 2016).

Bailey, J. (2012) *From Ward to Whitehall: The disaster at Mid-Staffs.* Stafford: Cure the NHS.

Beacock. S., Borthwick, R., Kelly, J., Craine, R. and Jelfs, E. (2015) *Learning Disabilities: Meeting education needs of nursing students.* London: UK Learning and Intellectual Disability Nursing Academic Network and the UK Council of Deans of Health.

Bottle, A., Jarman, B. and Aylin, P. (2011) Strengths and weaknesses of hospital standardised mortality ratios. *British Medical Journal* **342**, c7116.

Care Quality Commission (2013) *Time to Listen in NHS Hospitals: Dignity and nutrition inspection programme.* London: Care Quality Commission. www.cqc.org.uk/sites/default/files/documents/time_to_listen_-_nhs_hospitals_main_report_tag.pdf (accessed 3 January 2016).

Cavendish, C. (2013) *The Cavendish Review: An independent review into health care assistants and support workers in the NHS and social care settings.* www.gov.uk/government/uploads/system/uploads/attachment_data/file/236212/Cavendish_Review.pdf (accessed 3 January 2016).

Chancellor of the Exchequer (2015) *Chancellor George Osborne's Spending Review and Autumn Statement 2015 Speech.* www.gov.uk/government/speeches/chancellor-george-osbornes-spending-review-and-autumn-statement-2015-speech (accessed 3 January 2016).

DH (Department of Health) (2012) *Compassion in Practice: Midwifery and care staff. Our vision and strategy.* London: DH.

DH (2013) *Patients First and Foremost: The initial Government response to the report of the Mid-Staffordshire NHS Foundation Trust public inquiry.* London: DH.

Dewar, B. and Christley, Y. (2013) A critical analysis of Compassion in Practice. *Nursing Standard* **28** (10), 46–50.

Donnelly, L. and Sawer, P. (2013) 13,000 died needlessly at 14 worst NHS trusts. *Daily Telegraph* 13 July 2013 www.telegraph.co.uk/news/health/heal-our-hospitals/10178296/13000-died-needlessly-at-14-worst-NHS-trusts.html; www.gov.uk/government/publications/nhs-bursary-reform/nhs-bursary-reform (accessed 3 January 2016).

Duncan S., Thorne, S. and Rodney, P. (2015) Evolving trends in nurse regulation: what are the policy impacts for nursing's social mandate? *Nursing Inquiry* **22** (1), 27–38.

Francis, R. (2010) *Independent Inquiry into Care Provided by Mid-Staffordshire NHS Foundation Trust January 2005–March 2009, 2 Volumes.* London: Stationery Office.

Francis, R. (2013) *Report of the Mid-Staffordshire NHS Foundation Trust Public Inquiry Volumes 1–3.* London: Stationery Office.

Gillett, K. (2012) A critical discourse analysis of British national newspaper representations of the academic level of nurse education: too clever for our own good? *Nursing Inquiry* **19** (4), 297–307.

Gillett, K. (2014). Nostalgic constructions of nurse education in British national newspapers. *Journal of Advanced Nursing* **70** (11), 2495–2505.

Griffiths, P., Ball, J., Murrells, T., Jones, S. and Rafferty, A. M. (2015). Registered nurse, health care support worker, medical staffing levels and mortality in English Hospital Trusts: a cross-sectional study. *BMJ Open* **6**(2), 1–16.

Healthcare Commission (2009) *Investigation into Mid-Staffordshire NHS Foundation Trust.* http://webarchive.nationalarchives.gov.uk/20110504135228/www.cqc.org.uk/_db/_documents/Investigation_into_Mid_Staffordshire_NHS_Foundation_Trust.pdf (accessed 3 January 2016).

Hughes, D. and Clarke, V. (2016) Thousands of NHS nursing and doctor posts lie vacant. London, BBC www.bbc.co.uk/news/health-35667939 (accessed 3 January 2016).

Keogh, B. (2013) *Review into the Quality of Care and Treatment Provided by 14 Hospital Trusts in England: Overview report.* 2013. London: DH.

King's Fund (2016) *Quality Monitoring Report – February 2016.* http://qmr.kingsfund.org.uk/2016/18/?gclid=CN7u5eP0n8sCFQtAGwodKWcPpw (accessed 3 January 2016).

Kirkup, J. and Holehouse, M. (2012) David Cameron: There is a real problem with nursing in our hospitals *Daily Telegraph*, 6 January 2012. www.telegraph.co.uk/health/healthnews/8996771/David-Cameron-There-is-a-real-problem-with-nursing-in-our-hospitals.html (accessed 3 January 2016).

NICE (National Institute for Health and Care Excellence) (2014) *Safe Staffing for Nursing in Adult Inpatient Wards in Acute Hospitals.* NICE guidelines [SG1]. London: NICE.

NHS Employers (2015) *Care Certificate* www.nhsemployers.org/your-workforce/plan/education-and-training/care-certificate (accessed 3 January 2016).

NHS England (2016) *Valuing Mental Health Equally with Physical Health or 'Parity of Esteem'* www.england.nhs.uk/mentalhealth/parity/ (accessed 3 January 2016).

Nuffield Trust, Health Foundation and King's Fund (2015) *The Spending Review: What does it mean for health and social care?* www.health.org.uk/sites/default/files/Spending-Review-Nuffield-Health-Kings-Fund-December-2015_spending_review_what_does_it_mean_for_health_and_social_care.pdf (accessed 3 January 2016).

NMC (Nursing and Midwifery Council) (2013) *NMC Response to the Francis Report* www.nmc.org.uk/globalassets/sitedocuments/francis-report/nmc-response-to-the-francis-report-18-july.pdf (accessed 3 January 2016).

Paley, J. (2014) Cognition and the compassion deficit: the social psychology of helping behaviour in nursing. *Nursing Philosophy* **15** (4), 274–287.

Patient's Association (2009) *Patients … not numbers, People … not statistics* www.patients-association.org.uk/wp-content/uploads/2014/08/Patient-Stories-2009.pdf (accessed 3 January 2016).

Prime Minister's Office (2016) Prime Minister pledges a revolution in mental health treatment (press release) www.gov.uk/government/news/prime-minister-pledges-a-revolution-in-mental-health-treatment (accessed 3 January 2016).

Rolfe, G. and Gardner, L. D. (2014) The compassion deficit and what to do about it: a response to Paley. *Nursing Philosophy* **15** (4), 288–297.

Royal College of Nursing (2013) *Mid-Staffordshire NHS Foundation Trust Public Inquiry Report: Response of the Royal College of Nursing* www.nmc.org.uk/globalassets/sitedocuments/francis-report/nmc-response-to-the-francis-report-18-july.pdf (accessed 3 January 2016).

Royal College of Nursing (2015) *RCN Comments on Proposed Changes to Nurse Tuition Funding.* www.rcn.org.uk/news-and-events/news/rcn-comments-on-proposed-changes-to-nurse-tuition-funding (accessed 3 January 2016).

Salvage, J. and Heijnen, S. (1997) Nursing and midwifery in Europe. In *Nursing in Europe: A Resource for Better Health.* Salvage, J. and Heijnen, S. (eds). Copenhagen: World Health Organization, pp. 21–123.

Snelling, P. C., Lipscomb, M., Lockyer, L., Yates, S. and Young, P. (2010) Time spent studying on a pre-registration nursing programme module: an exploratory study and implications for regulation. *Nurse Education Today* **30** (8), 713–719.

Spiegelhalter, D. (2013) Have there been 13,000 needless deaths at 14 NHS trusts? *British Medical Journal* **347**, f4893.

Traynor, M., Stone, K., Cook, H., Gould, D. and Maben, J. (2014) Disciplinary processes and the management of poor performance among UK nurses: bad apple or systemic failure? A scoping study. *Nursing Inquiry* **21** (1), 51–58.

Unison (2015) *Axing Student Bursaries Will Deter Many from Careers in Nursing.* www.unison.org.uk/news/press-release/2015/12/plans-to-axe-student-bursaries-will-deter-many-from-careers-in-nursing-says-unison/ (accessed 3 January 2016).

Willis, P. (2012) *Quality with Compassion: The future of nursing education.* www.williscommission.org.uk (accessed 3 January 2016).

Willis, P. (2015) *The Shape of Caring Review (Raising the Bar).* London: Health Education England www.hee.nhs.uk/our-work/developing-our-workforce/nursing/shape-caring-review (accessed 3 January 2016).

2

PROFESSIONAL ISSUES

Janet Holt

LEARNING OUTCOMES

After reading and reflecting on this chapter, you should be able to:

- explain the importance of accountability for professional practice;
- identify the role and functions of professional regulation;
- outline the role of the Nursing and Midwifery Council;
- discuss how the Nursing and Midwifery Council calls nurses to account.

INTRODUCTION

Nursing has a long and distinguished history, but it is only within the last 100 years or so that it has emerged as a distinct profession. The progression of health care in modern times has caused nursing to evolve continually alongside other professional groups, while remaining distinct from them. This chapter considers issues of the place of nursing as a profession in the modern health care system, and is divided into three parts.

In Part 1, the history of nursing and its emergence as a profession is outlined, and there is discussion about how professional issues are linked to ethical and legal considerations guiding professional practice.

In Part 2, the question of whether nursing can be fully considered to be a profession is explored. Professional regulation is discussed, and the ways in which this is undertaken by the Nursing and Midwifery Council are explained.

In Part 3, a more critical approach is taken, and critiques of *The Code* are explored.

PART 1: OUTLINING PROFESSIONAL ISSUES

Case 2.1

Mairi is a newly qualified staff nurse working on a busy medical ward. In addition to the patients she is already caring for, the ward manager asks her to also look after an elderly woman admitted following a cerebrovascular accident (CVA). The patient is conscious but confused, and on Mairi's assessment, needs a considerable amount of nursing care. The patient is having intravenous medication through a pump that she is unfamiliar with. Mairi asks the ward manager either to allocate this patient or some of her other patients to another nurse as she feels unable to address her needs adequately. The ward manager tells Mairi that she cannot allocate the patient to another nurse and that she will just have to prioritise and do the best she can.

Health care is changing rapidly for many reasons, including the development of new technologies and the emergence of an ageing population with multiple health needs. Nursing is fundamental to the delivery of good health care, and while this has been the case for many hundreds of years, the concept of nursing as a distinct *profession* started about 150 years or so ago. The pace of change has accelerated, particularly in the last decade, and looks set to continue as policy develops in response to changing and challenging health care needs.

Development of the nursing profession

The history of nursing is long and complex, and in recent years there have been a number of substantial changes in the development of the profession. In the Middle Ages, care was undertaken in the home or by religious orders, hence the title 'Sister', which has persisted since this time. Florence Nightingale (1820–1910) is usually credited with initiating the reform of nursing and nursing education (Abbott and Wallace 1998). While she only had a small amount of training herself, she came from a well-connected and wealthy family and in 1854 was asked by the Minister of War, Sidney Herbert, to oversee the introduction of female nurses into the military hospitals of Turkey. The military hospitals were full of casualties from the Crimean War and it is for this work that Nightingale is perhaps best remembered. She was single-minded in pursuing policies that today may be recognised as fundamental to nursing care, prioritising cleanliness and nutrition. In 2 years the death rate fell from 40 per cent to 2 per cent (Porter 1997), and when she returned home in 1856 she was already a national hero. A public appeal produced the funds to establish a school of nursing at St Thomas', London. While Nightingale appreciated the need for training, she did not regard nurses as autonomous practitioners, but as working under the direction of doctors. For Nightingale, male doctors controlled the activities of female nurses.

According to McGann (2004), 1887 was the turning point in the emergence of the profession of nursing, with the formation of the British Nurses' Association (BNA), which campaigned for the formation of a register of nurses. In 1905, the Select Committee on the Registration of Nurses recommended 3 years' education and registration, but this failed to gain Government support. Along with other important social changes, World War I

(1914–1918) acted as the main catalyst to progress. The Nurses' Registration Act became law in 1919, setting up the first General Nursing Council with the following duties (Baly 1995):

- To complete a syllabus of instruction.
- To compile a syllabus for subjects for examination.
- To compile a register of qualified nurses.

Being accountable means being required to give reasons for your actions.

The International Council of Nurses (ICN) began work on a code of ethics for nurses in 1923, but it was not finally accepted until 1953 (Fry and Johnstone 2002). The clause in this code that required obedience to the doctor was only removed in 1973, at the behest of some student nurses from Canada (Chiarella 2002). The UK published its first Code of Conduct in 1983 and in 2002, the Nursing and Midwifery Council (NMC), the body that regulates nursing and midwifery, was established replacing the United Kingdom Central Council for Nursing Midwifery and Health Visiting (UKCC).

The profession of nursing continues to change and develop. In 2013, nursing in England became an all-graduate profession, in line with other health professionals and countries including Scotland, Wales and Eire. Many nurses routinely undertake tasks that until recently were considered to belong in the domain of medical practice such as venepuncture, cannulation, the performance of minor operations, and the prescription of almost all medicines. Consequently, the practice of nursing is increasingly complex and requires highly developed skills for which a knowledge base is required. While this knowledge base will include relevant anatomical, physiological and psychological information, any nurse working in current health care practice also needs an understanding of responsibility and accountability.

It has been suggested that accountability is 'one of those delightfully paradoxical words because no-one knows what it means' (Jacobs 2004, p. 21). However, even if the precise nature of accountability is problematic, its application needs to be straightforward. It is a real issue for nurses and patients and clients and to a large extent governs practice. The concept of **being accountable** is discussed by Fletcher and colleagues (1995), but as will be explained in this chapter, for nurses in practice there are different types of accountability. The cornerstone of accountability is *professional* accountability to the regulatory body, and the NMC provides some practical advice and guidance as well as the means by which nurses can be held to account for their actions or omissions.

There is much more to being professionally accountable than following professional advice, however authoritative it appears to be. There are other sources that guide action and can be referred to where accountability is required, and these can be categorised in a number of different ways. In this book the different facets of accountability are discussed not only in this chapter, but also in the two following chapters exploring ethics and law in professional practice. These three influences on practice often correspond, as represented in the Venn diagram (Figure 2.1).

A clause in *The Code* requires registrants to 'keep to the laws of the country in which you are practising' (NMC 2015a, Clause 20.4). However, this may not be quite as straightforward as it seems, as different criteria may be used to judge different actions. For example, professional criteria are contained within *The Code* and other publications from the NMC, legal requirements can be found within the law, but ethical standards can originate from a number of sources. Take for example the medical procedure of termination of pregnancy. In England, Wales and Scotland abortion is unlawful except

FIGURE 2.1
The relationship
between ethics,
law, and
professional
accountability

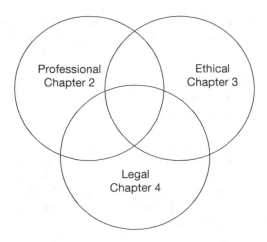

under the circumstances laid down in the Abortion Act 1967 (amended by the Human Fertilisation and Embryology Act 1990). Despite being lawful in certain circumstances, some individuals and 'pro-life' organisations believe abortion to be morally wrong irrespective of circumstances or the law. The law gives health care professionals, including nurses, the right to refuse to participate on grounds of conscientious objection, although it should be noted that this is not an absolute right, (that is, one that cannot be overridden in any circumstance) and there are limits placed on this as demonstrated in a recent case in the Supreme Court (Supreme Court 2014). Hence, an abortion may be lawful, but a nurse may consider it to be an immoral act and may, with the support of the NMC, refuse to participate in most circumstances (NMC 2015b).

This example shows the complex nature of professional accountability even when the initial edict, adherence to the law, appears on the face of it to be straightforward. The case study at the beginning of the chapter presents a similar dilemma for the nurse.

FIGURE 2.2
Standards
informing nursing
practice

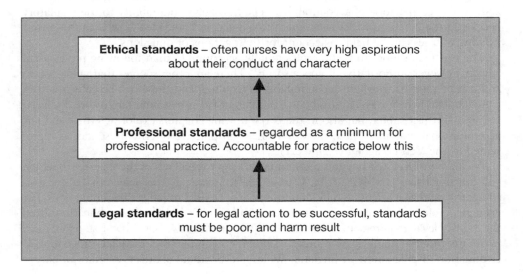

On one hand she has a professional duty of care (based in law) for the delivery of care to all of the patients she is responsible for. However, Mairi also has concerns about her ability to deliver care of an adequate standard. While the repercussions of compromising care can result in the nurse being called to account in a professional or legal capacity, the heart of Mairi's concerns in this case is probably neither professional or legal in nature but based upon the ethical concern of how best to care for people. Nevertheless, nurses will be held professionally accountable for their actions. Even if the influences are mutually supportive, their standards are not the same. Legal standards are the lowest, professional standards are higher and ethical standards higher still (Lesser 2014) (see Figure 2.2).

Activity 2.1

Write a list of contemporary nurses that appear in TV dramas like *Holby City* and *Casualty*. Are they good role models for you as a student nurse? Can you think of any instances where their professional behaviour might be questioned?

PART 2: EXPLAINING PROFESSIONAL ISSUES

The profession of nursing

The term 'professional' is not restricted to health care professions or others such as doctors or lawyers traditionally thought of as belonging to the professions. For example plumbers may offer a 'professional plumbing service' and sportsmen and -women such as footballers, golfers and athletes are also described as professionals. These forms of professionalism differ from its understanding in health care. The term 'professional' is used in sport simply to mean that individuals are paid for their services, and if a plumber offers a professional service, you could reasonably expect the work to be completed efficiently and competently. While some professions such as medicine and the law have been long established, there is much speculation over whether nursing can be accurately described as a profession. Professional identity has traditionally focused on the traits or characteristics that professionals were expected to demonstrate. The traits or characteristics defining a profession include:

- altruism;
- trustworthiness;
- specialist skills;
- a body of knowledge;
- competence;
- professional autonomy.

In addition, professions organise themselves into associations (such as Royal Colleges) and have a culture and etiquette that bind professionals together guided by codes of conduct. Professions are also seen to have power through their influence on policy making (Finlay 2000). Other accounts of professionalism have been described as functionalist, that is focusing on the role played by the professionals rather than their characteristics.

Janet Holt

In functionalist accounts, professions such as medicine directly help to maintain the social order by what Morrall (2001) describes as 'controlling entry to the sick role' (p. 83).

Both trait and functionalist accounts of professionalism are criticised by Morrall (2001) because 'they appear to reflect what those who consider themselves to be professionals believe are the characteristics of a profession. Therefore there is a strong element of self-justification in describing the professions in this way' (p. 83). While acknowledging the improved social status of nursing, Morrall (2001) is unconvinced of the professional status of nursing because he considers power to be central to the understanding of professions. In comparison to the power exercised by medicine, nursing appears to be powerless. There are also numerous occasions where, despite claims of professional autonomy, nursing activity is directed by doctors. Thus, on this account, nursing is regarded as a semi-profession complicated by unequal power relations.

An alternative approach to explaining professional identity in health care is examined by Colyer (2004), who discusses the five stages of professionalisation identified by Wilensky (1964). This process begins with the emergence of an occupational group, the establishment of a training and selection programme, the formation of a professional association, the development of a code of ethics, and political activity to establish recognition and protection of professional work. Using this definition, nursing can accurately be considered a profession as there is a clearly defined professional group, a training and selection programme, and a code of conduct overseen by the NMC. The recognition and protection of professional work is governed by the Nurses and Midwives Act (1979) and its subsequent amendment in 1992. There is also a professional

BOX 2.1 The Royal College of Nursing

The Royal College of Nursing (RCN) was established in 1916 and currently has around 420,000 members including health care assistants and students. The RCN represents about half of registered nurses in the UK. The RCN's homepage claims that it 'represents nurses and nursing, promotes excellence in practice and shapes health policies'. So it is more than just a trade union, which has narrower interests, though the RCN also fulfils this function, offering indemnity insurance, individual representation, and other membership benefits, similar to other trade unions representing nurses. In addition, it offers guidance on practice issues, accredited distance-learning courses from a number of institutions and has a research institute based at the University of Warwick. There is a student section at the RCN, the Association of Nursing Students. The most senior officer is the Chief Executive and General Secretary, but the College is governed by a representative council.

association, the Royal College of Nursing, which represents approximately half of the registered nurses in the UK (Box 2.1). Other nurses are represented by trade unions such as Unison.

The question of whether nursing can be truly considered to be a profession on an equal basis with medicine remains largely unresolved. Furthermore, the assumption that the professionalisation of nursing is necessarily beneficial to both society and to nursing has also been questioned. In the pursuit of professionalisation, nurses could be in danger of becoming elitist and subsequently compromise their inclusive, caring philosophies (Gerrish *et al.* 2003). Despite this lack of consensus, there are some elements of professional identity that are clearly evident in the organisation of nursing. One of the most important of these is the concept of professional regulation.

The Professional Standards Authority for Health and Social Care is the statutory body co-ordinating the regulatory bodies of all health professions.

Professional regulation

Professional regulation, through the establishment of regulatory bodies, is usually a feature of professions that have potential to cause harm to individuals or groups of people (Pearson 2005). There are a number of regulatory bodies in the UK that provide guidance and set standards for the profession they regulate (Table 2.1). Nurses and midwives are regulated by the NMC. The operation of each regulatory body varies, but their main function is to protect the public.

The work of the statutory bodies that regulate health and social care professionals such as the NMC is overseen by the **Professional Standards Authority for Health and Social Care** (PSA). The functions of this authority include assessing the performance of the regulators, conducting audits, scrutinising their decisions and reporting to Parliament. All decisions taken by the Conduct and Competence Committee of the NMC are referred to the PSA, which reviews overall performance and reports to Parliament

The Nursing and Midwifery Council

Nurses from all four branches of nursing, specialist community public health nurses and midwives are regulated by the NMC. The NMC states that

> We regulate nurses and midwives in England, Wales, Scotland and Northern Ireland. We exist to protect the public. We set standards of education, training, conduct and performance so that nurses and midwives can deliver high quality health care throughout their careers.
>
> We make sure that nurses and midwives keep their skills and knowledge up to date and uphold our professional standards. We have clear and transparent processes to investigate nurses and midwives who fall short of our standards. We maintain a register of nurses and midwives allowed to practise in the UK.
>
> (NMC 2015c)

The organisation is known as the Nursing and Midwifery Council, and the word 'Council' also refers to the board, which governs the activity of the NMC. Appointed by the Privy Council through an application process, the Council is made up of 12 members comprising a chair, 6 registrant and 5 lay members including a member from each of the UK four countries. Council meetings are held in public and minutes and associated documents are published on the NMC website

Janet Holt

TABLE 2.1 Professional regulatory bodies in the United Kingdom

Professional body	Professions regulated
General Chiropractic Council (GCC)	Chiropractors
General Dental Council (GDC)	Dentists, dental nurses, dental technicians, clinical dental technicians, dental hygienists, dental therapists and orthodontic therapists
General Medical Council (GMC)	Doctors
General Optical Council (GOC)	Dispensing opticians and optometrists
General Osteopathic Council (GOsC)	Osteopaths
General Pharmaceutical Council (GPhC)	Pharmacists and pharmacy technicians
Health and Care Professions Council (HCPC)	Arts therapists Biomedical scientists Chiropodists/podiatrists Clinical scientists Dietitians Hearing aid dispensers Occupational therapists Operating department practitioners Orthoptists Paramedics Physiotherapists Practitioner psychologists Prosthetists/orthotists Radiographers Social workers in England Speech and language therapists
Nursing and Midwifery Council (NMC)	Nurses and midwives
Pharmaceutical Society of Northern Ireland (PSNI)	Pharmacists in Northern Ireland

There are four committees of the Council, which explore issues in depth affecting the NMC, nurses, midwives and public protection and report back to Council. These committees are:

1 The Appointments Board
2 Audit Committee
3 The Midwifery Committee
4 The Remuneration Committee.

Activity 2.3

Spend some time navigating the NMC website, including biographies of Council members, Standards, Guidance and fitness to practise information and cases.

In addition, there are two further committees that deal with fitness to practise:

1   The Conduct and Competence Committee
2   The Health Committee.

The NMC Chief Executive and Registrar is an appointed position, accountable to the Council, with responsibility for leading and managing the Council's professional, business and financial affairs. The NMC, through the workings of its committees, the Council members and appointed members of staff, upholds the standards of nursing and midwifery practice and can call to account those deemed to have compromised standards of care. For professional regulation to be effective, regulatory bodies must be impartial and the needs of patients and clients must clearly be observed to be paramount to those of practitioners. The Conduct and Competence Committee for example generally holds hearings in public, in the belief that openness of the proceedings reflects the NMC's public accountability.

To achieve its core function of protecting the public, the NMC has four key aims:

1   To maintain a register of nurses and midwives allowed to practise in the UK.
2   To set standards of education, training, conduct and performance.
3   To have clear and transparent processes to investigate nurses and midwives who fall short of the required standards.
4   To ensure nurses and midwives keep their skills and knowledge up to date and uphold professional standards (see Chapter 19).

Maintain a register of nurses and midwives eligible to practise in the UK

Maintenance of the professional register is an important task and recognised as central to the professional aspirations of nurses 100 years ago. The most recent data published by the NMC shows 686,782 nurses and midwives on the register, of which over 28,00 registered for the first time and would mainly consist of students registering at the end of their programme of study (NMC 2015d). Only an individual who is registered as a nurse with the NMC is entitled to describe themselves as a registered nurse, and it is a criminal offence falsely to claim registration.

The word 'nurse' was used more frequently previously when health care workers who assisted nurses were often given the title 'auxiliary nurse'. Today these workers are more often entitled 'health care assistants', and more qualified workers are often entitled 'assistant practitioners' or 'associate practitioners'. Although these individuals may undertake tasks and procedures recognised as nursing care such as washing and dressing patients and clients, the use of the word 'nurse' does not appear in job titles, job descriptions or name badges. Recent plans announced by the Government in December 2015 indicate strengthening these roles with the creation of a new Band 4 'associate nurse' designed to bridge the gap between senior assistant practitioners and registered nurses. Due to be piloted in 2016, this initiative has received a mixed response with some nurse leaders in practice considering it to be a useful way to address nursing shortages, but the RCN Chief Executive describing the plans as a retrograde step (Merrifield 2015). For patients and clients, who may be bewildered by the range of different professionals contributing to their care, this helps to clarify that the term 'nurse' refers to registered nurses working within agreed standards of professional practice.

To set standards of education, training, conduct and performance

There are a number of standards published by the NMC on, among other things, medicines management (discussed in detail in Chapter 18), to support learning in practice, and social networking, and these serve as guides for practice. The most important of these is *The Code* (NMC 2015a)

The Code: Professional Standards of Practice and Behaviour for Nurses and Midwives

An important feature of professions is the existence of a code of ethics. The NMC regards *The Code* as a key document, which summarises the duties and obligations of registered nurses and midwives. The first Code of Conduct for UK nurses was published in 1983 by the UKCC. It has been revised several times and following the establishment of the NMC, a new version was produced in 2002. Further amendments were made in 2004 and 2008, and the latest version published in 2015. The Code was revised as one of a number of measures taken by the NMC in response to Sir Robert Francis's inquiry into Mid-Stafford-shire FNHST (Francis 2013). The recommendations of this report are far reaching and include the recruitment, education and training of nurses, continued professional development, fitness to remain on the register, effectiveness of raising concerns and whistle blowing, all of which necessitated a revised Code. Following a process of consultation, the new Code became effective in March 2015 and launched with an extensive media campaign for the general public as well as the profession. As well as giving more detailed explanation of issues present in previous versions such as respecting confidentiality or obtaining consent, the 2015 version includes new clauses concerning the duty of candour, use of social media and end of life care. There is also a greater emphasis placed on compassionate care, raising concerns, record keeping, delegation and accountability.

The Code is divided into four sections:

- Prioritise people
- Practise effectively
- Preserve safety
- Promote professionalism and trust.

Within each section there are a number of standard statements that nurses and midwives have a duty to uphold. In the first section, the issues are directed towards patient care such as treating people as individuals, upholding their dignity, listening to preferences, respecting confidentiality, meeting physical, psychological and social needs and always acting according to best interests. The standards of the second section are focused on effective practice and include evidence-based practice, communication skills, team working, record keeping and accountability for delegation. Section three details the obligations of the registrant to maintain patient safety including recognising the limits of competence, the duty of candour, acting in an emergency, escalating concerns where patient safety or public protection is potentially compromised particularly with vulnerable people. The final section is concerned with not bringing the profession into disrepute and requires registrants to uphold the reputation of the profession, fulfil registration requirements, exercise leadership in ensuring delivery of quality care and to cooperate with investigations and complaints. *The Code* is reproduced in full at the end of this chapter.

Codes of conduct generally are either aspirational or prescriptive (Johnstone 2009). Aspirational codes tend to be directed at virtue, stating aims rather than prescribing behaviour and subsequently concentrating on the characteristics of individuals. Prescriptive codes are more orientated to duties. The NMC Code can be said to be a prescriptive code; its language is directive, telling registrants what they *must* do, for example, 'you *must* respect a person's right to privacy in all aspects of their care' (NMC 2015a, clause 5.1). In this sense the code sets out *minimum* standards, below which registrants run the risk of censure and being called to account.

Case 2.1 (continued)

Mairi thinks that it is unfair on her and more importantly her other patients to be asked to care for the new admission. In her discussions with the ward manager she quotes from *The Code*, in particular the following clauses:

13.3 ask for help from a suitably qualified and experienced health care professional to carry out any action or procedure that is beyond the limits of your competence.

(NMC 2015a, p. 11)

16.1 raise and, if necessary, escalate any concerns you may have about patient or public safety, or the level of care people are receiving in your workplace or any other health care setting and use the channels available to you in line with our guidance and your local working practices.

(NMC 2015a, p. 12)

16.2 raise your concerns immediately if you are being asked to practise beyond your role, experience and training.

(NMC 2015a, p. 12)

16.3 tell someone in authority at the first reasonable opportunity if you experience problems that may prevent you working within the Code or other national standards, taking prompt action to tackle the causes of concern if you can.

(NMC 2015a, p. 12)

The ward manager, also a nurse, recognises these concerns, but the hospital is full and she has been required to accept the patient. Together they telephone the duty manager to explain that the transfer is not safe and that the patient will be at risk. They agree that this will be followed up with a letter as soon as it is possible. Mairi does make it clear, however, that she cannot operate the IV pump, because she doesn't know how it works. *The Code* states that: 'you must recognise and work within the limits of your competence' (NMC 2015a, clause 13, p. 11).

Standards for nurse education

The NMC is required to validate all courses leading to registration as a registered nurse. When students complete these validated courses, they are able to apply to be admitted to the register. Institutions offering the educational award are regularly audited by the NMC or other organisations acting on behalf of the NMC, and any changes to courses must be approved. Validated courses must be able to demonstrate how the standards for pre-registration nursing are met. The NMC, through its *Standards to Support Learning and Assessment in Practice* (NMC 2008) also stipulates who is able to assess students in practice, and universities are required to demonstrate their processes in meeting these standards. The regulation of courses evolves over time and there is no national curriculum as such, though there are *Standards for Pre-Registration Nursing Education* (NMC 2010), which now also apply to all nurses as *Standards of Competence* (NMC 2015e). Universities decide the content and assessment for their courses and through initial and periodic validation and the imposition of extra rules and regulation the NMC takes an active role in the regulation of nursing and midwifery education.

However, nurse education has been subject to scrutiny from observers both inside and outside the profession. In 2012 the Royal College of Nursing commissioned Lord Willis of Knaresborough to lead an independent enquiry into pre-registration education (RCN 2012). The report listed 32 recommendations across 6 themes and addressed issues such as patient-centred care, degree level education, mentorship, a sustainable funding model, the importance of patient safety, and in nursing education, evaluation of and research into nursing education to ensure programmes are fit for purpose, and the need to encourage a diverse range of applicants to nursing programmes.

The findings of the Francis Report (2013) had inevitable consequences for nurse education and subsequently Health Education England (HEE) and the NMC jointly commissioned Lord Willis to chair a further review focusing on the education of care staff and registered nurses. This Shape of Caring Review reported in a document 'Raising the Bar' in March 2015 setting out 34 recommendations in 8 themes (Willis 2015). At the time of writing, HEE is in an engagement phase gathering views from stakeholders on the recommendations through consultation, live events and Twitter chats.

Guidance on raising concerns

The NMC makes it clear in guidance about raising concerns in practice (NMC 2013a) that students have a duty to take action if they have concerns that a practitioner is not fit to practise because of a health or character issue, or if they have witnessed poor practice or a risk to public protection. Furthermore they should also report if they have concerns about the education provided by a university employee or a registrant. Recent changes to legislation offer protection to students from retaliation or victimisation when they raise concerns. From April 2015 students in practice settings as part of their educational programme will be given the same level of protection that already exists for nurses and midwives under the Public Interest Disclosure Act.

As part of its Quality Assurance Framework for education (NMC 2015f) the NMC requires universities to have a clearly defined policy for students to raise and escalate concerns and that together with practice placement partners, universities can demonstrate an agreed proactive approach to this. An additional requirement relates to student awareness and as part of each practice placement induction students should be informed of the process for raising and escalating concerns when on practice (NMC 2015f). However while the additional protection under the law is welcomed, the difficulties of raising concerns should not be minimised. As noted in a recent paper

> While there is a drive to promote openness in health care settings and an expectation that staff will raise concerns the reality is that the decision to do this can be very difficult. This is the case for some student nurses.
>
> (Ion *et al.* 2015, p. 900)

Students should familiarise themselves with NMC guidance and policies from their university and placement provider.

RESEARCH FOCUS 2.1

Factors influencing student nurse decisions to report poor practice witnessed while on placement

Research carried out by Ion *et al.* (2015) and published in the journal *Nurse Education Today*, aimed to explore influences on student decisions about whether or not to report poor clinical practice, which is a result of deliberate action and which is witnessed while on placement. Qualitative interviews with 13 pre-registration nursing students from the UK were undertaken. Participants included both adult and mental health nurses with an age range from 20 to 47. Qualitative analysis identified key themes. Category integrity and fit with data were confirmed by a team member following initial key findings: 4 themes were identified, 1 supporting reporting, and 3 that caused difficulties.

1 *'I had no choice'* described the personal and ethical drivers that influenced students to report. This was split into two subthemes reflecting the students' own moral standards, and the NMC requirement to report articulated in the Code. One student reported that 'it was disturbing my sleep . . . it was bothering me even when I wasn't there' (p. 902).

The remaining categories concerned difficulties in reporting.

2 *'Consequences for self'* describing the personal and professional consequences of reporting, including the fear of 'making a name for yourself' and a fear of failing the placement. Though this was identified none of the participants actually suffered adverse consequences apart from a sense of guilt for causing problems for other health care professionals.

3 *'Living with ambiguity'* giving an account of why some students struggle to report including whether what they had seen was actually poor practice. One student reported that: 'I began to wonder if I was over reacting . . . my mentor just brushed it off and got on with things . . . it seemed normal to her and also to the auxiliary who was helping' (p. 903).

4 *'Being prepared'* concerned how the university prepared students for raising concerns. Most felt well supported but some less so.

The study concluded that students have varying awareness of their responsibilities and processes for raising and escalating concerns. A number of reasons for not reporting were offered, but those who did report did so out of moral commitment to practice, and the study concluded by suggesting that strengthening this aspect of education may ensure that students and practitioners are better equipped 'to deal with the moral dilemmas that increasingly characterise nursing work' (p. 904).

To have clear and transparent processes to investigate nurses and midwives who fall short of the required standards

Caulfield (2005) describes professional accountability as the first pillar of accountability, 'at the heart of nursing practice . . . [and] . . . based on promoting the welfare and well-being of patients through nursing care' (p. 4). While being accountable may be broadly understood as being responsible for something or to someone, this is a somewhat simplistic account, and before the process by which the NMC holds nurses to account is considered, further discussion about the concepts of responsibility and accountability is required.

Responsibility

While as citizens we all have responsibilities in society such as paying taxes, upholding the law and keeping promises, health professionals have special responsibilities as part of their professional role. For example, according to *The Code* (NMC 2015a), nurses are expected to respect an individual's right to confidentiality, and recognise and work within the limits of their competence. This type of responsibility has been described by Hart (1968) as role responsibility. Hart suggested that if a person occupies an office or distinctive place within society, such as a nurse, then they are responsible for fulfilling whatever duties are recognised as part of that role. The duties attached to the role of the nurse may vary according to the area of clinical practice that they work in. For example, the duties expected of a nurse working in an intensive care unit might be quite different from those expected of a nurse practising in the community. Nevertheless, each nurse will have a role with corresponding responsibilities attached to it determined either by the NMC or the nurse's employer.

While duties determined by the nurses' employers are likely to be contractual responsibilities, role responsibility may have legal or moral implications. In many respects contractual duties are straightforward, relating to, for example, hours of work and holiday entitlement. In addition, depending on the level of seniority, the nurse will have other more specific contractual obligations. A ward manager, for example, will have leadership and management responsibilities not expected of a more junior member of the ward team. However, the idea of nursing as a moral activity is a recurring theme in the nursing literature (McCarthy and Gastmans 2015; Gallagher 2007; Gastmans 1999; Nortvedt 1998), and this implies a moral dimension to role responsibility. Therefore the morally responsible nurse does not just carry out what they are contractually or legally required to do, but also as Pattison (2001) suggests has 'an eye to the larger and more universal ethical principles applying to human existence and behaviour' (Pattison 2001, p. 7). This is a much more stringent form of responsibility, which can cause difficulties and conflict for the practitioner. An example of this can be seen in the case study at the beginning of the chapter where the nurse is concerned about the level of care that she can offer the new patient.

Other situations can arise that are equally difficult to resolve, but may be more directly related to the nurse's contractual responsibilities.

Case 2.2

Suppose that John, a student nurse, has asked Robert his mentor to spend some time with him to complete records of evidence for his portfolio of clinical practice. Robert knows that it is important that John completes this today. When he made the arrangements with Robert several days ago, John informed him that they need to be submitted to the university for verification. However, the clinical area has been exceptionally busy, and John has not been able to meet with his mentor prior to their shift ending. John tells Robert he is able to stay behind to complete the documents, but Robert wants to go shopping. He has decided to buy a new laptop and has just enough time to get there before the shop closes.

Robert may feel that as John's mentor he has a responsibility to agree to stay after work to help him and while this is clearly not a contractual responsibility (as Robert has completed the required working hours), it may be argued that Robert has a moral responsibility to help John succeed. The NMC Code states that a nurse must 'support students' and colleagues' learning to help them develop their professional competence and confidence.' (NMC 2015a, clause 9.4), so if Robert does not help John on this occasion he could be considered to be in breach of his professional requirements. Robert could simply walk away from the situation, or he may feel that he does have some moral responsibility to help John succeed and decide to postpone his shopping trip. We can see in this example that having a moral responsibility can be more onerous for the individual than legal or contractual responsibilities. Here Robert is just postponing a shopping trip, but what if he needed to collect his children from school or had made a promise to a patient rather than a student? In these situations the nurse may find it difficult if not impossible to fulfil moral responsibilities. Nevertheless, nurses need to define as closely as possible what legal, contractual and moral responsibilities are required of them because it is for these that they will be held to account.

Accountability

Being called to account means being required to give reasons for your actions (Fletcher *et al.* 1995), and nurses may be held to account in a number of ways and by different individuals or bodies such as patients and clients, employers or the NMC. Accountability therefore assumes being answerable to another person or group of people, and as discussed above, nurses are responsible for carrying out the duties expected as part of their professional role and thus are accountable for their actions in carrying out such duties. The NMC regards nurses as personally accountable for actions and omissions in professional practice and expects practitioners to be able to justify decisions they have made. Generally speaking, nurses are accountable to:

- patients and clients – through complaints and legal processes;
- their employers – through contractual responsibilities;
- the NMC – through *The Code*.

Accountability in law

Nurses, including student nurses are expected to act within the law and the NMC makes it clear that 'conduct is important in upholding the reputation of the professions, both when you are studying and in your personal life' (NMC 2015g). Therefore a nurse who is convicted of an offence in their personal life (such as driving over the permitted alcohol limit) will in addition to the punishment given to them by the courts be reported to the NMC. There has been a recent case where a nurse was removed from the register for numerous traffic offences and a conviction for damage to property (NMC 2015h). Like all other citizens, nurses are accountable under criminal law, and if a nurse is found to have committed a crime punishable by the state they would be called to account through the courts. Examples of criminal acts are murder, manslaughter, theft and drug-related offences. It is rare for any health care professional to be accused or found guilty of criminal behaviour for negligent practice, and health care professionals are more commonly held to account through the law of tort. The law of tort relates to civil actions or disputes between individuals where actions for compensation are brought in the civil courts. A complaint of wrongdoing could be made against a nurse and if proven compensation could be awarded.

Case 2.1 (continued)

If Mairi operated the intravenous pump wrongly and the patient suffered some complications as a result, she could be called to account by the patient or their relatives through the courts for her actions (see Chapter 4). Simply stating that she had been instructed to operate the pump by the ward manager would not be a defence for a professional in a court of law.

Accountability to employers

Nurses may be employed in the NHS, the private sector, through agencies or be self-employed. Any nurse in employment will have a contract of employment setting out the duties of both the employer (such as paying wages, health and safety responsibilities) and the employee. In addition there will be a number of policies and protocols to which the employee is expected to conform. Some policies and protocols may directly relate to the patient, such as a tissue viability policy, maintaining confidentiality, or health and safety issues. A nurse who does not adhere to what is required of them by their employer, either through their contractual responsibilities or those required by policies and protocols, may be subject to investigation and discipline through their employer's disciplinary procedures. In the case study at the beginning of the chapter, the nurse could also find herself being called to account by her employer. Suppose the patient's relatives made a formal complaint to the hospital about the care the woman had received. The hospital would investigate this in accordance with their complaints policy and a nurse could be asked to detail and explain their actions. If found to have breached any hospital policies and/or protocols, the nurse could face disciplinary action. Mairi has acted according to *The Code*, but others may not have been so clear about their actions.

Accountability to the NMC

The most significant aspect of accountability for nurses is that of professional accountability to the professional body. The core responsibility of the NMC is to protect patients and clients by ensuring that nurses receive a suitable educational programme that enables them to be both fit for purpose and fit for registration and furthermore that they are deemed to be fit for practice. The NMC sets the standards of professional behaviour required from nurses and these standards are set out in the *The Code*. Anyone can complain to the NMC about a registered nurse and complaints are made against practitioners by service users and carers, colleagues, employers or the police, though the NMC expects registrants to declare police charges, cautions or convictions themselves.

Complaints about fitness for practice

The procedure for calling practitioners to account is detailed in 'Advice and information for employers of nurses and midwives' (NMC 2015i). There are several categories of fitness to practise allegations:

- *misconduct* such as physical or verbal abuse, dishonesty, failure to provide adequate care or poor record keeping
- *lack of competence* such as lack of skill or knowledge, poor judgement, poor communication or team-working skills;

- *criminal behaviour* such as cautions or convictions, dishonesty or accessing illegal material from the Internet;
- *serious ill health* where long-term untreated or unacknowledged physical or mental health conditions impair the nurse's ability to practise.

If the NMC receives a complaint about a nurse the first thing that happens is an initial investigation by NMC Case Examiners who determine if there is a case to answer. On some occasions this results in the allegation being considered not sufficiently serious to require regulatory action and the case will be closed. If however, the initial investigation confirms that there is a case for the nurse to answer it will be referred to the Conduct and Competence Committee or the Health Committee, depending on the nature of the allegations. Committee panels are made up of registered nurses, midwives and lay members. At least one member of the panel must have expertise in the same area and be registered on the same part of the register as the person against whom the allegation has been made. For example, if the allegation is against a mental health nurse working in forensic psychiatry, then one of the panel members must also be a registered mental health nurse with expertise in that area of mental health.

Meetings of the Conduct and Competence Committee are usually public and a member of the NMC legal team will be in attendance to advise on points of law. During a hearing, the panel will consider written evidence, as well as hearing from witnesses and from the nurse against whom the allegations have been made. The nurse may be represented by a trade union official, or have legal representation from a solicitor or a barrister. If the panel decides that the nurse's fitness to practise has been impaired it may decide (rarely) that no action is necessary. If the panel decides that action is necessary, it can issue the following orders:

- Issue a caution that does not prevent a nurse from practising but that can last between one and five years (a caution order).
- Impose conditions of practice for a specified period of time between 1 and 3 years (a conditions of practice order).
- Suspend the nurse's registration for up to 1 year (a suspension order).
- Remove the person from the register for 5 years (a striking-off order).

The NMC publishes guidance about how these sanctions should be implemented (NMC 2012). This document states that a striking-off order is likely to be appropriate when the behaviour is fundamentally incompatible with being a registered professional, which may involve any of the following (this list is not exhaustive):

- Serious departure from the relevant professional standards as set out in key standards, guidance and advice.
- Doing harm to others or behaving in such a way that could foreseeably result in harm to others, particularly patients or other people the nurse or midwife comes into contact with in a professional capacity, either deliberately, recklessly, negligently or through incompetence, particularly where there is a continuing risk to patients.
- Abuse of position, abuse of trust, or violation of the rights of patients, particularly in relation to vulnerable patients.
- Any serious misconduct of a sexual nature, including involvement in child pornography.

Janet Holt

- Any violent conduct, whether towards members of the public or patients, where the conduct is such that the public interest can only be satisfied by removal.
- Dishonesty, especially where persistent or covered up.
- Persistent lack of insight into seriousness of actions or consequences.
- Convictions or cautions involving any of the conduct or behaviour set out above.

(NMC 2012, pp. 14–16)

Health Committee panels are of a similar composition to the Conduct and Competence Committee, but because confidential medical evidence may be considered, the meetings are held in private. This committee makes decisions about whether a nurse's fitness to practise is impaired on the grounds of physical or mental ill health and if the case is proven they may impose the following sanctions to protect the public:

- Issue a caution for a period of between 1 and 5 years.
- Impose conditions of practice for a period of up to 3 years.
- Suspend registration for up to 1 year.

The NMC publishes annual reports (NMC 2015d) giving information about cases that have been referred, investigated and heard under fitness for practice procedures. Details about numbers of referrals, investigation and hearings can be found in Figure 2.3. Full reports of the hearings of each case including the final decisions are available on the NMC website.

The annual reports and detailed case reports make uncomfortable reading, but the publication of the reports demonstrates the NMC's commitment to transparency in its duty to protect the public. While it is clearly important that the public is protected from incompetent, unsafe or dangerous practitioners, the whole process of professional regulation is also important to the growth and development of the nursing profession.

Standard of proof

In law there are two standards of proof that can be applied to the facts of a case. In civil cases involving disputes between persons, the standard of proof is 'on the balance of probability'. In criminal cases a more stringent standard of proof is used, 'beyond reasonable doubt' (see Chapter 4). NMC panels use the less stringent civil standard of proof to decide whether the facts of an allegation are proven. This means that a panel will consider the facts of a case proven if they find it is more likely than not to have happened.

Accountability and students

A common misconception is that students are not accountable for their actions. It is the case that students cannot be held to account for their actions by the NMC, as they are not registered practitioners. Students are supervised in clinical practice and if necessary, the NMC would call to account the registered practitioners with whom the student was working, and not the student. This is in keeping with Hart's definition of role responsibility, discussed earlier (Hart 1968). Part of the role of registered nurses is an obligation to 'support students' and colleagues' learning to help them develop their professional competence and confidence' (NMC 2015a, clause 9.4). If the registered nurse fails to supervise the student adequately or delegates a task beyond that expected of them at that

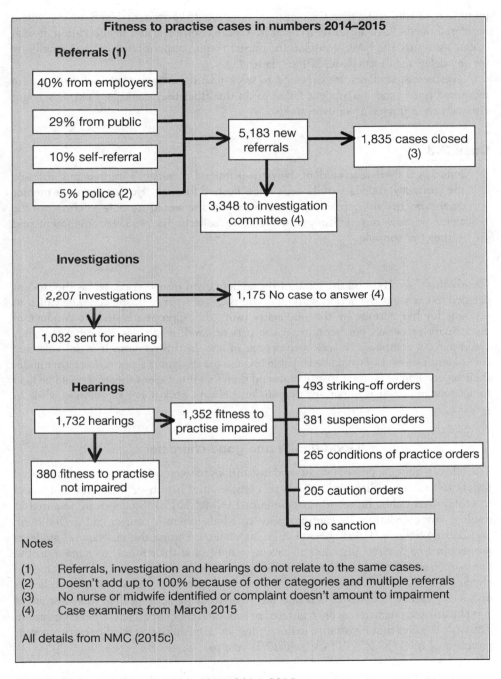

Fitness to practise cases in numbers 2014–2015

Referrals (1)

40% from employers

29% from public

10% self-referral

5% police (2)

5,183 new referrals

1,835 cases closed (3)

3,348 to investigation committee (4)

Investigations

2,207 investigations

1,175 No case to answer (4)

1,032 sent for hearing

Hearings

1,732 hearings

1,352 fitness to practise impaired

380 fitness to practise not impaired

493 striking-off orders

381 suspension orders

265 conditions of practice orders

205 caution orders

9 no sanction

Notes

(1)   Referrals, investigation and hearings do not relate to the same cases.
(2)   Doesn't add up to 100% because of other categories and multiple referrals
(3)   No nurse or midwife identified or complaint doesn't amount to impairment
(4)   Case examiners from March 2015

All details from NMC (2015c)

FIGURE 2.3 Fitness to practise in numbers 2014–2015

point in their education, then the registered nurse would be accountable. Similarly, where registered nurses have authority to delegate tasks to non-regulated health care staff such as care assistants, the NMC considers the nurse to retain responsibility and accountability for any delegated tasks (NMC 2015a, clause 11).

Nevertheless, students are expected to work under the appropriate supervision of a registered nurse, and if a student failed to do this then they could be held to account either by their university or even in law.

Case 2.3

Jenna is a third-year student. Having examined a patient's intravenous cannula she (correctly) judges that it needs to be flushed through. Having seen her mentor do this on several occasions, Jenna feels that she would be able to carry out the action without any difficulty and therefore collects the required equipment and flushes the cannula.

Clearly this task is beyond the remit of the student even if supervised, but as the student decided to carry out the action without consulting her supervisor, she could be called to account for her actions by the university using the appropriate student conduct or disciplinary processes. Furthermore, if the patient's well-being was compromised, they could make a complaint or seek recompense in law. In this scenario it is unlikely that the student's supervisor would be culpable because the student was not acting either under their supervision or on their instructions and therefore the student themself could be held to account in law. It is important that students always work under supervision while in practice.

Good health and good character

The NMC requires approved educational institutions to rigorously implement an approved fitness to practise policy and process to consider any health or character issues and to ensure that public protection is maintained (NMC 2015j). Students are required to disclose any convictions or cautions prior to admission to a course, and a Disclosure and Barring Service (DBS) check will be undertaken. During the programme, students are required to disclose any cautions or convictions, and their fitness to remain on the programme may be considered by the university fitness for practice panel. However, good character is more than an absence of convictions; any other behaviour that indicates dishonesty can be considered. Students are regularly required to declare that they are of good health and character, as are registered nurses, each time they renew their registration. *The Code* requires that registrants 'maintain the level of health you need to carry out your professional role' (NMC 2015a, clause 20.9), and to

tell both us and any employers as soon as you can about any caution or charge against you, or if you have received a conditional discharge in relation to, or have been found guilty of, a criminal offence (other than a protected caution or conviction).

(NMC 2015a, clause 23.2)

In accordance with the pre-registration nursing and midwifery standards, universities must assess the health and character of each student on completion of the course and sign a declaration of good health and good character. The NMC issues guidance to universities in making such decisions (NMC 2015j). The guidance aims to:

- ensure that relevant factors are considered and irrelevant ones are not considered when assessing whether applicants to the register are of sufficient character and health to be capable of safe and effective practice;
- ensure that decisions about admission to the register are consistent and made with reference to objective criteria; and
- ensure fairness and transparency in the decision-making process.

Use of social media

One area that has attracted the attention of the NMC is how practitioners use social media both in their professional and personal life. Social media such as Facebook and Twitter can be very useful for nurses both in practice and in education, but *The Code* requires that you must 'use all forms of spoken, written and digital communication (including social media and networking sites) responsibly . . . ' (NMC 2015a, clause 20.10). There is no doubt that rapid methods of communication can be beneficial in health care environments, such as the use of telehealth initiatives to communicate with patients. But sharing of personal information can raise ethical questions and compromise professional standards as illustrated in the following case.

In September 2015, the NMC Competence Committee heard the case of a registered nurse who admitted to posting inappropriate comments and photographs on Facebook (NMC 2015k). The charges included referring to her place of work as an asylum, complaining about her contract and threatening to go to the press, referring to elderly patients as gremlins, posting photographs, which included documents clearly identifying her place of work and suggesting she was about to go to work with a hangover. Following a disciplinary process, the nurse was dismissed from her employment for bringing the Trust into disrepute and subsequently referred by her employers to the NMC. The panel decided that the case was serious enough to warrant a sanction and issue an 18-month caution order to show the nurse, the public and the profession that such misconduct was unacceptable and must not be repeated. In this case, the nurse did not lose her registration, but did lose her job and has to live with the embarrassment of being named on a publicly searchable website. A similar case resulted in a suspension order, which was subsequently changed to a striking-off order (NMC 2013b, 2015l). The NMC *Guidance on Using Social Media Responsibly* clearly states that 'nurses may put their registration at risk, and students may jeopardise their ability to join our register, if they act in any way that is unprofessional or unlawful on social media' (NMC 2015m, p. 3).

PART 3: EXPLORING PROFESSIONAL ISSUES

What is of more importance than the existence of a code of ethics or conduct is its effectiveness in practice. This has been a subject of comment and research for over 10 years and was considered to be a sufficiently important topic to be the focus of one of the papers selected for the thirtieth anniversary issue of the *Journal of Advanced Nursing* in 2006. Esterhuizen's paper 'Is the professional code the cornerstone of clinical nursing practice?' was published in the 1996 volume of the *Journal of Advanced Nursing* (Esterhuizen 1996). In this paper Esterhuizen concludes that codes of nursing do provide the base for nursing actions and are necessary for professional accountability. Ten years later in the anniversary issue, the paper was reproduced with three commentaries from contemporary authors. While acknowledging the methodological limitations of Esterhuizen's review, the question is still considered to need further research (Gastmans and Verpeet 2006; Leino-Kilpi 2006). Leino-Kilpi (2006) points out that there is little evidence to suggest that nurses who put ethical codes into practice provide better nursing care than those who do not, especially since in countries that do not have ethical codes nurses still appear to care competently for patients.

Codes of ethics?

Whether *The Code* is, or even should be, a code of ethics or a set of standards is a matter of debate. Pattison (2001) pertinently asks 'Are nursing codes of practice ethical?' and concludes that although written in ethical language, professional codes do not develop or support independent critical judgement, which Pattison deems necessary for good professionalism. The latest version of *The Code* does not specifically mention ethics or ethical practice, but in keeping with former versions, it continues to be written in ethical language insofar as ethics is concerned with distinguishing between good and bad actions. However, *The Code* can more accurately be considered to be a code of conduct rather than a code of ethics (Snelling and Lipscomb 2004).

The Code does not give the nurse an indication of what they must do to act morally: it simply states the standard of behaviour to which the nurse is required to conform. For example, a nurse is expected to gain informed consent before they begin any treatment or care. This is a legal as well as a professional requirement, and should a nurse fail to do this, they could be called to account for their actions. However, it is possible for the nurse to approach the patient and obtain informed consent without any sense of the moral imperative of the act. The nurse would be acting in accordance with *The Code*, but may not (or indeed not need to) justify their actions morally. If the nurse was asked why they were obtaining informed consent, they could simply say because *The Code* requires them to do so, without explaining or justifying why this is morally the right action. Gastmans and Verpeet (2006) discuss how a decade earlier, Esterhuizen's (1996) paper pointed out that the most important feature of codes is their normative function rather than their disciplinary, legal or professional functions. However, to achieve this codes would need to be designed to be both useful and effective in bringing about ethical practice (Meulenbergs *et al.* 2004).

Following this theme, Pattison (2001) raises the concern that professional codes do not develop the independent critical thought needed for good moral and professional judgement, nor do they detail why the values and principles addressed in the codes have been selected. A code of ethics has been regarded as an essential characteristic of a profession and *The Code* is the central document used by the NMC in making judgements about fitness to practise. However, whether the latest version will be of help is open to debate. Snelling (2015), for example, contends that the new code does not meet its central purpose of giving guidance for action compounded by the reduction in additional explanatory guidance previously published by the NMC. Thus, codes may be considered simply as useful tools for social recognition, as an indicator of professional status or as instruments to control the activities of practitioners (Meulenbergs *et al.* 2004). Whether they provide guidance on ethical practice or develop a sense of ethical conduct in practitioners is open to debate. The NMC expects practitioners to act in the best interests of patients and clients, but how this may be best achieved in the many encounters with service users across a broad spectrum of practice is left to the practitioner to discern.

Good character and conduct

The NMC clearly expects practitioners not only to practise competently but also to be of good character. Students are required to make a self-declaration that they are of good health and good character, but before being admitted to the register, the NMC also requires that this is supported by a statement from a registered nurse involved in pre-registration education. Therefore, as well as completing the theoretical and clinical requirements of the programme, the student must also convince the person signing this declaration of good character (usually a designated member of the university staff) that they are a suitable candidate for inclusion on the register of nurses.

An assessment of good character requires consideration of conduct, behaviour or attitudes that are not compatible with professional registration in addition to any convictions or cautions. However, as Sellman (2007) discusses, NMC guidance for those making such character assessments is not explicit but requires the applicant to intend to comply with *The Code*, not have relevant criminal convictions, or not to have been found guilty of misconduct. Furthermore, to assess a person's character is to make a moral judgement about the person based upon the available evidence. Without this signed declaration, the application for registration as a nurse with the NMC will not be accepted. Consequently any wrongdoing on your part, which may be construed as not demonstrating good character and conduct, could prevent you from being admitted to the professional register even though you may have successfully completed the programme of study. Once you are registered as a nurse, how you behave in your personal life as well as when in practice will be subject to scrutiny, as demonstrated in a case brought before the Conduct and Competence Committee in 2011, where a nurse had been convicted of Class B controlled drug with intent to supply. Having already received a custodial sentence, a striking-off order was also issued. In this case, the panel found that the nurse's fitness to practise was impaired by reason of his misconduct compounded by the fact that he showed no insight into the seriousness of his misconduct (NMC 2011).

CONCLUSION

In this chapter, the concepts of responsibility and accountability have been explored. As a registered nurse you will be expected to adhere to the standards of practice required by the NMC and detailed in their publications, most notably in *The Code*. The primary function of the NMC is to protect the public, and it fulfils this responsibility by ensuring that nurses who are on the professional register are fit for practice and by imposing sanctions on nurses who do not meet the required standards. However, as discussed, there are different facets to accountability, and a nurse may be called to account by patients and clients through legal processes, or by their employers according to their terms and conditions of employment. Despite the changes in the regulation of practitioners and the emphasis put on careful recruitment and selection of students in the post-Francis era, some nurses may demonstrate poor practice, but never be challenged to give reasons for their actions. While the mechanisms of accountability are important, what lies at the heart of this issue is the integrity, honesty and trustworthiness of the practitioner, and hence a sense of the moral responsibility you have to the patients and clients in your care, your colleagues and to the profession as a whole.

Another important issue addressed in this chapter is the need to separate the issues of responsibility and accountability so you know what is expected of you in your professional role. As well as any specific aspects of practice, you will also be responsible for making judgements about what is and what is not within your scope of practice. As shown in the case study at the beginning of the chapter, if you accept responsibility for the care required by patients and clients, then this is what you are accountable for to the patient or client themselves (or their relatives), your employers and the NMC. Accountability may also extend to your personal life as well as regulating your professional life.

Nurses in the UK do not work in isolation, and if you are unsure of what to do in a given situation, it is important that you seek advice from more senior colleagues, though simply following the advice does not absolve you of personal accountability. You should also ensure that you keep clear records in case you need to refer to them at a later date. Professional responsibility and accountability is onerous for practitioners, but ensuring that only those practitioners who remain fit to practise have responsibility for patient care is the consequence of belonging to a profession with the privilege of self-regulation.

SUGGESTED FURTHER READING

The major source for further information about professional issues is the Nursing and Midwifery Council's website, www.nmc-uk.org. All of the documents referred to in this chapter are publicly available. Navigation around the site takes a little while to master, but patience is rewarded. The material there is invaluable to understanding your responsibilities as a nurse. In addition the Department of Health website contains much useful information, especially the Chief Nurse's page. www.england.nhs.uk/2015/08/26/cno-bull-sept-15/

There are links from here to relevant documents, and you can arrange for regular newsletters to be sent.

The following books explore professional issues and accountability in more depth:

Caulfield, H. (2005) *Accountability*, Oxford: Blackwell.
    A basic introductory textbook.
Chiarella, M. (2002) *The Legal and Professional Status of Nursing*, Edinburgh: Churchill Livingstone.
    This is a fascinating account of how the profession of nursing is defined in a number of different ways through judgments made in legal cases throughout the English-speaking liberal democracies.
Gallagher, A. and Hodge, S. (eds). (2012) *Ethics, Law, and Professional Issues: A practice based approach for health professionals*. Basingstoke: Palgrave Macmillan.
    This is a short, accessible and practice-focused book.
Tilley, S. and Watson, R. (eds). (2014) *Accountability in Nursing and Midwifery*, (2nd edn). Oxford: Blackwell.
    Contains an impressive discussion of accountability within a range of settings.

REFERENCES

Abbott, P. and Wallace, C. (1998) Health visiting, social work, nursing and midwifery: a history. In *The Sociology of the Caring Professions* (2nd edn), Abbot, P. and Meerabeau, L. (eds). London: UCL Press, pp. 20–53.

Baly, M. E. (1995) *Nursing and Social Change* (3rd edn). London: Routledge.

Caulfield H. (2005) *Accountability*. Oxford: Blackwell.

Chiarella, M. (2002) *The Legal and Professional Status of Nursing*. Edinburgh: Churchill Livingstone.

Colyer, H. M. (2004) The construction and development of health professionals: where will it end? *Journal of Advanced Nursing* **48** (4), 406–412.

Esterhuizen, P. (1996) Is the professional code still the cornerstone of clinical nursing practice? *Journal of Advanced Nursing* **23** (1), 25–31.

Finlay, L. (2000) The challenge of professionalism. In *Critical Practice in Health and Social Care*, Brechin, A., Brown, H. and Eby, M. A. (eds). London: Open University Press, pp. 73–95.

Fletcher, N., Holt, J., Brazier, M. and Harris, J. (1995) *Ethics, Law and Nursing*. Manchester: Manchester University Press.

Francis, R. (2013) The Mid-Staffordshire NHS Foundation Trust Public Inquiry. www.midstaffs publicinquiry.com/

Fry, S. T. and Johnstone, M.-J. (2002) *Ethics in Nursing Practice: A Guide to Ethical Decision-Making* (2nd edn). Oxford: Blackwell.

Gallagher, A. (2007) The respectful nurse. *Nursing Ethics* **14** (3), 360–371.

Gastmans, C. (1999) Care as a moral attitude in nursing. *Nursing Ethics* **6** (3), 214–223.

Gastmans, C. and Verpeet, E. (2006) 30th anniversary commentary of Esterhuizen, P. (1996) Is the professional code still the cornerstone of clinical nursing practice? *Journal of Advanced Nursing* **53** (1), 111–112.

Gerrish, K., McManus, M. and Ashworth, P. (2003) Creating what sort of professional? Master's level nurse education as a professionalising strategy. *Nursing Inquiry* **10** (2), 103–112.

Hart, H. L. A. (1968) *Punishment and Responsibility*. Oxford: Oxford University Press.

Ion, R., Smith, K., Nimmo, S., Rice, A. M. and McMillan, L. (2015) Factors influencing student nurse decisions to report poor practice witnessed while on placement. *Nurse Education Today*, **35** (7), 900–905.

Jacobs, K. (2004) Accountability and clinical governance in nursing: a critical overview of the topic. In *Accountability in Nursing* (2nd edn), Tilley, S. and Watson, R. (eds). Oxford: Blackwell, pp. 21–37.

Johnstone M.-J. (2009) *Bioethics: A Nursing Perspective* (5th edn). Sydney: Churchill Livingstone.

Leino-Kilpi, H. (2006) 30th anniversary commentary of Esterhuizen, P. (1996) Is the professional code still the cornerstone of clinical nursing practice? *Journal of Advanced Nursing* **53** (1), 112–113.

Lesser, H. (2014) An ethical perspective: negligence and moral obligations. In *Nursing Law and Ethics* (4th edn), Tingle, J. and Cobb, A. (eds). Oxford: Blackwell, pp. 118–127.

McCarthy, J. and Gastmans, C. (2015) Moral distress: a review of the argument-based nursing ethics literature. *Nursing Ethics* **22** (1), 131–152.

McGann, S. (2004) The development of nursing as an accountable profession. In *Accountability in Nursing* (2nd edn), Tilley, S. and Watson, R. (eds). Oxford: Blackwell, pp. 9–20.

Merrifield, N. (2015) Exclusive: new band 4 'associate nurse' role set to be created. *Nursing Times*, 30 November 2015. www.nursingtimes.net/roles/healthcare-assistants/exclusive-new-associate-nurse-role-set-to-be-created/7000747.fullarticle (accessed 17 December 2015).

Meulenbergs, T., Verpeet, E., Schotsmans, P. and Gastmans, C. (2004) Professional codes in a changing nursing context: literature review. *Journal of Advanced Nursing* **46** (3), 331–336.

Morrall, P. (2001) *Sociology and Nursing*. London: Routledge.

Nortvedt, P. (1998) Sensitive judgement: an inquiry into the foundations of nursing ethics. *Nursing Ethics* **5** (5), 385–386.

NMC (2008) *Standards to Support Learning and Assessment in Practice* (2nd edn) London: Nursing and Midwifery Council [online] www.nmc.org.uk/globalassets/sitedocuments/standards/nmc-standards-to-support-learning-assessment.pdf (accessed 17 December 2015).

NMC (2010) *Standards for Pre-Registration Nursing Education.* London: Nursing and Midwifery Council [online]. www.nmc.org.uk/globalassets/sitedocuments/standards/nmc-standards-for-pre-registration-nursing-education.pdf (accessed 17 December 2015).

NMC (2011) *Reasons from the Substantive Hearing of the Conduct and Competence Committee Panel – Adekunle Ola Jibona.* London: Nursing and Midwifery Council [online] www.nmc.org.uk/globalassets/sitedocuments/ftpoutcomes/cop2011/20110513-reasons-cccsh-jibona-24288.pdf (accessed 17 December 2015).

NMC (2012) *Indicative Sanctions Guidance to Panels.* London: Nursing and Midwifery Council [online] www.nmc.org.uk/globalassets/sitedocuments/ftp_information/indicative-sanctions-guidance.may-12.pdf (accessed 17 December 2015).

NMC (2013a) *Raising Concerns: Guidance for Nurses and Midwives.* London: Nursing and Midwifery Council [online] www.nmc.org.uk/globalassets/sitedocuments/annual_reports_and_accounts/raising-concerns-10-june-2015–2.pdf (accessed 17 December 2015).

NMC (2013b) *Conduct and Competence Committee Substantive Hearing – Allison Marie Hopton.* London: Nursing and Midwifery Council [online] www.nmc.org.uk/globalassets/sitedocuments/ftpoutcomes/2013/sep/reasons-cccsh-public-hopton-035146.pdf?_t_id=1B2M2Y8AsgTpgAm Y7PhCfg%3d%3d&_t_q=Facebook&_t_tags=language%3aen%2csiteid%3ad6891695–0234–4 63b-bf74–1bfb02644b38&_t_ip=86.161.44.198&_t_hit.id=NMC_Web_Models_Media_ DocumentFile/_274b1dd1–23e4–43aa-94f2–15ec6322ee89&_t_hit.pos=8 (accessed 17 December 2015).

NMC (2015a) *The Code: Standards of Conduct, Performance and Ethics for Nurses and Midwives.* London: Nursing and Midwifery Council [online] www.nmc.org.uk/standards/code/ (accessed 17 December 2015).

NMC (2015b) *Conscientious Objection by Nurses and Midwives.* London: Nursing and Midwifery Council [online] www.nmc.org.uk/standards/code/conscientious-objection-by-nurses-and-midwives/ (accessed 17 December 2015).

NMC (2015c) *Our Role* [online] www.nmc.org.uk/about-us/our-role/ (accessed 17 December 2015).

NMC (2015d). *Annual Fitness to Practise Report 2014–2015.* London: Nursing and Midwifery Council [online] www.nmc.org.uk/globalassets/sitedocuments/annual_reports_and_accounts/ftpannualreports/annual-ftp-report-2014–2015.pdf (accessed 17 December 2015).

NMC (2015e) *Standards of Competence for Registered Nurses.* London: Nursing and Midwifery Council [online] www.nmc.org.uk/standards/additional-standards/standards-for-competence-for-registered-nurses/(accessed 17 December 2015).

NMC (2015f) *Quality Assurance Framework for Nursing and Midwifery Education and Local Supervising Authorities.* London: Nursing and Midwifery Council [online] www.nmc.org.uk/education/quality-assurance-of-education/qa-framework-for-education/ (accessed 17 December 2015).

NMC (2015g) *Guidance for Students.* London: Nursing and Midwifery Council [online] www.nmc.org.uk/education/becoming-a-nurse-or-midwife/when-studying-to-be-a-nurse-or-midwife/guidance-for-students (accessed 17 December 2015).

NMC (2015h) *Conduct and Competence Committee Substantive Hearing – Perkis Kugura.* London: Nursing and Midwifery Council [online] www.nmc.org.uk/globalassets/sitedocuments /ftpoutcomes/2015/aug/reasons-kugura-cccsh-38107–20150807.pdf (accessed 17 December 2015).

NMC (2015i) *Advice and Information for Employers of Nurses and Midwives.* London: Nursing and Midwifery Council [online] www.nmc.org.uk/globalassets/sitedocuments/ftp_information/advice-for-employers-15-october-2015.pdf (accessed 17 December 2015).

NMC (2015j) *Character and Health Decision-Making Guidance.* London: Nursing and Midwifery Council [online] www.nmc.org.uk/globalassets/sitedocuments/registration/character-and-health-decision-making-guidance.pdf (accessed 17 December 2015).

NMC (2015k) *Conduct and Competence Committee Substantive Hearing – Claire Booker McLean*. London: Nursing and Midwifery Council [online] www.nmc.org.uk/globalassets/site documents/ftpoutcomes/2015/sep/reasons-mclean-cccsh-44789–20150911.pdf (accessed 17 December 2015).

NMC (2015l) *Conduct and Competence Committee Substantive Order Review Hearing – Allison Marie Hopton*. London: Nursing and Midwifery Council [online] www.nmc.org.uk/globalassets/site documents/ftpoutcomes/2015/mar/reasons-hopton-cccsor-35146–20150305.pdf?_t_id=1B2M 2Y8AsgTpgAmY7PhCfg%3d%3d&_t_q=Facebook&_t_tags=language%3aen%2csiteid%3ad 6891695–0234–463b-bf74–1bfb02644b38&_t_ip=86.161.44.198&_t_hit.id=NMC_Web_ Models_Media_DocumentFile/_336822f0–3756–48f4–8f28–5b09f3788f84&_t_hit.pos=44 (accessed 17 December 2015).

NMC (2015m) *Guidance on Using Social Media Responsibly*. London: Nursing and Midwifery Council [online] www.nmc.org.uk/globalassets/sitedocuments/nmc-publications/social-media-guidance-30-march-2015-final.pdf (accessed 17 December 2015).

Pattison, S. (2001) Are nursing codes of practice ethical? *Nursing Ethics* **8** (1), 5–18.

Pearson, A. (2005) Registration, regulation and competence in nursing. *International Journal of Nursing Practice* **11** (5), 191–192.

Porter, R. (1997) *The Greatest Benefit to Mankind: A Medical History of Humanity from Antiquity to the Present*. London: HarperCollins.

Royal College of Nursing (RCN) (2012) *Quality with Compassion: The Future of Nursing Education*. Report of the Willis Commission on Nursing Education. London: RCN.

Sellman, D. (2007) On being of good character: nurse education and the assessment of good character. *Nurse Education Today* **27** (7), 762–767.

Snelling, P. C. (2015) Can the revised UK code direct practice? *Nursing Ethics*. Published online before print November 30, 2015, doi: 10.1177/0969733015610802

Snelling, P. C. and Lipscomb, M. (2004) Academic freedom, analysis, and the Code of Professional Conduct. *Nurse Education Today* **24** (8), 615–621.

Supreme Court (2014) Greater Glasgow Health Board (Appellant) v Doogan and another (Respondents) (Scotland).

Wilensky, H. L. (1964) *Industrial Society and Social Welfare: The Impact of Industrialisation on the Supply of Social Welfare Services in the United States*. New York: Russell Sage Foundation.

Willis, P. (2015) *Raising the Bar. Shape of Caring: A Review of the Future Education and Training of Registered Nurses and Care Assistants*. London: HEE [online] www.hee.nhs.uk/sites/default/files/documents/2348-Shape-of-caring-review-FINAL.pdf (accessed 17 December 2015).

Appendix: The Code

Professional Standards of Practice and Behaviour for Nurses and Midwives

Quoted in full from nmc-uk.org with permission. Excludes footnotes. For full text go to www.nmc.org.uk/standards/code/.

PRIORITISE PEOPLE

You put the interests of people using or needing nursing or midwifery services first. You make their care and safety your main concern and make sure that their dignity is preserved and their needs are recognised, assessed and responded to. You make sure that those receiving care are treated with respect, that their rights are upheld and that any discriminatory attitudes and behaviours towards those receiving care are challenged.

1   *Treat people as individuals and uphold their dignity.* To achieve this, you must:
   1.1   treat people with kindness, respect and compassion
   1.2   make sure you deliver the fundamentals of care effectively
   1.3   avoid making assumptions and recognise diversity and individual choice
   1.4   make sure that any treatment, assistance or care for which you are responsible is delivered without undue delay, and
   1.5   respect and uphold people's human rights.
2   *Listen to people and respond to their preferences and concerns.* To achieve this, you must:
   2.1   work in partnership with people to make sure you deliver care effectively
   2.2   recognise and respect the contribution that people can make to their own health and well-being
   2.3   encourage and empower people to share decisions about their treatment and care
   2.4   respect the level to which people receiving care want to be involved in decisions about their own health, wellbeing and care
   2.5   respect, support and document a person's right to accept or refuse care and treatment, and

2.6 recognise when people are anxious or in distress and respond compassionately and politely.

3 *Make sure that people's physical, social and psychological needs are assessed and responded to.* To achieve this, you must:

3.1 pay special attention to promoting well-being, preventing ill health and meeting the changing health and care needs of people during all life stages

3.2 recognise and respond compassionately to the needs of those who are in the last few days and hours of life

3.3 act in partnership with those receiving care, helping them to access relevant health and social care, information and support when they need it, and

3.4 act as an advocate for the vulnerable, challenging poor practice and discriminatory attitudes and behaviour relating to their care.

4 *Act in the best interests of people at all times.* To achieve this, you must:

4.1 balance the need to act in the best interests of people at all times with the requirement to respect a person's right to accept or refuse treatment

4.2 make sure that you get properly informed consent and document it before carrying out any action

4.3 keep to all relevant laws about mental capacity that apply in the country in which you are practising, and make sure that the rights and best interests of those who lack capacity are still at the centre of the decision-making process, and

4.4 tell colleagues, your manager and the person receiving care if you have a conscientious objection to a particular procedure and arrange for a suitably qualified colleague to take over responsibility for that person's care.

5 *Respect people's right to privacy and confidentiality.* As a nurse or midwife, you owe a duty of confidentiality to all those who are receiving care. This includes making sure that they are informed about their care and that information about them is shared appropriately. To achieve this, you must:

5.1 respect a person's right to privacy in all aspects of their care

5.2 make sure that people are informed about how and why information is used and shared by those who will be providing care

5.3 respect that a person's right to privacy and confidentiality continues after they have died

5.4 share necessary information with other healthcare professionals and agencies only when the interests of patient safety and public protection override the need for confidentiality, and

5.5 share with people, their families and their carers, as far as the law allows, the information they want or need to know about their health, care and ongoing treatment sensitively and in a way they can understand.

PRACTISE EFFECTIVELY

You assess need and deliver or advise on treatment, or give help (including preventative or rehabilitative care) without too much delay and to the best of your abilities, on the basis of the best evidence available and best practice. You communicate effectively, keeping clear and accurate records and sharing skills, knowledge and experience where appropriate. You reflect and act on any feedback you receive to improve your practice.

6 *Always practise in line with the best available evidence.* To achieve this, you must:
   6.1 make sure that any information or advice given is evidence-based, including information relating to using any health care products or services, and
   6.2 maintain the knowledge and skills you need for safe and effective practice.
7 *Communicate clearly.* To achieve this, you must:
   7.1 use terms that people in your care, colleagues and the public can understand
   7.2 take reasonable steps to meet people's language and communication needs, providing, wherever possible, assistance to those who need help to communicate their own or other people's needs
   7.3 use a range of verbal and non-verbal communication methods, and consider cultural sensitivities, to better understand and respond to people's personal and health needs
   7.4 check people's understanding from time to time to keep misunderstanding or mistakes to a minimum, and
   7.5 be able to communicate clearly and effectively in English.
8 *Work cooperatively.* To achieve this, you must:
   8.1 respect the skills, expertise and contributions of your colleagues, referring matters to them when appropriate
   8.2 maintain effective communication with colleagues
   8.3 keep colleagues informed when you are sharing the care of individuals with other health care professionals and staff
   8.4 work with colleagues to evaluate the quality of your work and that of the team
   8.5 work with colleagues to preserve the safety of those receiving care
   8.6 share information to identify and reduce risk, and
   8.7 be supportive of colleagues who are encountering health or performance problems. However, this support must never compromise or be at the expense of patient or public safety.
9 *Share your skills, knowledge and experience for the benefit of people receiving care and your colleagues.* To achieve this, you must:
   9.1 provide honest, accurate and constructive feedback to colleagues
   9.2 gather and reflect on feedback from a variety of sources, using it to improve your practice and performance
   9.3 deal with differences of professional opinion with colleagues by discussion and informed debate, respecting their views and opinions and behaving in a professional way at all times, and
   9.4 support students' and colleagues' learning to help them develop their professional competence and confidence.
10 *Keep clear and accurate records relevant to your practice.* This includes but is not limited to patient records. It includes all records that are relevant to your scope of practice. To achieve this, you must:
   10.1 complete all records at the time or as soon as possible after an event, recording if the notes are written some time after the event
   10.2 identify any risks or problems that have arisen and the steps taken to deal with them, so that colleagues who use the records have all the information they need
   10.3 complete all records accurately and without any falsification, taking immediate and appropriate action if you become aware that someone has not kept to these requirements

10.4 attribute any entries you make in any paper or electronic records to yourself, making sure they are clearly written, dated and timed, and do not include unnecessary abbreviations, jargon or speculation

10.5 take all steps to make sure that all records are kept securely, and

10.6 collect, treat and store all data and research findings appropriately.

11 *Be accountable for your decisions to delegate tasks and duties to other people.* To achieve this, you must:

11.1 only delegate tasks and duties that are within the other person's scope of competence, making sure that they fully understand your instructions

11.2 make sure that everyone you delegate tasks to is adequately supervised and supported so they can provide safe and compassionate care, and

11.3 confirm that the outcome of any task you have delegated to someone else meets the required standard.

12 *Have in place an indemnity arrangement, which provides appropriate cover for any practice you take on as a nurse or midwife in the United Kingdom.* To achieve this, you must:

12.1 make sure that you have an appropriate indemnity arrangement in place relevant to your scope of practice.

For more information, please visit: www.nmc-uk.org/indemnity.

PRESERVE SAFETY

You make sure that patient and public safety is protected. You work within the limits of your competence, exercising your professional 'duty of candour' and raising concerns immediately whenever you come across situations that put patients or public safety at risk. You take necessary action to deal with any concerns where appropriate.

13 *Recognise and work within the limits of your competence.* To achieve this, you must:

13.1 accurately assess signs of normal or worsening physical and mental health in the person receiving care

13.2 make a timely and appropriate referral to another practitioner when it is in the best interests of the individual needing any action, care or treatment

13.3 ask for help from a suitably qualified and experienced health care professional to carry out any action or procedure that is beyond the limits of your competence

13.4 take account of your own personal safety as well as the safety of people in your care, and

13.5 complete the necessary training before carrying out a new role.

14 *Be open and candid with all service users about all aspects of care and treatment, including when any mistakes or harm have taken place.* To achieve this, you must:

14.1 act immediately to put right the situation if someone has suffered actual harm for any reason or an incident has happened that had the potential for harm

14.2 explain fully and promptly what has happened, including the likely effects, and apologise to the person affected and, where appropriate, their advocate, family or carers, and

14.3 document all these events formally and take further action (escalate) if appropriate so they can be dealt with quickly.

15 *Always offer help if an emergency arises in your practice setting or anywhere else.* To achieve this, you must:

15.1 only act in an emergency within the limits of your knowledge and competence

15.2 arrange, wherever possible, for emergency care to be accessed and provided promptly, and

15.3 take account of your own safety, the safety of others and the availability of other options for providing care.

16 *Act without delay if you believe that there is a risk to patient safety or public protection.* To achieve this, you must:

16.1 raise and, if necessary, escalate any concerns you may have about patient or public safety, or the level of care people are receiving in your workplace or any other healthcare setting and use the channels available to you in line with our guidance and your local working practices

16.2 raise your concerns immediately if you are being asked to practise beyond your role, experience and training

16.3 tell someone in authority at the first reasonable opportunity if you experience problems that may prevent you working within the Code or other national standards, taking prompt action to tackle the causes of concern if you can

16.4 acknowledge and act on all concerns raised to you, investigating, escalating or dealing with those concerns where it is appropriate for you to do so

16.5 not obstruct, intimidate, victimise or in any way hinder a colleague, member of staff, person you care for or member of the public who wants to raise a concern, and

16.6 protect anyone you have management responsibility for from any harm, detriment, victimisation or unwarranted treatment after a concern is raised.

For more information, please visit: www.nmc-uk.org/raisingconcerns.

17 *Raise concerns immediately if you believe a person is vulnerable or at risk and needs extra support and protection.* To achieve this, you must:

17.1 take all reasonable steps to protect people who are vulnerable or at risk from harm, neglect or abuse

17.2 share information if you believe someone may be at risk of harm, in line with the laws relating to the disclosure of information, and

17.3 have knowledge of and keep to the relevant laws and policies about protecting and caring for vulnerable people.

18 *Advise on, prescribe, supply, dispense or administer medicines within the limits of your training and competence, the law, our guidance and other relevant policies, guidance and regulations.* To achieve this, you must:

18.1 prescribe, advise on, or provide medicines or treatment, including repeat prescriptions (only if you are suitably qualified) if you have enough knowledge of that person's health and are satisfied that the medicines or treatment serve that person's health needs

18.2 keep to appropriate guidelines when giving advice on using controlled drugs and recording the prescribing, supply, dispensing or administration of controlled drugs

18.3 make sure that the care or treatment you advise on, prescribe, supply, dispense or administer for each person is compatible with any other care or treatment they are receiving, including (where possible) over-the-counter medicines

18.4 take all steps to keep medicines stored securely, and

18.5 wherever possible, avoid prescribing for yourself or for anyone with whom you have a close personal relationship.

For more information, please visit: www.nmc-uk.org/standards.

19 *Be aware of, and reduce as far as possible, any potential for harm associated with your practice.* To achieve this, you must:
   19.1 take measures to reduce as far as possible, the likelihood of mistakes, near misses, harm and the effect of harm if it takes place
   19.2 take account of current evidence, knowledge and developments in reducing mistakes and the effect of them and the impact of human factors and system failures
   19.3 keep to and promote recommended practice in relation to controlling and preventing infection, and
   19.4 take all reasonable personal precautions necessary to avoid any potential health risks to colleagues, people receiving care and the public.

PROMOTE PROFESSIONALISM AND TRUST

You uphold the reputation of your profession at all times. You should display a personal commitment to the standards of practice and behaviour set out in the Code. You should be a model of integrity and leadership for others to aspire to. This should lead to trust and confidence in the profession from patients, people receiving care, other healthcare professionals and the public.

20 *Uphold the reputation of your profession at all times.* To achieve this, you must:
   20.1 keep to and uphold the standards and values set out in the Code
   20.2 act with honesty and integrity at all times, treating people fairly and without discrimination, bullying or harassment
   20.3 be aware at all times of how your behaviour can affect and influence the behaviour of other people
   20.4 keep to the laws of the country in which you are practising
   20.5 treat people in a way that does not take advantage of their vulnerability or cause them upset or distress
   20.6 stay objective and have clear professional boundaries at all times with people in your care (including those who have been in your care in the past), their families and carers
   20.7 make sure you do not express your personal beliefs (including political, religious or moral beliefs) to people in an inappropriate way
   20.8 act as a role model of professional behaviour for students and newly qualified nurses and midwives to aspire to
   20.9 maintain the level of health you need to carry out your professional role, and
   20.10 use all forms of spoken, written and digital communication (including social media and networking sites) responsibly, respecting the right to privacy of others at all times.
   For more guidance on using social media and networking sites, please visit: www.nmc-uk.org/guidance.
21 *Uphold your position as a registered nurse or midwife.* To achieve this, you must:
   21.1 refuse all but the most trivial gifts, favours or hospitality as accepting them could be interpreted as an attempt to gain preferential treatment
   21.2 never ask for or accept loans from anyone in your care or anyone close to them
   21.3 act with honesty and integrity in any financial dealings you have with everyone you have a professional relationship with, including people in your care

21.4 make sure that any advertisements, publications or published material you produce or have produced for your professional services are accurate, responsible, ethical, do not mislead or exploit vulnerabilities and accurately reflect your relevant skills, experience and qualifications

21.5 never use your professional status to promote causes that are not related to health, and

21.6 cooperate with the media only when it is appropriate to do so, and then always protecting the confidentiality and dignity of people receiving treatment or care.

22 *Fulfil all registration requirements.* To achieve this, you must:

22.1 meet any reasonable requests so we can oversee the registration process

22.2 keep to our prescribed hours of practice and carry out continuing professional development activities, and

22.3 keep your knowledge and skills up to date, taking part in appropriate and regular learning and professional development activities that aim to maintain and develop your competence and improve your performance.

For more information, please visit: www.nmc-uk.org/standards.

23 *Cooperate with all investigations and audits.* This includes investigations or audits either against you or relating to others, whether individuals or organisations. It also includes cooperating with requests to act as a witness in any hearing that forms part of an investigation, even after you have left the register. To achieve this, you must:

23.1 cooperate with any audits of training records, registration records or other relevant audits that we may want to carry out to make sure you are still fit to practise

23.2 tell both us and any employers as soon as you can about any caution or charge against you, or if you have received a conditional discharge in relation to, or have been found guilty of, a criminal offence (other than a protected caution or conviction)

23.3 tell any employers you work for if you have had your practice restricted or had any other conditions imposed on you by us or any other relevant body

23.4 tell us and your employers at the first reasonable opportunity if you are or have been disciplined by any regulatory or licensing organisation, including those who operate outside of the professional healthcare environment, and

23.5 give your NMC Pin when any reasonable request for it is made.

24 *Respond to any complaints made against you professionally.* To achieve this, you must:

24.1 never allow someone's complaint to affect the care that is provided to them, and

24.2 use all complaints as a form of feedback and an opportunity for reflection and learning to improve practice.

25 *Provide leadership to make sure people's well-being is protected and to improve their experiences of the health care system.* To achieve this, you must:

25.1 identify priorities, manage time, staff and resources effectively and deal with risk to make sure that the quality of care or service you deliver is maintained and improved, putting the needs of those receiving care or services first, and

25.2 support any staff you may be responsible for to follow the Code at all times. They must have the knowledge, skills and competence for safe practice, and understand how to raise any concerns linked to any circumstances where the Code has, or could be, broken.

3

ETHICS

Paul Snelling

LEARNING OUTCOMES

After reading and reflecting on this chapter, you should be able to:

* explain the importance of ethics to nursing practice;
* describe the four principles of bioethics and their application to individual cases;
* outline critiques of the four principles approach;
* identify the differences between justice and care orientations to ethics;
* discuss the importance of both ethical analysis and caring disposition in ethical nursing practice.

INTRODUCTION

All of us have ideas and feelings about the rightness or wrongness of actions and use them in formulating and discussing our opinions, but ethical nursing practice requires more than unstructured feelings to guide right action. This chapter cannot hope to cover all of the ground of the ethical considerations that confront nurses in their everyday practice, but it is hoped that it will provide an introduction to the topic. Examples taken from current ethical problems and issues are used to illustrate more general points.

The chapter is divided into three parts. Part 1 will outline the nature of ethics and the reasons why it is so important for nursing practice.

Part 2 will begin to explain ethics further. The four principles approach will be used to discuss some of the most important ethical issues in health care.

Part 3 will explore a number of critiques of the four principles, and alternative and opposing approaches of care ethics will be discussed.

Ethics, in theory and practice, is concerned about what is good and right; how we ought to live our lives.

PART 1: OUTLINING ETHICS

Case 3.1

Peter, a registered nurse, is working the night duty on a busy medical ward caring for, among others, Mr Smith, who was admitted with a chest infection and is known to be a heavy drinker. During the night he becomes distressed and argumentative with staff, who refuse to take him outside so that he can have a cigarette. Peter is reluctant to allow him to go outside unaccompanied because he needs oxygen to maintain his saturation levels. He has been prescribed a sedative by medical staff but he refuses to take it, saying that sedatives make him sleepy the next day. Peter knows that he hasn't taken the prescribed sedative before; it is a new drug known to have very few side effects. He frequently states that he is desperate to go to sleep, and Peter also knows that a good night's sleep will be beneficial for his recovery. As the night progresses he wakes other patients in the bay. He asks for a cup of tea and a colleague suggests that Peter add the liquid preparation of the prescribed sedative. It would solve the problem for Peter and be beneficial for Mr Smith as well as the other patients, some of whom are becoming upset that their needs aren't being met because the nurses are spending a lot of time with Mr Smith. Despite the obvious attractions, Peter hesitates. Is it the right thing to do?

The word ethics is derived from the Greek word *ethos*, meaning custom or convention, the same meaning as the Latin word *mores*, from which the terms moral and morality are derived (Thompson *et al.* 2006). Some texts (for example, Thompson *et al.* 2006) attempt to differentiate between the terms ethics and morals. For them, morals refer to standards of behaviour, while ethics refers more specifically to the study of morals and morality. Others (Johnstone 2016, Seedhouse 2009) claim that there is no significant difference in the words and use them interchangeably. There do seem to be conventions in common usage. We speak of 'nursing ethics' rather than 'nursing morals'. There is probably little to be gained from such detailed debates. In simple terms, **ethics**, in theory and practice, is concerned about what is good and right; how we ought to live our lives.

In a wide sense we can pick up a newspaper or magazine and see ethical elements in many stories, not just obvious ones involving war or crime. Is it right for banks to make huge profits? for schools to exclude unruly pupils? for footballers to be paid such vast sums? for parents to smack their children? or to lie to a friend in order to avoid an unpalatable truth? It has even been claimed that sitting in an armchair is a moral issue in the sense that you could be doing something more worthwhile, and choose not to (Seedhouse 2009).

There is more to professional ethics, especially in the health care professions, than following our common morality, which might be relied upon in coffee shop or saloon bar discussions on these questions. There are a number of reasons for this, including:

- In professionally caring for our patients, we are obliged to act in certain ways, which might be considered optional in other settings.
- Patients are generally vulnerable (Sellman 2005) and this has moral significance, for example, in the potential for harm.
- Nurses and other health professionals are accountable for their actions, and this requires justified reasons other than 'gut feeling' or unjustified opinion.

- Because of the nature of their work, nurses are faced with many obviously moral problems, more so than would be expected in other walks of life.
- The complexity of problems commonly encountered, for example, in developing technologies concerning assisted conception, requires ethical analysis in order to avoid inconsistency.

It is sometimes suggested that there is no right or wrong, and disagreement in moral matters seems justifiable in many cases. In a general sense, for example, there are valid reasons for arguing both in favour and against the legalisation of euthanasia, or the criminalisation of abortion. We cannot appeal to a single, provable (true) law of ethics to help us decide what our opinions should be or what we ought to do in the same way that we can appeal to scientifically verifiable fact (empirical knowledge), or the law (formal knowledge) (Allmark 2005). We *know* that giving a large dose of potassium chloride is likely to kill a person, and we also *know* that it is against the law to administer it with the intention of causing death. Still it does not follow from this that it is wrong for the drug to be administered. We might want to take the view, and many people do, that it is always wrong. Or we might take the view that *sometimes* it would be the right thing to do. These views on morality may in turn influence our views about the legality of the act, whether euthanasia should be legalised, or abortion criminalised. These are opinions, not matters of fact. But saying that opposing viewpoints can both be valid is not the same as saying that everything is right, that we can all do as we feel or think without any attempt at justification. This would lead to inconsistencies and result in patients and colleagues not knowing what they could expect of us or anyone else.

The Nursing and Midwifery Council (NMC) requires that nurses practise within an ethical and legal framework. We can point at the legal framework (see Chapter 4), and also to a professional framework set out in *The Code* (NMC 2015a) (see Chapter 2). However, *The Code* does not function as a recognised ethical framework. There is nothing – at least that we can point to as some sort of 'official' ethical framework – that tells nurses, in all cases, what they ought to do and why. There have been attempts to identify decision-making models (Greipp 1992, Seedhouse 2009), but these offer frameworks for analysis of an issue or problem, rather than a prescription for its resolution. Perhaps the most established framework in bioethics is the four principles approach, and though this is not without its vociferous critics, it is useful in both analysing individual problems and identifying important ethical issues about which there is a deeper consensus. There is also evidence that students find decision-making frameworks helpful (Cameron *et al.* 2001).

Activities

The activities in this chapter should ideally be undertaken in small facilitated groups, rather than alone. This is because the nuances of ethical positions are best considered by debate. In this way your positions can be challenged and amended. Having weaknesses or contradictions in your position pointed out, and seeking these in a colleague's position can help to strengthen reasoning. However, caution is required. Often the most interesting and difficult debates concern areas, such as abortion, about which people may have strong feelings and/or personal experience. Rigorous debate needs to take account of these possibilities and care is needed in expressing opinions.

Paul Snelling

> **Activity 3.1**
>
> Discuss your initial feelings in groups. Should the medication be given concealed in Mr Smith's tea? What reasons can be given to support your conclusions?

PART 2: EXPLAINING ETHICS

The four principles approach to ethics

The four principles approach to ethics, known more simply as 'principlism', was popularised by the publication, in 1978, of the book *Principles of Biomedical Ethics*, by two American authors, Tom Beauchamp and James Childress. The book is now in its seventh edition (2013), and remains highly influential. A more accessible book, which retains the systematicity of the original and applies it to nursing practice was published by Steven Edwards in 1996 (Edwards 2006, 2009). The approach highlights four levels of ethics (Figure 3.1).

In a general sense, ethics is concerned with types of actions or situations. Is stealing wrong, and for what reasons? More specifically, the question is whether a certain individual action is right or wrong. Is it right for Mrs Jones to steal a loaf of bread at 5 pm in the afternoon in order to feed her hungry children? We might agree that generally speaking stealing is wrong, but that in this case it is acceptable. Perhaps the baker makes excessive profits, or the bread is about to be thrown away at the end of the day, or perhaps the children have not eaten all day. The point here is the relationship, if any, between the view that generally, stealing is wrong (a rule or principle) and the view that in this or that particular case it is acceptable. Morality is more than simply applying general rules to everyday situations. Black-and-white analyses are easy, but most of life occurs in shades of grey.

Level 1: individual moral judgements

We are often reminded of the moral nature of the situation that we find ourselves in when we understand it in terms of a dilemma. This means that we are unsure about what we should *do* in a particular situation. Two forms of moral dilemma can be identified (Beauchamp and Childress 2013):

1 *Where there are good reasons for thinking that an act is both morally right and morally wrong, but where the evidence is inconclusive.* The example of a woman grappling with a decision on whether or not to have an abortion is offered as an example of this. It

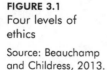

FIGURE 3.1
Four levels of ethics

Source: Beauchamp and Childress, 2013.

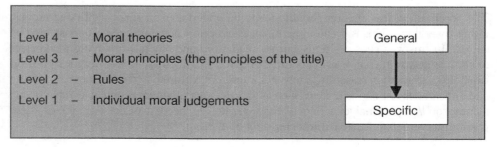

Level 4	–	Moral theories	General
Level 3	–	Moral principles (the principles of the title)	
Level 2	–	Rules	
Level 1	–	Individual moral judgements	Specific

need not be a difficult decision for everybody, however. Many would be quite clear about the resolution of this particular dilemma for themselves and some would seek to impose their opinion on everyone else.

2   *Where somebody thinks that two things are morally required but they are mutually exclusive.* For example, suppose you have promised to accompany a sick friend to an appointment. You are driving to the hospital, when you come upon an accident. You think that you ought both to keep your promise to your friend and offer assistance to the accident victim. You cannot do both, and your dilemma is which obligation to break. It need not be a difficult dilemma; it would depend on the circumstances.

Case 3.1 (continued)

The case study might be considered a dilemma because the nurse is thinking about *doing* something. Peter is apparently undecided. There are many options open to him, but the one we are discussing is whether or not he should give the prescribed medication covertly. The case study seems to fall within the first category of moral dilemma. Peter feels that there are moral reasons for both giving and not giving the medication. To help him untangle these reasons, and decide between them, Peter refers the dilemma to higher levels.

Level 2: rules

Beauchamp and Childress (2013) 'draw only a loose distinction between rules and principles. Both are general norms which guide action' (p. 14). Rules are more specific. Beauchamp and Childress offer the following:

- *Veracity.* This rule requires truth in relationships with patients (Collis 2006).
- *Privacy.* Respecting privacy involves a number of issues concerned with protecting an individual's freedom from interference. These include informational privacy (restricting information), physical privacy (focusing on personal space), decisional privacy (concerning personal choices), and relational privacy (concerning family and other relationships). A nurse who intrudes unnecessarily on a family attempting to come to terms with bad news would breach the rule of privacy.
- *Confidentiality.* There is some overlap between the rules of privacy and confidentiality; keeping a confidence is part of respecting privacy. Breaking a confidence occurs when information is disclosed to a third party. This rule is part of many professional codes – priests must not disclose confessional secrets, and some journalists have gone to prison protecting the identity of their sources. In nursing, keeping confidences is very important in the nurse–patient relationship. The obligation is not absolute, but should only be broken in exceptional circumstances (confidentiality is discussed more fully in Chapter 4).
- *Fidelity.* This rule is concerned with the requirement to act in good faith, keeping promises and maintaining relationships (Beauchamp and Childress 2013).

These are prima facie (at first sight) rules, meaning that they are not meant to be followed slavishly and can be overridden by other obligations. They should inform rather than direct action and can be overruled but only with justification. Nor is the list exhaustive; many further prima facie rules can be contained within them, for example,

Paul Snelling

a rule that nurses should not steal from patients is contained within the rule of fidelity. However, the rules cover the wide ground of nurse–patient relationships, and a fuller list of derivative rules would be of little value.

Case 3.1 (continued)

Applying these rules to the case study at the beginning of the chapter, we can see that giving the sedative covertly probably breaches the rules of veracity and privacy, but some would claim that this is justified. Applying the rules in this way doesn't seem to help much in this particular dilemma – if it can be resolved by simply invoking a prima facie rule, it cannot have been much of a dilemma.

In order to throw more light on the dilemma and the reasons we might advance for deciding either to give or not give the medication in this way, the dilemma can be analysed with reference to the four principles from which the rules are derived. The principles are:

- respect for autonomy
- nonmaleficence
- beneficence
- justice.

Level 3: principles

Respect for autonomy

The principle is that, generally, autonomy should be respected, but there are many problems with this. Autonomy is a complex concept and there is evidence that the term is used in different ways by individual nurses (Aveyard 2000). The word *autonomy* derives from the Greek words for *autos* (self) and *nomos* (rule, governance or law). First understood as the right of a community to self-government, modern accounts see it as relating to personal independence in some way. There are many definitions and nuances in the literature, but simply, **autonomy** is the ability to be able to make decisions for oneself, and respecting autonomy requires that we accept and where possible facilitate the choices of others.

Within the many definitions and accounts of autonomy, two features are common: liberty and agency (Beauchamp and Childress 2013). Liberty means freedom from controlling influences. An extreme example would be a confession extracted under torture, but more subtle controlling influences, based in part on power imbalance in nurse–patient relationships, are possible (Henderson 2003). A decision made by a patient under pressure, either from a nurse or doctor or by an overbearing relative, is not autonomously made. Liberty is part of autonomy but not all of it. Animals can be thought of as free but not as autonomous. Nurses should be aware of the potential for influences and take action to minimise them, for example, by enabling discussion of treatment options to take place away from relatives.

Agency means having the capacity to decide. Capacity is reduced in many ways; by illness, learning disability and in childhood. Autonomy is relational in the sense that a capacity to make decisions depends on the nature of the decision being made. For example, a person with a learning disability or a child may lack the capacity to decide whether to undertake chemotherapy, but be perfectly able to decide on meal choices. An individual's capacity to decide can also vary in time; a patient who is mildly confused because of infection, or postoperative hypoxia, may not be able to decide whether or not to take medication one day, but be perfectly capable the next.

Respecting autonomy cannot simply be reduced to agreeing with and implementing patients' choices. Respecting autonomy can be analysed in terms of **rights**, which can be defined as 'justified claims' (Beauchamp and Childress 2013, p. 368) made upon others and on society. A right to autonomy, like other rights, can be either a **liberty right** or a **claim right**. Liberty, mentioned above as an almost universally agreed component of autonomy, is associated with negative or passive rights – that is the right not to be prevented from doing something. By contrast, a claim right requires someone else to do something, imposing a duty upon another person – it is a positive, active right.

The distinction can be illustrated by discussing Do Not Attempt Resuscitation (DNAR) orders. Assuming capacity, any patient can refuse treatment, and this includes resuscitation, despite medical, nursing, or family opinion that resuscitation would be of benefit, and therefore should be performed. In declining treatment the patient is claiming a negative right – the right to be left alone. This is a strong claim, and according to the principle of respect for autonomy should be honoured. A different scenario is of a terminally ill patient who asks to be resuscitated despite medical and nursing opinion that invasive and intrusive procedures would not succeed or not be beneficial. In this case, the patient is claiming a positive right, and if accepted, this puts an obligation on someone else to do something, that is it obliges a nurse to initiate resuscitation. This is a weaker claim; health care professionals cannot be required to undertake a procedure that they believe not to be in the patient's interests. In some sensitive areas like DNAR orders it may be justified to accede to the patient's wishes, but this cannot be an obligation (Resuscitation Council 2014).

Some people are obviously unable to make a decision, for example if they are semiconscious, and health care professionals should not follow wishes expressed while in this state. It is not an autonomous decision. A 3-year-old child cannot be expected to make a decision concerning radiation therapy; any more than a severely hypoxic and confused patient can properly decline oxygen therapy. If the patient has sufficient capacity to make a decision, it must be respected. If the patient is not able to make the decision, someone must make it for them. Clearly this is difficult where there is some doubt as to whether the patient is able or not able to make the decision. This judgement is significant because different actions (or inactions) follow directly from it. There must be a robust method of assessing the ability of the patient to make the decision.

This crucial question forms part of the Mental Capacity Act, which is discussed in detail in Chapter 4. It should be noted that the test is not a measure of capacity in itself, but rather a judgement, however crude, of a patient's ability to make a particular decision at a particular time. Following the principle of respecting autonomy, as well as the law, the presumption is in favour of capacity. The legal case that informed the legal test involved a client within a secure hospital diagnosed with paranoid schizophrenia, who was nevertheless assessed by a judge as being capable to decide whether or not his leg should be amputated, illustrating the point that patients who are not fully rational can remain capable of making a major life or death decision.

If the patient has been assessed as lacking capacity, someone else must make decisions for him. It is sometimes assumed in practice that this duty falls to the next of kin,

A **right** is a justified claim. A **liberty right** requires that the right holder simply be left alone, not interfered with. A **claim right** requires someone to do something for the right holder.

a position reinforced in the past by the practice of asking next of kin to sign consent forms. Legally, the duty of deciding in the patient's best interests falls to the medical team, led by the consultant, though it is becoming more recognised that the senior clinician in certain circumstances may be a suitably qualified nurse or other health care professional. This is not to suggest that relatives should not be consulted or their views dismissed. However, respecting autonomy requires that the *patient's* wishes are considered, and it is not always the case that the patient's wishes are the same as the next of kin's. When discussing decisions with patients' families, as well as being mindful of confidentiality, it should be remembered that asking what the patient would want is not the same question as asking what the relative wants for the patient. There may be tensions. In some cases patients have left detailed instructions about treatment options in certain eventualities – these are known as advance decisions. There are also now legal arrangements for patients to nominate another individual to make decisions on their behalf when incapacitated (see Chapter 4), known as lasting power of attorney (LPA). Both of these arrangements are justified by the important moral duty to respect autonomy.

Paternalism might be considered as the opposite of respecting autonomy. A nurse acts paternalistically if she does not respect a patient's autonomous decision because she believes it to be against his interests. The word 'paternalism' is based on the concept of 'fatherhood', choosing for one's children in their interest. A distinction has been drawn between weak and strong paternalism (Ikonomidis and Singer 1999). Weak paternalism occurs when an agent (or the state) intervenes on the grounds of beneficence or nonmaleficence on behalf of a person without capacity, even if they are able to express a preference. Strong paternalism occurs where an intervention overrides or disregards the wishes of a person with capacity. Strong paternalism in policy terms has been justified. Certain choices are not available to citizens. Declining to wear a seatbelt is punished by the retrospective levying of fines, and the state acts positively to prevent citizens from using heroin, even when the decision is autonomously made. The justification (Glover 1977) is:

1   that the suffering is very great;
2   that there is very little uncertainty that suffering will occur;
3   that the process of heroin addiction after initial use is not readily reversible, and restricts future freedom of choice.

One way in which nurses might be accused of being paternalistic is in implementing smoking bans. Hospitals of all types have increasingly introduced bans, which not only apply to public indoor areas following legislation, but also to outside areas, where the ban is justified not to prevent harm to others through second hand smoke, but to the smoker himself. Nurses are in a difficult position here. Facilitating autonomous choice may indeed threaten the health of the patient, but both failing to facilitate choice and actively seeking to prevent it are paternalistic acts. In some areas, the decision of whether to facilitate a smoker's choice is complicated further by policies, which threaten staff with disciplinary action if they do (Snelling 2016). These coercive policies additionally threaten a nurse's professional autonomy so that doing what might be considered the right thing in respecting autonomy may come at some significant personal cost. The most obvious practical manifestation of the principle of respecting autonomy is in requirement for informed consent. This is covered in more detail in Chapter 4.

Case 3.1 (continued)

Mr Smith declined to take the offered sedation. His decision might have been taken on the basis of incomplete information; a major reason for his declining the medication seems to be that sedatives he has taken in the past have made him sleepy, and Peter suspects that the newer ones prescribed will not have this effect. This means that in order to reassess his decision, Mr Smith simply needs more information, it does not affect his capacity to make the decision. Depending on the cause and nature of his agitation, and remembering that the starting presumption is that people are capable of making decisions unless deemed otherwise, Peter assumes that he does have capacity. Respecting his autonomy requires that Mr Smith's refusal to take the sedation be respected.

The principle of **nonmaleficence** requires that health care professionals should not harm patients.

It might be considered that Mr Smith is being unwise, but to overrule him and give him the medication would be a case of strong paternalism. It might be considered that if he is capable of making the decision, then he is also capable of understanding the consequences of it, not only for himself, but also for the other patients in the ward. Giving the sedation covertly might be justified not in his interests, but in everyone else's. In this case it would not be considered paternalistic; perhaps authoritarian would be a more accurate description. Following the principle of respecting autonomy requires you not to give the medication.

Nonmaleficence

The principle of **nonmaleficence** requires that health care professionals should not harm patients. On the face of it, this seems straightforward, associated with the maxim (often mistakenly attributed to the Hippocratic Oath): *Primum non nocere* (first, do no harm). Nurses and others do not require this principle to tell them that they should not punch a patient or steal from them, but the concept of harm is more complex than this, and there are some problems associated with this principle. First is the problem that many health care interventions have harmful as well as beneficial effects. Drugs have side effects; operations require painful incisions. These harms are justified in the pursuit of the overall good, and the need to balance good with harm in this way has led some to argue that the principles of nonmaleficence (avoiding harm) and beneficence (doing good) should be regarded together as a single principle

Second is the problem of defining harm, and the most striking examples of this problem occur at the end of life. Normally, killing would be seen as the most grievous harm that can be visited on a person, resulting in murder being regarded as the most serious of crimes. Yet there have been a number of cases where 'mercy killing' has been treated leniently by the courts.

A powerful argument against euthanasia is that killing a person, even at their express wish, causes them harm. However, for some people near the end of life, the harm, *from their point of view*, lies not in being killed but by remaining alive because their suffering is so great as to be considered, by them, as worse than being dead. Whether or not the idea of death being better than life is accepted, there remains the problem of who decides whether harm has been or will be done. Part of the power of the argument in favour of euthanasia derives from the claim that it is for the patient to decide whether harm has occurred; following the principle of respect for autonomy as well as illustrating that the notion of harm is subjective rather than objective.

59

When the end of life approaches, the focus of health intervention shifts from cure to care. It is recognised that treatments that would be considered beneficial for some patients, such as resuscitation or invasive surgery, would be regarded as harmful for others because of the lack of benefit provided. In addition, dosages of drugs that would normally be considered harmful are routinely given to persons as they approach the end of life, in the knowledge that death may be hastened as a result. This is common practice, considered permissible under the doctrine of double effect.

The doctrine of double effect

The doctrine of double effect (DDE) was originally formulated in the Middle Ages by Catholic theologians to describe the circumstances in which evil is permitted in the overall pursuit of good. It allows an 'evil' to occur so long as it is not intended, even though it may be foreseen. The DDE is used to justify the use of very large dosages of opiate analgesia and other drugs (Jansen 2010) in terminally ill persons, even though it is known that the side effects of the drugs may shorten life.

Much of the defence for the DDE is based on religious morality, mainly Catholic but also supported by other denominations and religions (Keown and Keown 1995). The DDE has been criticised for its religious roots by Quill et al. (1997), who question whether it is right for this tradition to be reflected in the law of multicultural society, in their case, the United States of America. The formulation of the DDE is often merely stated rather than argued. Generally, there are four conditions for an act to be justified using the DDE (Schwarz 2004), and details of how the parts of the doctrine are applied to the case of the administration of large doses of opiate drugs near the end of life are added in italics below.

- The act considered separately from its consequences must not be intrinsically wrong. *Giving analgesia near the end of life would be considered morally acceptable, even obligatory.*
- With both a good and a bad effect of a single act, the bad effect must not be intended but simply permitted, even where it is foreseen. *Here the 'bad' effect of the act is the shortening of life. For the DDE to be correctly applied, this must not be an intention. It's an important distinction, which separates the use of opiates from (for example) potassium chloride. It would be difficult to argue that there is no intention to end life by giving this drug as it has no analgesic properties.*
- The good effect must be sufficiently desirable to offset permitting the bad effect. *Here the bad of shortening life must be compared with the good of analgesia. In end of life decisions the good of relief from severe pain outweighs the shortening by hours or days of a life of poor quality. It would not outweigh relief from mild pain where life of a reasonable quality was shortened by a longer period.*
- The good effect must not be brought about by the bad effect. *This means that the good effect of painlessness must not be brought about only by the bad effect of shortening life.*

Some formulations of the DDE (for example, Perkin and Resnik 2002) add a fifth criterion, that there should be no other way of producing the intended effect.

Problems with the DDE include difficulties with intention. There is evidence to show that intention is not always as stated (Quill et al. 1997). A further difficulty is the notion that we are somehow not responsible for consequences of our actions that are foreseen but can be claimed to be unintentional. It has been described as a 'very dubious and shifty' argument (Warnock 1998, p. 41) and its survival is perhaps a result of its pragmatism rather than its morality (Shaw 2002). Practitioners appear more ready to accept it than philosophers (Dickenson 2000). UK law enshrines the DDE even if it does not actually state it. It has been described by judges on a number of occasions, famously in the case of *R v Adams*, where Dr Adams was acquitted of murdering his patients by giving them increasingly large dosages of opiates. The patients were incurably but not terminally ill. In his summing up the trial judge said that 'the doctor is entitled to relieve pain and suffering even if the measures he takes may incidentally shorten life' (Dimond 2001, p. 1480).

The principle of **beneficence** requires health care professionals to act to promote the general well-being of others.

Case 3.1 (continued)

The good effect of giving the sedation could be that he goes to sleep and the bad that his autonomy has been overruled. The bad effect is intended, and it causes the good effect, so the doctrine of double effect could not be applied. Would Mr Smith be harmed by being given a sedative against his wishes? Certainly physical harm would be unlikely. Overriding his wishes might be considered harmful, especially by him, and giving the medication in this way will also probably harm the trust relationship between Mr Smith and the nurses caring for him.

Beneficence

The principle of **beneficence** requires health care professionals to act to promote the general well-being of others. Beauchamp and Childress (2013) discuss two forms of the principle.

First, positive beneficence requires that nurses provide benefits to their patients. Without making claims about the character and motivation of nurses, it is safe to assume that a desire to help people is part of the continuing appeal of nursing and other health care professions, but it is less clear what the nurse is obliged to do for patients, and what they might justifiably do. For example, consider if you were rostered for an early shift, and a number of your colleagues reported sick for the late shift. You might consider that you ought to stay and do a double shift, even if you had tickets to the theatre. If you followed this course of action, you might be considered to have done a good thing, but can you be criticised if you fail to do the double shift? Acting 'above and beyond' the call of duty might be a common occurrence in nursing and other health care provisions, but it cannot be an obligation (Edwards 2009). There are also problems here in balancing the amount of good that you are able to do for one patient when compared with the competing needs of others. This is discussed in the section on justice.

Second, utility requires that nurses balance the good and bad effects of their actions, as discussed in the section on nonmaleficence. Just as harm is difficult to define, so is well-being, and deciding where a person's best interests lie. Even where a nurse overrides the wishes of a patient and coerces treatment, for example in giving a Jehovah's Witness a blood transfusion against their autonomously stated wishes, this is not done out of spite or malice, but in the belief that acting in this way is beneficial. Many of the conflicts between principles occur between beneficence and respect for autonomy, and key to resolving these is understanding that a seemingly obvious and objective benefit, like a life-saving blood transfusion, may not be viewed as such by everyone.

Paul Snelling

Justice
is a complex
concept, but at a
simple level, it can
be regarded as
treating people
fairly.

Case 3.1 (continued)

Giving Mr Smith a sedative disguised in tea might be considered a beneficent act, because the resulting rest will be good for him. Perhaps this justification is more attractive to Peter trying to justify giving it this way than to Mr Smith who doesn't want it.

Justice

Justice is a complex concept, but at a simple level, it can be regarded as treating people fairly. This is seen in matters of distribution (distributive justice) and punishment (retributive justice). Justice in health care is largely concerned with the distribution of resources. Newsworthy debates about resource allocation commonly concern the availability or otherwise of drug treatments for cancer, but the same analysis applies to more everyday matters such as a nurse allocating their time. Common to all theories of justice is a minimum formal requirement traditionally attributed to Aristotle: 'Equals must be treated equally, and unequals must be treated unequally'.

It might be suggested that none of us are exactly the same. I have an identical twin brother, and though our genetic material is identical, even we are not *exactly* the same. He is slightly taller and yet less heavy, and wears his hair a little longer. We can point to differences between all of us, men and women, black and white, heterosexual and homosexual, but applying Aristotle's requirement doesn't mean that we should all be treated differently. Justifying treating people differently requires a *morally relevant* difference. Difficulty arises in discussing and deciding what constitutes a morally relevant difference. At this time, almost all would agree that gender, skin colour and sexual orientation are not relevant, though all would have been considered relevant in the not too distant past, and there remains a minority who continue to see the distinction as relevant. There is more debate about whether age is relevant (Shaw 1994), with even a significant minority of older people agreeing that it is right that older people give way to younger people on a heart surgery waiting list (Bowling *et al.* 2002).

There are many ways of attempting fairness in the distributions of health care including:

- To each person an equal share.
- To each person according to need.
- To each person according to effort.
- To each person according to contribution.
- To each person according to merit.
- To each person according to free market exchanges.

Beauchamp and Childress, 2001, p. 250

All of these can be challenged, but it is distribution according to need that is nearest to nursing's values and the core principles of the NHS that are set out in the NHS constitution (NHS for England 2013). A challenge to the intuitively attractive requirement that resources should be directed at those who need them is that often those who need treatment most will not benefit from it. An alternative understanding of need that addresses this point is need as capacity to benefit. One way in which the needs of different groups and individuals can be compared is by using the quality-adjusted life year (QALY). This is a system whereby quality of life is assessed on a scale from 0 (death) to 1 (normal health). Improvement in health status following treatment can be assessed on the same scale, and the gain in health, multiplied by the length of time for which the improvement remains, gives a QALY score for a particular treatment for a particular condition. This score can then be divided by the cost to give a 'cost per QALY' with the implication that the treatments with the lowest cost per QALY are most cost-effective and therefore prioritised (see Box 3.1).

There are a number of problems associated with QALYs, not least difficulties in calculating the scores. If the public is involved in setting the scores, the perceived democratising benefit of making resource allocation more visible is offset by the fact that healthy members of the public do not have experience of being ill, and find it difficult to put a value on quality of life for certain conditions, which must be subjective. QALYs seem a rather detached way of assessing priorities, threatening a more caring approach valued by nurses (Hirskyj 2007), and QALYs inevitably disadvantage the old and the chronically sick. Regardless of the method of funding, cost-effectiveness is now an important aspect of nursing care, for example the introduction of new nursing roles (Kilpatrick *et al.* 2014), and also changes in the performance of old ones (see Research focus 3.1

A further problem for using need as a criterion for distribution is the difference between needs and wants. For example, when the drug Viagra was introduced offering a treatment

---

BOX 3.1 Quality-adjusted life years

Patient X has a serious, life-threatening condition.

> If he continues receiving standard treatment he will live for 1 year and his quality of life will be 0.4.
> If he receives a new drug he will live for 1 year 3 months (1.25 years), with a quality of life of 0.6.

A new treatment is compared with standard care in terms of the QALYs gained:

Standard treatment: 1 (year's extra life) × 0.4 = 0.4 QALY
New treatment: 1.25 (1 year, 3 months' extra life) × 0.6 = 0.75 QALY
Therefore, the new treatment leads to 0.35 additional QALYs (that is: 0.75–0.4 QALY = 0.35 QALYs).
The cost of the new drug is assumed to be £8,000, standard treatment costs £3000.
The difference in treatment costs (£5,000) is divided by the QALYs gained (0.35) to calculate the cost per QALY. So the new treatment would cost £14,285 per QALY.
NICE generally regards interventions costing the NHS less than £20,000 per QALY as cost-effective, though treatments costing up to £30,000 per QALY may also be regarded as cost-effective. Where other significant benefits can be identified these are also taken into account in funding decisions.

NICE (2013)

Paul Snelling

RESEARCH FOCUS 3.1

Research cannot prove ethical 'facts', but it can illuminate opinions and judgements. For example, research that shows that a majority of the public finds that abortion is morally acceptable does not mean that it is permissible – only that a certain majority thinks that it is. Care is needed to separate the empirical (what can be measured) from the normative (what ought to be done). This distinction can be widely seen in ethical practice even where it might seem unlikely.

A paper in the *Journal of Advanced Nursing* (Marsden *et al.* 2015) about the cost-effectiveness of pressure ulcer prevention illustrates the point. The economic analysis compared two regimes for pressure ulcer prevention in an RCT conducted in Belgian nursing homes with individuals at high risk of developing a pressure ulcer. Two-hourly turns and alternating 2- and 4-hourly turns were compared, and the findings of the study showed fewer pressure ulcers in the 2-hourly group. Further data from other research about quality of life with and without pressure ulcers, and the additional nursing cost in performing more frequent turns were entered into an economic model, which calculated that the cost per QALY gained was nearly £2 million, and therefore not deemed cost-effective. This research informed NICE guidelines that adults at high risk of developing a pressure ulcer should be offered help to change their position at least every four hours (NICE 2014).

The model aims to ensure that resources are distributed justly, but there are acknowledged weaknesses in the calculation. Recommending less frequent turns while acknowledging that this will likely result in an additional pressure sore for an unknown patient assumes that the time saved is profitably used elsewhere. The analysis and recommendation do not make it ethically acceptable always to reduce the frequency of turns, but it can help to inform your decisions.

for erectile dysfunction, the Government issued guidance about which conditions it could be prescribed for, and also that normally one treatment per week was allowed (NHSE 1999). The patent for Viagra expired in 2013 meaning that much cheaper generic Sildenafil is now available, but the weekly limit remains (for example, Dorset Clinical Commissioning Group 2014). Whether enabling a weekly sex act counts as a need or a want is open for discussion, as are other treatments, like cosmetic plastic surgery. Does the desire for bigger breasts constitute a shallow capitulation to societal expectations obsessed with appearance, or a treatment to cure deep psychological insecurity profoundly affecting quality of life? The distinction between needs and wants is of interest both between and within treatments.

There appears to be some appetite among the general population for penalising those who are in some way responsible for their health needs (Dolan and Shaw 2003) and so the idea of distribution according to merit requires consideration. In one study 42 per cent of respondents among the general public agreed with the statement that 'people who contribute to their own illness – for example through smoking, obesity or excessive drinking – should have a lower priority for their health care than others' (Bowling 1996). There is little recent academic research on this point, which is perhaps surprising in light of the current financial difficulties of the NHS, though the media periodically suggest that NHS Trusts are denying treatment to smokers and that many health care professionals support this (Barker 2012). See Sharkey and Gillam (2010) for an exploration of the issue.

64

Case 3.1 (continued)

Some of the other patients in the ward might not regard it as fair that their sleep is being disturbed by Mr Smith, and that their needs are not being attended to as quickly as they would like. It might be considered that he does not need so much care, but that he is choosing to monopolise it by being argumentative. He wants a cigarette, he does not need one. The other patients may feel that it is unjust that Mr Smith is receiving more of a resource (the nurse's time) than he is justly entitled to. It might be considered that in order to redress this unfair distribution, the principle of justice justifies giving the sedative covertly.

Level 4: moral theories

The highest level in the classification is moral theories. Theories provide general methods for resolving problems, and guides for right action (Upton 2003). Beauchamp and Childress (2013) claim that the moral principles they propose are included in most classical theories, and so rules and principles can serve as starting points for analysis, regardless of which moral theory is favoured. If theories agree that their main features are encapsulated within the principles, it might be suggested that there is little point in studying them; much less attempting to apply them to practice-based moral problems. Respecting autonomy is important to two of the most important moral theories, but for different reasons. Why then study moral theory at all?

One answer to this question is that studying moral theories illuminates our reasons for thinking the way we do, and helps us to be clear about the sorts of things that are most important to us. Two important approaches assessing the morality of an act are duty-based and consequence-based moral theories.

Duty-based moral theory (deontology)

Deontology is based on the philosophy of Immanuel Kant (1724–1804). Kant argued that intention was all important, and that the good action was the one that followed our duty. In order to determine what our duty is, we should apply the categorical imperative

Activity 3.2

Consider the following scenario.

A passenger plane with 200 passengers on board taking off from Heathrow airport has been hijacked, and it is now flying up the Thames towards Canary Wharf, where 5,000 people are working. You have every reason to believe that the hijackers intend to emulate the attacks on the World Trade Center in New York (the 9/11 attacks) by crashing the plane into the building. A fully armed fighter jet is on patrol and can get to the area in time to shoot the airliner down.

It is your decision whether to shoot the airliner down. First, write down your initial reaction. Should you shoot it down? Then take 10 minutes, alone or preferably in small groups, to write down the arguments both for and against shooting the airliner down. Some suggestions are given below.

'I ought never to act except in such a way that I can also will that my maxim become a universal law'.

This means that in the same circumstances, everyone should act in the same way, universally and impartially. This is reformulated as 'One must act to treat every person as an end and never a means only'.

Under this formulation, every person is to be respected and treated with dignity. The details are complex, but among the important features of deontology are that it provides absolute rules, and that appeals to the bad consequences of applying the rules simply are not permitted.

Consequence-based moral theory (consequentialism)

The most important figure for consequentialism is John Stuart Mill (1808–1873). There are a number of different versions, of which his utilitarianism is the most recognised. In consequentialism, it is the consequences of an act that are important. The best thing to do is the thing that gives the best outcomes. This means calculating the probable outcomes for all the different options in any given scenario, and choosing the one that gives the best (or least bad) outcome. There are different versions about the sorts of things that can be included in the calculations, and how the calculations can be made. The important contrasting difference between consequentialism and deontology (sometimes referred to as non-consequentialism) is the consideration of consequences. This can mean that the same act can be allowed or not allowed in different circumstances, depending on the calculations. In the end of life decisions discussed earlier, consequentialism sees no difference between giving potassium chloride or giving an opiate at the end of life. The distinction of intention, vital for application of the DDE, is less important for consequentialists. For them the outcomes of giving the two drugs are the same, and so the morality is the same. If it is acceptable to give the opiate, it is also acceptable to give the potassium.

Case 3.1 (continued)

There are so many complications and nuances in the abstract moral theories that simply applying them to complex real-life situations is probably unhelpful for Peter. However, thinking about whether and to what extent we are using consequentialist or non-consequentialist thinking can help in clarifying issues. A deontologist would not give the concealed medication to Mr Smith because it would involve deceit. A consequentialist might give the medication, depending on the details of the case, and the type of consequentialism, but if many other patients were being disturbed, and there was very little risk to Mr Smith, giving the medication concealed in tea could probably be defended on consequentialist grounds.

Returning to Activity 3.2.
Reasons for shooting the airliner down include:

1   Fewer people would be killed – 200 on the airliner against 5,000 in the building (c).
2   It would minimise the sense of victory for hijackers, demonstrating the resolve of government (c).

Reasons against shooting the airliner down include:

3   It is wrong to kill innocent passengers (d).
4   It might crash onto another building killing more people (c*).
5   It might not be hijacked at all – it might be a mistake (c*).
6   The passengers might overpower the hijackers (c*).

The obvious consequentialist position is given in point 1, and the deontological position is given as point 3. No amount of arguing for these positions will satisfy the other – the deontologist's position holds even if a million people were in the building, and an appeal to the fact that the passengers would die anyway is met with the response that it is the hijackers that would be killing them, not the fighter pilot. It is not so simple to say that consequentialists would shoot down the plane, and deontologists would not – the reasons marked (c*) are appeals for more information. If there was a good chance that there were only 300 in the building, but that the only place to shoot down the aeroplane would result in 1,000 additional deaths, the consequentialist would not shoot. In classroom discussion of this problem, shooting the airliner down is by far the most popular action, and yet this is an intuitively difficult position. Appeals for more information seem to stem from reluctance to fire on the airliner, but the appeals remain consequentialist in nature; people are attempting to make the calculation more accurate. If opposition to firing on the airliner was the result of a deontological view that it is wrong, appeals to likely consequences are simply not relevant. Apart from valuable dissection and discussion of a pressing moral problem, the value of the exercise lies in identifying the different approaches, helping us to understand why we think in the way that we do.

Applying the principles to the case study

Not all of the principles have equal prominence when applied to individual scenarios. However, applying the principles in Mr Smith's case gives the following reasons for giving or not giving the sedative (Figure 3.2).

In real-life scenarios similar to this, there may be other factors to consider. For example, Mr Smith may tell you that if you do not accompany him for a cigarette he will have one by the bedside, and you may feel that this constitutes a fire hazard because of his use of oxygen. There may also be other options outside the 'give or do not give' dilemma. You may feel that the best thing all round for Mr Smith (and the other patients) might be to take him for a cigarette after all; it would depend on the level of his agitation and his need for oxygen, and in taking him you might also want to consider some other issues such as a nurse facilitating a habit known to be harmful to health. The application of the principles can be amended according to the changed circumstances; the devil is always in the detail. Applying the principles of respect for autonomy and nonmaleficence to a decision about taking a patient with respiratory impairment for a cigarette could provide some interesting and contrasting views.

Applying the four principles has given some insight into the sorts of things that are seen as valuable, and also helped deconstruct the dilemma presented so that it is easier to see which elements are important. What it does not do is tell you what you should do, and this lack of action guidance is one of the critiques of the approach, which will be considered in Part 3.

TABLE 3.1 Applying the four principles to Mr Smith

	Give the sedative	Do not give the sedative
Respect autonomy		Respect for autonomy requires that Mr Smith not be given the sedative covertly as it overrides his autonomous choice not to take it
Nonmaleficence		Harm to the professional relationship might follow if the sedative is given covertly
Beneficence	A good night's sleep will benefit Mr Smith. He will feel much better for having the sleep rather than being agitated all night	
Justice	Justice is served because all of the other patients will get a better night's sleep if Mr Smith is sedated. It is unfair for them to be kept awake when he could be asleep	

Professional issues

It was noted in Chapter 2 that there is considerable overlap between ethical and professional considerations of practice issues. Peter may have his views about whether giving the medication disguised in the tea is right or wrong, but he should also consider the professional implications. NMC guidance on covert administration of medication has been withdrawn but the NMC *Standards for Medicines Management* make it clear that whatever the moral arguments in favour are, covert administration is not good practice:

> As a general principle, by disguising medication in food or drink, the patient or client is being led to believe they are not receiving medication, when in fact they are. The NMC would not consider this to be good practice. The registrant would need to be sure what they are doing is in the best interests of the patient, and that they are accountable for this decision.
>
> (NMC 2007, p. 32)

Though this statement does not take account of the capacity of the person receiving the medication, the scenario here assumes that Mr Smith does have capacity and the assumption must be that a nurse would be very unwise to act by giving the medication in this way.

PART 3: EXPLORING ETHICS

Critiques of principlism

There are a number of critiques of principlism. These can broadly be categorised in three headings:

1   The insufficient philosophy critique.
2   Procedural critiques.
3   The critique from agent-centred ethics.

The insufficient philosophy critique

This critique highlights the fundamental differences in approach that will be discussed shortly. In a famous paper from the *Journal of Medicine and Philosophy* it is argued that the principles do not constitute a coherent moral theory, but rather are 'tantamount to using two, three or four conflicting moral theories to decide a case' (Clouser and Gert 1990, p. 221). In applying the principles, 'the agent is unwittingly using several diverse and conflicting accounts rather than simply applying a well developed unified theory' (1990, p. 223). One problem here is that moral theories tend to be regarded as a 'historical relic' (1990, p. 233), rather than an 'ongoing attempt to explain and justify our common moral intuitions' (1990, p. 233).

The rigid application of Kant and Mill to modern health care problems both lead to some implausible positions, but it doesn't follow from this that moral theory in itself, or the attempt to formulate one, is unhelpful. A problem with the absence of an underlying theory is that a moral agent does not know why he is doing the things that the principles tell him he should do. We might agree that respecting and promoting autonomy is important, even that it is the most important principle, but simply following the principle does not tell us *why* it is important. A similar critique could be levelled at other principle or rules-based systems, even *The Code*. Principlism operates at the level of a useful checklist, a function about which most of its critics seem to agree (for example, Harris 2003). Beauchamp and Childress (2013) acknowledge and discuss these critiques in later editions of their work.

Procedural critiques

A number of 'procedural' critiques have been grouped into this section, and there is some overlap between them:

- Principlism does not tell you what to do. Beauchamp and Childress (2013) do not give any indication about which principle should have precedence where there is a conflict, though other supporters of principlism are more specific, holding that respect for autonomy is the most important (Gillon 2003), and that therefore it trumps the rest. The autonomy-weighted version has been referred to as an immodest version, with Beauchamp and Childress's (2013) version being described as modest because it doesn't weigh the principles (Edwards 2006). The former version has more action-guiding properties, but as we have seen, autonomy can be a difficult concept and the requirement to respect it is clearest where a capable person refuses treatment.
- Following on from this, it is suggested that autonomy is overvalued, representing a predominantly individualised (Callahan 2003) and Western view of the good. In the presented case study, for example, privileging the application of the principle of respect for autonomy seems a little unfair; respecting Mr Smith's autonomy comes at a price paid by other patients. Other moral theories and other cultures take a wider view of moral action.

- It has been criticised as being both too simple and too complex. Too simple because it is difficult to reduce complex moral issues to four principles (Edwards 2009), or even whether ethical principles apply at all (Johnstone 2016). Too complex because of the use of jargon, a point often made by students trying to pronounce and spell the principles.

The critique from agent-centred ethics

However, the major critique is not against the principles themselves so much as against the whole idea that the correct way to decide on the morally good is to analyse it from the question, what should I do? This is the starting point for the act-centred moral theories (deontology and consequentialism) introduced earlier. These theories, also known as 'the ethics of justice', assume that the best way to resolve a moral dilemma is to have a good think about the problem, using reason and calculation, seeing the problem from outside. However, if we try to conjure up an image of a really good person, it is unlikely to be one who focuses right action solely on the ability to reason and calculate. We are more likely to think of someone who has some element of goodness within them, as part of their character, reflecting an ancient way of looking at morality, set out most importantly by Aristotle. In describing virtue ethics, Aristotle concentrated not on what people should do, but how they should be. The differences in approaches are summarised in Figure 3.2.

Virtue ethics

Virtue ethics emphasises the character of the agent – who the person is as well as what they do. It is an *agent*-centred approach to ethics. Good people do good things (as opposed to the possibility of bad people doing good things) because they possess virtues, traits of character or disposition. Courage, compassion and generosity are all virtues. After a long period in decline, the popularity of virtue ethics has increased in recent years. Many nurses are attracted to an account of virtue ethics (Armstrong 2007, Sellman 2011) largely because a description of the good nurse as one who simply calculates what her duty is, or what the consequences would be, coldly and dispassionately offers only an impoverished account. It seems to matter that nurses be caring, compassionate people rather than calculating automatons. Of course this is not to suggest that there is a crude dichotomy between act- and agent-centred ethical approaches; a complete account includes both character and action (Paley 2006). The desirability of good character is recognised by the NMC. Before students can register with the NMC having completed an approved course, a signed declaration of good character is required (NMC 2015b). The NMC Code (NMC 2015a) requires that nurses must treat people with kindness, respect and compassion, reinforcing the idea that character and some emotional engagement is important for good nursing practice, though the regulatory as opposed to philosophical view of good character involves declaring that no crimes have been committed (Sellman 2007).

Care and the ethics of care

The concepts of care and caring are central to nursing. Tschudin (2003) starts her book *Ethics in Nursing: The caring relationship* with the observation that 'Caring is not unique to nursing, but it is unique in nursing' (p. 1). Other professions 'look after' or 'treat' patients, but only the profession of nursing has care and caring at its core. One problem in understanding the concepts involved is that the word 'care' is used in a number of different ways. We care *for* all sorts of things in nursing; the word can be used to describe everything that we do. A book chapter might describe the care of a person undergoing myocardial infarction, and it would describe the sorts of things that need to be undertaken in caring for the patient. They might need reassurance, information, assistance with hygiene, and certain technical tasks to be performed. In this sense we are describing, as much as anything, technical competence. A different sense of the word is deployed in caring *about*, which implies an emotional component or attachment to something or some person. Care is the first of the '6 Cs' upon which the Department of Health's nursing strategy is based (Department of Health 2012). There is, however, wide use of the term, and even commercial organisations claim to 'care about' their customers. For example, in their habit of displaying old photographs, Facebook claims that 'we care about you and the memories that you share . . . '

There is some debate about whether or not care can be considered a virtue (Allmark 1998). However, unlike virtue, and despite its centrality in the vocabulary and understanding of good nursing, care in this sense defies easy definition or even description. In an important critique of the body of research, which attempts to define the meaning of care, Paley (2001) points out that many studies attempting to discern what nurses understand by caring simply produce a list of synonyms, including empathy, compassion and kindness. This list is virtually indistinguishable from the lists of synonyms to be found in any thesaurus, leading him to call this 'thesaurus knowledge' (Paley 2001, p. 191).

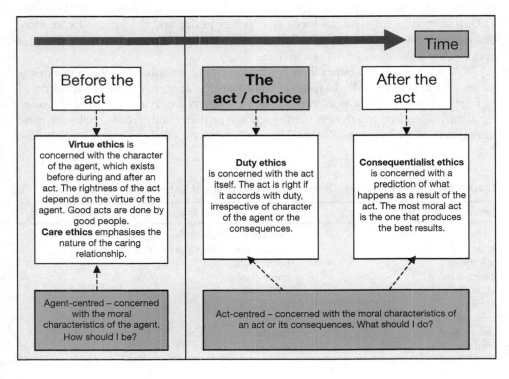

FIGURE 3.2
Diagram showing different types of moral theory

The paper is unusual in that it elicited a full paper in response the following year (Deary et al. 2002), followed by a slightly tetchy series of shorter ripostes thereafter. As an example of rigorous debate about what counts as knowledge about a central tenet of nursing, this exchange is highly recommended.

Understanding of care as the basis for ethical action has its root in the debates between Kohlberg (1981) and Gilligan (1982). In studying the moral development of children, Kohlberg claimed that they progressed through a series of stages of development, the highest of which involved abstract reasoning based on universal principles. Gilligan, who was a former pupil and collaborator of Kohlberg's, responded with the influential book *In a Different Voice*. She found that women's values were at the middle stages of Kohlberg's hierarchy, and rather than accepting that the development of women's morality was somehow inferior, she argued that women think in different ways, that they have a different moral understanding and language, which emphasises the importance of relationships and care (Hugman 2005).

The debate developed from empirical findings rather than any notion of arguments about how people *ought* to be or behave. The feminist ethics of care grew from this debate, and it found an eager home within nursing ethics, which was attempting to move on from its place as a subset of medical ethics (Fry 1989). The care ethics perspective cannot be understood in abstract or hypothetical terms, but only in actions stemming from caring relationships between people. Despite some understanding of a professional nursing relationship as somehow emotionally detached, a care ethics perspective must include emotional aspects (Scott 2000) and even love. If this sounds rather aspirational, perhaps beyond the call of duty, it should be remembered that TLC (tender loving care) is a term used by many nurses, usually to communicate that medical treatment has been withdrawn from the patient as they approach the end of life (Kendrick and Robinson 2002). Walker (1998) referred to the different views of ethics of justice and the ethics of care more descriptively as 'theoretical-juridical', and 'expressive-collaborative'. Some differences between the approaches are set out in Table 3.2.

Table 3.2 is illustrative rather than definitive. It is not suggested that the justice orientation is exclusive to male doctors, nor that the care approach to ethics is restricted to female nurses. In medicine, at least as far as numbers are concerned, there is a more equal mix of genders, and though nursing remains predominantly female, males are more heavily represented in certain areas. The distinctions are more than mere stereotype –

TABLE 3.2 Differences between ethics of care and ethics of justice

Ethics of justice tend to be . . .	Ethics of care tend to be . . .
theoretical-juridical	expressive-collaborative
impartial, detached	partial, based on relationships
top down	bottom up
generalisable	contextual
objective	subjective
male	female
rational	emotional
reductionist	holistic
medical	nursing

there is some evidence that nurses and doctors think differently about moral matters (Elder *et al.* 2003, Oberle and Hughes 2001).

Case 3.1 (continued)

Peter has analysed the issue of Mr Smith's medication using the four principles approach, but he feels that it is inadequate to help him decide. He spent a considerable amount of time the previous night getting to know him. Mr Smith explained how exhausted he was with his social circumstances and how desperate he was for a good rest. Mr Smith complimented Peter on how he alone of the nursing staff seemed to make time to listen to him and to understand him. Peter felt that he could understand what Mr Smith really wanted was some sleep and was beginning to consider that covert medication could be the most caring way to help him.

There are problems for both sides of this illustrative dichotomy. While a reliance on abstract deductive reasoning to resolve ethical issues dispassionately does not capture the essence of nursing, relying only on an emotional, contextual and individual way of seeing ethical practice also seems problematic. Its critics suggest that the ethics of care is 'hopelessly vague' (Allmark 1995, p. 19), but this lack of consistency is accepted by Nel Noddings (2003), an influential feminist philosopher:

> Clearly I do not intend to advocate arbitrary and capricious behaviour . . . such an ethics [of care] does not attempt to reduce the need for human judgement with a series of 'thou shalts' and 'thou shalt nots'. Rather it recognises and calls forth human judgement across a wide range of fact and feeling and it allows for situations and conditions in which judgement (in the impersonal, logical sense) may properly be put aside in favour of faith and commitment.
>
> (p. 25)

An account of nursing ethics that sees the good nurse as someone who cares about the patients and is also able to analyse and justify decisions, taking account of both sides of this rather crude binary analysis (Kuhse 1997). Indeed, most people use both orientations at the same time, in varying degrees (Flanagan and Jackson 1987). An accessible review of the contrast is provided by Botes (2000).

Lastly, the dichotomy poses a problem for nursing education. The analytical approach to ethics can be taught and learnt in much the same way as any other form of knowledge; it is a subject to know and understand, much like anatomy or physiology. However, possession of knowledge and understanding of moral theory does not in itself mean that the possessor of such knowledge will act in a good way, or be a good person. A pressing question for educators and students is how to facilitate the development of character so that student nurses become moral, sensitive and perceptive carers. These things cannot be taught by lectures and seminars, but they may be developed, largely in practice, by discussion, reflection, communication and observation of experienced nurses and mentors, and by practising ethical nursing; that is, by having the will to become a good nurse (Begley 2006).

RESEARCH FOCUS 3.2

In research undertaken at an ethics conference in the United States, Smith and Godfrey (2002) asked 53 registered nurses to answer two open-ended questions. (1) A good nurse is one who . . . and (2) how does a nurse go about doing the right thing? The two questions are posed from the positions of describing the characteristics of the good nurse (agent-centred – question 1) and describing how a nurse might go about doing the right thing (act-centred – question 2). After analysis of the answers, and to the researchers' surprise, the responses to the two questions fell into the same seven categories. These are:

1   Personal characteristics
2   Professional characteristics
3   Knowledge base
4   Patient-centredness
5   Advocacy
6   Critical thinking
7   Patient care.

The researchers conclude that 'this finding supports the position that the traditional justice or care dichotomy for explaining nurses' ethical decision-making is far too confining' (Smith and Godfrey 2002, p. 309). Many empirical studies of this sort are undertaken in the US, where the health care environment is very different, but there are also enough similarities in, for example, professional roles to make this finding supportive of the intuitive understanding that the binary distinction is insufficiently explanatory.

CONCLUSION

The analysis using the four principles approach should help identify some important issues for consideration, helping you weigh them up in arriving at a decision about right action. However, the principles cannot help you come to a view on how your decision will be enacted. This will require a willingness to engage with Mr Smith as a person, with perception and sensitivity to see the whole person with desires, concerns, wishes and feelings; an attempt to empathise with him; to communicate effectively; to understand why he is behaving the way that he is. In short, to care for him, and all the other patients in your care

SUGGESTED FURTHER READING

Recommended journals

Nursing Ethics
Journal of Advanced Nursing
Nursing Philosophy
Journal of Medical Ethics
Nursing Inquiry

Textbooks

Beauchamp, T. L. and Childress, J. F. (2013) *Principles of Biomedical Ethics* (7th edn), Oxford: Oxford University Press. This book is medically and philosophically orientated, and American in origin, but it is very comprehensive.

Davis, A. J., Tschudin, V. and de Raeve, L. (eds) (2006) *Essentials of Teaching and Learning in Nursing Ethics*, Edinburgh: Churchill Livingstone. This book contains chapters by different eminent authors. It does not cover issues (such as euthanasia) as such, but rather approaches to ethics.

Edwards, S. D. (2009) *Nursing Ethics: A principle-based approach* (2nd edn), Basingstoke: Macmillan. This is a shorter and more accessible application of the four principles approach.

Gallagher, A. and Hodge, S. (eds). (2012) *Ethics, Law and Professional Issues: A practice-based approach for health professionals*. Basingstoke: Palgrave Macmillan.

Johnstone, M. J. (2016) *Bioethics: A nursing perspective* (6th edn) Sydney: Churchill Livingstone. This Australian textbook is comprehensive and well written.

Kuhse, H. (1997) *Caring: Nurses, women and ethics*, Oxford: Blackwell. This book is among the best, in my view. It's not about ethics in the general sense, but it explores the role of women in caring and nursing, and is very good on the care–justice debate.

REFERENCES

Allmark, P. (1995) Can there be an ethics of care? *Journal of Medical Ethics* **21** (1), 19–24.

Allmark, P. (1998) Is caring a virtue? *Journal of Advanced Nursing* **28** (3), 466–472.

Allmark, P. (2005) Can the study of ethics enhance nursing practice? *Journal of Advanced Nursing* **51** (6), 618–624.

Armstrong, A. (2007) *Nursing Ethics: A virtue-based approach*. Basingstoke: Palgrave Macmillan.

Aveyard, H. (2000) Is there a concept of autonomy that can usefully inform nursing practice? *Journal of Advanced Nursing* **32** (2), 352–358.

Barker, D. (2012) Doctors back demands to deny NHS treatment for smokers and the obese. *Daily Mail*. April 29 2012 www.dailymail.co.uk/health/article-2136999/No-treatment-smokers-obese-Doctors-measures-deny-procedures-unhealthier-lifestyles.html (accessed 22 January 2016).

Beauchamp, T. L. and Childress, J. F. (2001) *Principles of Biomedical Ethics* (5th edn). Oxford: Oxford University Press.

Beauchamp, T. L. and Childress, J. F. (2013) *Principles of Biomedical Ethics* (7th edn). Oxford: Oxford University Press.

Begley, A. M. (2006) Facilitating the development of moral insight in practice: teaching ethics and teaching virtue. *Nursing Philosophy* **7** (4), 257–265.

Botes, A. (2000) A comparison between the ethics of justice and the ethics of care. *Journal of Advanced Nursing* **32** (5), 1071–1075.

Bowling, A. (1996) Health care rationing: the public's debate. *British Medical Journal* **312** (7032), 670–674.

Bowling, A., Mariotto, A. and Evans, O. (2002) Are older people willing to give up their place in the queue for cardiac surgery to a younger person? *Age and Aging* **31** (3), 187–192.

Callahan, D. (2003) Principlism and communitarianism. *Journal of Medical Ethics* **29**, 287–291.

Cameron, M. E., Schaffer, M. and Park, A. E. (2001) Nursing students' experience of ethical problems and use of ethical decision-making models. *Nursing Ethics* **8** (5), 432–447.

Clouser, K. D. and Gert, B. (1990) A critique of principlism. *Journal of Medicine and Philosophy* **15** (2), 219–236.

Collis, S. P. (2006) The importance of truth telling in health care. *Nursing Standard* **20** (17), 41–45.

Deary, V., Deary, I. J., McKenna, H. P., McCance, T. V., Watson, R. and Hoogbruin, A. L. (2002) Elisions in the field of caring. *Journal of Advanced Nursing* **39** (1), 96–102.

Department of Health (2012) *Compassion in Practice: Nursing midwifery and care staff. Our vision and strategy*. London: Department of Health.

Dickenson, D. L. (2000) Are medical ethicists out of touch? Practitioner attitudes in the US and UK towards decisions at the end of life. *Journal of Medical Ethics* **26** (4), 254–260.

Dimond, B. (2001) Legal aspects of consent 18: issues relating to euthanasia. *British Journal of Nursing* **10** (22), 1479–1481.

Dolan, P. and Shaw, R. (2003) A note on the relative importance that people attach to different factors when setting priorities in health care. *Health Expectations* **6** (1), 53–59.

Dorset Clinical Commissioning Group (2014) Briefing: changes to legislation on drugs for erectile dysfunction www.dorsetccg.nhs.uk/Downloads/aboutus/medicines-management/Other%20 Guidelines/Briefing%20on%20ED%20changes.pdf (accessed 22 January 2016).

Edwards, S. D. (2006) A principle-based approach to nursing ethics. In *Essentials of Teaching and Learning in Nursing Ethics*, Davis, A. J., Tschudin, V. and de Raeve, L. (eds). Edinburgh: Churchill Livingstone, pp. 55–66.

Edwards, S. D. (2009) *Nursing Ethics: A principle-based approach* (2nd edn). Basingstoke: Macmillan.

Elder, R., Price, J. and Williams, G. (2003) Differences in ethical attitudes between registered nurses and medical students. *Nursing Ethics* **10** (2), 149–164.

Flanagan, O. and Jackson, K. (1987) Justice, care and gender: the Kohlberg–Gilligan debate revisited. *Ethics* **97** (3), 622–637.

Fry, S. T. (1989) The role of caring in a theory of nursing ethics. *Hypatia* **4** (2), 88–103.

Gilligan, C. (1982) *In a Different Voice: Psychological theory and women's development*. Cambridge, MA: Harvard University Press.

Gillon, R. (2003) Ethics needs principles – four can encompass the rest – and respect for autonomy should be 'first among equals'. *Journal of Medical Ethics* **29** (5), 307–312.

Glover, J. (1977) *Causing Death and Saving Lives*. London: Penguin.

Greipp, M. E. (1992) Greipp's model of ethical decision making. *Journal of Advanced Nursing* **17** (6), 734–738.

Harris, J. (2003) In praise of unprincipled ethics. *Journal of Medical Ethics* **29** (5), 303–306.

Henderson, S. (2003) Power imbalances between nurses and patients: a potential inhibitor of partnership in care. *Journal of Clinical Nursing* **12** (4), 501–508.

Hirskyj, P. (2007) QALY: an ethical issue that dare not speak its name. *Nursing Ethics* **14** (1), 72–82.

Hugman, R. (2005) *New Approaches in Ethics for the Caring Professions*. Basingstoke: Palgrave Macmillan.

Ikonomidis, S. and Singer, P. A. (1999) Autonomy, liberalism and advance care planning. *Journal of Medical Ethics* **25** (6), 522–527.

Jansen, L. A. (2010). Disambiguating clinical intentions: the ethics of palliative sedation. *Journal of Medicine and Philosophy*, **35** (1), 19–31.

Johnstone, M.J. (2016) *Bioethics: A nursing perspective* (6th edn). Sydney: Churchill Livingstone.

Kendrick, K. D. and Robinson, S. (2002) 'Tender loving care' as a relational ethic in nursing practice. *Nursing Ethics* **9** (3), 291–300.

Keown, D. and Keown, J. (1995) Killing, karma and caring: euthanasia in Buddhism and Christianity. *Journal of Medical Ethics* **21** (5), 265–269.

Kilpatrick, K., Kaasalainen, S., Donald, F., Reid, K., Carter, N., Bryant-Lukosius, D. *et al.* (2014). The effectiveness and cost-effectiveness of clinical nurse specialists in outpatient roles: a systematic review. *Journal of Evaluation in Clinical Practice*, **20** (6), 1106–1123.

Kohlberg, L. (1981) *Essays in Moral Development: Volume I, the psychology of moral development*. San Francisco, CA: Harper & Row.

Kuhse, H. (1997) *Caring: Nurses, women and ethics*. Oxford: Blackwell.

Marsden, G., Jones, K., Neilson, J., Avital, L., Collier, M. and Stansby, G. (2015). A cost-effectiveness analysis of two different repositioning strategies for the prevention of pressure ulcers. *Journal of Advanced Nursing*, **71** (12), 2879–2885.

NHSE (National Health Service Executive) (1999) *Treatment for Impotence. Health Service Circular 1999/148*. London: DH (www.dh.gov.uk).

National Health Service for England (2013) *NHS Constitution*. London: Department of Health (www.nhs.uk).

NICE (National Institute for Health and Clinical Excellence) (2013) *How NICE Measures Value for Money in Relation to Public Health Interventions* London: NICE (www.nice.org.uk).

NICE (National Institute for Health and Clinical Excellence) (2014) *Pressure Ulcers: Prevention and management NICE guidelines [CG179]*. London: NICE (www.nice.org.uk).

Noddings, N. (2003) *Caring: A feminine approach to ethics and moral education* (2nd edn). Berkeley, CA: University of California Press.

NMC (Nursing and Midwifery Council) (2007) *Standards for Medicines Management*. London: NMC (www.nmc-uk.org).

NMC (2015a) *The Code: Professional standards of practice and behaviour for nurses and midwives*. London: NMC (www.nmc-uk.org).

NMC (2015b) *Character and Health Decision-Making Guidance*. London: NMC (www.nmc-uk.org).

Oberle, K. and Hughes, D. (2001) Doctors' and nurses' perceptions of ethical problems in end-of-life decisions. *Journal of Advanced Nursing* **33** (6), 707–715.

Paley, J. (2001) An archaeology of caring knowledge. *Journal of Advanced Nursing* **36** (2), 188–198.

Paley, J. (2006) Past caring: The limitations of one to one ethics. In *Essentials of Teaching and Learning in Nursing Ethics*, Davis, A. J., Tschudin, V. and de Raeve, L. (eds). Edinburgh: Churchill Livingstone, pp. 149–164.

Perkin, R. M. and Resnik, D. B. (2002) The agony of agonal respiration: is the last gasp really necessary? *Journal of Medical Ethics* **28** (3), 164–169.

Quill, T. E., Dresser, R. and Brock, D. W. (1997) The rule of double effect: a critique of its role in end-of-life decision-making. *New England Journal of Medicine* **337** (24), 1768–1771.

Resuscitation Council (2014) *Decisions relating to Cardiopulmonary Resuscitation* (3rd edn). London: Resuscitation Council UK.

Schwarz, J. K. (2004) The rule of double effect and its role in facilitating good end of life palliative care: a help or a hindrance? *Journal of Hospice and Palliative Nursing* **6** (2), 125–133.

Scott, P. A. (2000) Emotion, moral perception, and nursing practice. *Nursing Philosophy* **1** (2), 123–133.

Seedhouse, D. (2009) *Ethics: The heart of health care* (3rd edn). Chichester, UK: John Wiley & Sons.

Sellman, D. (2005) Towards an understanding of nursing as a response to human vulnerability. *Nursing Philosophy* **6** (1), 2–10.

Sellman, D. (2007) On being of good character: nurse education and the assessment of character. *Nurse Education Today* **27** (7), 762–767.

Sellman, D. (2011) *What Makes a Good Nurse: Why the virtues are important for nurses*. London: Jessica Kingsley.

Sharkey, K. and Gillam, L. (2010). Should patients with self-inflicted illness receive lower priority in access to health care resources? Mapping out the debate. *Journal of Medical Ethics*, **36** (11), 661–665.

Shaw, A. B. (1994) In defence of ageism. *Journal of Medical Ethics* **20** (3), 188–191, 194.

Shaw, A. B. (2002) Two challenges to the double effect doctrine: euthanasia and abortion. *Journal of Medical Ethics* **28** (2), 102–105.

Smith, K. V. and Godfrey, N. S. (2002) Being a good nurse and doing the right thing: a qualitative study. *Nursing Ethics* **9** (3), 301–311.

Snelling, P. C. (2016) Rounding on the smokers: The myth of evidence based (nursing) policy. In Lipscomb, M. (ed.), *Exploring Evidence-Based Practice: Debates and challenges in nursing*. Abingdon, UK: Routledge.

Thompson, I., Melia, K. M. and Boyd, K. M. (2006) *Nursing Ethics* (5th edn). Edinburgh: Churchill Livingstone.

Tschudin, V. (2003) *Ethics in Nursing: The caring relationship*. Edinburgh: Butterworth Heinemann.
Upton, H. (2003) Ethical theories and practical problems. *Nursing Philosophy* **4** (2), 170–172.
Walker, M. U. (1998) *Moral Understandings: A feminist study in ethics*. New York: Routledge.
Warnock, M. (1998) *An Intelligent Person's Guide to Ethics*. London: Duckworth.

4

LAW

Richard Thomas and Paul Snelling

LEARNING OUTCOMES

After reading and reflecting on this chapter, you should be able to:

- trace the fundamental basis of law in England and Wales;
- outline the notion of reasonableness, reasonable practice and duty of care;
- discuss the principles involved in consent to treatment and how these are manifest in acceptable clinical practice;
- consider the Mental Capacity Act (2005) and its role in clarifying the duty of care owed and imperatives in nursing practice;
- outline confidential relationships and discuss their application to patient care;
- consider how human rights legislation applies to nursing care and treatment and how issues such as withholding and withdrawing treatment and euthanasia are influenced by this legislation;
- state the principles of negligence and discuss these principles in relation to clinical practice.

INTRODUCTION

The Code (NMC 2015) makes it clear that nurses must have knowledge of the law for their practice. To remain within the law nurses need to understand what is required, justified and forbidden within their practice. However, it could be argued that the law only provides support and guidance and expects nurses to exercise discretion within a logical, defensible approach. It is therefore important to consider how the law judges nurses as to what is reasonable and as to what is an acceptable standard of practice.

The chapter is divided into three parts. In Part 1, we outline the fundamentals of law, how it is made and administered, and emphasise the importance of good record keeping.

In Part 2, we explain some of the legislation that governs nursing practice. A chapter of this size cannot hope to cover all of the ground, but important aspects are explained, including consent to treatment and the Mental Capacity Act (2005), Confidentiality and the Human Rights Act (1998).

In Part 3, we discuss negligence and explore the issues that courts would take into account if an action in negligence is brought by a patient or relative.

PART 1: OUTLINING THE LAW

Case 4.1

Rhiannon is a student nurse working on a surgical ward. Mr Adams, a widower aged 83, is admitted because of bleeding from a gastric ulcer that he has had for some years. In addition to his ulcer he has arthritis and heart failure and describes his health as very poor. Major surgery is planned to repair the ulcer and the surgical registrar comes hurriedly to the ward to 'consent him'. Mr Adams' daughter is present while the registrar tells Mr Adams that he has got to have the operation to 'fix his tummy'. During the consultation, she asks questions and interrupts her father when he says that he just 'wants to be left alone'. Mr Adams tires and mumbles during the consultation and his daughter signs the consent form on his behalf. Rhiannon is asked to take Mr Adams to theatre for the operation, but as she approaches his bed, he tells her clearly that he doesn't want an operation, that he has 'had enough' and wants to be left alone. He says that 'you can't take me to theatre'. The consent form is signed, and the operating theatre is waiting. Without the operation, he will probably die, but Rhiannon feels very uneasy as she accompanies him down the corridor. Have the legal processes been properly followed?

The fundamental basis of law in England and Wales

The law and legal processes in the UK have evolved over hundreds of years and the right of the sovereign to make and administer the law has been split into two, Parliament and the judiciary with, in general, Parliament predominant. The two types of law are:

1   *statute law*, which follows from Acts of Parliament and statutory instruments (enacted from the power of Parliament), including European Union laws. These are known as statutory sources and take precedence over other laws; and
2   *common law*, known also as judge-made law or case law.

Statute, set down in Acts of Parliament, is supreme and overrides any uncertainty or conflict in common law, but it is impossible for legislators to cover every eventuality in the laws enacted through Parliament. Common law sets out areas of law not covered by Acts of Parliament, and interprets the statutes in individual cases. 'Judge-made law' as it is also called sets precedents that are followed by subsequent judgments. Hence previous case law decisions will guide opinion and a judge will rely in part on previous judgments in arriving at their opinion, applying them to the particular case in question and completing the opinion with final weighing up and legal argument. This is guided throughout by precedence and a logical and legal interpretation of the events.

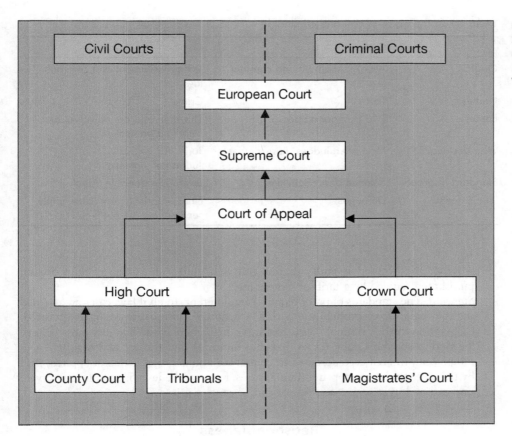

FIGURE 4.1
Simplified structure
of court hierarchy
in England and
Wales

Courts in England and Wales are hierarchical (see Figure 4.1). Under certain circumstances appeals can be made to courts higher in the hierarchy and lower courts must be guided by decisions made in higher ones. Important decisions of the courts are reported, recorded and published in resources such as the *All England Law Reports* available via Internet databases (e.g. www.lexisnexis.co.uk and www.westlaw.com) making them available for students and for subsequent court guidance and rulings. The law is administered in civil and criminal courts. The differences between civil and criminal law (summarised in Table 4.1, p. 82) include the following:

- *Origin*. Both criminal and civil law can be derived from Acts of Parliament. Judges interpret the law and develop it as common law.
- *Names*. A civil 'wrong' is a tort. A criminal 'wrong' is a crime.
- *Parties*. Cases under civil law involve a dispute between two or more parties, a common example being divorce. Criminal law involves the state, acting on behalf of the monarch and the people, prosecuting an individual for wrongdoing, or for an offence against the state.
- *Who decides*. Most civil cases are decided by a judge or judges, though juries are employed in certain circumstances. Criminal cases above magistrates' courts are heard before a jury normally of 12 people, who decide on the facts of the case, that is,

TABLE 4.1 Comparison of civil and criminal law

	Civil	Criminal
Origin	Act of Parliament and common law	Act of Parliament and common law
Names	Tort	Crime
Parties	Two or more parties	The state and an individual or (rarely) organisation
Who decides	Most often judges. Rarely juries	Juries for verdict Judge for sentence
Standard of proof	Balance of probabilities	Beyond reasonable doubt
'Punishment'	Damages	Fines, imprisonment, community service

whether the accused is guilty or not guilty. If guilty, the judge decides on the punishment guided by a tariff of sentencing.

- *Standard.* The standards of proof required are different. In civil law, cases are decided on the 'balance of probabilities'; that is what is most likely to have occurred. Conviction in the criminal courts requires a higher standard. The jury must believe 'beyond reasonable doubt' (or so that they are sure) that the accused is guilty.
- *Punishment.* In civil cases, orders can be granted and damages levied or applied, paid by the loser to the winner. In criminal cases, fines can be levied, community service imposed and in serious cases, people can be sent to prison.

Reasonableness

A significant principle governing legal aspects of clinical practice is that of reasonableness. The word 'reasonable' is used extensively throughout law: for example, a person may use reasonable force in self-defence, and the Disability Discrimination Act (DDA) requires educational institutions (in some circumstances) to make reasonable adjustments. However, despite its importance there is no clear definition of what 'reasonable' means, because it is a subjective adjective. A dictionary definition includes the following 'having sound judgement, sensible, not asking too much' (Oxford English Dictionary 2008). So in the case of the DDA, an institution would be expected to do more than install a cursory temporary ramp to gain access, but less than a complete rebuilding of a lecture theatre. What counts as reasonable can ultimately be decided on in court, and this is of necessity retrospective, of little help to a nurse attempting to decide on what a reasonable decision is. To put it another way, an action may be compared to what a 'reasonable' person would have done, this person being, in the famous phrase, 'the man on the Clapham Omnibus', a metaphor for an average person. 'Respectable' and 'responsible' have also been used to describe what supports the notion of 'reasonable'.

Perhaps a better way of deciding what is reasonable, and where there is no clear case law, is simply to ask how defensible the decision is. There is no compulsion for everyone to do the same thing, but what was done in the circumstances must be reasonable, and considered acceptable by colleagues, employers and regulatory bodies. Authority for decisions can be derived from evidence (hence evidence-based practice), which can be in the form of policy, protocol, directives or guidelines allied with perhaps evidence in the form of research or other sources. It could be argued that it is possible and lawful to be wrong in a given situation as long as the nurse is reasonably wrong, and could not reasonably be expected to have done differently, that is, what was wrong was not obviously wrong. When asked to judge another nurse's actions you could ask yourself 'Would I have done the same thing?' You may answer 'Yes'. If you answer 'No', you may want, then, to ask yourself 'Can I see why it was done? Do I find it acceptable?' For it to be reasonable and acceptable you might not agree with what was done but is it acceptable practice and that is what is considered reasonable. So, by definition there are different ways of behaving and courts are mainly interested in whether these are reasonable in their circumstances.

Activity 4.1

Reflect upon one or two clinical decisions you have seen made in practice. Can these decisions withstand a rigorous critique and examination?

Record keeping

It is sometimes asserted that health records are legal documents. In fact, all documents are legal documents, insofar as they can be presented as evidence in court. However, when there is a patient complaint or legal action, investigation will start with health records. For this reason (and for many others) keeping good records is an essential part of nursing, although it is sometimes regarded as a chore (McGeehan 2007, Prideaux 2011). *The Code* (NMC 2015, clause 10) requires that you must 'keep clear and accurate records relevant to your practice'. There is some elaboration, but previously available NMC advice on documentation has been withdrawn:

10 Keep clear and accurate records relevant to your practice

To achieve this, you must:

10.1 complete all records at the time or as soon as possible after an event, recording if the notes are written some time after the event;

10.2 identify any risks or problems that have arisen and the steps taken to deal with them, so that colleagues who use the records have all the information they need;

10.3 complete all records accurately and without any falsification, taking immediate and appropriate action if you become aware that someone has not kept to these requirements;

10.4 attribute any entries you make in any paper or electronic records to yourself, making sure they are clearly written, dated and timed, and do not include unnecessary abbreviations, jargon or speculation.

Courts of law tend to the view that 'if it is not recorded it has not been done'. Records fulfilling the above criteria are able to represent what was done, and why it was done,

A material fact is one that if it were withdrawn would make a difference.

Consent is giving permission for somebody to do something. To be valid, consent must be given voluntarily by a person who has capacity and sufficient information.

showing that acts and omissions were reasonable in their context. In law it is necessary to consider what is material and how **material facts** can be considered in health care decisions. An example of a material fact is that a policy or protocol exists. Professional nurses, utilising and relying upon a body of opinion, are empowered and required to exercise discretion and judgement, but this must normally be within policy, and so nurses should be aware what policies exist. Decisions by nurses must be based on and supported by NMC standards and guidance and can also include national, regional and local policy and other relevant codes and requirements, including legal obligations. Any action or omission outside the policy must be defended as reasonable. An investigation (legal or otherwise) will attempt to discover the truth and to determine responsibility, and health records are very important in evidencing what care was given.

PART 2: EXPLAINING THE LAW

In many cases the practice of nurses and other health care professionals is directly governed by law. The law informs the individuals and institutions what they are:

- *required to do*, for example, nurses are required to report certain illnesses – this means that they are at fault if they do not do this;
- *justified or allowed to do*, for example, nurses with prescribing powers are allowed to prescribe, according to their clinical judgement. It is also lawful in certain circumstances to withhold treatment 'in the patients' best interests';
- *forbidden to do*, for example, nurses (and all others) are forbidden to give drugs at the end of life with the intention of shortening the life.

A chapter of this length cannot deal with all areas of health care law. However, the following areas of law are very important, and are covered in more detail:

- consent to treatment – including the Mental Capacity Act (2005);
- the Mental Health Act (1983 and 2007);
- confidentiality, including the Data Protection Act (1998) and the Freedom of Information Act (2000); and
- the Human Rights Act (1998).

Consent to treatment

It is a fundamental ethical, legal and professional principle that valid **consent** must be obtained before starting any treatment, investigation or even giving care to a patient. In ethics this is the most obvious manifestation of the principle of respect for autonomy, requiring that nurses and other health care professionals recognise the right of individuals to determine as far as possible what happens to their own bodies. Without consent, touching a patient can amount to the crime of assault and the tort of battery, and if this seems extreme and unlikely, performing a procedure without consent, or deliberately misleading the patient has resulted in legal action. Brazier and Cave (2011) report the Canadian case of Allan v Mount Sinai Hospital [1980] where a woman expressed a wish to be injected in her right arm. The doctor injected her left, and lost the case in battery.

The days of patients passively acquiescing in treatment and care decided for them by health care professionals are thankfully long gone. The giving of valid consent is an expression of the partnership between professional and patient. The Department of Health (DH) has published a series of guides about consent, including an excellent reference guide (DH 2009). This can be downloaded and saved as a pdf file, and should be considered required reading. This document starts with the following:

> For consent to be valid, it must be given voluntarily by an appropriately informed person who has the capacity to consent to the intervention in question (this will be the patient or someone with parental responsibility for a patient under the age of 18, someone authorised to do so under a Lasting Power of Attorney (LPA) or someone who has the authority to make treatment decisions as a court appointed deputy.) Acquiescence where the person does not know what the intervention entails is not 'consent'.
>
> (DH 2009, p. 9)

From this definition, the following necessary features of valid consent can be identified:

- It must be voluntary.
- The patient must be appropriately informed.
- The patient must have the capacity to consent.

Each of these will be discussed and related to Case 4.1, which was presented at the beginning of the chapter.

It must be voluntary

Nurses must be aware of the potential for coercion and the way that this can influence a person's decisions. Historically, the clichéd manifestation of this was the powerful doctor, retinue in tow, who would merely decide a course of treatment and assume that the patient would agree. Today, perhaps, influences are more subtle. Overbearing relatives might attempt to influence a treatment, or a choice of home care, and nurses who suspect that this is the case should consider discussing options with the patient in private. Nurses also wield a considerable amount of power (Henderson 2003), and need to be aware of this; when we or the colleagues that we are supervising offer to wash a patient, can we really be sure that he is not merely acquiescing because he can see that we are busy? Or perhaps this 'busyness' has resulted in us applying a subtle pressure to the patient to agree?

Case 4.1 (continued)

There are a number of issues that may have resulted in Mr Adams feeling pressurised. His daughter interrupts him constantly, and in fact signs the consent form for him. The doctor's explanations are hurried and this may apply pressure for Mr Adams to make up his mind quickly. In these circumstances, it seems unlikely that initial consent is voluntarily given, and Rhiannon is right to feel uneasy.

The patient must be appropriately informed

A patient must be provided with sufficient information to be able to make a decision about treatment or care. For routine care decisions this does not seem to be difficult, but as decisions and options increase in their complexity, more information is required, and the interpretation of relevant information and the evidence base for the treatment needs to be presented in a manner appropriate for each individual patient. Written material explaining operations and procedures is often available and can help patients understand what is being proposed. Many complex decisions will be about medical treatment and here the responsibility lies with the medical team or senior nurses. However, the principles are the same for all decisions.

The law does not tell us exactly what patients must be told. Instead there have been a number of cases where patients have sued for negligence and these rulings set precedents detailing the amount of information considered reasonable for patients to expect. These cases often result from the occurrence of a known complication of a procedure, where patients sue on the grounds that they would not have consented to the procedure had they known the risks of the complication occurring. In a case heard in 1999, Mrs Pearce was two weeks overdue on delivering her sixth child, and discussed the risks of induction or caesarean section. She was not told of the small risk (1 in 1000) of stillbirth associated with waiting for a vaginal delivery. The child was stillborn. Mrs Pearce sued and subsequently lost her case. The judge said that the doctor should inform the patient of 'a significant risk which would affect the judgement of a reasonable patient' (Brazier and Cave 2011, DH 2009). Mrs Pearce was distressed at the time, and it was judged reasonable not to disclose this risk. By contrast, in an Australian case (*Rogers v Whittaker* 1992), a patient won a case for negligence because she was not informed of a 1 in 14,000 chance of blindness following surgery, despite voicing her concerns about losing her sight. So it is not possible to specify that risks above a certain likelihood must be disclosed. The law is currently evolving in this area, but, consistent with law and policy in other areas of practice, the discretion of the health care professional to decide what is best for the patient, including how much to tell them about their treatment, is diminishing.

A case in point here is *Montgomery v Lanarkshire Health Board* [2015] UKSC 11. Nadine Montgomery claimed she had the right to know that her small stature and diabetes enhanced the risk of complications during birth. Her son was asphyxiated when his shoulder got stuck, had to be resuscitated and suffered brain damage. The obstetrician involved was aware of the risk of shoulder dystocia but decided not to discuss it with Montgomery, who said she would have had a caesarean if she had known the risks involved. The court in this case supported the view that doctors (including health care professionals) have a duty to discover what the 'reasonable patient' wants to know and to be reasonably aware of what a patient might attach significance to. So, there appears to be a move towards the patient deciding on the level of acceptable risk to them rather than a paternalistic view. Again, this area of law continues to evolve (Griffith 2015a).

The consent form in use in the UK, downloadable from the Department of Health website, requires the doctor, or whoever is seeking consent, to sign to say that they have explained the intended benefits, serious or frequently occurring risks, and any extra procedures that may become necessary during the procedure, including blood transfusion. On the face of it, detailed information is a good thing although there is some evidence that these complex forms can conflict with patients' needs for personal communication and advocacy (Akkad *et al.* 2004). The Cochrane Library has produced a detailed review of interventions to promote informed consent (Kinnersley *et al.* 2013).

Case 4.1 (continued)

There is little detail in the case study about exactly what information was given, and as in all cases, much depends on the detail. However, the operation appears to be life-saving and Mr Adams would need to understand this and also the risks of the anaesthetic and the likely outcome of the operation, for example, whether a stoma is likely. Telling Mr Adams that the operation is necessary to 'fix his tummy' does not appear to satisfy the minimum requirement for information.

Good and lawful practice includes:

- giving sufficient information for the patient to understand in broad terms the nature of a procedure (DH 2009), and other options, including doing nothing;
- giving information about anaesthesia if appropriate;
- disclosing details of any 'material' or 'significant' risks;
- disclosing whether students will be participating in care or treatment;
- answering questions fully and honestly;
- making records about what has been discussed. This is also important when patients do not want to know the details of their treatment.

Activity 4.2

Get a copy of the consent form that you use in your clinical area, or from the Department of Health website. From your experience of observing or participating in the gaining of consent, has the form always been correctly completed?

The patient must have capacity to consent

Seeking consent for treatment is the cornerstone of the partnership between patient and health professional, but a difficulty arises where a patient is unable to make a decision about their treatment. It is clear that the law absolutely allows people to make decisions that health care professionals may think unwise or even irrational but this only applies when the patient is able to make the decision. **Mental capacity** 'is the ability to make a decision' (Ministry of Justice 2007, p. 41). This definition refers to having the *cognitive* ability to make decisions and communicate them, rather than the absence of any other restrictions, for example, the power relationships discussed earlier. Capacity can be restricted for a number of reasons, including physical and mental illness and cognitive impairment. Examples include:

- stroke or other brain injury;
- a mental health problem;
- dementia;
- a learning disability;
- confusion or drowsiness;
- substance misuse (including alcohol).

Mental capacity is the ability to make a decision.

The issue of capacity often arises where there is disagreement about treatment options, where, for example, the nurse thinks that a patient needs oxygen therapy, and the patient says he does not want it. After hearing an explanation of the reasons why the nurse thinks that oxygen therapy is necessary, a patient declining to have the therapy may be making a considered judgement based on the information given, or be confused by hypoxia or sedatives, such that pushing away the oxygen mask is not a meaningful act, but just a reflex action. In the former case a patient with capacity has made what might be considered an unwise decision, which must be respected. In the latter, an incapable patient is not able to make a decision at all, and to respect this 'refusal' would be to put the patient at risk of harm. The nurse must look after the patient's best interests and these cannot be served by allowing the refusal of oxygen therapy. Instead the nurse is obliged to make all reasonable attempts at finding an alternative way of giving the therapy which the patient will tolerate, even to the point, perhaps, of sitting with them and holding the mask so that they are unable to push it away.

What this example illustrates most of all is that lawful action depends largely on the issue of whether or not a patient is considered to have capacity, and this applies to all decisions. Since the issue of capacity will frequently arise in health care, there is a need for a clear process of assessing whether a person has capacity or not, and a clear legal framework of what should be done when a person is considered to lack capacity. These frameworks are provided by the Mental Capacity Act 2005 (MCA), which came into force during 2007. There are excellent, easy to read guides about the MCA, and these can be downloaded free from the Ministry of Justice website. Guide number 3 (Office of the Public Guardian 2007) in particular should be considered essential reading. A full code of practice is also available free to download (Ministry of Justice 2007). The requirement to be aware of legislation regarding mental capacity is stated in *The Code* (NMC 2015, clause 4.3). The five principles of the MCA are:

1   *A presumption of capacity.* Every adult has the right to make his or her own decisions and must be assumed to have the capacity to do so unless it is proved otherwise.
2   *Individuals being supported to make their own decisions.* A person must be given all practicable help before anyone treats them as not being able to make their own decisions.
3   *Unwise decisions.* Just because an individual makes what might be seen as an unwise decision, they should not be treated as lacking the capacity to make the decision.
4   *Best interests.* An act done or a decision made under the Act for or on behalf of a person who lacks capacity must be done in their best interests.
5   *Least restrictive option.* Anything done for or on behalf of a person who lacks capacity should be the least restrictive of their basic rights and freedoms.

Assessing capacity

The presumption is always in favour of the view that the person has capacity. The patient does not have to show that they have capacity, the health care professional must assume that this is the case, unless it can be shown that they do not. It cannot be assumed that just because someone has a particular condition, for example dementia, they can never make any decisions, and neither can assumptions be made about capacity based on age, appearance, or eccentricities of a person's behaviour. The assessment of capacity is always about a particular decision to be taken at a particular time, not made in the general sense for all decisions at all times. Some people are able to make simple decisions but not complex ones, and some people's ability to make decisions fluctuates so that they may have capacity one day and not the next.

The MCA puts into statute a test for capacity, which has been in use since 1994, deriving from the case of *Re C* [1994]. In this case, Mr C, a 68-year-old man, who was detained in a psychiatric hospital because of paranoid schizophrenia, developed serious leg problems. Doctors treating his leg considered him to have a 15 per cent chance of survival without an amputation, but he refused consent, and sought an injunction to prevent doctors from performing the amputation without his consent. Despite the fact that he was seriously mentally ill, suffering from delusions, the judge found that he was nevertheless able to make this particular decision (Brazier and Cave 2011). The test for capacity arising from that case is now contained within the MCA (2005), as a two-stage test. The first stage is to decide whether there is impairment of, or disturbance in the functioning of, the patient's mind or brain. If impairment is present, the second stage considers whether it results in the person being able to make a specific decision when they need to. A person is unable to make a decision if they cannot:

1 understand information about the decision to be made (the Act calls this 'relevant information');
2 retain that information in their mind;
3 use or weigh that information as part of the decision-making process; or
4 communicate their decision (by talking, using sign language or any other means).

(Ministry of Justice 2007, p. 45)

If the application of this process concludes that the patient does have capacity, then refusal of treatment must be accepted, however unwise it seems to health care professionals. On rare occasions this might even lead to a patient's death, and the refusal of Jehovah's Witnesses to consent to a blood transfusion is a commonly cited example of this (McInroy 2005). *Re S* and *Re T* are relevant legal cases. The more serious the decision to be taken, the more formal the application of this test needs to be, and the greater the requirement for sound documentation.

If the patient is not capable of making the decision, then clearly this falls to someone else, normally the doctor, nurse or social worker. It is sometimes assumed that in the absence of capacity the next of kin has legal responsibility, but in the absence of a lasting power of attorney this is not the case. Decisions must be made 'in the best interests' of the patient. This is not as simple as it may seem, and the code of practice (Ministry of Justice 2007) gives detailed advice on what factors should be taken into consideration. In making the decision, the decision-maker should (see Figure 4.2):

- encourage participation;
- identify all relevant circumstances;
- attempt to find out the patient's views;
- avoid discrimination;
- assess whether the patient might regain capacity;
- not be motivated by a desire to bring about the patient's death;
- consult others;
- avoid restricting the patient's rights.

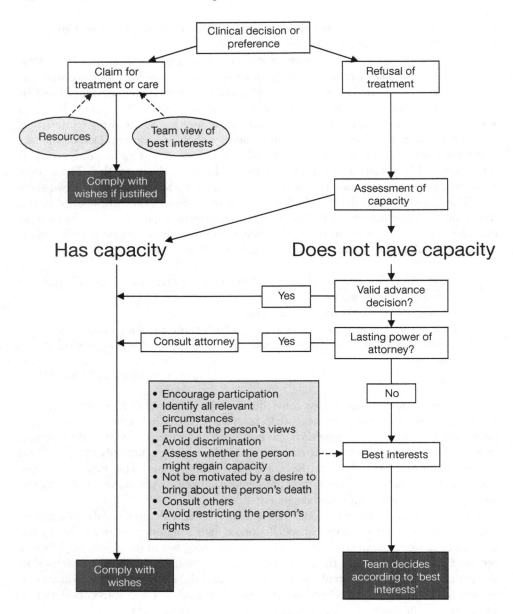

FIGURE 4.2 Flow chart for decisions about capacity

Case 4.1 (continued)

The case study shows that a number of errors have been made in consenting Mr Adams for his operation. There seems to have been no assessment of his capacity, it appears to have been assumed that he lacks capacity since his daughter has signed the consent form unlawfully. The details are important, but there does not seem to have been any consideration at all of his views, nor was it apparently considered that Mr Adams' capacity to make the decision may improve with more conservative treatment after, for example, he has had some fluid, oxygen and analgesia. When Rhiannon went to Mr Adams to take him to theatre and he told her he didn't want to have the operation, at the very least this is an indication for an assessment of his capacity, which may have improved since the consent form was (unlawfully) signed. If it cannot be shown that Mr Adams does not have capacity, then his wishes not to have the operation must be respected. An operation undertaken in these circumstances is probably unlawful.

Lasting power of attorney
allows a person to appoint somebody else to make health and welfare decisions on their behalf should they lose their capacity in the future.

An **advance decision** is a mechanism whereby a person can specify in advance that they do not want certain treatment at a future time when they lack capacity to make the decision.

Lasting power of attorney and advance decisions

There are two other areas of the Mental Capacity Act (2005) that enable decisions to be made for those lacking capacity. First, **lasting power of attorney** (LPA) allows a person to appoint somebody else to make health and welfare decisions on their behalf should they lose capacity in the future. There are specific processes that must be followed to give these appointments legal force, including registration with the Office of the Public Guardian. Second, the Act clarifies the arrangements for **advance decisions** that previously derived their legal status from common law. An advance decision is a mechanism whereby a person can specify in advance that they do not want certain treatment, ensuring that a person's wishes are adhered to at a future point when they are no longer able to make or communicate decisions. This is important when it can be predicted that the person will lose capacity. Again, there are specific rules attached to their operation and there are further details in the MCA Code of Practice.

- The advance decision must be valid – the person must not have withdrawn it, made an LPA, or acted in a way inconsistent with the advance decision.
- It must be applicable to the treatment in question, explaining the circumstances that the refusal applies to.
- Advance decisions do not apply where people are lawfully detained under the Mental Health Act.
- People cannot ask for their life to be ended.
- People cannot use advance decisions to ask for treatment, only to refuse it. This is a very important distinction.

Advance decisions, properly made, are legally binding on health professionals. They do not have to be written in a certain way, or on a certain form, to be binding. However, where the decision refuses life-sustaining treatment, it must be in writing, signed and witnessed, and specifically state that the decision is to be applied even if life is at risk. Some charities, for example, the Alzheimer's Society (no date) provide useful templates. Others, for example Age UK provide useful factsheets, which are worth reading because they are written for a wide audience (Age UK 2015). Some have taken extreme measures

Richard Thomas and Paul Snelling

Implied consent is when a patient demonstrates by their actions that they consent to treatment, for example, rolling up a sleeve and putting their arm out when they see a nurse approaching with a sphygmomanometer.

Words are important in describing people under 18. The Children Act (1989), and the law in general, refers to a person under 18 as 'a child'. The Mental Capacity Act (2005) refers to an individual under 16 as a 'child' and an individual of ages 16 or 17 as a '**young person**'.

Gillick competence allows a child under the age of 16 to consent to treatment if he or she has sufficient understanding and intelligence to enable him or her to understand fully what is proposed.

to communicate their wishes, for example a woman who had her instructions tattooed on her chest. Though apparently unambiguous and demonstrating a feisty determination to make her wishes known, these tattoos in themselves would not constitute a valid advance decision, because it is not signed or witnessed and does not specify the circumstances in which it applies. The woman in question did have a valid advance decision in her notes and had made her wishes known to the local hospital (Lawn and Bassi 2008).

As a balance to these provisions of treating people who lack capacity, there are now regulations regarding the protection of such people. These are designed to deal with persons who fail to care and treat such people reasonably. Section 44 of the Mental Capacity Act (2005) provides for up to 5 years in prison for ill-treatment or wilful neglect of patients who 'lack capacity'. Since April 2015, against the background of the Francis Report and the prosecutions arising from the Winterbourne View events and serious case review, there is now a new criminal offence of ill-treatment or wilful neglect in health and social care. Sections 20–25 of the Criminal Justice and Courts Act 2015 sets out the new offences. Though the MCA (2005) concerns itself with persons who lack capacity these new offences do not discriminate according to type of patient (lacking or with capacity). These new offences cover both individual workers and also provider organisations. The individual care provider is identified as 'an individual who "ill-treats or wilfully neglects" another individual of whom he has care "by virtue of being a care worker" (Section 20 of the Criminal Justice and Courts Act 2015) (Griffith, 2013, 2015b).

Documenting consent

Most nurses will be familiar with the signing of consent forms prior to procedures, and this is an obvious manifestation of the process of gaining consent. However, valid consent does not require a signature on a form, though this is considered best practice for many procedures. Valid consent can be obtained without a signature, and where a signature is present, it does not of itself demonstrate that the consent was valid. Consent can also be given orally or by implication. **Implied consent** is when a patient's actions imply that they have consented to what is being proposed, for example, by rolling up a sleeve at the approach of a nurse with a sphygmomanometer. Implied consent can be regarded as an 'integral component of the nurse–patient relationship, taking account of the on-going relationship between both parties and the nature of nursing care' (Aveyard 2002, p. 202). There is a danger in confusing implied consent with acquiescence, and Aveyard (2002) suggests that verbal consent should be obtained prior to a nursing care procedure.

Consent and young people

The discussion on consent above specifically applies to adults over the age of 18. Different arrangements apply for young people under the age of 18. The Family Law Reform Act 1969 allows **young people** aged 16 or 17 to consent for their own treatment, and as for adults this is only the case where there is capacity. Under common law, children under 16 are also able to consent for treatment where 'the child has sufficient understanding and intelligence to enable him or her to understand fully what is proposed'. This statement has become known as '**Gillick competence**' arising from the famous case of *Gillick v West Norfolk and Wisbech AHA and Department of Health and Social Service (DHSS)*. Mrs Gillick challenged the lawfulness of a memorandum of guidance from the DHSS that supported

---

RESEARCH FOCUS 4.1

The law and its application to nursing practice do not seem to present many opportunities for undertaking research. A question concerning what is lawful and what is not can only be settled by referral to the appropriate legal processes, not by undertaking or consulting empirical research. However, research can illuminate other concerning aspects of practice that may have legal implications.

One of the groups of practitioners who are frequently required to decide on capacity are those staff working in emergency departments, so it is to be hoped that their level of knowledge supports good and lawful practice. Evans *et al.* (2007) gave a short questionnaire about capacity and consent to 86 doctors, nurses and paramedics working in an accident department in Birmingham. The first question asked; 'what three points would you look for in assessing one's capacity to give valid consent?' (The correct answers are: (1) To take in and retain information; (2) believe it; and (3) to weigh the information, balancing risks and needs). Questionnaires that gave 2 out of 3 correct responses were deemed correct, but despite this, 33 per cent of the doctors, 90 per cent of the nurses and 100 per cent of the ambulance staff gave incorrect or incomplete answers. The responses to the closed questions that completed the short questionnaire were more promising, but remember that the only available responses were yes/no/don't know. The first question asked 'If a competent adult refuses treatment, can you still treat them under common law? (correct answer = NO): 90 per cent of the doctors, 67 per cent of the nurses, and 91 per cent of the ambulance staff answered correctly. Some of the nurses were untrained, but even allowing for this, 5 registered nurses from the 19 answering the questionnaire (26 per cent) were wrong about this fundamental tenet of the legal system, which is also clearly articulated in the version of the Code of Professional Conduct current at the time of the research. The research was conducted prior to the implementation of the Mental Capacity Act (2005), and noted that the implementation of the Act was not accompanied by any strategy to train those who should be using it. However, this research demonstrates a worrying lack of knowledge of basic legal processes. This paper was one of many considered by an integrative review (Lamont *et al.* 2013), which concluded that there are inconsistencies in practice.

---

the principle that a doctor could lawfully prescribe contraception to a girl under 16 years old without parental consent. Mrs Gillick challenged this on the grounds that the advice contained in the memorandum was:

- wrong and unlawful;
- harmed or potentially harmed the welfare of her children;
- affected her rights as a parent;
- interfered with her duty to care for her children.

Mrs Gillick considered that the principle within the guidelines effectively put her outside of the law and interfered with her ability and duty to protect her children. She was not suggesting that this treatment would never go ahead, but it should require her prior knowledge and consent. Mrs Gillick eventually lost. It was ruled that in exceptional circumstances it would be lawful to provide contraceptive advice and treatment to a girl under 16 without parental consent. This ruling led to the notion of Gillick competence and the detailed ruling concerning contraception is known now as the Fraser Guidelines after Lord Fraser, who stated that the exceptional circumstances are:

1   The girl would (although under 16 years old) understand the doctor's advice.
2   The doctor could not persuade her to inform her parents that she was seeking advice and treatment or allow him to do so.
3   The girl was very likely to have sexual intercourse with or without this advice and treatment.
4   Unless she received this contraceptive advice and/or treatment her physical or mental health (or both) were likely to suffer.
5   The girl's best interests requires the doctor to provide contraceptive advice, treatment or both without parental consent.

On the face of it this could be criticised as condoning unlawful sexual activity. Supporting a girl under the age of 16 in this way perhaps needs to be seen as the least bad option in the circumstances and it must be remembered that not all children have positive relationships with their parents. This aspect of clinical practice can be seen as a human rights issue and it is the right of the child to be assessed as to the suitability for health care or medical treatment, in this case contraceptive advice or treatment.

The test of Gillick competence is applied to all treatment decisions in children under 16. The test is whether the child had sufficient understanding and intelligence to enable them to understand what is proposed. The test is usually applied by doctors, and a more holistic approach has been advocated (Parekh 2006). If the test is passed, then the child's consent to treatment is valid. In applying the test, nurses should be aware that:

- There is no specific age at which a child becomes competent to consent.
- Each child and each procedure must be considered on his/her/its own merits.
- The seriousness and complexity of the proposed procedures may be such that a child may be capable of consenting to some procedures but not to others.
- Attempts should be made to persuade the child to confide in his/her family.

The discussion above concerns children's and young people's ability to consent to treatment, but not to refuse it. This is a very important distinction, as the legal right of the young person to control what happens to their body is clear only insofar as they *agree* to what is being proposed. A *refusal* of treatment proposed by others can be overridden, leading Brazier and Cave (2011) to conclude that 'adolescent autonomy is little more than a myth' (p. 451). A number of cases support this view, including where refusal of treatment by young people has been challenged in court. The judge in the case of *Re E*, a 15-year-old Jehovah's Witness who attempted to refuse a blood transfusion, supported by his parents, commented that 'although parents may martyr themselves, the court should be very slow to allow an infant to martyr himself' (Woolley 2005, p. 717). There is no hard and fast guidance, and it is not suggested that a refusal of treatment by a child or young person can *always* legitimately be overruled by a parent, or a health care professional. Refusal of consent by a young person may be overruled by one or both parents, or where the parents agree with the young person, by health care professionals through the courts. Good practice depends on the individual circumstances, which will include the age and ability of the child, and the nature of the treatment under consideration. The Department of Health offers the following guidance as part of the reference guide to consent (DH 2009), concerning young people and Gillick-competent children:

- No definitive guidance on appropriateness to overrule has been given, but it has been suggested that it should be restricted to where there is 'grave and irreversible mental or physical harm' (p. 34, para. 14).
- Even where those with parental responsibility wish to overrule refusal, consideration should be given to applying to the court for a ruling prior to treatment.
- A breach of confidentiality allowing information concerning the nature of the decision to be given to parents may be justifiable where there is serious risk to the child.
- Refusal by a competent child and all persons with parental responsibility can be overruled by the court if the welfare of the child requires it.
- Where there is a life-threatening emergency, the courts have stated that doubt should be resolved in favour of preservation of life (p. 35, para. 18).

Nurses and other health care professionals wanting a definitive list of what is lawful and what is not will be doomed to continual disappointment; such a list does not and cannot exist. It is impossible to cover every eventuality as the law considers each case on its individual merits. However, considerable guidance is covered by official publications, and this should be sufficient for nurses to be able to make reasoned opinions, and to contribute to multi-professional decisions that can withstand scrutiny as part of professional accountability. Immediate decisions are seldom necessary and legal advice, even court rulings, can be obtained at short notice where necessary.

Consenting for children

Previous discussions on consent apply only to young people and children who are Gillick competent. Where younger children or those not Gillick competent are treated, consent must be obtained from someone with parental authority or by the court. The Children Act (1989) sets out persons who have parental responsibility (DH 2001), and this includes:

- the child's mother;
- the child's father, if he was married to the mother at the time of birth;
- unmarried fathers, who can acquire parental responsibility in several different ways:
  - for children born before 1 December 2003, unmarried fathers will have parental responsibility if they marry the mother of their child or obtain a parental responsibility order from the court;
  - register a parental responsibility agreement with the court or by an application to court;
  - for children born after 1 December 2003, unmarried fathers will have parental responsibility if they register the child's birth jointly with the mother at the time of birth (Under section 111 of the Adoption and Children Act 2002, unmarried fathers who register their child's birth jointly with the mother will automatically acquire parental responsibility);
  - re-register the birth if they are the natural father;
  - marry the mother of their child or obtain a parental responsibility order from the court;
  - register with the court for parental responsibility.

- the child's legally appointed guardian;
- a person in whose favour the court has made a residence order concerning the child;
- a local authority designated in a care order in respect of the child.

In everyday situations consenting for a child is often straightforward, but numerous complexities can arise. The rights of parents to consent and to refuse treatment for their children are limited and can be challenged. Brazier and Cave (2011) point out that many cases show that where the interests of children are concerned, courts tend to favour medical over parental opinion, and in addition the courts have made it clear that certain procedures, for example sterilisation, should not be performed without a court order. Courts can also be asked to decide where there is disagreement between parents.

It has been perhaps assumed so far that the child will comply willingly with the treatment proposed, but nurses and parents reading this chapter will know that this is not always the case. A small child aged 3 or 4 may be carried kicking and screaming into the practice nurse's room to have inoculations, but as children get older their views should at least be taken into consideration. This might be considered good lawful practice rather than the dry application of principles and case law, and it is not suggested that objections should be decisive, even of course where there is Gillick competence. The level to which a child objects to a procedure is one factor that has to be weighed up when considering best interests, and treatment performed forcibly requires justification (Brazier and Cave 2011).

Lastly, in this section, the issue of emergency treatment needs clarity. Where a child requires treatment in an emergency, and no one is available to give consent, the law is clear that it is permissible to proceed with the treatment, on the basis that it is in the child's best interests. Indeed not to give emergency treatment because no one is available to consent may well be indefensible.

A further Department of Health publication, *Seeking Consent, Working with Children* (DH 2001) is available free to download from the Department of Health website, and again this should be considered required reading for those whose practice involves caring for children, and to those of us who care for our own children.

The Mental Health Act (1983 and 2007)

The Mental Health Act (1983) (MHA) governs compulsory admission and treatment of certain individuals with a mental disorder, though the majority of patients within the mental health system are not detained under the MHA and will have sought admission or treatment with consent (Dimond 2015). The main purpose of the MHA (2007) is to amend the MHA (1983).

Compulsory detention

A strict process seeks to ensure that only those who appear to be suffering from a mental disorder and are actively seeking to avoid admission to hospital are compulsorily detained (see Box 4.1). In all other circumstances, informal admission under Section 131 of the MHA (1983) is more appropriate (Griffith and Tengnah 2008). The definition of mental disorder from Section 1(2) MHA (1983) is 'any disorder or disability of the mind'. However, a person with a learning disability cannot be compulsorily admitted for treatment or guardianship unless their disability is associated with abnormally aggressive or seriously irresponsible conduct (MHA 1983; Section 1(2A)). In itself, dependency upon alcohol or drugs cannot be considered a mental disorder under the MHA.

The use of powers under the MHA is required to be the least restrictive. Three groups of people are primarily involved in the processes:

- the approved mental health professional (AMHP);
- a registered medical practitioner;
- the patient's nearest relative.

The AMHP can be a nurse or social worker who has a duty to conduct an interview with a person prior to any application for detention. The AMHP is seen as providing protection from the misuse of powers.

The opinions of two medical practitioners must be sought (only one in an emergency). One doctor must be approved and recognised by the primary care trust. The medical opinion must confirm that the person is suffering from a mental disorder of a *nature* or *degree* that indicates compulsory admission. The *nature* is the prognosis, person's past history, previous admissions and compliance with treatments. The *degree* of disorder is its current severity. Only one criterion has to be satisfied (Griffith and Tengnah 2008).

The nearest relative is a 'statutory friend' and is drawn from a hierarchy of relatives (see MHA 1983; Section 26). Since 1 December 2007 this includes civil partners.

The care of the patient will be supervised by an approved clinician. This can be a consultant psychiatrist but under the MHA (2007) reforms, clinical psychologists, consultant nurses and occupational therapists can also be approved clinicians. Clinicians can supervise treatment, grant leave, renew detention orders and discharge patients from hospital.

A code of practice for the MHA is available at the DH website (DH 2015). At over 400 pages, it is a lengthy document, though it is easy to navigate.

BOX 4.1 Compulsory admission provisions or sections within the MHA

- *Section 2* Ordinary admission to hospital for up to 28 days for assessment. The application made by an approved mental health professional (AMHP) based on two medical recommendations, one of which is from an approved clinician. Not renewable.
- *Section 3* Admission to hospital for up to 6 months for treatment. The application made by an AMHP based on two medical recommendations, one of which is from an approved clinician. Can be renewed for a further 6 months, then yearly.
- *Section 4* Admission on an emergency basis for up to 72 hours. The application made by an AMHP or nearest relative founded upon one medical recommendation. Can convert to a Section 2 if a second medical opinion is presented.
- *Section 37* Hospital order by a court for 6 months, renewable for 6 months and then yearly.
- *Section 37* Guardianship order by the court. 6 months, renewable for 6 months then yearly.
- *Section 37/41* Hospital order with restriction. Without time limit, with discharge and leave granted by the Home Office.

Holding power of the nurse under Section 5(4) of the MHA (1983)

The nurse must be 'prescribed' under the MHA (1983), meaning that they are trained in mental health or learning disability nursing. Section 5(4) provides for a prescribed nurse to hold a patient for up to 6 hours if they consider the patient to be at risk (Houlihan 2005). This means that the nurse can lawfully prevent an informal patient from leaving the hospital using the minimum force necessary. However:

- The patient must be an inpatient receiving treatment for mental disorder.
- The prescribed nurse must have evidence that the patient is suffering from mental disorder of such a degree that it is necessary for their health or safety or for the protection of others for them to be immediately restrained and prevented from leaving the hospital.
- It is not possible to immediately secure the attendance of a practitioner who could exercise powers under Section 5(2) of the MHA.

The MHA only applies to care and treatment for mental disorder. If a patient detained under the MHA requires treatment for physical illness, valid consent by the patient is required and where capacity is absent, the provisions of the MCA (2005) are applied. The MHA (2007) also amends the MCA (2005). Changes to the MCA (2005) provide for procedures to authorise the deprivation of liberty of a person resident in a hospital or care home who lacks capacity to consent. The MCA (2005) principles of supporting a person to make a decision when possible, and acting at all times in the person's best interests and in the least restrictive manner, will apply to all decision-making in operating the procedures. The changes in relation to the MCA are in response to the 2004 European Court of Human Rights judgment (*HL v UK* (Application No.45508/99), the 'Bournewood judgment') involving an autistic man (HL) who was kept at Bournewood Hospital by doctors against the wishes of his carers. The European Court of Human Rights found that admission to and retention in hospital of HL under the common law of necessity amounted to a breach of Article 5(1) ECHR (deprivation of liberty) and of Article 5(4) (right to have lawfulness of detention reviewed by a court).

Confidentiality

A duty of confidence arises when one person discloses information to another (e.g. patient to clinician) in circumstances where it is reasonable to expect that the information will be held in confidence. Confidentiality is:

- a legal obligation that is derived from case law;
- a requirement established with professional codes of conduct; and
- must be included within NHS employment contracts as a specific requirement linked to disciplinary procedures.

(DH 2003)

The Code (NMC 2015, clause 5) requires that:

- You must respect people's right to confidentiality.
- You must ensure people are informed about how and why information is shared by those who will be providing their care.

- You must disclose information if you believe someone may be at risk of harm, in line with the law of the country in which you are practising.

A patient has a right to expect information about them is confidential, and this right is recognised in professional codes of practice and in law. This right places a duty on all professionals and employees to work within the rules of confidentiality and to be aware as to what this duty means for them. Detailed guidance is available from the Department of Health (2003). The Department of Health (2003) proposes a model with four requirements (see Figure 4.3):

1 *Protect*: look after the patient's information.
2 *Inform*: ensure that patients are aware of how their information is used.
3 *Provide choice*: allow patients to decide whether their information can be disclosed or used in particular ways.
4 *Improve*: always look for ways to protect, inform and provide choice.

Confidentiality does not simply cover not discussing confidential details of patients, but also protecting the information. For example if it relates to care and treatment, it is reasonable for nurses to discuss patients between themselves, but care should be taken that these conversations cannot be overheard. Curtain screens around beds are not soundproof. Confidentiality is a duty for many professions, such as journalists, priests and lawyers, and the nature of the duty differs between them. In the area of health care, the duty is not absolute and can legitimately be breached in at least the following circumstances:

1 *With the consent of the patient*. An example of this is seeking permission from a patient to disclose information to their relatives. It should not be assumed that patients always give consent to allow disclosure to spouses and children about the nature and prognosis of their illnesses, care and treatment.

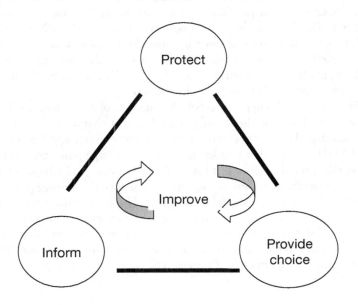

FIGURE 4.3
Confidentiality model
Source: DH 2003.

2   In some cases there is a *legal requirement* to disclose and failure to do so may result in an offence, or contempt of court. For example, statutory duty to disclose is part of the Road Traffic Act 1988 (as amended) and under terrorism legislation.

3   *In the public interest.* Public interest is defined by the Department of Health (2003) as

> exceptional circumstances that justify overruling the right of an individual to confidentiality in order to serve the broader social interest. Decisions about the public interest are complex and must take account of both the potential harm that disclosure may cause and the interest of society in the continued provision of confidential health services.
>
> (DH 2003, p. 6)

The Department of Health further notes that

> under common law, staff are permitted to disclose personal information in order to prevent and support detection, investigation and punishment of serious crime and/or to prevent abuse or serious harm to others where they judge on a case by case basis that the public good that would be achieved by the disclosure outweighs both the obligation of confidentiality to the individual patient concerned and the broader public interest in the provision of a confidential service.
>
> (DH 2003, p. 34)

It is worthwhile to quote at length from the NHS code of practice on confidentiality as it illustrates a number of important issues. There seems to be something of a conflict with *The Code* (NMC 2015), which requires rather than permits disclosure where the nurse believes someone may be at risk of harm (not serious harm), though the relevant paragraph does require action to be 'in line with the laws relating to the disclosure of information' (NMC 2015, clause 17.2, Snelling 2015). Disclosure must be justified on a case by case basis – blanket justification, for example, in the case of a certain disease is not supported. These decisions can be very complex (Beech 2007), not least in the requirement that health care professionals must also consider wider societal interests of retaining a confidential health service; if patients knew that breaches of confidentiality were made regularly, they might be less likely to divulge information, leading to a detrimental effect on people's health and treatment.

The DH statement also appears to beg the question of the distinction between crime and serious crime. Like the discussion in Part 1 of this chapter about reasonableness, it must be noted that the adjective 'serious' must be subjectively applied. The Department of Health (2003) suggests that murder, rape, treason, kidnapping and child abuse are all serious, and theft, fraud or damage to property would not generally justify disclosure. It is a further illustration, if one was needed, that exhaustive lists are not possible and nurses must be able to justify their reasonable decisions. The risks of harm to others associated with infection control, for example, where a sexual partner is unaware of HIV infection, can also justify disclosure (Dimond 2004). It should be clear that cases are often finely balanced, and a full discussion within the health care team is advisable (GMC 2009). Legal advice can also be obtained if necessary.

Activity 4.3

Based on the limited information available, consider how strong the case for disclosure is in the following cases. Imagine that you are involved in a multidisciplinary discussion about whether or not confidentiality should be breached. Giving reasons, what action would you advocate?

- A patient confesses to abusing a child 10 years ago.
- A patient known to have HIV infection has been admitted for treatment of chest infection. It becomes clear that his partner does not know about the HIV infection.
- After being diagnosed with epilepsy, a young woman makes it clear that she will not inform the DVLA of her condition.

Freedom of Information Act (2000)

An individual has the right to apply for access to all types of recorded information held by public authorities regardless of the date of the information. There are 23 exceptions to this right and some of these are based upon a public interest test; that is, the public body must consider if it is in the public interest to withhold the information or to release the information. There are also absolute exemptions where the public interest test does not apply, for example, information provided in confidence and personal information where the applicant is the subject, which is covered by the Data Protection Act (1998). Most exemptions fall within the category where the public interest test does apply and this includes personal information and audit functions. Accessible further information can be found on the Ministry of Justice website.

Data Protection Act (1998)

This Act gives right of access to people who have data held about them (known as data subjects). This includes health records and within this would be nursing records. The Act allows data subjects to:

- know if personal information is processed;
- have a description of the data held, purpose of processing and where and to whom it can be disclosed;
- receive a copy of the information;
- have details of the source of the information.

The data subject also has the right to have records corrected and apply to the court or information commissioner for an enforcement notice. Data can be corrected, prevented from being released or destroyed, or a true record inserted. The subject can seek compensation if they consider they have been harmed by the incorrect or inaccurate records.

Withholding information under the Data Protection Act

The right of access to information is a conditional rather than absolute right. The Data Protection (Subject Access Modifications) (Health) Order. Statutory Instrument 2000 No. 413 makes certain provisions allowing withholding of information:

- If access 'would be likely to cause serious harm to the physical or mental health or condition of the data subject or any other person (which may include a health care professional)'.
- If access is requested by someone other than the subject (perhaps a parent about a child) this access can be denied if the subject expected it not to be disclosed and does not give their permission.
- If giving access to the subject will reveal the identity of another person then access can be denied. If the third party has given their permission then it can be disclosed or if it is reasonable and indicated to comply with the subject's request without the third party consent. Health care professionals are not included in this provision unless it can be shown that they are likely to suffer serious harm to their physical or mental health.

Human Rights Act (1998)

The Human Rights Act (1998) (HRA) made rights from the European Convention on Human Rights enforceable in UK courts (see Box 4.2). The HRA imposes a direct legal obligation on NHS Trusts to ensure they respect European Convention rights in all that they do (McHale *et al.* 2001). This means that NHS Trusts need to consider the human rights implications of all of their policies and practices. Any person who feels that an NHS Trust has breached their human rights may be able to take the Trust to court or use human rights arguments in other processes.

An example of a failed attempt to apply the provisions of the HRA is in the case of Mrs Diane Pretty, a 42-year-old woman with motor neurone disease. She wished to take her own life with the assistance of her husband as she was physically incapable of doing it herself. Mrs Pretty was confined to a wheelchair and paralysed from the neck down. Citing articles 2, 3, 8, 9 and 14, she applied for a declaration from the court that her husband would not be prosecuted if he assisted her suicide. In losing the case, the court ruled that, for example, Article 2 (The right to life) did not include the right to die.

This contrasts with the case of Miss B, a 43-year-old former social care professional who was quadriplegic and required artificial ventilation to live. She asked that her ventilation be discontinued in the knowledge that she would die. As an adult with capacity it was ruled that she could insist that treatment be stopped by withdrawing her consent. After a move to another hospital, ventilation was withdrawn and Miss B died. Subsequent debate about the cases of Miss B and Mrs Pretty argued that both women wished to determine their own fate and control their lives, but the differences in outcome did not reflect a moral difference (Singer 2002). Because Miss B required medical treatment to keep her alive and could refuse it, she could exercise her rights. Mrs Pretty could not because she needed assistance to exercise her rights and did not need immediate medical treatment that could be refused and thus withdrawn (McHale and Gallagher 2003).

BOX 4.2 Articles of the European Convention on Human Rights (ECHR)

Schedule 1 of the Human Rights Act 1998

Article 2 Right to life
Article 3 Prohibition of torture
Article 4 Prohibition of slavery
Article 5 Right to liberty and security
Article 6 Right to a fair trial
Article 7 No punishment without law
Article 8 Right to respect for private and family life
Article 9 Freedom of thought, conscience and religion
Article 10 Freedom of expression
Article 11 Freedom of assembly and association
Article 12 Right to marry
Article 14 Prohibition of discrimination
Article 16 Restrictions upon political activity of aliens
Article 17 Prohibition of abuse of rights
Article 18 Limitation on use of restrictions on rights.

PART 3: EXPLORING THE LAW

Registered nurses are accountable in law for their actions and omissions. Student nurses are also accountable, though there has in the past been a misunderstanding that a student is immune in some way from the responsibility associated with mistakes or errors that amount to negligence or recklessness in practice. It is a matter of fact that nurses (student or registered) are accountable in full for all of the things for which they are responsible. The key for all nurses is to work out what they are responsible for. Where there is shared responsibility, each nurse is 100 per cent accountable for their part.

Case 4.2

Mrs Jones, a thin emaciated woman, was admitted to a medical ward one evening. She was considered to be at risk of developing a pressure sore, and an assessment showed that she should be moved to a special pressure-relieving mattress. The special mattress came to the ward at midnight, but Alice, the nurse in charge, decided not to transfer her because she feared that she would wake the other patients. The staff were very busy that night and Mrs Jones did not get turned. In the morning she was turned and it was discovered that a pressure ulcer had formed. She was transferred to the pressure-relieving mattress but the pressure ulcer became infected: it took a long time to heal and caused considerable pain and discomfort. After she finally went home, Mrs Jones sued the hospital for negligence, claiming that she should have been transferred to the special bed when it arrived on the ward.

103

Accountability under the law can generally be considered as being under the criminal or civil law.

Criminal

Health care staff are rarely charged with criminal offences as a result of their clinical practice, but due to the nature and effect of their practice they might become involved in cases of murder, manslaughter or assault. Criminal law can be seen as a set of rules issued on behalf of the state. These rules act as a deterrent to people who are aware that they will be punished for breaking these rules. It is extremely unlikely that any of the nurses in the scenario will face criminal charges, unless the patient died and it is considered that they intentionally attempted to harm the patient or their acts were grossly reckless.

Civil

Civil law allows individuals redress or remedy against each other when legal rights of the individual have been, or are considered likely to have been, affected. The successful outcome to civil litigation is a court order requiring or preventing an action (an injunction) or an award of money (damages). In clinical negligence claims against a nurse, a patient will seek monetary compensation for any loss suffered. The court's findings will have mainly financial implications, but liability in court can damage a nurse's professional reputation, and their employer and professional body will also be interested in what the courts decide when considering disciplinary or professional action against the nurse.

Clinical negligence

In 2014 The NHS Litigation Authority stated that it had made provision for nearly £25.6 billion for future compensation claims against the NHS. This is a record high. The number of negligence claims rose to 11,495. In 2013, £1.2 billion was paid in damages. The NHS in England in 2013 published figures of more than 300 patients dying each month from medical errors. The National Patient Safety Agency (now part of the NHS Commissioning Board Special Health Authority) publishes figures regarding incidents reported to it. These figures are available on their website (Dimond 2015, p. 45).

Clinical negligence is claimed when a patient is dissatisfied by the care received. When people say that they are 'going to sue' it is likely that they will be taking civil action alleging negligence and seeking damages. For a claim of negligence to succeed the following must be demonstrated:

- There must be a duty of care.
- There is a breach in the duty of care (that is the care is substandard).
- Harm has resulted.

Each of these criteria will be explored in turn in relation to the case involving Mrs Jones in Case 4.2

There must be a duty of care

The claimant must demonstrate that there is a duty of care owed to them personally. In the NHS there will be little difficulty in establishing the duty owed by the hospital to the patients admitted to it (Brazier and Cave 2011). It is more complex in private medicine, where the duty is part of a contract. As far as treatment out of hospital is concerned, there are as yet no laws in the UK that require a nurse to go to someone's aid, unless the victim has an existing professional relationship with the nurse or the nurse caused the situation that resulted in injury. Apart from these circumstances, if harm results from failure to assist a bystander, there can be no negligence because there is no duty of care. If a nurse does go to a bystander's assistance then a duty is accepted, and a claim of negligence is possible. If this seems to discourage nurses from assisting bystanders in peril of their health, it should be remembered that the NMC regard this as a professional if not a legal duty and so a nurse declining assistance unreasonably may find herself professionally accountable (NMC 2015, clause 15).

Case 4.2 (continued)

There clearly is a duty of care owed to Mrs Jones as she is a patient in an NHS hospital being cared for by nurses employed by the NHS.

There is a breach in the duty of care

In order to be successful in a claim of negligence, the care must be substandard in some way. In some cases the fact that the care has been substandard is obvious from the facts, for example, where a swab has been left inside a patient, or where a patient has been given the wrong tablets. This is known as *res ipsa loquitor* (the thing speaks for itself). In many cases there is room to believe that the care was not substandard, or that it was the best that could be done under the circumstances. In these cases the judge will come to a view about whether or not the care breached the duty. If it did not, the case fails. If it did the case at least has a chance of success. Most judges have limited medical and nursing experience, and cannot decide using their own knowledge. So there are legal tests applied, and in applying these, the views of other practitioners are sought. Essentially, there is a process whereby nurses are judged against the actions and standards of their peers. Any legal investigation will seek to compare the facts against what is currently considered adequate practice and from this make a judgement regarding responsibility and blame where there is substandard care.

The Bolam Test is used to determine whether what was done in the circumstances was acceptable and reasonable. Mr Bolam was receiving electroconvulsive therapy (ECT) and there were, in the 1950s, two 'schools of thought' about how patients should be managed and treated during the procedure. One method recommended that relaxant drugs should be used and the other that they should not as there is a risk of fractures to the patient during the treatment. The claimant (Mr Bolam), was not warned of the risk of fractures, had not been given the relaxant drugs, and had not been restrained to pre-vent injury. He suffered a fractured hip and he alleged negligence. In directing the jury (at that time these cases were heard before juries), the judge said that:

A doctor is not guilty of negligence if he has acted in accordance with a practice accepted as proper by a responsible body of medical men skilled in that particular act . . . Putting it the other way round, a doctor is not negligent, if he is acting in accordance with such a practice, merely because there is a body of opinion that takes a contrary view.

Bolam v Friern Hospital Management Committee [1957] 2 All ER 118

Though this case concerned doctors, the same test of comparing a practice claimed to be a breach in the duty of care to practice accepted by a group of practitioners can be applied to nurses and other health care professionals. It has been argued that in the years after the Bolam case was decided in favour of the doctors, the test was used to allow 'judgement by colleagues to substitute for judgement by the courts' (Brazier and Miola 2000, p. 89), forming part of a general deference to doctors by the courts.

The House of Lords has modified or developed understandings of Bolam in the case of Bolitho [1997]. Cases subsequent to *Bolam* used different adjectives to describe the 'body of medical opinion', such as 'responsible', 'reasonable' and 'respectable'. A case in 1997 (though the events took place in 1984) clarified the test. Patrick Bolitho, aged 2, was admitted to hospital suffering from respiratory difficulty. He had a collapse, followed by respiratory arrest and subsequently died. The defendant, the paediatric registrar, was summoned but failed to attend the emergency, and admitted that this was a breach of duty. However, negligence was denied on the grounds that even if she had attended she would not have intubated Patrick, and this was required to prevent the subsequent disastrous respiratory arrest. Expert witnesses gave evidence to support both intubation and non-intubation before the collapse, and since a responsible body of medical opinion agreed that she should not have intubated (even if she had attended), then her absence could not have caused the death. So the case failed on lack of causation. On appeal to the House of Lords, their Lordships found that the court does not have to find for the doctor if a responsible body of opinion supports the practice questioned: 'the court has to be satisfied that the exponents of the body of opinion relied upon can demonstrate that such opinion has a logical basis'.

Case 4.2 (continued)

In the case of Mrs Jones the question would be whether failure to transfer her to a special bed was a breach of duty. Staff Nurse Smith had decided against because she did not want to disturb Mrs Jones or the rest of the patients. Perhaps witnesses would be called to agree or disagree with this course of action, and the precise details would be very important. It could have been reasonable not to transfer her to the bed if she was turned regularly. Perhaps she was turned regularly, but does the documentation or other evidence support this? Any deviation from normal practice in exceptional circumstances needs to be justified and documented.

Harm has occurred

It is possible that both of the other conditions required for a successful claim for negligence are satisfied, without harm having occurred. So in the case of Mrs Smith, if the nursing staff had acted appallingly by not moving the patient onto the bed because they could not be bothered, but no harm occurred, the case will not succeed and no damages are payable. This does not mean that they would not be held to account in other ways, by their employer and/or professional body. In other cases, mainly for reasons of bad luck, severe harm has been caused. There is a principle within law of 'thin skull', illustrated by the case of *Smith v Leech Brain & Co. Ltd*, in which a worker was splashed on the lip with molten metal and eventually died. The company admitted liability for the original accident but denied that they were to blame for the unfortunate death from cancer of the victim. The judge in the case ruled that the test in this case was not whether it is foreseeable that the victim would be harmed and that he would die, it was whether the original event was foreseeable. What happens to the victim after this was directly related to the 'constitution of the victim'. The widow was able to win damages. Nurses should be aware that even though they could not see or reasonably predict that serious harm would occur they would be expected to see that their act or omission would cause the initial event (Dimond 2015). Even if the infection in the pressure ulcer was not foreseeable, the fact that a pressure ulcer could form probably was.

The harm has to be reasonably foreseeable. A reasonable person is not expected to predict unknown risks. Unforeseeable risks cannot be anticipated and failing to protect against them would not be negligent. In *Roe v Minister of Health* [1954] the claimant (patient) suffered pain and permanent paralysis from the waist down, after being injected with a spinal anaesthesia (nupercaine). This nupercaine had been stored in glass ampoules, which had been placed in a phenol solution, a disinfectant. Evidence was produced at the trial that minute and invisible cracks had formed in the glass ampoules, allowing some of the nupercaine to be contaminated by the phenol, which then damaged the patient. It was accepted at the trial that such an occurrence was reasonably unforeseeable and that such a phenomenon had not previously been detected or anticipated. It could not therefore be guarded against and so the defendants escaped liability for negligence. However, the law would expect the health care system to learn from these mistakes and if a similar event were to occur it could be seen as negligence as it should have been anticipated. Safe systems of work need to be introduced so that incidents like this can be reported and disseminated.

Vicarious liability is when one person, or organisation, is liable for the negligent acts of another person.

Case 4.2 (continued)

In the case of Mrs Jones, the question would be whether the failure to put her on the bed caused the pressure ulcer. If her position had been changed regularly throughout the night, it may be difficult to demonstrate causation; perhaps the damage had already been done, and transferring her to the special bed would not have made any difference. To succeed in the case, Mrs Jones would have to show that she should have been transferred, *and* that the failure to transfer caused the pressure ulcer. If she can do this, on the balance of probabilities, she could win the case and be awarded damages.

Damages

Legal action can be very expensive, especially if a decision is appealed to a higher court, and damages can be substantial. Nurses are required by the NMC to have professional indemnity insurance (NMC 2015, clause 12) and this is offered by trade unions and professional bodies. Previously the possibility of having to bear costs may have deterred potential litigants, but in recent years many firms of solicitors have operated a 'no win, no fee' system whereby solicitors' costs are payable only if the case is settled, removing risk but reducing payout, and having at least the potential to increase the numbers of litigants. In some cases claimants can also sue the employer through **vicarious liability**, and so the costs are against the NHS, rather than to individual nurses or their insurers. Vicarious liability arises if certain criteria are satisfied, and if the negligent act occurred during the course of employment. Generally it would be in the interests of the claimant to pursue vicarious liability as, despite their tight financial position, NHS Trusts are better placed to settle claims than individuals.

Employment

As an employee, a nurse has a duty to her employer to obey reasonable and lawful instructions and to take all reasonable care and skill in carrying out duties. This principle is based upon the view of courts, unless proven otherwise, that implied terms exist (conditions or terms that exist even though not explicitly written or discussed) in a contract of employment. Indeed, a job description only reflects a small proportion of duties and responsibilities of the employee; the fine details are implied and relate to the area of practice. It would be impossible to list all duties of an employee and that there is a need for flexibility. This does not, however, give the employer the right to vary terms of employment without consultation.

A nurse will be held personally liable by their employer and subject to disciplinary action, if they fail to take care or fall below a reasonable standard of practice while giving care. Under these circumstances the employer has a right to intervene. In fact they might consider this a duty to protect both the public and the nurse. This intervention can range from verbal or written warning through to suspension, compulsory re-training, demotion or possibly dismissal.

CONCLUSION

Nurses' practice has always been governed and supported by law. In a sense this is self-evident as all citizens are required to follow the law, and are at risk of censure and punishment if it is broken. The standards of proficiency for pre-registration nursing education require that nurses have knowledge of the relevant legislation, and this requirement has been incorporated explicitly in the latest version of *The Code* (NMC 2015, clause 4.3), which refers to the legislation concerning mental capacity. This chapter has given details about some of the important areas

of legislation, notably concerning consent to treatment, an area of law that governs practice every time a nurse touches a patient. A common theme running through the chapter is that codified law cannot tell a nurse what to do in every situation, and in this regard at least, legal accountability has similarities to professional accountability. *The Code* makes it very clear on a number of occasions that the law must be followed in the country in which the nurse is practising, and to do this the nurse must know what that lawful practice requires, and also know the processes that are followed when actions or omissions are challenged. This challenge is the basis of accountability, both legal and professional. Nurses must be able to defend their actions and omissions, and while both legal and professional redress are rarer than many people seem to think, the habit of defending actions to others, to peers, colleagues, in supervision and in audit can only advance practice. As long as a nurse follows the law where it is clear and can defend reasonable actions where it is not, they have nothing to fear from the law.

BOX 4.3 Cases referred to in the text

These cases are in England unless specifically mentioned otherwise. Other jurisdictions such as Canada and Australia can be quoted in English legal judgments. The numbers and letters refer to where the cases are reported. For example, the case of *Bolam v Friern Hospital Management Committee* is reported in volume 2 of the 1957 editions of the *All England Law Report* starting at page 118. These references can be used to access a full report of the case, including full judgments, via legal databases.

- *Allan v New Mount Sinai Hospital* [1980] 109 DLR (3d) 634 (Canadian High Court)
- *Bolam v Friern Hospital Management Committee* [1957] 2 All ER 118
- *Bolitho v City and Hackney Health Authority* [1998] AC 232
- *Gillick v West Norfolk and Wisbech AHA and DHSS* [1985] 3 All ER 402
- *Montgomery v Lanarkshire Health Board* [2015] UKSC 11.
- *Pearce v United Bristol Healthcare Trust* [1991] PIQRP 53
- *Pretty v United Kingdom* [2002] (Application 2346/02) European Court of Human Rights
- *Re C (An Adult: refusal of medical treatment)* [1994] 1 All ER 819, (1993) 15 BMLR 77
- *Re E (A Minor) (Wardship: Medical treatment)* [1993] 1 FLR 386
- *Re S (An Adult: refusal of medical treatment)* [1992] 4 All ER 671
- *Re T (An Adult: refusal of medical treatment)* [1992] 4 All ER 649
- *Roe v Minister of Health* [1954] 2 QB 66
- *Rogers v Whitaker* [1992] 67 ALJR 47 (Australian High Court)
- *Smith v Leech Brain & Co. Ltd*; QBD [1961] All ER 1159

SUGGESTED FURTHER READING

There are a number of textbooks covering health care law in general and the law as it affects nurses in particular.

Brazier, M. and Cave, E. (2011) *Medicine, Patients and the Law* (5th edn), London: Penguin.
Dimond, B. (2015) *Legal Aspects of Nursing* (7th edn), London: Pearson.
Mason, J. K. and McCall Smith, A. (2005) *Mason and McCall Smith's Law and Medical Ethics*, Oxford, New York: Oxford University Press.

Journals

Journal of Health Politics, Policy and Law
Medical Law Review
Medical Law Reports
Medical Law Monitor

Richard Thomas and Paul Snelling

Websites

Websites of reputable origin are valuable resources and free. Websites of charities often offer legal resources in their particular field. The value of 'official' websites should not be underestimated, for example, a wide range of resources about the Mental Capacity Act and the Human Rights Act can be found on government websites at the Department of Health and Ministry of Justice, respectively.

REFERENCES

Age UK (2015) Advance decisions, advance statements and living wills. www.ageuk.org.uk/documents/en-gb/factsheets/fs72_advance_decisions_advance_statements_and_living_wills_fcs.pdf?dtrk=true (accessed 18 December 2015).

Akkad, A., Jackson, C., Kenyon, S., Dixon-Woods, M., Taub, N. and Habiba, M. (2004) Informed consent for elective and emergency surgery: questionnaire study. *British Journal of Obstetrics and Gynaecology* **111** (10), 1133–1138.

Alzheimer's Society (n.d.) Advance decisions and advance statements. www.alzheimers.org.uk/site/scripts/download_info.php?fileID=2659 (accessed 18 December 2015).

Aveyard, H. (2002), Implied consent prior to nursing care procedures. *Journal of Advanced Nursing* **39** (2), 201–207.

Beech, M. (2007) Confidentiality in health care: conflicting legal and ethical principles. *Nursing Standard* **21** (21), 42–46.

Brazier, M. and Miola, J. (2000) Bye-bye Bolam: a medical litigation revolution? *Medical Law Review* **8** (1), 85–114.

Brazier, M. and Cave, E. (2011) *Medicine, Patients and the Law* (5th edn). London: Penguin.

Criminal Justice and Courts Act (2015) Sections 20–25. www.legislation.gov.uk/ukpga/2015/2/contents/enacted (accessed 18 December 2015).

DH (Department of Health) (2001) *Seeking Consent: Working with children*. London: DH. http://webarchive.nationalarchives.gov.uk/20130107105354/http:/www.dh.gov.uk/prod_consum_dh/groups/dh_digitalassets/@dh/@en/documents/digitalasset/dh_4067204.pdf (accessed 18 December 2015).

DH (2003) *Confidentiality: NHS code of practice*. London: DH. www.gov.uk/government/uploads/system/uploads/attachment_data/file/200146/Confidentiality_-_NHS_Code_of_Practice.pdf (accessed 18 December 2015).

DH (2009) *Reference Guide to Consent for Examination or Treatment* (2nd edn). London: DH. www.gov.uk/government/uploads/system/uploads/attachment_data/file/138296/dh_103653__1_.pdf (accessed 18 December 2015).

DH (2015) *Mental Health Act – Code of Practice: Revised edition*. London: DH. www.gov.uk/government/uploads/system/uploads/attachment_data/file/435512/MHA_Code_of_Practice.PDF (accessed 18 December 2015).

Dimond, B. (2004) A patient is told that he is HIV positive and he asks for this to be kept a secret from his wife: what should you do? *Nursing Times* **100** (45), 18.

Dimond, B. (2015) *Legal Aspects of Nursing* (7th edn). Harlow: Pearson.

Evans, K., Warner, J. and Jackson, E. (2007) How much do emergency workers know about capacity and consent? *Emergency Medicine Journal* **24** (6), 391–393.

General Medical Council (GMC) (2009) Confidentiality: disclosing information about serious communicable diseases. London: General Medical Council. www.gmc-uk.org/Confidentiality_disclosing_info_serious_commun_diseases_2009.pdf_27493404.pdf (accessed 18 December 2015).

Griffith R. (2013) Extending the scope of wilful neglect will result in paternalistic nursing care. *British Journal of Nursing* **22** (20), 1190–1191.

Griffith, R. (2015a). Duty to warn of risks moves to a prudent patient approach. *British Journal of Nursing* **24** (7), 408–409.

Griffith R. (2015b) Patient protection: ill-treatment and wilful neglect. *British Journal of Nursing* **24** (11), 600–601.

Griffith, R. and Tengnah, C. (2008) *Law and Professional Issues in Nursing.* Exeter, UK: Learning Matters.

Henderson, S. (2003) Power imbalances between nurses and patients: a potential inhibitor of partnership in care. *Journal of Clinical Nursing* **12** (4), 501–508.

Houlihan, G. D. (2005) The powers and duties of psychiatric nurses under the Mental Health Act 1983: a review of the statutory provisions in England and Wales. *Journal of Psychiatric and Mental Health Nursing* **12** (3), 317–324.

Kinnersley, P., Phillips, K., Savage, K., Kelly, M. J., Farrell, E., Morgan, B., Whistance, R., Lewis, V., Mann, M. K., Stephens, B. L. and Blazeby, J. (2013) Interventions to promote informed consent for patients undergoing surgical and other invasive health care procedures. *The Cochrane Library* **7**, CD009445.

Lamont, S., Jeon, Y. H. and Chiarella, M. (2013) Health-care professionals' knowledge, attitudes and behaviours relating to patient capacity to consent to treatment: an integrative review. *Nursing Ethics* **20** (6), 684–707.

Lawn, A. and Bassi, D. (2008) An unusual resuscitation request. *Resuscitation* **78** (1), 5–6.

McGeehan, R. (2007) Best practice in record keeping. *Nursing Standard* **21** (17), 51–55.

McHale, J. and Gallagher, A. (2003) *Nursing and Human Rights.* London: Butterworth Heinemann.

McHale, J., Gallagher, A. and Mason, I. (2001) The UK Human Rights Act 1998: implications for nurses. *Nursing Ethics* **8** (3), 223–233.

McInroy, A. (2005) Blood transfusion and Jehovah's Witnesses: the legal and ethical issues. *British Journal of Nursing* **14** (5), 270–274.

Ministry of Justice (2007) *Mental Capacity Act Code of Practice.* London: The Stationery Office. www.gov.uk/government/uploads/system/uploads/attachment_data/file/224660/Mental_Capacity_Act_code_of_practice.pdf (accessed 18 December 2015).

NMC (2015) *The Code: Standards of conduct, performance and ethics for nurses and midwives.* London: Nursing and Midwifery Council. www.nmc.org.uk/standards/code/ (accessed 18 December 2015).

Office of the Public Guardian (2007) *Making Decisions: A guide for people who work in health and social care* (3rd edn). www.gov.uk/government/publications/health-and-social-care-workers-mental-capacity-act-decisions (accessed 18 December 2015).

Oxford English Dictionary (2008) http://dictionary.oed.com/entrance.dtl (accessed 18 December 2015).

Parekh, S. A. (2006) Child consent and the law: an insight and discussion into the law relating to consent and competence. *Child Care, Health and Development* **33** (1), 78–82.

Prideaux, A. (2011) Issues in nursing documentation and record-keeping practice. *British Journal of Nursing,* **20** (22), 1450–1454.

Singer, P. (2002) Ms B and Diane Pretty: a commentary. *Journal of Medical Ethics* **28** (4), 234–235.

Snelling, P. C. (2015) Can the revised UK code direct practice? *Nursing Ethics.* Published online before print November 30, 2015, doi: 10.1177/0969733015610802

Woolley, S. (2005) Children of Jehovah's Witnesses and adolescent Jehovah's Witnesses: what are their rights? *Archives of Disease in Childhood* **90** (7), 715–719.

5

HEALTH POLICY

Iain Snelling

LEARNING OUTCOMES

After reading and reflecting on this chapter, you should be able to:

- discuss the way in which health care policy is made and implemented;
- outline the way in which health care policy influences the management of health care services;
- discuss the relevance of health care policy to nursing practice;
- explain how you are able to update your knowledge and understanding.

INTRODUCTION

The establishment and maintenance of the National Health Service (NHS) is rightly considered one of the major achievements of our nation and the intensity of political debate about the NHS and its future direction is clear evidence of its importance. The NHS is the largest employer in Europe, employing approximately 1.3 million people. Health policy is more than *just* political policy about *just* the NHS. However, NHS spending accounts for the vast majority of all spending on health care, and the way that the NHS is funded and managed are primarily political questions. The chapter is divided into three parts.

In Part 1, health policy is outlined, the concept of health policy is introduced, and the role of politicians in running the NHS is discussed.

In Part 2, the current reforms of the NHS are placed in a historical context. Details about structures of the NHS and how these facilitate reform are explained along with how these put the patient at the centre of the NHS.

In Part 3, the role of research in evaluating and influencing health policy is explored.

PART 1: OUTLINING HEALTH POLICY

Case 5.1

Brian, a recently qualified staff nurse, attended a ward meeting today. The Director of Nursing came to talk about the hospital's finances, which need to be improved. Lengths of stay were too high, and joint working with community services and general practitioners could be improved. Some work might be moved out of the hospital. The hospital also had to reduce infections, and make people want to have their treatment there, because otherwise they might go somewhere else. Brian had to leave before the end because there weren't enough nurses on the ward. Brian's colleagues think that they should understand what is driving all these changes so that they can decide how to develop their careers and help to improve services. Brian is not sure that they shouldn't just try to keep things as they are, and try to get a few more staff. Everyone seemed very concerned that the Care Quality Commission are coming next month for an inspection.

What is health policy and how is it made?

Right at the start of this chapter we should emphasise that our discussion is about England, not the UK as a whole. Health policy for Scotland, Wales and Northern Ireland is made in those nations, and devolution within England is also a developing theme, which we will return to.

Health policy is the statement of priorities relating to health issues and the broad means through which these priorities will be addressed. It is determined by the Government, principally through the Department of Health (DH) in England, although as far as the availability of resources is concerned, the Treasury will have the major influence.

Government policy is made by ministers who are appointed by the Prime Minister. The senior minister at the DH is the Secretary of State for Health. He or she is a member of the Cabinet, which is the highest decision-making body in government, chaired by the Prime Minister, who also appoints all of its members. There are also five junior ministers in the DH. Ministers of State are a higher rank than Parliamentary Under Secretaries. In January 2016 the junior ministerial posts were:

- Minister of State for Community and Social Care;
- Parliamentary Under Secretary of State for Care Quality;
- Parliamentary Under Secretary of State for Public Health;
- Parliamentary Under Secretary of State for Life Sciences;
- Parliamentary Under Secretary of State for NHS Productivity.

Each minister has a specific portfolio of responsibilities, detailed on the DH website. Ministers have a range of duties but their primary purpose is to be accountable to Parliament for the work of the department. Ministers are Members of Parliament either of the House of Commons (hence the initials MP) to which they will have been elected, or the House of Lords. One member of the ministerial team will be a member of the House of Lords representing the whole department there. Accountability means having the responsibility to explain (account for) policies and their implementation, usually through oral and written questions. Where health policy requires a change in the law, ministers present legislation to parliament. Increasingly, accountability has a more public face, with ministers being interviewed through the media to explain policies directly to the population.

Activity 5.1

Find out from the Department of Health website who the current health ministers are, and what their duties are.

Each government department has a Permanent Secretary, the highest civil servant in the department, who advises the Secretary of State, and is responsible for the management of the department. There is a clear division in government between making policy, which is the responsibility of ministers, and for carrying it out, which is the responsibility of the civil service. Civil servants remain accountable to the Cabinet Secretary – the head of the civil service – rather than ministers in their own department.

The DH has a Permanent Secretary but it also has a Chief Executive of the NHS who has equal status, reflecting the importance of the NHS in carrying out health policy. The body accountable for the running of the NHS in England is NHS England, which is separate from the DH. The Chief Nursing Officer is a Board member of NHS England.

Although a definition of policy has been given, and a distinction made between policy-making and implementation, in reality things are more complex. Ham notes that 'although many writers have attempted to define policy, there is little agreement on the meaning of the word' (Ham 2009, p. 131). He makes five points about the study of policy:

1   *Policy includes both decisions and actions.* We can study formal decisions, and the process through which the decisions were made, but 'what happens in practice may be different from what was intended by decision makers' (Ham 2009, p. 132). Understanding how policy is implemented is as important as understanding the policy itself.
2   *Policy may not be expressed as a single decision, but as a series of decisions taken by different groups of people.* A policy may not have a single clear definition: 'It tends to be defined in terms of a series of decisions which, taken together, comprise a more or less common understanding of what the policy is' (Ham 2009, p. 132).
3   *Policy changes evolve over time in a dynamic process rather than a series of discrete steps.* An explanation of current policy can be given in terms of how it has evolved through a number of developments, each drawing from the experience of what has gone before. Some of these developments represent discrete changes, while others may involve changes in the pace or style of implementation.
4   Studying how policy is made can ignore the role of maintaining the status quo: 'non decision-making', the political process of resisting change. This may be particularly important when policy is developing quickly, raising the importance of opposition, in terms of both the formal process of decision-making and its implementation. For example, in 2001 Dr Richard Taylor, a retired consultant physician, was elected as an independent MP after a local campaign to downgrade the facilities at Kidderminster Hospital. He was re-elected in 2005 but lost his seat in 2010. This

highlights the significance of processes designed to stop change rather than promote it.

5   *Finally, policy 'can be seen as actions without decisions'* (Ham 2009, p. 132). We normally think of policy as 'top-down' from the Government to those who implement it. Policy can also be made 'bottom-up', where the actions of those who deliver services or who lead them, can be said to have made policy.

So, although health policy is at one level a reasonably clear concept, there are complications. It is not as simple as deciding what to do, and then deciding how it should be done. It is a complex evolving process, involving many individuals and groups. Ministers have overall responsibility but do not simply impose decisions. Many reasons for a particular policy reflect wider changes in society, such as the development of improved information and communication technology, changes in the law (including European law), and the development of consumerism. Learning about health policy is not just about learning what it is; it requires developing understanding of the wider context of health care provision and how it will affect you, your career and your patients.

Health policy and health and social care policy

The title of this chapter is 'Health policy'. The learning outcomes relate to 'health care policy'. Health policy, which is concerned with all matters relating to health, is wider than health care policy, which relates to the health care system, how it is financed and delivered. This focus on health care reduces the emphasis on social care, which has a major effect on health care and on patients and service users. In England, social care is not publicly funded for everyone. It is means tested and funded by local authorities for those who meet strict eligibility criteria operated locally, so access varies across the country. For many patients, especially those with complex needs, the way that health services and social care

---

POLICY FOCUS 5.1

Official government policy documents

A White Paper is a formal statement of government policy, published 'by command of Her Majesty'. The author of a White Paper is a government minister, who presents it to parliament, hence the author reference is the relevant minister and a command number is included. For example:

> Secretary of State for Health (2010) *Equity and Excellence: Liberating the NHS* Cm 7881. London: The Stationery Office.

In many cases, a White Paper requires legislation before its provisions can be implemented. White Papers are published by the Stationery Office, and can be downloaded free of charge from the DH, although hard copies can only be purchased. These documents tend to be long, but usually have an executive summary.

The DH publishes many significant policy papers. For these the author is usually the Department itself. These papers do not require legislation; they usually explain the implementation of policy. These papers can also be downloaded free of charge. An example is: DH (2015) *Delivering the Forward View: NHS Planning guidance 2016/17–2020/21.*

---

services work together is crucial. The interface between health and social care often has a high profile when patients cannot be discharged from hospital because social care packages are not ready, but this is not the only issue. In many cases hospital admission may have been avoided in the first place if social care had been better integrated with primary care (Purdy 2010). Recent reductions in social care are likely to have an effect on NHS usage, but this is difficult to demonstrate and quantify (Ismail *et al.* 2014).

The NHS is the main vehicle through which health care policy is implemented. Over the past 25 years or so the NHS has gone through significant changes, many of them controversial. A key reference document for understanding current policy and future direction is the White Paper published in June 2008 close to the sixtieth anniversary of the founding of the NHS on 5 July 1948. *High Quality Care for All* (Secretary of State for Health 2008) is often referred to as the Darzi review, since the work of detailed planning and consultation that preceded it was led by Lord Darzi, a Minister for Health who is also an eminent NHS surgeon. *High Quality Care for All* made the case for a written constitution for the NHS.

> The NHS must continue to change. But the fundamental purpose and values of the NHS can and must remain constant. Setting this out clearly, along with the rights and responsibilities of patients, the public and staff, will give us all greater confidence to meet the challenges of the future on the basis of a shared understanding and common purpose.
>
> (Secretary of State for Health 2008, p. 77)

A draft constitution was published with the Darzi Review, and after consultation *The NHS Constitution for England* was published in January 2009. A revised version was published in 2015. It has seven key principles that 'guide the NHS in all it does' (DH 2015a, p. 3). The principles are given in Policy focus 5.2. The principles reflect the aims of policy for the NHS, written in various documents over a number of years, but *The NHS Constitution* clarifies them, giving them an enhanced practical status.

POLICY FOCUS 5.2

The NHS Constitution: principles that guide the NHS

- The NHS provides a comprehensive service, available to all . . . (and) it has a wider social duty to promote equality through the services it provides . . .
- Access to NHS services is based on clinical need, not an individual's ability to pay.
- The NHS aspires to the highest standards of excellence and professionalism.
- The patient will be at the heart of everything the NHS does.
- The NHS works across organisational boundaries and in partnership with other organisations in the interest of patients, local communities and the wider population.
- The NHS is committed to providing best value for taxpayers' money and the most effective, fair and sustainable use of finite resources.
- The NHS is accountable to the public, communities, and patients that it serves.

(DH 2015, pp. 3–4)

Activity 5.2

In small groups discuss these principles, and consider the extent to which you think the NHS meets them, illustrating your discussion with examples from your nursing practice.

PART 2: EXPLAINING HEALTH POLICY

The Triple Aim

The framework used to consider health policy in this chapter is the *Triple Aim* (Berwick *et al.* 2008). These goals were suggested for the American health care system in 2008, as a system of 'linked goals . . . improving the individual experience of care; improving the health of populations; and reducing the per capita cost for populations' (Berwick *et al.* 2008, p. 760). These goals are not independent. Pursuing the Triple Aim requires balance, as improving performance on one of the goals may affect one or other of the other ones. In particular, quality and cost are often seen in competition, that increasing the quality of care will also increase the cost. That relationship may not always be true. There are situations where poor quality increases cost, such as with the costs incurred in treating hospital acquired infections. If quality is improved by reducing hospital acquired infections it is likely that this would also lead to reduced costs.

The Commonwealth Fund (Davis *et al.* 2014) has produced international rankings, based on indicators taken from the three elements of the Triple Aim. The summary shown in Figure 5.1 is taken from their report, which shows that the UK system ranked first in the 2014 rankings.

The one area where the UK was not highest ranked or in the top three was healthy lives, where three indicators were considered: mortality amenable to health care, infant mortality, and healthy life expectancy at age 60. Population health will depend on a range of factors other than the health care system, such as lifestyle, income, a range of public services and genetic differences between populations, although the health care system and health policy in general have significant roles. Public health is considered in more detail in Chapter 15. The measure of equity, in which the UK is ranked third, refers to the way that health care services are accessible to the population, and particularly whether there are differences between those earning above average income and those earning below average income.

There is no indicator in this table for inequalities in health outcomes – the extent to which health outcomes are distributed among the population. The issue most often considered is socio-economic group; there are significant differences in health outcomes between richer and poorer people. Health inequalities, discussed in Chapter 10, are also seen between ethnic groups. This chapter will be concerned mainly with the cost and quality elements of the Triple Aim.

Before considering quality and cost in turn a very brief history of the NHS will provide some context and consider the way in which policy evolves and develops over time. It is often difficult to appreciate current policy without some historical perspective, particularly relating to recent history. A brief explanation of the structure of the NHS is

COUNTRY RANKINGS

Top 2*
Middle
Bottom 2*

	AUS	CAN	FRA	GER	NETH	NZ	NOR	SWE	SWIZ	UK	US
OVERALL RANKING (2013)	4	10	9	5	5	7	7	3	2	1	11
Quality Care	2	9	8	7	5	4	11	10	3	1	5
Effective Care	4	7	9	6	5	2	11	10	8	1	3
Safe Care	3	10	2	6	7	9	11	5	4	1	7
Coordinated Care	4	8	9	10	5	2	7	11	3	1	6
Patient-Centered Care	5	8	10	7	3	6	11	9	2	1	4
Access	8	9	11	2	4	7	6	4	2	1	9
Cost-Related Problem	9	5	10	4	8	6	3	1	7	1	11
Timeliness of Care	6	11	10	4	2	7	8	9	1	3	5
Efficiency	4	10	8	9	7	3	4	2	6	1	11
Equity	5	9	7	4	8	10	6	1	2	2	11
Healthy Lives	4	8	1	7	5	9	6	2	3	10	11
Health Expenditures/Capita, 2011**	$3,800	$4,522	$4,118	$4,495	$5,099	$3,182	$5,669	$3,925	$5,643	$3,405	$8,508

Notes: * Includes ties. ** Expenditures shown in $US PPP (purchasing power parity); Australian $ data are from 2010.
Source: Calculated by The Commonwealth Fund based on 2011 International Health Policy Survey; 2012 International Health Policy Survey of Sicker Adults; 2013 International Health Policy Survey of Primary Care Physicians; 2013 International Health Policy Survey; Commonwealth Fund National Scorecard 2011; World Health Organization; and Organization for Economic Cooperation and Development, *OECD Health Data, 2013* (Paris: OECD, Nov. 2013).

FIGURE 5.1 Overall ranking of international health care systems

Source: The Commonwealth Fund.

necessary to understand policy, particularly in its implementation. Changing structures and organisations in the NHS is something of a recurring theme in health care policy.

A brief history of the NHS

The NHS was founded in 1948 as part of the welfare state created after World War II. The hospital service including municipal hospitals run by local authorities and voluntary hospitals was nationalised. Their employees, including medical staff, became employees of the state, although the right of consultants to maintain private practice was retained. General practitioners (GPs), on the other hand, remained independent, contracting to provide services for the NHS. This distinction between primary care provided by GPs and secondary and tertiary care in hospitals remains substantially in place today.

Reorganisations of the NHS in 1974 and 1982 changed the management structure but left the essential infrastructure intact. In the late 1980s however, there was a series of service crises. A review was followed by publication in 1989 of a White Paper, *Working for Patients* (Secretary of State for Health 1989), which proposed far-reaching changes, much more radical than previous reorganisations and resulting in an 'explosion of opposition' (Klein 2013, p. 152). At the heart of the proposals was the establishment of an internal market, establishing what was known as the purchaser–provider split. The internal market introduced the policy of competition between health care providers for contracts for services that purchasers (mainly District Health Authorities) would manage.

The internal market never really developed into an effective marketplace. In 1990 John Major replaced Margaret Thatcher as Prime Minister and his approach was less radical. The Major Government launched the *Patients' Charter*, part of a wider citizens' charter initiative, which gave explicit rights to patients, such as the first maximum waiting time guarantee. However, the reforms of the early 1990s did establish market principles in the NHS.

Development of the NHS was a key area of the 1997 general election with an apparent choice of market principles on the one hand (Conservatives), against the re-establishment of a national, planned service on the other (Labour). Labour won the election and promised to end the internal market. The Labour Party manifesto promised that 'Our fundamental purpose is simple but hugely important: to restore the NHS as a public service working co-operatively for patients, not a commercial business driven by competition' (New Labour 1997). Since 1997, there have been a number of landmark publications through which the development of health policy can be traced. The first Labour policy statement on the NHS, *The New NHS. Modern. Dependable* (Secretary of State for Health 1997) announced changes, but also retained the basic structure of the NHS. Over the succeeding years of the Labour Government, the internal market was not abolished but strengthened.

The NHS Plan, published in 2000 (Secretary of State for Health 2000), is widely regarded as a key point for the NHS. *The NHS Plan* was the starting point for recent policy because it developed two themes, which were influential for most of the first decade of the twenty-first century, summed up in its subtitle: 'A plan for investment, a plan for reform'. As well as identifying that additional resources were required, *The NHS Plan* expressed the firm view that as far as delivering services was concerned the basic model had not really changed since the 1940s. Services were organised from the perspective of the organisations and professions providing them rather than according to the needs and preferences of the people using them. Inefficient appointment systems, waiting lists, poor

Primary care is given in the community and is something patients themselves choose to access. Primary care is provided and primarily managed by general practitioners.
Secondary care is more specialised, usually based in a local hospital and requiring a referral.
Tertiary care is more specialised still, usually requiring a referral from secondary care, for example, specialised surgical services in a regional centre.

119

communication, frequent visits to large impersonal hospitals, and strictly demarcated professional roles were all features of this view. *The NHS Plan* stated therefore, that the NHS was to be 'redesigned' around the needs and preferences of patients. *The NHS Plan* contained many targets and pledges designed to improve the patient focus of the NHS. The targets that had the highest profile and caused the most difficulty were waiting time targets, which have subsequently been made shorter still. The reforms evolved into new directions not envisaged at the time, such as changes to the organisational structure of the NHS, but every new policy initiative had, as a central aim, improving the patient focus of the NHS, not just through structural changes but more importantly through changing culture. As discussed in Chapter 6, this is a recurring theme, particularly relevant to improving the quality of services after the Francis Reports.

In 2010 in the wake of the financial crisis, the increase in resources that had produced sustained increases in expenditure for the health service stopped, and the difficult financial environment facing the NHS over the foreseeable future became much more important. In 2009 David Nicholson, then the NHS Chief Executive, said that in the period between 2010 and 2015 the NHS would need to make between £15 billion and £20 billion of efficiency savings. This was known as the Nicholson Challenge, or the Quality, Innovation, Productivity and Prevention (QIPP) initiative, which became an umbrella term for a range of national and local schemes (Appleby *et al.* 2014). His argument was that there would be no more big increases in resources available and that additional demands on the service would need to be funded by efficiency savings. This level of efficiency savings, about 4 per cent per year, had never been achieved before. The programme to achieve the savings had three broad elements: 40 per cent from national initiatives including pay restraint; 40 per cent on provider efficiency through reducing each year the value of payments made to NHS providers; and 20 per cent through changes in the way that services are provided.

> [F]or example by providing care closer to home for diabetes or chronic obstructive pulmonary disease (COPD), or by changing the pattern of acute services for major trauma or stroke. These will be the most challenging changes to achieve, requiring joined-up local planning and strong clinical engagement, but changes of this kind are vital to meeting the QIPP challenge.
>
> DH 2011, p. 2

Although the Nicholson Challenge was introduced in 2009 when the Labour Government was still in office it was the coalition Government elected in 2010 that oversaw the development of the NHS after the period of investment following *The NHS Plan*. As well as the financial challenge, there was a second factor that dominated the development of NHS policy as the Government changed in 2010. At Mid-Staffordshire NHS Foundation Trust, appalling standards of care from 2005 had been discovered and subsequent investigations including an inquiry by Robert Francis had highlighted many weaknesses in the system. The Francis Inquiry published its report just before the general election in 2010. One of its recommendations was to hold another inquiry to consider in more depth how the terrible events at Mid-Staffordshire were allowed to happen (Francis 2010). This was made a public inquiry, which has a higher status, and it reported in 2013 (Francis 2013). By then many changes in the system had already been introduced. The period of austerity following the financial crisis and concerns about quality of services provide the context to health policy developments since 2010. These issues reflect both elements of the Triple Aim, which we are concentrating on.

The coalition Government's White Paper, *Equity and Excellence: Liberating the NHS* (Secretary of State for Health 2010) was published in July 2010, just two months after the election result. During the period when the Bill was debated in Parliament, there was an unusual pause while some of the key provisions were debated more fully in the service and the country, in a process known as the Future Forum (Field 2011). In 2012 the Health and Social Care Act came into force. This act is often referred to as 'the Lansley reforms' after the Secretary of State for Health at the time, Andrew Lansley. One reason that the reforms were controversial was that the coalition agreement between the Conservatives and the Liberal Democrats stated that: 'We will stop the top-down reorganisations of the NHS that have got in the way of patient care' (HM Government 2010, p. 24). However, the Health and Social Care Act was widely perceived as such a top-down reorganisation. It made a number of changes in the way that the health and social care system operated. A key theme was that the NHS would become 'liberated' through a much more clinically led service and the key commissioning organisations described below were reorganised with many NHS managers being made redundant in the process. Responsibility for public health was transferred from the NHS to local authorities, and new bodies called Health and Wellbeing Boards, hosted by local authorities, were established to be key local forums where leaders of health and social care would work together to improve the health and well-being of their populations, including tacking health inequalities.

A National Commissioning Board, NHS England, was established. This is the body responsible for overseeing the NHS, and each year it will be given a mandate by the Government setting out its aims and resources. NHS England has established outcomes frameworks that reflect the terms of the mandate and that identify priorities for service, especially relating to quality. At the national level, there is now clear separation between the DH and the NHS, although the Secretary of State still has plenty of scope to intervene in the detailed running of the NHS.

The King's Fund published two reports on the coalition Government's record on the NHS just before the general election in 2015, one on the reforms and the other on NHS performance (Appleby *et al.* 2015, Ham *et al.* 2015). On the NHS reforms, the report was hard-hitting:

> Historians will not be kind in their assessment of the coalition Government's record on NHS reform. The first half of the 2010–2015 Parliament was taken up with debate on the Health and Social Care Bill, the biggest and most far-reaching legislation in the history of the NHS ... The second half of the parliament was devoted to limiting the damage caused by the Bill and dealing with the effects of growing financial and service pressures in the NHS.
>
> (Ham *et al.* 2015, p. 4)

In October 2014 NHS England published a *Five Year Forward View* (NHS England 2014). This paper gave the NHS a renewed commitment to prevention and public health, ensuring patients have greater control in their own care, and removing barriers between organisations and teams in how care is provided. It acknowledged that new models of care are required, but that it wasn't possible to impose a single model across the whole of England. A particular aim was to improve primary and 'out of hospital' care. In 2015, 50 'vanguard' sites were chosen, which were to take the lead in developing new models of care for the NHS. The vanguard sites have access to a transformation fund to support their work. All regions of England are represented in five new care models:

- *Integrated primary and acute care systems* – joining up GP, hospital, community and mental health services.
- *Multispecialty community providers* – moving specialist care out of hospitals into the community.
- *Enhanced health in care homes* – offering older people better, joined-up health, care and rehabilitation services.
- *Urgent and emergency care* – new approaches to improve the coordination of services and reduce pressure on A&E departments.
- *Acute care collaborations* – linking hospitals together to improve their clinical and financial viability.

(NHS England 2015a)

This programme signals a commitment to pilots and evaluations, and locally determined and implemented change, through 'diverse solutions and local leadership' (NHS England 2014, p. 28).

The *Five Year Forward View* also acknowledged that if there was no extra funding for the NHS until 2020/2021, and no efficiency savings, then the extra demands would require another £30 billion per year. This £30 billion figure had a high profile in the general election of 2015. The NHS element of it was set at £22 billion per year to be achieved by efficiency savings, in the order of 2–3 per cent per year, a figure similar to that of the earlier 'Nicholson Challenge'. After the election, fulfilling an election pledge, the Government agreed to find the other £8 billion per year, and subsequently agreed to make £10 billion per year available before 2020, with most of the additional resources coming early to help fund developments (King's Fund 2015). However, in 2015/2016 many NHS organisations experienced financial difficulty, and so it seems that the NHS has started badly in its renewed search for efficiency savings.

In summary, recent years have seen the introduction of market principles, a period of investment and modernisation, and a period of financial challenge all of which were accompanied by significant organisational change.

The structure of the NHS in England

Figure 5.2 is a simplified version of the structure of the NHS in England. A more detailed version is available on NHS Choices' website (NHS Choices 2015). This is the website that gives patients information about the NHS and NHS providers (www.nhs.uk). It is important to differentiate between three types of NHS organisations:

- commissioning organisations;
- provider organisations; and
- regulators.

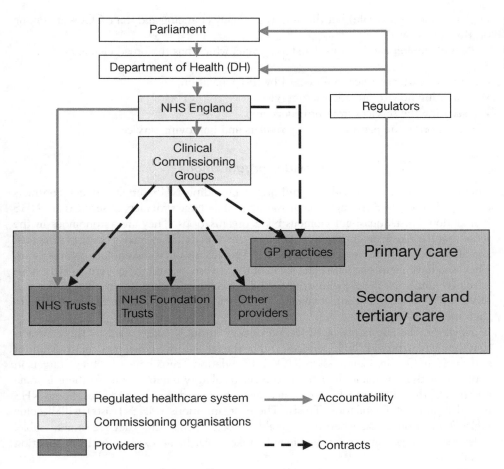

FIGURE 5.2
The simplified
structure of the
NHS in England

Commissioning of Primary Care has transferred in some places from NHS England to Clinical Commissioning Groups

Commissioning organisations

Commissioning involves buying services from health care providers, which might include primary care and hospitals. It is a process that includes needs assessment, planning and joint working with other agencies. Following the Health and Social Care Act 2012, the main commissioners are Clinical Commissioning Groups (CCGs) which have responsibility for commissioning a range of services for their population. There are over 200 CCGs in England, covering an average population of around 230,000, although there is wide variation. They are responsible for commissioning hospital services and community health services. Some more specialist services are commissioned by NHS England. When CCGs were first established they were not responsible for commissioning primary care (NHS

Iain Snelling

Commissioning involves buying services from health care providers, which might include primary care and hospitals. It is a process that includes needs assessment, planning and joint working with other agencies.

England took on this role) but this is now gradually changing and some CCGs are taking on this role as well.

Commissioning can be considered as a cycle, which has the broad elements of

- assessing what services are needed by the population;
- planning how to provide these services;
- securing the services from providers; and
- monitoring the performance of providers and improving services.

Provider organisations

There are a range of provider organisations providing NHS services under contracts developed and agreed through commissioning. Most large providers of services are NHS Foundation Trusts, quasi-autonomous NHS organisations. They are autonomous in the sense that the Government doesn't manage them directly. They have a board of directors, and also governors who represent staff and the public as well as stakeholder organisations. They also have members, who elect some of the governors, and the governors elect non-executive directors. People who work for a Trust or are a patient or who live in the area served by a Trust can become a member. Foundation Trusts are therefore accountable to their members.

However, the autonomy of NHS Foundation Trusts is constrained by the contracts that they sign to provide NHS services, and by the regulatory regime, particularly Monitor and the Care Quality Commission (CQC). Foundation Trusts have to achieve targets in contracts within available finances, and meet regulatory requirements, so there is some question of the extent to which they can really be regarded as autonomous. Some NHS providers are not Foundation Trusts. These organisations (NHS Trusts) will become NHS Foundation Trusts when they are able to demonstrate that they are sound, viable, independent organisations, or they may be taken over by an existing NHS Foundation Trust.

Other organisations may provide NHS services. These include private sector organisations or third sector organisations, which are neither public sector nor private sector, including charities and social enterprises. In some cases these organisations will have won contracts for NHS services, and in others they may be chosen by patients to be providers of their NHS services. All services that provide NHS care need to be registered with the CQC and most need to be licensed by Monitor.

Regulators

There are a number of regulators of health care, but the two most important are the CQC and Monitor. The CQC was established in 2009, as a successor to a number of other regulators, including the Health Care Commission. The CQC's role, according to its website is:

> We monitor, inspect and regulate services to make sure they meet fundamental standards of quality and safety and we publish what we find, including performance ratings to help people choose care.

> (CQC 2016a)

The CQC is responsible for regulating all health care and social care providers. They have a number of powers to enforce their regulation including, ultimately, to remove registration, which would mean that the organisation would not be able to provide services. The CQC hosts Healthwatch England, which is formally a statutory committee of the CQC. Healthwatch is the 'consumer champion' for the NHS and there are also a series of local Healthwatch organisations that work with patients and the public. The purpose of Healthwatch locally and nationally is to 'understand the needs, experiences and concerns of people who use services and to speak out on their behalf' (Healthwatch 2014, p. 5).

Monitor started as the independent regulator of NHS Foundation Trusts and retains this role. In addition, after the Health and Social Care Act 2012, it has taken on the role of health care sector regulator. As well as regulating NHS Foundation Trusts, Monitor has additional roles of licensing most NHS providers, making sure that essential services are maintained if an NHS provider fails, regulating the NHS payment system that determines how much NHS Commissioners pay providers for their services, and making sure that the system works in the best interests of patients, for example, by ensuring that there is choice of services available, and that procurement of services by commissioners is effective (Monitor 2014). In 2015, Monitor and a body responsible for NHS Trusts who had not become Foundations Trusts, the NHS Trust Development Authority, together became known as NHS Improvement.

When a Foundation Trust is established, it is granted a licence, which sets out the services it must provide. Any changes to the services must be agreed by Monitor. Monitor has a number of powers it can use when the finances of a Trust are beginning to show signs of weakening. These range from more frequent monitoring to removal of board members or ultimately removal of the licence of the NHS Foundation Trust, in which case it would revert to being an NHS Trust. Monitor works closely with the CQC, so that, for example, Foundation Trusts regarded by the CQC as failing to meet standards can be placed in 'special measures', a formal sanction applied by Monitor. Although a Foundation Trust is regulated by Monitor it remains accountable to its members, as discussed above.

Regulation is discussed in more detail below, as it has significant roles in developing and implementing policy concerned with the two elements of the Triple Aim that form the focus of the chapter, namely quality and cost. There are other regulators with specific objectives. The National Institute for Health and Care Excellence (NICE) is a significant regulator, which provides advice and guidance for the NHS. This can cause controversy because NICE is the organisation that recommends whether new treatments should be available on the NHS. Consideration of regulators for the NHS should also include the professional regulators, including the Nursing and Midwifery Council, as discussed in Chapter 2.

Current health policy

As discussed below and in Chapter 1, events at Mid-Staffordshire have had a significant effect on health policy. The effect of financial targets and the ambition of the hospital to achieve Foundation Trust status were significant issues, as was the regulatory regime in place at the time, which was based primarily on self-assessment. In this section current policy is considered in three sections: how quality is considered in the NHS mandate, how quality is regulated and how integrated care is a central idea in improving quality. Discussion of funding health services will follow the section on quality.

Quality

Each year the Government sets the NHS objectives in a mandate. In the 2016/2017 mandate there are seven objectives. The first is: 'Through better commissioning, improve local and national health outcomes, particularly by addressing poor outcomes and inequalities' (DH 2016, p. 8). The Government expects:

> NHS England to demonstrate improvements against *The NHS Outcomes Framework*, and work with CCGs to reduce variations in quality of care and outcomes at a local level. NHS England must secure measurable reductions in inequalities in access to health services, in people's experience of the health system, and across a specified range of health outcomes.
>
> (DH 2016, p. 8)

Other objectives are to address quality issues, including improving cancer services, improving services for people with dementia and improving out of hospital services, particularly for people with mental health problems, learning disabilities and autism.

Quality in health care is difficult to assess, because there are so many ways in which it can be considered and measured. The Darzi Review (Secretary of State for Health 2008) identified three elements of quality: safety, effectiveness, and experience. These three elements of quality are reflected in *The NHS Outcomes Framework*, established in 2010 as part of the process of the reforms. There are five domains in the *Outcomes Framework*, which are used to assess the performance of the NHS. The domains are:

- preventing people from dying prematurely;
- enhancing quality of life for people with long-term conditions;
- helping people to recover from episodes of ill health or following injury;
- ensuring that people have a positive experience of care;
- treating and caring for people in a safe environment and protecting them from avoidable harm.

> (DH 2014a)

Separate outcomes frameworks are published for public health and social care.

The outcomes framework contains a number of indicators in each domain, such as mortality rates, the proportion of people being supported to manage their condition, emergency readmissions, patient experience data and incidences of health care acquired infections. At the end of each year, the targets for the previous year are reviewed, both by NHS England itself in its annual report, and by the DH. In 2015, NHS England gave details of the performance of the NHS against the mandate in the 2014/2015, and the DH undertook its own assessment (NHS England 2015b, DH 2015b). The results, expressed by the Secretary of State in the DH publication, were that:

> I agree with the assessment in your annual report for 2014–2015 that NHS England has made good progress against the mandate. In a challenging year, your organisation has made progress on the majority of the mandate objectives. The majority of the 68 indicators of the NHS outcomes framework, which is used to help assess whether NHS England has achieved its objectives, show improvements in outcomes over the past year.
>
> (DH 2015b, p. 3)

The *Outcomes Framework* is intended to focus on accountability for outcomes. The Labour Governments of 1997–2010 were criticised for having too many process targets, such as waiting time targets, and the Lansley reforms aimed to concentrate on outcomes when considering how the NHS is performing. However, targets have not disappeared. Some are included in *The NHS Constitution*, detailed in its handbook. For example, the handbook states that you have the right to:

- start your consultant-led treatment within a maximum of 18 weeks from referral for non-urgent conditions; and
- be seen by a cancer specialist within a maximum of 2 weeks from GP referral for urgent referrals where cancer is suspected.

(DH 2015c, p. 32)

There are further targets including other cancer targets and the 4-hour target for admission or discharge from Accident and Emergency. These targets are monitored by regulators, particularly Monitor. Each NHS Trust and Foundation Trust has to publish quality accounts each year alongside its financial accounts, and the NHS Choices website includes a number of indicators including information about nurse staffing levels. Both NHS Trusts and Foundation Trusts are covered, and patients are able to leave their own reviews and ratings.

Regulation of quality – The Care Quality Commission

The regulation of quality in the NHS has developed significantly over recent years, in response to the events at Mid-Staffordshire. Immediately after the final report of the Public Inquiry was published in 2013, the Medical Director of the NHS, Sir Bruce Keogh, was asked to review the quality of care provided by 14 Trusts in England who had high mortality rates (Keogh 2013). Some lessons from the review process informed the development of the CQC's regulatory system. The process was based on principles of patient and public participation, listening to the views of staff, openness and transparency, and co-operation between organisations, and included information analysis and visits by a team involving patients, doctors, nurses, managers, and regulators.

The CQC has a set of fundamental standards, which 'reflect the recommendations made by Robert Francis following his inquiry into care at Mid-Staffordshire NHS Foundation Trust' (CQC 2015a, p. 5). These fundamental standards that are given in full in regulations and law, are shown in Box 5.1 and explained on the CQC website.

Breaching some of these standards constitutes a criminal offence. The CQC has an enforcement policy (CQC 2015b), which explains how it uses its powers. All providers of health and social care need to be registered with the CQC, and the registration process requires providers to demonstrate that they will be able to meet standards set out in the regulations. The CQC can require improvement through requirement notices or warning notices, force improvement through enforcement powers such as imposing conditions to registration or special measures, 'or hold providers or individuals to account for failure' (CQC 2015b, p. 14). In 2014/2015, 1,179 enforcement actions were taken. The vast majority were warning notices (1,037) but there were also 27 urgent procedures for suspension, variation or conditions of registration, and 5 prosecutions in social care and primary care. Twenty-one hospitals and 10 primary medical services were placed in special measures (CQC 2015b).

BOX 5.1

The CQC describes the fundamental standards as: the standards below which your care must never fall. *Everybody* has the right to expect the following standards:

Person-centred care

You must have care or treatment that is tailored to you and meets your needs and preferences.

Dignity and respect

You must be treated with dignity and respect at all times while you're receiving care and treatment.

This includes making sure:

- You have privacy when you need and want it.
- Everybody is treated as equals.
- You are given any support you need to help you remain independent and involved in your local community.

Consent

You (or anybody legally acting on your behalf) must give your consent before any care or treatment is given to you.

Safety

You must not be given unsafe care or treatment or be put at risk of harm that could be avoided.

Providers must assess the risks to your health and safety during any care or treatment and make sure their staff have the qualifications, competence, skills and experience to keep you safe.

Safeguarding from abuse

You must not suffer any form of abuse or improper treatment while receiving care.

This includes:

- neglect;
- degrading treatment;
- unnecessary or disproportionate restraint;
- inappropriate limits on your freedom.

Food and drink

You must have enough to eat and drink to keep you in good health while you receive care and treatment.

Premises and equipment

The places where you receive care and treatment and the equipment used in it must be clean, suitable and looked after properly.

The equipment used in your care and treatment must also be secure and used properly.

Complaints

You must be able to complain about your care and treatment.

The provider of your care must have a system in place so they can handle and respond to your complaint. They must investigate it thoroughly and take action if problems are identified.

Good governance

The provider of your care must have plans that ensure they can meet these standards.

They must have effective governance and systems to check on the quality and safety of care. These must help the service improve and reduce any risks to your health, safety and welfare.

Staffing

The provider of your care must have enough suitably qualified, competent and experienced staff to make sure they can meet these standards.

Their staff must be given the support, training and supervision they need to help them do their job.

Fit and proper staff

The provider of your care must only employ people who can provide care and treatment appropriate to their role. They must have strong recruitment procedures in place and carry out relevant checks such as on applicants' criminal records and work history.

Duty of candour

The provider of your care must be open and transparent with you about your care and treatment.

Should something go wrong, they must tell you what has happened, provide support and apologise.

Display of ratings

The provider of your care must display their CQC rating in a place where you can see it. They must also include this information on their website and make our latest report on their service available to you.

(CQC 2016b)

The CQC monitors providers, and also has a regular inspection process. The inspection process gives a comprehensive assessment of quality by asking five questions. Is the service:

- safe?
- effective?
- caring?
- responsive to people's needs?
- well-led?

Iain Snelling

The same framework is used for all services inspected: hospitals and community health care services (NHS and independent), mental health services, primary care (GP practices and out-of-hours services and dentists), ambulance services, and adult social care. The CQC website includes provider handbooks for all types of services, giving details of how the inspection process runs with specific questions that will be asked (key lines of enquiry), and statements that give descriptions of the ratings. At the end of the process providers are given an overall rating of:

- outstanding;
- good;
- requires improvement; or
- inadequate.

Individual areas are also given one of these ratings, if applicable, against each of the five questions, so the organisations have an individual scorecard. All reports are available on the CQC website. Each year the CQC publishes a state of health care and adult social care report. The 2015 reports give a breakdown of the ratings by sector (CQC 2015c). The overall rating by sector of the 5,439 organisations inspected and rated up until 31 May 2015 are shown in Figure 5.3 (CQC 2015c, p. 12).

The CQC has had its own difficulties in maintaining its performance. In 2015 the House of Commons Committee of Public Accounts published a report that highlighted that it was behind on its inspection programme, that there was often a considerable delay in producing reports. The CQC had originally set out that it would inspect all acute hospitals by the end of 2015, and all social care and GP providers by the end of February 2016. These targets were not achieved, in part because of difficulty in recruiting staff (House of Commons Committee of Public Accounts 2015).

FIGURE 5.3
Breakdown of inspection ratings by sector, 2015

Sector	Number of organisations inspected	% rated outstanding	% rated good	% rated requires improvement	% rated inadequate
Adult social care	4,294	1	59	33	7
Primary medical services	976	3	82	11	4
Hospitals	169	2	37	54	8

Activity 5.3

Go to the CQC website and locate the report for your placement. When you have read it, discuss it with your colleagues and mentor and consider how it has affected the delivery of care, including morale in your placement area.

Integrated care

Integrated care is a term widely used to describe care that is not affected by boundaries between organisations or teams. The idea has been around for many years but it has been

130

difficult to address in practice (Glasby and Dickinson 2014). In the years of the Labour Governments there were a number of initiatives and pilots, but sustained improvements were elusive. There are fundamental contradictions between policies designed to promote competition and choice on the one hand and collaboration and integration on the other. For many service users, particularly those with complex conditions, services are received from a number of organisations within health care, and between health care and other organisations, particularly social care. Integrated care might mean that teams work in the same organisation, or that they work so closely with each other that the total service, as experienced by the service user, is 'seamless'.

The interface between health care and social care has often been cited as a significant obstacle in improving services. Social care is funded separately from the NHS through local authorities and is means tested. Local authorities have had significant reductions in their budgets since the financial crisis, a position much worse than the NHS. Adult social care includes services such as care homes, reablement services, day care, domiciliary services and support for carers. In 2014, a National Audit Office briefing gave some key facts on adult social care (NAO 2014). These included:

- £19 billion was spent by local authorities in 2012/13 on adult social care, including £2.5 billion user contributions.
- An estimated £10 billion was spent privately on care and support, in 2010/2011.
- There are 5.4 million unpaid informal carers, providing an estimated £55 billion's worth of care and support, in 2011.
- The number of adults receiving local authority-funded care has reduced from 1.79 million in 2008/2009 to 1.33 million in 2012/2013. The number of adults over 65 in these numbers were 1.22 million to 0.9 million.
- There are 1.5 million people working in adult social care, which is higher than the NHS workforce (and doesn't include informal carers).

In 2014 the Care Act was passed, which consolidated the legislative framework in a number of areas and introduced some significant reforms. Additional duties were placed on local authorities, including integrating services with NHS services. Funding arrangements for social care were reformed in the Care Act, through the introduction of a cap on the costs of care that an individual has to meet privately, and an increase in the levels of personal savings allowed before an individual is required to fund their own social care needs. These changes were due to have been implemented from April 2016 but were delayed until 2020 because of financial pressures (Carers UK 2015).

Integrated care was hardly mentioned in the White Paper that announced the 2012 reforms (Secretary of State for Health 2010), but it was developed as a theme by the Future Forum (2011), which made a number of recommendations. In 2013 it was announced that a Better Care Fund would be established from 2015/2016 with the aim of achieving 'better, more joined-up services to older and disabled people, to keep them out of hospital and to avoid long hospital stays' (HM Treasury 2013, p. 22). This fund drew from existing resources, mainly from the NHS, to create pooled budgets for health and social care to support integrated care. In 2016/2017, £3.9 billion will be allocated to the Better Care Fund from the NHS, with local flexibility to allocate additional resources (DH and Department for Communities and Local Government 2016). The Government will make additional resources available to local authorities from 2017/2018. Local plans need to be agreed by Health and Wellbeing Boards.

Integrated care has in recent years caught the imagination of policy makers, although it has been an aim for many years. Further developments are to be expected. The Government's Autumn Statement and Spending Review in 2015 set out

> an ambitious plan so that by 2020 health and social care are integrated across the country. Every part of the country must have a plan for this in 2017, implemented by 2020. Areas will be able to graduate from the existing Better Care Fund programme management once they can demonstrate that they have moved beyond its requirements, meeting the government's key criteria for devolution
>
> (Chancellor of the Exchequer 2015, p. 34)

The Autumn Statement of 2015 also stated that, in contrast to the health care reforms of the coalition Government, the current Government will not impose how the NHS and local government deliver integration. Like the new care models discussed in the *Five Year Forward View*, it seems that local approaches will be supported. Integrated Care Pioneers have also been established to develop local programmes and approaches, although they don't have access to the Transformation Fund. A National Collaboration for Integrated Care and Support, which shows how existing structures can be used to support integration has been established. The framework was developed by 12 national partners, including the DH, social services and care organisations, and regulators including CQC and Monitor. It was produced in association with National Voices, a national coalition of health and social care charities (National Collaboration for Integrated Care and Support 2013). This is an important resource for considering integrated care.

Activity 5.4

The discussion above outlines a number of initiatives to improve quality. This is a fast-moving policy area, and by the time you are reading this chapter, many of the initiatives and process discussed will be out of date. Most references given are to official documents and websites, so it is possible to keep track of developments, although it takes time and patience. In groups, take one topic each and brief each other on recent developments in the following areas:

- The Five Year Forward View Vanguards.
- The CQC process of regulation and state of health and social care reports.
- The Better Care Fund.
- Progress against indicators in the NHS Outcomes Framework and the Social Care and Public Health Outcomes Frameworks.

Personalisation

The areas discussed above are mainly concerned with organisations and processes, for example accountability and regulation, but retaining focus on the individual is of great importance. Foot *et al.* (2014) identify eight forms of individuals' involvement in their own care. This does not include collective forms of engagement or where individuals take on roles not directly related to their own care. The eight forms are:

- engaging people in keeping healthy;
- shared decision-making;
- supported self-management;
- having a personal health or social care budget;
- involving families and carers;
- choosing a provider;
- taking part in research as part of treatments;
- evaluating services through feedback.

Many of these forms of engagement can be pursued through good leadership, particularly through clinical leadership, as a number of these areas are implemented through clinical practice, and are evident in *The Code* (NMC 2015), other Nursing and Midwifery Council documents and *The NHS Constitution*. Other forms require some policy or infrastructure development. Having a personal budget for health and social care, for example, has required more significant changes to practice. This policy is spreading from adult social care into other services (Needham and Glasby 2014). *The Adult Social Care Outcomes Framework*, which was referred to earlier, includes a measure of the proportion of people using social care who receive direct payments. The Government target is 70 per cent, which was achieved by fewer than half of local authorities in 2013/2014 (DH 2014a).

Patient choice has been an element of personalisation for some time, for example, through choosing a general practitioner. There was a renewed emphasis on choice in policy in the early 2000s and patients now have a greater number of choices, for example in where to be referred to. The NHS publishes a choice framework to explain the choices that are available (DH 2015d). However, surveys show that patients are not always informed about the choices they have (Foot *et al.* 2014).

Funding health services

The organisation of health services is a key issue for health policy, but perhaps the biggest issue is how health services are funded and how much spending is devoted to them. Throughout the lifetime of the NHS, it has always been funded predominantly by general taxation.

Activity 5.5

Jot down your answers (or guesses!) to the following questions. If you do this quick exercise in a group, discuss the reasons for your individual answers.

- How much money does the government spend annually on the NHS in England? How much is total UK public expenditure on health? This includes all expenditure under the general heading of health including public health, regulators, education, etc. in the whole of the UK. How does health expenditure compare with other areas of public spending such as defence and education?

- How does the UK differ from other countries in terms of the percentage of total national expenditure that goes on health and the percentage of spending that comes from the government?

The answers are given at the end of this section.

The answers to these questions sum up important top-level health policy issues for government. They are expressed here in financial terms but really they are wider issues. For example, what balance should there be between individual and governmental responsibility for providing health services? How should health care relate to other government expenditure priorities, many of which will affect health, for example, housing and employment? There is a wide consensus in the UK that health care should continue to be funded mainly through taxation, with most services free at the point of use. However, there are other methods of funding, and most countries, including the UK, use a mix. Though the NHS is mainly funded through general taxation, some charges are levied, for example, for prescriptions (in England) and for dentistry. There is also a small private sector, funded mainly from insurance. Robinson (2011) identifies that funding methods include:

1   *Private insurance.* This is optional insurance, taken out by individuals, or companies on behalf of their employees.
2   *Taxation.* Funding health services through taxation also has a number of different possibilities since there are many ways that governments, national and local, raise funds through taxation, for example income tax and VAT.
3   *Social insurance.* This is a form of compulsory insurance, paid by individuals or employers.
4   *Charges and co-payments.* Sometimes this is known as 'out of pocket' charges to distinguish it from insurance.

As discussed above, there was a significant increase in health expenditure after *The NHS Plan*, which recognised that underfunding was a major problem in the NHS and committed to a real terms increase (i.e., after the effects of inflation have been taken into account) of one-third over 5 years. In 2002, the Treasury published a report by Derek Wanless (2002), which considered the resources required for the NHS over two decades, taking into account developments in a number of factors, such as changing expectations and health care needs and the possibilities offered by medical advances. A conclusion of the review was that health care spending needed to increase substantially over the period considered (up until 2023), particularly in the early years to 'catch up'; a real terms increase in excess of 7 per cent per annum for 5 years was recommended. These levels of increase were initially achieved, but as discussed above, the period of austerity after the financial crisis means that only very small real increases will be achieved in the decade between 2010 and 2020, and significant efficiency savings will be required. The Quality, Innovation, Productivity and Prevention (QIPP) challenge is difficult to assess. Central figures of contributions to the 'challenge' have not been published since 2012/2013, and productivity is difficult to measure (Appleby *et al.* 2015). The financial position of the NHS in 2015/2016 worsened considerably compared to the previous year with little evidence that big improvements in productivity have been achieved.

Answers to questions in Activity 5.5

- The Chancellor's Spending Review and Autumn Statement in 2015 outlined that the plan for NHS spending in England will rise from £101 billion in 2015/2016 to £120 billion in 2020/2021 (Chancellor of the Exchequer 2015). This is NHS England's budget. The Chancellor's budget in 2015 showed total government spending on health to be planned at £141 billion in 2015/16. This is all health expenditure in the UK. Other major areas of spending include social protection, which is made up of payments to individuals, such as pensions and benefits (£231 billion), education (£99 billion), defence (£45 billion) and personal social services, which includes publicly funded social care (£30 billion). Total planned government expenditure in 2008/2009 is £742 billion, so NHS expenditure accounts for around 19 per cent (HM Treasury 2015).
- The Organisation for Economic Co-operation and Development (OECD) is a group of 34 member countries committed to democracy and market economies. It provides a range of statistical services to support policy development. Its figures for 2013 show that health expenditure as a percentage of GDP (gross domestic product – the total national income) in the UK was 8.5 per cent (OECD 2015). Figure 5.4 shows public and private health expenditure in OECD countries. Overall the UK spends less in terms of per cent GDP than the OECD average, but with a higher proportion of public spending.

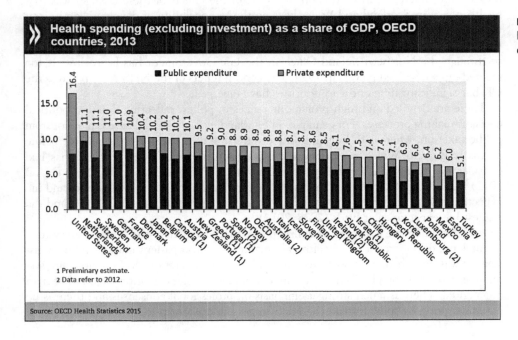

FIGURE 5.4
Health spending as share of GDP

Iain Snelling

Capital and revenue expenditure

Expenditure in the NHS is divided into two types – revenue and capital. **Revenue expenditure** pays for day-to-day running of services, and **capital expenditure** is for major investments, not only new hospitals costing millions of pounds, but also items such as medical equipment and maintenance. If more investment is required it is not easy to reduce day-to-day funding in order to pay for it. On the other hand, if more day-to-day spending is required it is easier to reduce investment.

A way of increasing investment without a big increase in public expenditure is to ask the private sector to fund development, which is then paid for over a long-term arrangement through the NHS leasing back the facilities. This policy, which began in the early 1990s across a wide range of government departments, is known as the Private Finance Initiative (PFI), or more recently Public/Private Partnerships. As well as increasing investment without increasing public expenditure, the policy was designed to improve planning by making sure that investment could be afforded in the long term.

Critics of PFI schemes (Pollock 2004) point out that the private investment is paid back over a long time and costs more than it would have to invest from public funds. Although controversial, many new hospitals have recently been almost entirely funded through PFI, and the scheme has helped achieve a major modernisation of health care facilities. Since the period of resource increase for the NHS ended in 2010 there have been fewer PFI agreements and the scheme has been substantially amended. Nevertheless, the cost of leasing health care buildings procured through the Private Finance Initiative is a contributor to financial difficulties in some areas.

National differences in the UK

In 1999 the Scottish Parliament and the Welsh Assembly took over their devolved powers, after referenda in both countries. One of the effects of these changes was that health policy in Scotland and Wales became the responsibility of devolved administrations. Northern Ireland has a longer tradition of devolved administration, but because of the political problems of recent years, the development of domestic policy in the province or through the Northern Ireland Office in the UK Government has been slow. It too secured more devolved powers in 1999. The central tenets of the NHS remain across the UK but significant differences in priorities have emerged.

There are detailed and high-profile differences in policy, reflecting different political decision-making processes. For example, in Scotland, personal social care is paid for from public taxation, whereas in England only the nursing element of care is paid for before means testing. In Wales, prescription charges have been abolished. England has had considerably more success in reducing waiting times. The National Audit Office (NAO 2012) identified differences in a number of key indicators including expenditure and life expectancy, with England having the lowest expenditure per head (2010/2011), and the highest life expectancy at birth (2008–2010).

A major difference concerns structures put in place to manage the health care system. In England, development of a health care market based on patient choice and commissioning was described, with some recent emphasis on integration. In Scotland, the system has gone in a completely different direction. Here services are integrated rather than fragmented. There is much stronger emphasis on professional consensus and there is no purchaser/provider split. Instead the NHS in Scotland is organised through 14 regional

NHS Boards responsible for managing the whole system of care. Wales initially maintained the purchaser/provider split, but has reorganised the NHS around regional health delivery bodies. Northern Ireland, alone of the four health systems, has integration of health and social care.

Health policy evolves rather than develops in discrete steps based on thorough evaluation. However, if policy divergences between the four systems in the UK continue, there will be an opportunity to evaluate differences more thoroughly, for example in the degree of success in changing the dominance of hospitals in health care delivery, and the effect of specific differences such as in the funding of personal social care (Baggott 2015). Whether evaluations are influential in producing more evidence-based policy making is likely to depend on the political policy-making process.

PART 3: EXPLORING HEALTH POLICY

What evidence is there to support health policies described in this chapter? The requirement for evidence-based practice by health care professionals is well understood, but should we expect policy makers to apply similar principles? For example, what evidence is there for expecting that clinically led commissioning will improve services, or that a regulatory regime based largely on inspection will be able to ensure standards in diverse providers?

A number of difficulties can be identified in developing an evidence base for the development and implementation of policy. A key issue is that 'there is usually more room for disagreement about outcomes in policy making than in medicine. In medicine, randomised control trials can (sometimes) clinch arguments about outcomes. This never happens in policy making' (Cookson 2005, p. 119). Context is important in developing an evidence base. This is particularly important when considering evidence from other countries, who have implemented similar policies. The social and political context cannot be controlled in the comparison. Policy depends 'crucially upon people's decision-making behaviour' (Cookson 2005, p. 119). Whether a policy succeeds in achieving its aims is important, but it is also important to understand how it works, and this depends on many people's decisions.

Policy making is essentially a political activity, which seeks to achieve a balance between various perspectives. What balance, for example, should be struck between the rights of professionals to autonomy and the rights of patients to a service that achieves reasonably standard outcomes? In the UK context, the constant demand on policy makers for improvements in health services means that time for researching effects of policy before changes are demanded is rarely available. For example, intentional rounding has been widely implemented following political intervention and in the absence of robust evidence in support, but now that it has been widely implemented, there are too few sites not doing it to make a randomised trial feasible (Snelling 2016). Politicians who make key decisions are also likely to have strong beliefs that lead to a specific point of view. Barriers to using research include the lack of personal contact between researchers and policy makers, the lack of timeliness or relevance of research and mistrust between policy makers and researchers (Innvaer *et al.* 2002).

This is not to say that evidence is not important in making policy, but compared with evidence-based clinical practice a different model of what constitutes evidence and how it is used is needed (Dobrow *et al.* 2004). The evidence, for example, may be unpublished evaluations supporting the development of policy through implementation, or stakeholder perceptions of policy outcomes. In some areas, evidence comes from high-profile public enquiries, as was the case in the development of policy in the wake of the Francis Reports. The demand for evidence is increased by greater pressures for transparency, accountability and efficiency in all areas of public policy (Cookson 2005). Improvements in information and communication technology increase both the volume of evidence available, and its communication.

Looking to the future

Earlier in the chapter the influence of a report by Derek Wanless, which considered the resources required for the NHS over the next two decades was noted. The report (Wanless 2002) concluded that resources required depended crucially on whether the public engaged in relation to their health, for example, by pursuing healthy lifestyles, and whether the NHS becomes more responsive and efficient, for example, in developing information and communication technology (ICT) and becoming more efficient. Wanless identified three scenarios:

- *Slow uptake.* There is no change in the level of public engagement: life expectancy rises by the lowest amount in all three scenarios and the health status of the population is constant or deteriorates. The health service is relatively unresponsive with low rates of technology uptake and low productivity.
- *Solid progress.* People become more engaged in relation to their health: life expectancy rises considerably, health status improves and people have confidence in the primary care system and use it appropriately. The health service is responsive with high rates of technology uptake and more efficient use of resources.
- *Fully engaged.* Levels of public engagement in relation to their health are high: life expectancy increases go beyond current forecasts, health status improves dramatically and people are confident in the health system and demand high-quality care. The health service is responsive with high rates of technology uptake, particularly in relation to disease prevention. Use of resources is more efficient.

The 'fully engaged' scenario envisaged a situation in 2022 where expenditure was £30 billion less than would be required under the 'slow uptake' scenario. The 'fully engaged' scenario, better health outcomes for considerably less resources, is clearly worth pursuing. Wanless was subsequently asked to consider how the fully engaged scenario could be achieved and his second report, published in 2004, set the scene for the development of public health policy (Wanless 2004). The key issue for Wanless was resources. The 'catch up' he recommended was achieved. His projections went forward until 2022/2023. In the 'solid progress' scenario, he estimated that by then we will need to spend 11.1 per cent of GDP on health. These increases could be achieved by increasing health spending at between 4.7 per cent and 2.7 per cent above inflation each year.

Although the era of significant additional resources for the NHS began in 2000 with the publication of *The NHS Plan* (Secretary of State for Health 2000), the Wanless report provided justification for maintaining and extending the increase in resources. In 2007, the King's Fund published a review of NHS funding and performance, led again by Derek Wanless (Wanless *et al.* 2007). The review concluded that the extra resources the 2002 report identified had been made available to the NHS, but that in other areas – outputs, outcomes and determinants of health, and productivity – progress is only on a path between slow uptake and solid progress.

The Wanless reports were perhaps a high point of optimism in recent health policy. He outlined a framework for health policy that included public health and the roles and responsibilities of individuals, as well as of the health care system to change and develop, particularly in the areas of health technology and information and communication technology and workforce development. The framework included sustained additional investment in the long term.

Increases in resources stopped because of the financial crisis and subsequent policies. The Nuffield Trust, the King's Fund and the Health Foundation jointly published a summary of the 2015 autumn statement and spending review and concluded that

> the NHS is halfway through the most austere decade in its history. Public spending on health in the United Kingdom as a proportion of GDP is projected to fall to 6.7 per cent by 2020/2021, leaving us behind many other advanced nations on this measure of spending.
>
> (King's Fund *et al.* 2015, p. 1)

This is a long way from the optimistic projections of the Wanless report. Recent policy developments as discussed above have addressed the two key issues of cost and quality, starting from the difficult positions of the legacy of the Francis Reports and the prospect of no growth in the resources.

National or devolved policy?

Recent developments in health policy have highlighted the importance of local development of health systems rather than top-down national systems. After the general election of 2015, the Government developed its plans for devolving responsibility for a range of services to local regions and cities. Before the election, the Chancellor agreed with the leaders of 10 local authorities in Manchester to transfer a range of government responsibilities and budgets, including responsibility for health and social care. Bids were invited for the transfer of powers locally, with discretion about what powers were being sought and what constituted the 'region', with local authorities able to combine. One requirement for devolved powers is the election of a Mayor. Around half of the 38 bids received are thought to have asked for some health and social care powers (King's Fund 2015, p. 5). This policy and process is still developing, and it is difficult to see how local health and social care provision will develop.

Alongside these changes in government structures, the *Five Year Forward View* process involves a range of different care models being developed locally. Here again there is emphasis on local development rather than mandated change from the Government. NHS England has recently asked NHS leaders to produce 5-year 'sustainability and transformation plans' (NHS England 2015c). The areas for these local plans are to be determined locally, and agreed nationally. The guidance gives three overarching questions for local plans:

- *How will you close the health and well-being gap?* This section should include your plans for a 'radical upgrade' in prevention, patient activation, choice and control, and community engagement (NHS England 2015c, p. 17).

- *How will you drive transformation to close the care and quality gap?* This section should include plans for new care model development, improving against clinical priorities, and roll-out of digital health care (NHS England 2015c, p. 18).
- *How will you close the finance and efficiency gap?* This section should describe how you will achieve financial balance across your local health system and improve the efficiency of NHS services (NHS England 2015c, p. 20).

These plans devolve substantial responsibility to local leaders and signal an emphasis on 'place-based' leadership and systems of care (Ham and Alderwick 2015) for all the NHS as well as those developing vanguards and those areas seeking new devolved powers. The NHS in 2020 will increasingly be shaped locally within significant financial constraints, a notable shift in health policy since the early years of the twenty-first century when sustained investment in a clear national direction were the key features.

CONCLUSION

Health policy is a complex area – it is developing all the time and a key challenge for many in the NHS is keeping up to date with all the changes. The distinction between health policy and health care policy is important. This chapter has dealt mainly with health care policy. Health policy includes a range of initiatives, relating to, for example, public health and inequalities that are wider than the health care system. Social policy and the provision of social care are also very important and have not been considered in as much detail as health care policy.

In this chapter current health care policy has been discussed, but when you read it there will have been changes. Recommendations for further reading have been provided and you will need to consider developments to gain a full and up-to-date understanding. The key challenges in health policy since 2010 have been to assure quality of services and deal with a significantly constrained financial position, which address two elements of the Triple Aim framework introduced earlier.

SUGGESTED FURTHER READING

A number of books on health policy are cited in the chapter. Unfortunately, because of delays in production, large parts of them are likely to be out of date. This is also the case with this chapter. Keeping up to date with policy developments requires more contemporary resources and the Internet and other media are key. Tutors will often caution you about your use of the Internet, but for understanding health policy you will need to know your way around some important sites.

- There are a number of professional journals, which include news sections and commentaries on contemporary issues, for example, the *Nursing Times* and *Nursing Standard*. The *Health Service Journal* is an important weekly publication aimed at NHS managers, which gives useful commentaries. These are very useful sources of information about policy, although you should be aware that they are often written from a particular perspective and for a particular audience.

- Because of the enormous public interest in health issues, the media – newspapers, magazines, television, radio and the Internet – are good sources of information, although again you have to be wary of specific perspectives. The 'quality' papers often have in-depth articles, and current affairs programmes on the television and radio often cover health issues. The BBC website has a health news section, which can be very useful. It is so up to date that a week or so after a development, the relevant information is not so easy to find! Other news organisations also provide useful information.
- The DH website (www.gov.uk/government/organisations/department-of-health) is a very useful resource. The DH publishes many documents setting out policy and giving guidance for those responsible for its implementation. These documents are often detailed, but they usually include an executive summary, which can be helpful in giving an overview and directing more detailed reading. Some particularly helpful documents are produced specifically for the public. DH documents are sometimes available free of charge in printed form. Details of how to order them are on the back cover of the electronic version.
- Devolved administrations in Scotland, Wales and Northern Ireland have their own web resources, with sections related to their health policies and structures:
  - In Scotland, the Scottish Executive: www.scotland.gov.uk/Topics/Health.
  - In Wales, the Welsh Assembly Government: http://gov.wales/topics/health/?lang=en.
  - In Northern Ireland, the DH, Social Services and Public Safety: www.dhsspsni.gov.uk.
- There are many bodies that have been set up to implement health policy. Their websites are often useful sources of information. For example, the Care Quality Commission, and the National Institute for Health and Clinical Excellence.
- Trade unions and professional bodies also produce useful resources, particularly where an issue has specific importance for its membership. For example, the Royal College of Nursing (www.rcn.org.uk) and Unison (www.unison.org.uk) both have useful resources, although you should be aware that they will take a particular perspective on issues.
- There are a number of research organisations and interest groups, which consider health issues and produce resources to support policy debates. Examples include:
  - The Health Foundation (www.health.org.uk)
  - The King's Fund (www.kingsfund.org.uk)
  - The NHS Confederation (www.nhsconfed.org)
  - The Nuffield Trust (www.nuffieldtrust.org.uk)
  - The Picker Institute (www.pickereurope.org).
- Social media, particularly Twitter, give access to many individuals and organisations who comment on health policy.

Spending a few hours familiarising yourself with these resources is likely to be very useful.

REFERENCES

Appleby, J., Galea, A. and Murray, R. (2014) *The NHS Productivity Challenge: Experience from the front line*. London: The King's Fund.

Appleby, J., Baird, B., Thompson, J. and Jabbal, J. (2015) *The NHS under the Coalition Government Part Two: NHS performance*. London: The King's Fund.

Baggott, R. (2015) *Understanding Health Policy* (2nd edn). London: Policy Press.

Berwick, D., Nolan, T. and Whittington, J. (2008) The Triple Aim: care, cost and quality. *Health Affairs* **27** (3), 759–769.

CQC (Care Quality Commission) (2015a) *Guidance for Providers on Meeting the Regulations*. London: CQC.

CQC (2015b) *Enforcement Policy*. London: CQC.

CQC (2015c) *The State of Health Care and Adult Social Care in England 2014/2015*. London: CQC.

CQC (2016a) *What We Do*. www.cqc.org.uk/content/what-we-do (accessed 19 February 2016).

CQC (2016b) *The Fundamental Standards*. www.cqc.org.uk/content/fundamental-standards (accessed 19 February 2016).

Carers UK (2015) Policy Briefing August 2015 http://socialwelfare.bl.uk/subject-areas/services-activity/social-work-care-services/carersuk/175424carers-uk-briefing-on-delay-to-cap-on-care-costs-implementation-august-2015.pdf (accessed 19 February 2016).

Chancellor of the Exchequer (2015) *Spending Review and Autumn Statement*. Cm 9162. London: The Stationery Office.

Cookson, R. (2005) Evidence-based policy making in health care: what it is and what it isn't. *Journal of Health Services Research and Policy* **10** (2), 118–121.

Davis, K., Stremikis, K., Squires, D. and Schoen C. (2014). *Mirror Mirror on the Wall: 2014 update*. New York: The Commonwealth Fund.

DH (Department of Health) (2011) *The Quarter: Quarter 1 2011/12*. London: DH.

DH (2014a) *The NHS Outcomes Framework 2015/2016*. London: DH.

DH (2014b) *The Adult Social Care Outcomes Framework 2015/2016*. London: DH.

DH (2015a) *The NHS Constitution*. London: DH.

DH (2015b) *Annual Assessment of the NHS Commissioning Board (known as NHS England) 2014–2015*. London: DH.

DH (2015c) *The Handbook to the NHS Constitution*. London: DH.

DH (2015d) *2015/16 Choice Framework*. London: DH.

DH (2016) *The Government's Mandate to NHS England for 2016–17*. London: DH.

DH and Department for Communities and Local Government (2016) *2016/17 Better Care Fund: Policy Framework*. London: DH.

Dobrow, M. J., Goel, V. and Upshur, R. E. G. (2004) Evidence-based health policy: context and utilisation. *Social Science and Medicine* **204** (58), 207–217.

Field, S. (2011) *NHS Future Forum: Summary report on proposed changes to the NHS*. London: DH.

Foot, C., Gilburt, H., Dunn, P., Jabbal, J., Seale, B., Goodrich, J., Buck, D. and Taylor, J. (2014) *People in Control of their Own Health and Care: The state of involvement*. London: The King's Fund.

Francis, R. (2010). *Independent Inquiry into Care Provided by Mid-Staffordshire NHS Foundation Trust January 2005–March 2009*. London: Stationery Office.

Francis, R. (2013) *Report of the Mid-Staffordshire NHS Foundation Trust Public Inquiry*. London: Stationery Office.

Future Forum (2011) *Integration: A report from the NHS Future Forum*. London: DH.

Glasby, J. and Dickinson, H. (2014) *Partnership Working in Health and Social Care: What is 'integrated care' and how can we deliver it?* (2nd edn). Bristol: The Policy Press.

Ham, C. (2009) *Health Policy in Britain* (6th edn). London: Palgrave.

Ham, C. and Alderwick, H. (2015) *Place-Based Systems of Care: A way forward for the NHS in England*. London: The King's Fund.

Ham, C., Baird, B., Gregory, S., Jabbal, J. and Alderwick H. (2015) *The NHS under the Coalition Government Part One: NHS reform*. London: The King's Fund.

Healthwatch (2014) *Healthwatch England Strategy 2014–2016*. www.healthwatch.co.uk/sites/healthwatch.co.uk/files/healthwatch-england-strategy_2014–2016.pdf (accessed 19 February 2016).

HM Government (2010) *The Coalition: Our programme for government.* London: The Stationery Office.

HM Treasury (2013) *Spending Round 2013.* London: The Stationery Office.

HM Treasury (2015) *Summer Budget 2015.* HC264. London: The Stationery Office

House of Commons Committee of Public Accounts (2015) *Care Quality Commission: Twelfth report of session 2015–16.* HC501. London: The Stationery Office.

Innvaer, S., Vist, G., Trommald, M. and Oxman, A. (2002) Health policy-makers' perceptions of their use of evidence: a systematic review. *Journal of Health Services Research and Policy* 7 (4), 239–244.

Ismail, S., Thorlby, R. and Holder, H. (2014) *Focus On: Social care for older people. Reductions in adult social services for older people in England.* London: The Health Foundation and the Nuffield Trust.

Keogh, B. (2013) *Review into the Quality of Care Provided by 14 Hospital Trusts in England: Overview report.* London: NHS England.

King's Fund (2015) *Devolution: What it means for health and social care in England.* London: King's Fund.

King's Fund, Health Foundation, and Nuffield Trust (2015) *The Spending Review: What does it mean for health and social care?* London: King's Fund.

Klein, R. (2013) *The New Politics of the NHS: From creation to reinvention* (7th edn). London: Radcliffe.

Monitor (2014) *Monitor's Strategy 2014–2017: Helping to redesign health care provision in England.* London: Monitor.

NAO (National Audit Office) (2012) *Health Care across the UK: A comparison of the NHS in England, Scotland, Wales and Northern Ireland.* London: NAO.

NAO (2014) *Adult Social Care in England: Overview.* London: NAO.

National Collaboration for Integrated Care and Support (2013) *Integrated Care and Support: Our shared commitment.* London: DH.

Needham, C. and Glasby, J. (2014) Taking stock of personalisation. In *Debates in Personalization.* Needham, C. and Glasby, J. (eds). (2014). Bristol: Policy Press, pp. 11–24.

New Labour (1997) *Because Britain Deserves Better.* www.politicsresources.net/area/uk/man/lab97.htm (accessed 19 February 2016).

NHS Choices (2015) *The NHS in England* www.nhs.uk/NHSEngland/thenhs/about/Pages/nhsstructure.aspx (accessed 19 February 2016).

NHS England (2014) *Five Year Forward View.* London: NHS England.

NHS England (2015a) *New Care Models: Vanguards – developing a blueprint for the future of NHS and care.* London: NHS England.

NHS England (2015b) *Our 2014/2015 Annual Report: Health and high quality care for all, now and for future generations.* London: NHS England.

NHS England (2015c) *Delivering the Forward View: NHS Planning guidance 2016/17–2020/21.* London: NHS England.

NMC (Nursing and Midwifery Council) (2015) *The Code: Professional standards of practice and behaviour for nurses and midwives.* London: NMC.

Organisation for Economic Co-operation and Development (OECD) (2015) *Focus on Health Spending.* Paris: OECD.

Pollock, A. M. (2004) *NHS plc: The privatisation of our health care.* London: Verso.

Purdy, S. (2010). *Avoiding Hospital Admissions: What does the research evidence say?* London: The King's Fund.

Robinson, S. (2011) Financing health care: funding systems and health care costs. In *Healthcare Management* (2nd edn), Walshe, K. and Smith, J. (eds). Maidenhead: Open University Press, pp. 37–62.

Secretary of State for Health (1989) *Working for Patients.* Cm 555. London: The Stationery Office.

Secretary of State for Health (1997) *The New NHS. Modern. Dependable.* Cm 380. London: The Stationery Office.

Iain Snelling

Secretary of State for Health (2000) *The NHS Plan*. Cm 4818-I. London: The Stationery Office.

Secretary of State for Health (2008) *High Quality Care for All: NHS next stage review final report*. Cm 7432. London: The Stationery Office.

Secretary of State for Health (2010) *Equity and Excellence: Liberating the NHS*. Cm 7881. London: The Stationery Office.

Snelling, P. C. (2016) Rounding on the smokers: the myth of evidence based (nursing) policy. In *Exploring Evidence-Based Practice: Debates and challenges in nursing*, Lipscomb, M. (ed.). London: Routledge, pp. 204–220.

Wanless, D. (2002) *Securing our Future: Taking a long term view*. London: HM Treasury.

Wanless, D. (2004) *Securing Good Health for the Whole Population*. London: HM Treasury.

Wanless, D., Appleby, A., Harrison, A. and Patel, D. (2007) *Our Future Health Secured?* London: King's Fund.

6

MANAGEMENT AND LEADERSHIP

Iain Snelling, Cathryn Havard and David Pontin

LEARNING OUTCOMES

After reading and reflecting on this chapter, you should be able to:

*   explain key issues in leadership and management and their application in a health care setting;
*   use conceptual and theoretical knowledge to support reflection on leadership and management practice;
*   appreciate critical perspectives on leadership and management.

INTRODUCTION

Increasingly, nurses are managers and leaders as well as deliverers of care. This doesn't mean that nurses are away at meetings all day, or spend all their time fulfilling bureaucratic functions. Management and leadership means much more than this. Being responsible and accountable for the actions of others in the health care team, which is a core function in the work of most nurses, means that you manage them.

The chapter is divided into three parts. In Part 1, we outline management and leadership and discuss how they are relevant for professional practice.

In Part 2, we explain how a manager running a department, ward or outpatient clinic, for example, might address their challenges. This will hopefully give you some scope to reflect on your experiences on placement.

In Part 3, we explore some critical perspectives on management and leadership.

PART 1: OUTLINING MANAGEMENT AND LEADERSHIP

Case 6.1

Lisa is a final-year student on placement on a surgical ward. She is worried about the ward. She observes that the shifts are very busy and chaotic. Although she can't point to anything that is really unsafe, or that the quality of care is not good enough, it just seems that it could be better. She has mentioned this to the ward manager, who sort of agreed, but said that there was no more money to improve things and that the staff 'should do their best'. If there were specific concerns they would be addressed, but otherwise, we should just get on with it. Although Lisa wants to concentrate on her nursing duties on placement, she reflects on the ward team and how the care it provides might be improved.

Why should I study management and leadership?

The environment for management and leadership in the NHS at all levels has changed significantly recently because of the events at Mid-Staffordshire NHS Foundation Trust. Between 2005 and 2009 the Trust consistently had a high mortality rate. Despite the poor quality of its care, which was subsequently held up to extraordinary scrutiny, the Trust was well rated by the Healthcare Commission, the quality regulator (which has been subsequently replaced by the Care Quality Commission), and achieved the coveted Foundation Trusts status, which gave it considerable autonomy. In 2008 concerns about the quality of its services led to a review by the Healthcare Commission (2009), which identified serious shortcoming. An inquiry was established by the Secretary of State, chaired by Robert Francis, which reported in 2010. The inquiry laid bare the extent of the failings in Mid-Staffordshire. It estimated that in the 3 years between 2005/6 and 2007/8 there had been 492 more deaths than expected, caused by poor care (Francis 2010, p. 361). The patient stories included in this report told of appalling standards of care, poor management with a focus on financial targets, a 'weak professional voice', a culture that tolerated poor standards and a lack of transparency. There were a number of recommendations specifically aimed at the Trust, and some aimed at levels in the system including regulators and the Department of Health. Subsequently a second inquiry, this time a Public Inquiry (which has a status in law) was held, also chaired by Robert Francis, to consider in more depth the 'commissioning, supervisory and regulatory bodies in relation to their monitoring role at Stafford Hospital with the objective of learning lessons about how failing hospitals are identified' (Francis 2013, p. 10).

Chapter 23 of the second inquiry considered nursing and chapter 24 considered leadership. Three key themes in chapter 24 were, first, that 'leadership and managerial skills are not the same, but both are required' (Francis 2013, p. 1545). Leadership skills in particular, needed to involve all levels in the organisation and staff at all levels needed to be empowered to provide the best possible care. Second, 'clinicians must be engaged to a far greater degree of engagement in leadership and management roles. The gulf between clinicians and management needs to be closed' (Francis 2013, p. 1545). Third, 'effective management and leadership development is essential to remedy these issues' (Francis 2013, p. 1545). The inquiry noted that a NHS Leadership Academy had already been established in 2012 and that it was already working towards improving leadership development processes in the NHS.

As part of the process for improving leadership development, the NHS Leadership Academy has published the Healthcare Leadership Model. This model 'describes the things you can see leaders doing at work and is organized in a way that helps everyone to see how they can develop as a leader' (NHS Leadership Academy 2013, p. 3). The model is organised around a series of statements, which will help you to reflect on your practice as a leader, and the NHS Leadership Academy's new range of development programmes supports leaders to develop their practice. The Healthcare Leadership Model is described in Box 6.1.

The significance of the events in Mid-Staffordshire for management and leadership are difficult to overstate. There were other implications too, including for nurse training and regulation, which are discussed in Chapter 1. As preparation for considering management and leadership, it would be very useful to be familiar with what happened at Mid-Staffordshire and the responses to it.

Why should you study leadership and management? The particular challenge here is to focus on the wider aspects of being a registered nurse. Students are asked: 'how do you think that you will *manage* in your future professional role?' In particular: 'how will you manage yourselves, manage other people, and manage in the context in which you work?' We will return to these questions later in the chapter.

We also want to encourage you to reflect on who inspires and challenges you – in other words, who you look to for leadership. In the following section, we look at ideas about leadership and management and how these relate to the work of newly qualified nurses. Our aim is to encourage you to think critically about your work and to identify the sorts of people skills needed to work with patients and clients, colleagues and other carers. We propose that an understanding of leadership and management practice and underpinning theories and concepts will help you develop greater personal, professional and organisational effectiveness.

How will this help me in my work?

Following initial registration as a nurse, many people's first priority is finding a job and settling in to a new role. This means finding out about the practical realities and responsibilities of the job. It also includes spending time and energy getting to know colleagues, the types of patient/client issues you will be facing and usual situations that arise. In short – managing yourself, managing others and managing in the context. You will find that there is an expectation within the workplace that the required competence level will be reached within an agreed time frame, and evidence will need to be produced to support the achievement of competence. Increasingly these will be prescribed by and linked with the requirements for the job, possibly within a preceptorship framework as discussed in Chapter 19.

Your progress towards achieving competence may be affected by the quality of preceptorship and leadership in your area and not all the skills and tasks may be achieved at the same point. However, there will come a time, perhaps 3 months, 6 months, or a year into the role, when you may find yourself in a situation where you not only have to manage events but function as a leader as well.

Leadership will increasingly be a key element of the role of all health care practitioners. The Healthcare Leadership Model, which was introduced briefly above and will be

Management deals with the pragmatic, logistical issues of resources, planning, monitoring and evaluating.

Leadership reminds you of why you wanted to become a nurse in the first place by kindling your aspirations and creativity.

The **authority of managers** comes from the formal roles they occupy within the organisation.

Influence is not formally linked to a role. Anyone may exert influence.

considered in more depth, applies to all staff and not only those in formal management positions.

Aren't management and leadership just different words for the same thing?

Activity 6.1

Consider the definitions of management and leadership given in the margin in relation to your placement experiences. Using the prompt questions below, take 5 minutes to write down as many examples as you can. Start with the most recent placement and work backwards in time.

- Who has inspired you and why?
- Who has challenged you? How were you challenged?
- Who has supported you? What did they do?

Look at your responses to Activity 6.1. Have you identified people in a formal **management** or **leadership** role in the organisation? There is a temptation to look only at people in authority roles for inspiration but you might find that you have been inspired by people who have recently qualified as a nurse or who have been nursing for a long time. They may not be nurses at all but workers in the wider health and social care team, perhaps a physiotherapist or a social worker. Who has challenged you? Perhaps it was a mentor who was a rigorous assessor but from whom you learned a great deal.

You may not be aware of the ways in which managers fulfil supporting roles. They are often working in the background, wrestling with targets and juggling resources. This buffering role of a manager provides shelter for clinical staff from wider internal and external forces, enabling them to focus on direct care activities. It is an essential function and often underestimated by nurses, especially if a manager is not highly visible. If you can, try to arrange to spend some time with a manager at your current placement and find out about their role and workload. It is important that you start to look outside your immediate practice area and widen your organisational horizons. Understanding the pressures and constraints of another person's role and work can be extremely helpful in promoting understanding and empathy rather than conflict and confrontation.

Distinctions between management and leadership

Rost (1993) identifies four main distinctions in the general literature between management and leadership (see Table 6.1).

The **authority of managers** comes from the formal roles they occupy within the organisation, which legitimates their power to act and requires other people to do as they are asked or told. **Influence** on the other hand is not formally linked to a role. Anyone may exert influence but they may not be able to compel someone to act. Leaders have to persuade people, either by word or deed, that they should follow their example or ideas; that is, there is a voluntary agreement to act. This is not to say that managers cannot be

TABLE 6.1 Distinctions between management and leadership

Management	Leadership
Authority relationship with others	Influence relationship with others
Roles classed as managers and subordinates	Roles classed as leaders and followers
Rationale is the production of goods/services for consumption and sale	Rationale is the intention to make observable changes in the work environment
The production of goods/services comes from the co-ordination of others' activities	The intention to make changes that reflect the shared purposes of colleagues or co-workers

Source: Rost 1993.

leaders, or vice versa. Effective managers are also leaders. Valerie Iles, for example, 'outlines a style of management . . . [called] real management . . . Real management straddles the divide drawn between management and leadership' (Iles 2005, p. 2). Whether individuals are acting as managers or leaders, or both, they do so in an organisational context, including the established structure.

The focus of the Healthcare Leadership Model is very much on leadership behaviour, rather than management competencies.

BOX 6.1 The Healthcare Leadership Model

The Healthcare Leadership Model was published by the NHS Leadership Academy in 2013 as part of the response to the Mid-Staffordshire NHS Foundation Trust inquiries. There was a leadership framework in place before the events at Mid-Staffordshire but the Francis Inquiry considered that it had insufficient emphasis on patient safety. The inquiry recommended improving the existing model with a greater emphasis on patient safety, and drawing up a list 'of all the qualities generally considered necessary for a good and effective leader. This could inform a list of competencies a leader would be expected to have' (Francis 2013, p. 1563).

The introduction to the model states that

> The Healthcare Leadership Model is to help those who work in health and care to become better leaders. It is useful for everyone – whether you have formal leadership responsibility or not, if you work in a clinical or other service setting, and if you work with a team of five people or 5,000. It describes the things you can see leaders doing at work and is organised in a way that helps everyone to see how they can develop as a leader. It applies equally to the whole variety of roles and care settings that exist within health and care.
>
> (NHS Leadership Academy 2013, p. 3)

In the model, leadership is understood as a role that all staff can take, rather than a role that is confined to management positions.

The model has nine dimensions of leadership behaviour. In each dimension there are a number of statements of behaviour, which 'are not meant to be answered with a simple yes or no. Instead they should help you explore your intentions and motivations, and see where your strengths and limitations lie' (NHS Leadership Academy 2013, p. 3). The behaviours are given at four levels: essential, proficient, strong and exemplary. The model doesn't give competencies to be 'achieved' but supports a continuous process of critical reflection about your leadership. The nine dimensions are:

- inspiring shared purpose;
- leading with care;
- evaluating information;
- connecting our service;
- sharing the vision;
- engaging the team;
- holding to account;
- developing capability;
- influencing for results.

As an example, the statements below are those in the 'inspiring shared purpose' domain, at the essential level. Inspiring shared purpose means 'valuing a service ethos', being 'curious about how to improve services and patient care' and 'behaving in a way that reflects the principles and values of the NHS' (NHS Leadership Academy 2013, p. 5).

The 'essential' statements of behaviour are:

- Do I act as a role model for belief in and commitment to the service?

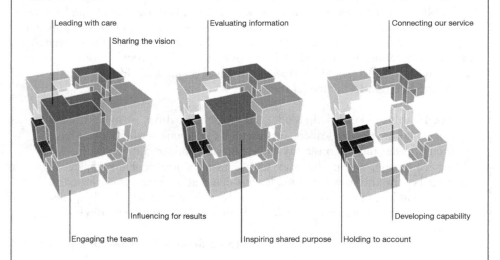

FIGURE 6.1 Healthcare Leadership Model

Source: NHS Leadership Academy 2013.

- Do I focus on how what I do contributes to and affects patient care or other service users?
- Do I enable colleagues to see the wider meaning in what they do?

The Healthcare Leadership Model will help you consider your own leadership behaviours and also to consider the leadership behaviours of others. The behaviours might also be used in training materials, appraisals or in person specifications in job descriptions. There is a self-assessment tool available for you to use, and a 360-degree appraisal tool.

The Healthcare Leadership Model's dimensions are shown in an image, with 'inspiring shared purpose' at the centre.

Activity 6.2

Download the Healthcare Leadership Model and consider again your answers to Activity 6.1 above when you considered who has inspired, challenged and supported you. Can you recognise the behaviours you observed in the people you considered from placement experiences in the Healthcare Leadership Model behaviour statements?

Organisational structures and roles

All health care organisations have a formal structure. It would be helpful if you could obtain a copy of the structure of an organisation you are working in or have worked in. You might find one on the website, or get one from the human resources (HR) department. The complicated work of the organisation will be organised very carefully so that all required tasks are completed. The structure shows how individuals in key roles work together so that everything that needs to be done is done effectively.

The organisational structure will have a number of levels. Usually it is shown from the top down, with the board of directors, and the Chief Executive and Chair at the top. Much of the literature about management and leadership is concerned with the activities of people who 'do' management and leadership, and perhaps have the word 'manager' or 'director' in their job title. In health care much of the management and leadership work is undertaken by clinicians, including nurses, many of whom maintain clinical practice. These roles, which combine management and leadership responsibility with clinical practice are sometimes called 'hybrid' roles and include ward managers, matrons and clinical directors. Sometimes, moving into these roles causes some difficulty in reconciling the clinical and managerial elements of the role (Croft *et al.* 2015) but it is important to acknowledge that management, as well as leadership, which was discussed above, is a professional issue as well as an issue for managers.

This chapter approaches management and leadership as activities and roles as part of understanding clinical practice rather than something concerned with activities outside clinical practice. You might find it useful though to consider what happens at the top of an organisation and attending a board meeting is a good way of gaining insight about how the organisation works.

BOX 6.2 Attending a board meeting

You will have experienced team management and operational management in your placements. To get a picture of how the top level of management and leadership works, you can attend a board meeting as a member of the public. At least some parts of board meetings are held in public; confidential issues are dealt with at the end of the meeting after the public has been excluded. Board papers are also available; agendas, minutes and supporting reports. These will be available on an organisation's website or from the chief executive's office.

PART 2: EXPLAINING MANAGEMENT AND LEADERSHIP

In this section, management and leadership will be explained in more detail. This will be structured around four areas:

1   managing self;
2   managing and leading others;
3   managing resources; and
4   managing in the context.

Managing self

Two related issues frequently identified as development needs are improving time management and coping with stress.

Time management

You can only do so much in the time available. The answer to pressure of tasks building up is not to increase the time available, for example by staying late, arriving early, or skipping breaks. To make the most effective use of your time, you need to do two things: prioritise your tasks and then undertake each task as efficiently as possible.

The first issue to consider is prioritisation – doing the right things. Tasks might be categorised in two dimensions: their urgency and their importance. A common problem is that urgent tasks, even relatively unimportant ones, take precedence over important ones. The grid in Table 6.2 suggests some strategies for prioritising tasks based on this categorisation.

There are some pitfalls in prioritising:

* Your personal priorities may not be the same as others.
* Staff priorities may not be patient priorities and vice versa.
* There may be different views within teams.
* There may not be anyone available to delegate to.

Prioritising tasks is not only key to managing yourself, it is also important in planning and delivering care.

152

TABLE 6.2 Prioritising strategies

Classification	Important	Not important
Urgent	Do it	Delegate it
Not urgent	Plan it	Leave it

The Health and Safety Executive defines **stress** as 'the adverse reaction people have to excessive pressure or other types of demand placed on them at work'.

Case 6.1 (continued)

Lisa observed that the ward was 'busy and chaotic'. She made a list of tasks that staff undertook routinely during their work and identified those that she thought they might be able to do more quickly without reducing the quality and those where if they had more time, the quality would be increased. She also used the urgent/important grid. Her first example was the handover between shifts. She marked this as urgent and important, but felt that it could be done more quickly if it was better organised.

For many tasks, there is a trade-off between time taken and quality. It takes longer to do something well than it does to do it badly. That may be true up to a point, but it is likely that after a while extra time devoted to a task adds very little, if any additional quality. Quality might even begin to fall after a while. Conversations or meetings might fall into this category. If you are involved in a meeting you might find that although it begins with energy and focus, after a while people become tired and think about other things they might be doing. New agenda items are not dealt with as well. Later still the meeting might become ineffective, as people leave or begin to get irritated with others' behaviour under the pressure of time.

Stress

The Health and Safety Executive (HSE 2015) defines **stress** as 'the adverse reaction people have to excessive pressure or other types of demand placed on them at work'. Some pressure at work is helpful – it stimulates and motivates – but after an optimum level of performance is reached, additional pressure reduces performance, and can lead to stress. According to the HSE, about 1 in 5 people find their work either very or extremely stressful. The primary risks for stress at work are:

- the demands of your job;
- your control over your work;
- the support you receive from managers and colleagues;
- your relationships at work;
- your role in the organisation;
- change and how it is managed.

(Mackay *et al.* 2004, pp. 91–112)

The HSE has developed management standards to cover these six areas and has a number of resources available on their website to support organisations to achieve best practice. For example, the standards relating to demands of the job are:

- employees indicate that they are able to cope with the demands of their jobs; and
- systems are in place locally to respond to any individual concerns.

(HSE 2009, p. 7)

The following 'should be happening' in organisations:

- the organisation provides employees with adequate and achievable demands in relation to the agreed hours of work;
- people's skills and abilities are matched to the job demands;
- jobs are designed to be within the capabilities of employees; and
- employees' concerns about their work environment are addressed.

(HSE 2009, p. 7)

One cause of stress that is particularly relevant to nursing and other health care professionals is emotional labour (Sawbridge and Hewison 2011, 2013). The term emotional labour was coined by Hochschild, who defined it as 'the management of feeling to create a publicly observable facial and bodily display' (Hochschild 2012, p. 7). This involves the suppression of 'feeling in order to sustain the outward countenance that produces the proper state of mind in others' (Hochschild 2012, p. 7). Hochschild was writing, originally in 1993, about flight attendants who are expected to maintain a civil and professional demeanour whatever the circumstances and provocation. Many workers will undertake emotional labour, but surely none more so than health care workers. Supporting nurses in their emotional labour is difficult, until the stress caused by excessive and unrecognised emotional labour causes illness (Sawbridge and Hewison 2013). Despite the difficulties of supporting nurses, which seem mainly to do with time and costs, it is an issue that is beginning to receive more attention. If you are feeling under stress, you should first try to understand the cause, and then discuss it with your manager.

Managing and leading others

It is when thinking about the way you relate to others that the distinction between management and leadership becomes most important. An element of the distinction relates to formal authority and accountability arrangements within the organisation. A managerial relationship is formal – each employee should be clear about who their line manager is. A leadership relationship is less formal.

The discussion about management and leadership in Part 1 identified that both are essentially to do with people. Management and leadership are social sciences drawing on a range of other disciplines, including sociology and psychology. This section will draw on a range of theories, but first it will be useful to consider what management theory is, and how it will help you think about your role as a nurse.

Think about infection control. There is a great deal of knowledge about how infections are spread, and how health care professionals can reduce the spread of infection. The development of knowledge in this area has a number of clear implications that for practical purposes are true, for example, in emphasising the importance of hand hygiene. You know what you should do (even though you may not need to know all the fine details of microbiology) and you know that if you follow the basic rules, the chances of you being responsible for the spread of infection will be reduced. In the sections below, theories will be introduced about, for example, how teams develop. The theories will have some key practical implications.

However, the theories are not 'true' in the same sense that theories about basic science are. Research in management and leadership does not identify basic truths, it offers likely explanations. Even if a theory offers a clear prescription, you should think about it and apply it to your situation and your experience. Application to practice will not necessarily give the results you want. For many reasons your practice may be more complex than the prescription might suggest. Applying theory to practice requires critical reflection, rather than just knowing what to do.

Delegation and accountability

Within any structure, the process of delegation is the key to effective provision of services. The chief executive is accountable for all the service that an organisation provides but he or she cannot be in charge of everything. So, responsibilities are **delegated** to individuals, who are **competent**, along with the **accountability** to achieve specific **objectives**, and the appropriate **authority**.

The highlighted terms are all important. Simple definitions are given in the margin. You might find it interesting to consider what you understand by these terms, as they are applied to your practice. Many have a specific professional meaning and application, as discussed in Chapter 2.

We have identified delegation in a broad and simple sense. There are many elements of good practice in delegation. Pearce (2006) has developed a 10-step guide for effective delegation, which is explained in Box 6.3. These steps are aimed at people who are delegating, but your experience of delegation may be as the person to whom the task is delegated. It should be clear that the process that Pearce outlines is mutually supportive and developmental, not just someone getting rid of their work. The principles apply to a chief executive delegating responsibility for nursing issues to the director of nursing, or a ward sister delegating a specific task to a staff nurse, or a third-year student nurse delegating care to others in their final placement.

Professional issues and positions

The Code (clause 11) states that you are accountable for your decisions to delegate tasks and duties to other people.

To achieve this, you must:

- only delegate tasks and duties that are within the other person's scope of competence, making sure that they fully understand your instructions;
- make sure that everyone you delegate tasks to is adequately supervised and supported so they can provide safe and compassionate care; and
- confirm that the outcome of any task you have delegated to someone else meets the required standard.

(NMC 2015, p. 10)

There are a number of colleagues who you could delegate to:

- someone who has an *equivalent* qualification, role and function (that is, someone from your own peer group);

Delegation is the process of passing on responsibility for a task to another person, in an agreed planned way.

A **competent** person is able to perform a specific task. What a person needs to know and understand and the skill required to perform a specific task are defined in a competency.

Accountability is individual responsibility for behaviour or the achievement of a specific objective. Accountability should include reference to the person or body to whom an individual is accountable.

Objectives are explicit statements of tasks to be performed or outcomes achieved.

Authority is an acknowledged right to influence or direct people. It is often related to the idea of power. Considering authority leads to questions about how the right to influence is acknowledged and where the limits of authority lie.

BOX 6.3 Ten steps to effective delegation

Step 1   Decide what you delegate.
Step 2   Be clear what you delegate.
Step 3   Decide who you delegate to.
Step 4   Inform other team members.
Step 5   Decide how to brief subordinates.
Step 6   Decide how to guide and develop subordinates.
Step 7   Assign responsibility and authority.
Step 8   Monitor performance.
Step 9   Give feedback.
Step 10   Evaluate the experience.

(Pearce 2006, p. 9)

- someone who has a *different* qualification, role and function, for example, doctors and other health care professionals, health care assistants, support workers, carers and students;
- someone who has *no formal* qualifications, for example patients and informal carers.

Assessing competence is very important in making sure that delegation is safe and effective.

Activity 6.3

Think of anything that you know you are good at – sport, hobby or activity.

- How do you know this?
- How could other people know this?
- What evidence would confirm this?

Now apply this to yourself in a work context and link with your self-assessment of current skill level. As mentioned previously, it is important that you are competent in the tasks being delegated so if you identify that there are gaps in your knowledge/skills, you will need to make a plan to fill them. Now apply this to working with other staff. When you do not know them or their background you may need to make an evaluation and assessment of them by:

- asking questions about their qualifications and asking for proof or evidence;
- exploring their previous experience;
- asking them to explain or demonstrate the elements of a skill or procedure that you wish them to undertake;
- observing their practice;
- evaluating standards of care.

156

This gets more complicated in practice, because of a range of contextual and cultural issues related to delegation including:

- high workload;
- fast throughput;
- variously qualified staff;
- variable numbers of staff;
- increasing ethnic diversity in staff and patients;
- increasing public expectations.

Because of the complexity of health care, it is crucial that registered nurses are able to critically appraise and evaluate evidence (from a range of sources) and supervise and evaluate the performance of others and self.

'A **team** is a small number of people with complementary skills who are committed to a common purpose, performance goals and approach for which they hold themselves mutually accountable' (Katzenbach and Smith 1993, p. 45).

Objectives

Setting objectives is particularly important. Thinking about what is to be delegated is the first step in deciding who it should be delegated to and whether they are competent and have the authority to carry it out. A popular guide for objectives is that they should be SMART:

- *Specific*: it should be possible to identify whether the objective has been achieved or not.
- *Measurable*: how the achievement is to be measured should be clear.
- *Achievable*: the objective should be achievable, which is not the same as saying it should be easy to achieve. Whether it is achieved will depend in large part on the performance of the person who has been set the objective.
- *Relevant*: to both the staff member and the organisation.
- *Time-bound*: to be achieved within a defined period.

Team working

Health care emphasises team working, and particularly interprofessional teams providing care. The terms 'clinical team', or 'management team' are often used, and 'project teams' are often formed for specific purposes. So, developing an understanding of how teams can improve their effectiveness is an important area for management research. This is important for those who lead teams, but also for those who are team members. The first issue to consider is 'what is a team?', and 'how does it differ from a collection of individuals, or a group?'

There is a great deal of research about team working that can be described only superficially here. Four areas of theory are briefly presented and an activity will ask you to consider how they may help you to understand better the development of teams. The four areas of theory are:

1 The team performance curve (Katzenbach and Smith 1993).
2 Stages of team development (Tuckman 1965).
3 Team roles (Belbin 1993).
4 Real teams and co-acting groups (Lyubovnikova *et al.* 2015).

157

I. Snelling, C. Havard and D. Pontin

Case 6.1 (continued)

Lisa used the team performance curve model to consider where the ward team might be on the team performance curve. She thought that it might be at the 'potential team' stage. There is a need for a team with 'a common purpose, performance goals and approach'. Issues like performance goals (standards) are discussed at ward meetings, but the discussions don't often seem to lead to new ideas. Some staff say that their job is just to complete their own work, suggesting that the team has not established mutual accountability.

FIGURE 6.2
The team
performance curve

Source: Adapted
from Katzenbach
and Smith 1993.

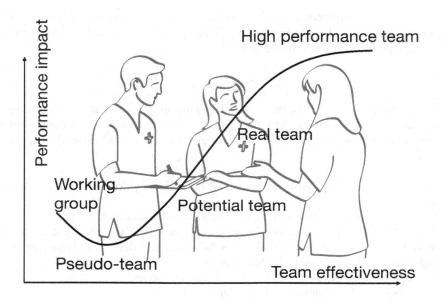

TABLE 6.3 Characteristics of identified points on team performance curve

Working group	No significant need that would require it to become a team Members interact primarily to share information Makes decisions to help each individual to perform within his or her area of responsibility No common purpose or joint-work products
Pseudo-team	There could be a need that would require it to become a team, but is not trying to achieve it
Potential team	There is a need that requires it to become a team, and it is trying to achieve it Requires more clarity of purpose, goals or work-products Has not established collective accountability
Real team	Team members have complementary skills and are equally committed to a common purpose, goals, and a working approach for which they hold themselves mutually accountable
High performing team	In addition to the features of the real team, has members who are deeply committed to one another's personal growth and success

The team performance curve helps teams to develop but it does not suggest that these are necessary stages in development. Tuckman's model (1965) suggests that during their establishment, new teams need to go through four phases before they become effective. Some teams that you are a member of may have been established for a long time before you joined them, but high turnover or a change in role may, in effect, push a team backwards in its development. The four stages are:

1 Forming
2 Storming
3 Norming
4 Performing.

The forming stage relates to that time when team members are getting to know each other and the purpose of the team. After this has been accomplished, teams develop into the storming phase, characterised by conflict. As team members get to know each other better they may be more willing to give opinions, especially about the task or purpose of the team. There may be an element of 'jockeying for position'. As these conflicts are resolved, the team will develop a way of working. This is the norming stage, where attention will be given to the group rather than the task. Finally, the team will develop to the performing stage, where it begins to work effectively.

TABLE 6.4 Team roles

Team roles	Description
Plant	Creative, imaginative, unorthodox, solves difficult problems
Resource-investigator	Extrovert, enthusiastic, communicative Explores opportunities Develops contacts
Co-ordinator	Mature, confident, a good chairperson Clarifies goals, promotes decision-making, delegates well
Shaper	Challenging, dynamic, thrives on pressure Has the drive and courage to overcome obstacles
Monitor evaluator	Sober, strategic and discerning Sees all options Judges accurately
Teamworker	Co-operative, mild, perceptive, and diplomatic Listens, build, averts friction, calms the waters
Implementer	Disciplined, reliable, conservative and efficient Turns ideas into practical actions
Completer	Painstaking, conscientious, anxious Searches out errors and omissions Delivers on time
Specialist	Single-minded, self-starting, dedicated Provides knowledge and skills in rare supply

Source: Belbin 1993.

Belbin's (1993) analysis concentrated on roles within a team. She identified that the most successful teams had nine identifiable roles. There are a number of questionnaires available, which can help people to identify what their naturally preferred roles are, but it is important to remember that these are roles and not people acting helplessly in the only role they are able to fulfil. Being aware of the need for different roles can help team members to adapt their natural behaviour. It does not mean that every team has to have at least nine members, each able to act in their own natural preference. The roles are listed in Table 6.4 with the descriptions given to them by Belbin (1993, p. 22).

Lyubovnikova *et al.* (2015) used data from the NHS staff survey to consider whether 'real teams' produce better results than 'co-acting groups', also called pseudo-teams. In the staff survey, staff were asked whether they worked in a team, and for those who reported that they did (the vast majority), three further questions were asked relating to whether the team had clear objectives, whether team members had to work closely together, and whether the team regularly discussed its effectiveness and how it could be improved (reflexivity). Those who answered yes to all three questions were categorised as working in a 'real team'. Those who answered no to at least one were categorised as working in a co-acting group. Staff also reported a range of other variables relating to their working experiences. The results of the study showed that staff working in real teams 'witnessed fewer errors and incidents, experienced fewer work related injuries and illness, were less likely to be victims of violence and harassment, and were less likely to intend to leave their current employment' (Lyubovnikova *et al.* 2015, p. 929). Organisations that had higher proportions of staff reporting real team membership had lower levels of patient mortality and lower levels of staff sickness. Each of the three variables had strong effects in the analysis, suggesting that these three characteristics of team working (shared objectives, close working relationships, and reflexivity) were associated with better patient care.

Case 6.1 (continued)

Lisa has observed that discussions at team meetings about standards didn't often lead to new ideas. One area where there was often progress was in infection control where there was a link nurse who was very passionate. Sue thought that she might be acting as a 'specialist' and that such a role might be missing for other areas where improvements could be made.

Activity 6.4

Having considered some ideas relating to teams and illustrated them through the case study, reflect on whether any of these ideas help you to understand any team that you are part of. For example, have you been part of a new team that has experienced conflict fairly soon after its establishment? Can you think what your preferred team role is and can you identify others' through observing their behaviours? You may find that different models are useful for different types of teams.

RESEARCH FOCUS 6.1

There is a substantial literature available on nurse leadership specifically, and more generally on clinical leadership. As in leadership and management studies, research on nurse leadership can come from both the quantitative and qualitative traditions. Leadership research in the quantitative tradition generally investigates statistical associations between a number of leadership variables relating, for example, to leadership style, or team working variables, and some measures of patient quality outcomes such as mortality or patient satisfaction. Wong et al. (2013) undertook a systematic review of studies to update a similar review they published in 2007. In total the two reviews identified 20 articles reporting original research, which examined statistically the relationship between nursing leadership and patient outcomes. All except five were conducted in America, and none in the UK. In all of the studies except one, leadership was assessed by asking followers to rate their formal leader. A number of different leadership theories were used to assess leadership, and outcomes were also assessed in different ways. In total 43 different statistical relationships between a measure of leadership and a measure of quality were included in the research reviewed. Twenty-seven demonstrated a significant relationship between leadership and improved quality, and one had a significant relationship in the opposite direction. Despite differences in the way that leadership and quality are measured across the studies, there is strong evidence linking nurse leadership with improved quality of care.

In the qualitative tradition, leadership is examined in more depth through methods such as interviews and observations. For example Martin and Waring (2013) interviewed 23 clinical leaders in 2 operating theatres, who had recently been given enhanced leadership roles and most of whom were nurses. While the leaders understood good leadership principles, in practice their ability to make changes was constrained by the existing managerial and professional hierarchies – in other words although they were formally leaders and understood how to lead, they were really only able to make changes which the existing general management or professional (medical) wanted. In the title of the paper, these leaders experienced 'constrained realities'.

In this research focus we have only examined one systematic review and one qualitative research report. Other research is referred to in the text of this chapter. There is plenty of research for you to examine as you develop your understanding of leadership. The NHS Leadership Academy has published a paper examining some research that supports the Healthcare Leadership Model (Storey and Holti 2013).

Managing resources

Both you and the people you work with are resources that have to be carefully managed, but in this section finance is considered. Budget management is an important area for NHS managers. 'Keeping within my budget' is regarded as a very important objective. In recent years, there has been significant pressure on NHS budgets and this looks set to continue. Even if a service manager considers their budget adequate and does not need to find ways of saving money, it remains important that a service runs efficiently. Inefficient services deny the opportunity to invest resources elsewhere. In this section, some of the key issues of financial management will be identified, which will hopefully help you to develop some insight into some of the actions and decisions that your managers might make.

If a service reduces its costs by buying the same things (staff and non-staff) for less money, it becomes more **economic**.

What is a budget?

Each service will have a budget, which is the amount of money available to it to spend in delivering a service. The budget should give a reasonable plan for the year in setting out some assumptions about what might happen. For example, a certain amount of sickness might be expected in a ward, or a certain number of admissions may be planned. In some cases, if one of the assumptions made when setting the budget proves incorrect during the year, adjustments can be made. If, for example, there are more admissions than planned, more money may be available to cover the extra costs incurred. However, in some other instances there may not be any more money available and therefore the area that holds the budget will have to try to reduce spending if there are signs in the year that spending is too high. Managing the budget is a problem that many managers find difficult, because it often involves making difficult choices. One issue that has had a high profile recently is the cost of agency staff, which has increased substantially. New rules were introduced by regulators (Monitor and Trust Development Agency 2015) to reduce the costs of agency staff but this issue cost a great deal of money. If the cost of agency staff goes up, which causes a budget overspend, this is likely to be a major issue. The organisation will need to decide to respond to this sort of cost pressure by, for example, agreeing to overspend, limiting the use of agency staff, or finding savings elsewhere. Pursuing financial control was one of the main causes of the appalling quality provided at Mid-Staffordshire NHS Foundation Trust, so issues like this are exceptionally sensitive and politically charged.

Financial management and control

How do managers spend the money available to deliver the services they are responsible for? An organisation will have strict processes for controlling how money is spent, to make sure that it is spent wisely and to prevent its managers spending too much. A key issue for financial control is levels of authorisation; who does the organisation allow to spend its money? Usually this will be a person who holds the budget, but for some items of expenditure additional authorisation might be required. The budget holder is responsible for ensuring that the budget is not overspent, and is used for the purposes for which it is intended. In practice some budgets are likely to be overspent. Decisions to address this should only be taken when the causes are known and the consequences of reducing spending in that budget area have been assessed.

Value for money

Value for money is a term that you will come across from time to time; another related term is cost-effectiveness. Producing as much benefit as possible from the money available (money, which, it should not be forgotten, comes from all of us in tax) is an important objective of management. How can you judge whether you can improve the cost-effectiveness of your service? The model below describes the NHS Production Pathway (Wanless *et al.* 2007, p. 11). It shows how cost-effectiveness measures how money produces benefits. This is broken down into three separate stages:

- The money *'buys resources'*. For the NHS these are mainly staff, but also equipment and supplies. Cost-effectiveness can be improved here by reducing the cost of these resources, becoming more **economic**.

- *The resources are used to produce activities*, which might, for example, be nursing interventions, or district nurse visits. Cost-effectiveness might be improved here by producing the same output with fewer resources (or more output with the same resources), which might mean, for example, fewer staff, becoming more **efficient or productive**.
- *The outputs of the process are not goals in themselves*. Goals are expressed in terms of outcomes, which in general are described as 'health' but might also include other desirable outcomes such as 'independence' or 'safety'. Cost-effectiveness might be improved here by producing the same outcome with fewer activities, becoming more **effective**.

If a service produces the same amount of work with fewer resources (staff and non-staff) it becomes more **efficient or productive**.

If a service gets better at achieving its goals, it becomes more **effective**.

The model is shown in Figure 6.3.

The important thing is that cost-effectiveness is maximised. Attempts to improve one part of the model may not increase cost-effectiveness overall.

Case 6.1 (continued)

Lisa thought about this model when a ward meeting was discussing how the ward could make savings, and someone had suggested that they could save on food because a lot was wasted. If the right portions were given to all patients, which resulted in less food being sent from the kitchen, there would be an increase in efficiency. However, the purpose of food is to maintain and enhance nutritional status, and a lot of wasted food may suggest that this was not being achieved. Perhaps increasing the quality of the food (and its cost) and helping patients to eat their food if they were having difficulty would lead to more food being eaten, and better achievement of the goal. In that case the process would become less economic and less efficient. It would become more effective. It would be difficult to know if the whole process had become more or less cost-effective.

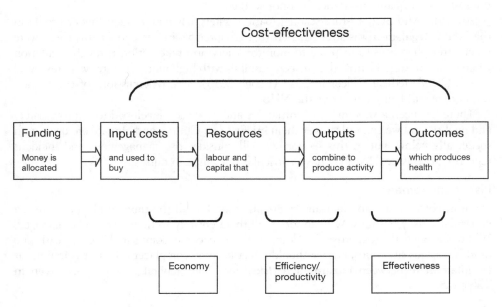

FIGURE 6.3
The NHS production pathway

I. Snelling, C. Havard and D. Pontin

Managing in the context

In this section, the context in which you work will be discussed. This is important because managers and leaders have to work in context – that is they must work within organisational systems and priorities, and other elements of their context. In the short term these elements of context are likely to be fixed and managers are likely to have to work within constraints. In the longer term priorities may change. The major issue of context considered here is the importance of leaders and managers taking responsibility for safety and quality.

Safety and quality

In the second half of the 1990s the realisation that health care organisations harmed people avoidably in the course of treating them began to be widely understood. In the NHS, clinical governance, introduced in 1997, established a statutory duty for quality of care. Previously the main duties on health services in the NHS were not to spend over their allocation.

Clinical governance created a set of systematic ways in which it should become increasingly difficult for an organisation to give poor quality service. As clinical governance was being developed over a number of years, some reports addressing scandals gave the issue added importance and urgency. The most important of these were the poor outcomes achieved in paediatric heart surgery at the Bristol Royal Infirmary between 1984 and 1995 (Kennedy 2001) and Dr Harold Shipman's murder of 215 patients between 1975 and 1998 (Smith 2002). In Bristol, although individual doctors were disciplined by the General Medical Council, it was the failings of the system that were identified as the main cause of the problem. In Shipman's case, although the deaths were the result of his action, the system he worked within allowed him to continue and he was only caught when he forged a patient's will. Clinical governance attempts to create *systems* of care, which reduce the likelihood of poor quality. The events at Mid-Staffordshire showed that the systems for quality assurance had not worked.

After the Mid-Staffordshire scandal, patient safety has had a much higher profile in the NHS. Regulation was strengthened (see Chapter 5) and as part of this there were much stronger processes in place to monitor safety and take action through regulation when concerns were identified. Fourteen hospitals with high mortality rates were reviewed by the Chief Medical Officer in 2013 (Keogh 2013). The repercussions of the Francis Inquiry are still being felt across the NHS.

There has been a wide range of initiatives and processes developed to improve safety and quality, and we can only cover them briefly here. Culture and climate are dealt with specifically below, but in this section we will consider risk management and incident reporting, two issues that may have particular relevance to nurses.

Risk management

Hazards, both natural and man-made, are all around us all the time and health care is a particularly risky business. We cannot avoid them entirely so they have to be managed. When we have the expertise for doing this we become comfortable, even with the most hazardous situations, but we should never become complacent. First it is important to differentiate between **hazards** and **risks**, and some general examples are given in Table 6.5.

TABLE 6.5 Examples of hazards and risks

Hazard	Risk
Wet floor	Slips and falls
Electrical equipment	Electrocution; burns
Hot water/baths/drinks	Scalds
Body fluids	Infection; cross-infection
Invasive procedures, e.g. catheterisation; biopsy	Infection; trauma
Surgical interventions	Peri- and post-operative complications
Blood transfusion	Adverse reactions
Sharps/needles	Injury; infection; cross-infection; inadvertent inoculation
Medicines	Errors; adverse drug reactions
Violent/abusive patients or visitors	Damage or trauma to staff
Major incidents/terrorism	Damage to property

Risk assessment is a systematic and effective method of identifying risks and determining the most cost-effective means to minimise or remove them (NPSA 2008).

Hazards are always present – you cannot just avoid them so hazard awareness is imperative and reporting of actual and potential hazards essential. What is needed is a strategy to manage and minimise risk and this starts with making an effective assessment.

Although managing risks is important in the provision of safe care, it is possible that an organisation can go too far. Managing risks has a cost, as well as implications for the actions of staff. In order to strike the right balance organisations will use systematic **risk assessment** processes.

Risks are assessed against two dimensions:

1   *Impact.* If the risk that has been identified actually happens, how serious would it be?
2   *Likelihood.* What are the chances of the risk happening?

These dimensions can be shown as a matrix (see Figure 6.4).

Assessing risk in this way will help managers to decide what to do about it. If a risk is very unlikely to happen, and even if it did the impact would be low, it might be decided that no action should be taken. If a risk is likely to happen, and if it did the impact would be very serious, the organisation may put great effort and significant resources into reducing the chances that it will happen, and reducing its impact if it does.

	Low likelihood	High likelihood
High impact		
Low impact		

FIGURE 6.4 Risk assessment matrix

Activity 6.5

Identify risks from your experience (in your personal and professional life) and use the matrix in Figure 6.4 to assess them.

While it is easy to determine priorities between low likelihood/low impact and high likelihood/high impact, the other two quadrants in the matrix are more difficult. What is more important: a risk that is unlikely to happen but with high impact, or one that is likely to happen but with low impact?

A systematic process for assessing and prioritising risk is required. If the impact and likelihood are given a numeric score against criteria to make sure that the scoring is consistent, then multiplying the scores together will give a single risk score. This will allow comparisons to be made, and help organisations decide where to put the most effort and resources to manage risk. Individual organisations will have in place detailed processes and procedures for identifying, assessing and managing risks.

Incident reporting and root cause analysis

There will also be procedures for incident reporting. Learning from adverse events is a key process for improving patient safety. Individual organisations have had their own incident-reporting systems for some time, but in 2003 a National Reporting and Learning System (NRLS) was established. This system developed a national database of incidents, and details for individual organisations in England and Wales are available through the NRLS website (NRLS 2015).

After a serious incident or near miss, there may be a root cause analysis (RCA). As the name suggests a RCA is an in-depth investigation into the causes of an incident. NHS England has published guidance (NHS England 2015), which, like the incident-reporting information discussed above was originally developed by the National Patient Safety Agency that was abolished in 2012.

One of the first policy documents in the NHS to deal with organisational learning regarding patient safety was *An Organisation with a Memory* (DH 2000). This report acknowledged that there were two ways of considering human error. The first and most common way is the 'person-centred' approach where an investigation will concentrate on finding out where individual errors were made. The second approach is the systems approach. 'This approach starts from the premise that humans are fallible and that errors are inevitable, even in the best-run organisations' (DH 2000, p. 21). When considering the causes of incidents the systems approach looks beyond finding an individual error and considers context and system conditions. One way of illustrating how system conditions can cause errors is called the 'Swiss cheese model' (Reason 1997) shown in Figure 6.5.

The model shows a number of slices of Swiss cheese, each one representing a defence against adverse incidents. These defences might include procedures for checking the administration of drugs or continuing professional development for staff. In different conditions, the holes in some of the slices will move and close, and open up elsewhere. For example, in a very busy ward with some staff missing, some procedures may be rushed because of pressures. One of the slices of Swiss cheese might relate to 'busyness'. This would be an example of a latent condition, a feature of the system, which in normal times doesn't cause error. Sometimes though, these latent conditions might shift and become more relevant in different contexts, and so in the illustration offered by the Swiss cheese model, the holes line up so light can be shined through all the defences. This is when an incident occurs, which could lead to catastrophic loss, including the death of a patient or patients.

The system approach led some to suggest a 'no blame' culture – that is to say seeing all errors as the responsibility of the system rather than individuals. However, it is important to maintain accountability. Although it may not be appropriate to find someone

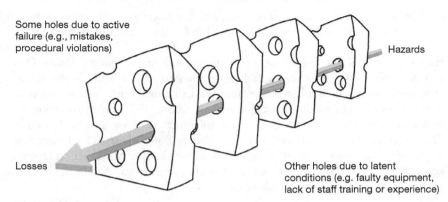

The 'Swiss cheese' model of accident causation

Some holes due to active failure (e.g., mistakes, procedural violations)

Hazards

Losses

Other holes due to latent conditions (e.g. faulty equipment, lack of staff training or experience)

Successive layers of defences, barriers and safeguards

FIGURE 6.5
The Swiss cheese model

Source: Department of Health 2000.

to blame for a specific incident, neither is it appropriate to have no sense of individual accountability. A 'just' culture might be an alternative. This is one element of an informed culture, which promotes safety. The other elements are as follows:

- A *reporting culture* – where people will report errors and incidents, including 'near misses'.
- A *just culture* – where individual accountability is balanced with recognition of system factors that contributed.
- A *flexible culture* – where staff are able to respond flexibly to changing demands.
- A *learning culture* – where there is a clear will, and processes, for the organisation to learn and adapt, from its own experiences and experiences elsewhere.

(Reason 1997, DH 2000)

Culture is discussed in more detail below.

The focus on patient safety in the last 20 years or so has drawn on the literature and research from 'high-reliability' industries such as the airline industry and the nuclear industry. The patient safety movement in the English NHS has been given great support from Martin Bromily, an airline pilot whose wife Elaine died in 2005 during a routine operation. He founded the Clinical Human Factors Group, a charitable organisation committed to making healthcare safer, drawing on a systems approach to patient safety. Their website (http://chfg.org/) contains excellent resources.

Activity 6.6

Watch the video on YouTube called 'Just a routine operation'.

- How did you feel when watching the video?
- What do you think are the key lessons to be learned from Elaine's case?

Culture and climate

Robert Francis' letter to the Secretary of State, which introduced the findings of the Public Inquiry into the failings at Mid-Staffordshire NHS Foundation Trust stated that

> the story it tells is first and foremost of appalling suffering of many patients. This was primarily caused by a serious failure on the part of a provider Trust Board. It did not listen sufficiently to its patients and staff or ensure the correction of deficiencies brought to the Trust's attention. Above all, it failed to tackle an insidious negative culture involving a tolerance of poor standards and a disengagement from managerial and leadership responsibilities. This failure was in part the consequence of allowing a focus on reaching national access targets, achieving financial balance and seeking foundation trust status to be at the cost of delivering acceptable standards of care.
>
> (Francis 2013, p. 9)

The failures at Mid-Staffordshire were caused in the main by the culture that was allowed to develop, and many of the recommendations for change in the Francis Report relate to changing the culture. The word culture is often preceded by an adjective describing an aspect of it, such as the explanation of Reason's 'informed culture' discussed previously. Other examples might be 'learning culture', 'toxic culture', 'blame culture', 'safety culture', and 'compassionate culture'. Talk of culture has become widespread in management and leadership.

Despite widespread use of the word culture there seems to be little agreement about its definition. Most definitions emphasise the values and beliefs that are held within groups (Davies and Mannion 2013). Culture is often used as 'organisational culture', which might suggest that the values and beliefs are held by the organisation as a whole. 'In everyday language, culture is "the way things are done around here"' (Davies and Mannion 2013, p. 3). In complex organisations such as health care organisations there are likely to be a number of cultures, or sub-cultures, among different groups, perhaps relating to particular professional groups, or on different sites managed by the same organisation.

Climate is a concept also used, and some scholars have differentiated between culture and climate. However, this too is contested. West *et al.* (2014) suggest that culture and climate are different ways of looking at the same phenomena, but climate is more associated with 'values in action' – the way that shared values are put into practice by the organisation – for example, through features such as procedures for managing staff and reporting safety concerns. Both climate and culture are used as metaphors to describe an organisation, but can also be seen as something that can be measured as a property of an organisation, perhaps a little like morale.

There is a substantial literature on organisational culture in health, addressing issues such as how culture can be assessed and measured, what the effects of culture are on performance, and how it can be changed. West *et al.* (2014) reviewed a number of relevant studies and concluded that a link between different types of culture and performance has been consistently demonstrated. However, as there are many ways of measuring both culture and performance there is no straightforward association. Even if it was demonstrated that certain forms of culture were associated with good performance, then achieving change in the culture in that direction would be difficult. There are several studies that link a number of variables, which might be considered as elements of 'climate' (values-in-action) with a number of different ways of measuring health care organisation performance and quality of care. For example, Aiken *et al.* (2012) showed working environment (as well as nurse staffing levels) was associated with higher quality of care, and West *et al.* (2011) showed links between elements of climate such as well-structured team environments and support from management, and indicators of quality. In short, although there are methodological difficulties in exploring links between climate and culture and organisational performance, particularly related to quality of care, there is a strong and developing evidence base that associates leadership, which is engaging and valuing of staff and service users, with good quality care. The NHS Leadership Academy has published a paper exploring the evidence supporting the Healthcare Leadership Model, considered in Box 6.2.

Leadership has a significant effect on culture and climate, although other factors are also significant that may not be so easily influenced, such as professional culture. When culture is understood as a contributor, perhaps the major contributor, to a major safety and quality issue there is impatience to make improvements and change the culture. However, culture cannot be changed quickly. 'Instead the emphasis needs to be on careful local nurturing' (Davies and Mannion 2013, p. 3), through local leadership and management.

Quality improvement

In recent years, particularly since the events at Mid-Staffordshire, the emphasis on quality improvement has been on leadership and developing cultures in which quality can improve. There is also an emphasis on quality improvement tools and techniques although this has had less prominence in recent years, and particularly since the NHS Institute for Improvement and Innovation was abolished in 2013. The Institute produced a range of resources, and led projects drawing on tools and techniques that have their origins in the Japanese car industry after World War II (Kenny 2008). The Productive Ward: Releasing Time to Care programme, for example, used techniques from Lean, which was a quality improvement process developed at Toyota, and often referred to as the Toyota Production System (NHS Institute for Innovation and Improvement 2010).

Two tools that have been widely used are process mapping and PDSA cycles. Both are based on the idea that in order to improve the quality of services provided, you need to understand in detail the work processes that have developed to undertake complex tasks.

Process mapping is a key technique to help teams identify suggestions for change, helping teams to develop a detailed understanding of the process that produces an outcome. When a team develops a process map, it is important that it records what actually happens, not what should happen, or what the most important person in the room thinks happens. The idea behind process mapping is that the system that has developed to complete a task may have evolved over many years, and is unlikely to be understood in detail by any person with a responsibility for improving the outcome of the system. Process mapping creates this understanding, and when it has been achieved, the process can be changed to improve its performance (Trebble *et al.* 2010).

After a process map has been completed in detail, it may be used to consider changes to the process, which will result in an improvement. The model for improvement (Langley *et al.* 1996) is widely used, and is shown in Figure 6.6. It is based on the plan–do–study–act (PDSA) cycle, where change ideas are tested on a small scale before

A process map is a diagram that shows all the tasks required to complete a process for a patient's care and treatment, in the sequence that they are completed.

169

FIGURE 6.6
The model for improvement

Source: Langley et al. 1996.

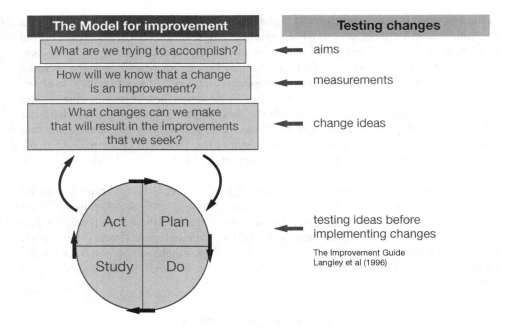

wider implementation. There are many cases studies in the literature of PDSA cycles being used. For example, Perry *et al.* (2014) report on its use to reduce times to assessment and diagnosis in a community memory assessment service.

Case 6.1 (continued)

Several patients from Lisa's ward had complained that when they were taken to X-ray, they were kept waiting for a long time in a cold corridor. A small team from the ward, the X-ray department, and the porters got together and completed a process map so that they could fully understand what the process was. The process involved requests being taken from the wards and being checked in the X-ray department before being put in a tray for the porters. There were several delays in the process, which led to problems, for example, the porter often found that the patient was not available. Because of these delays the porters tried to maintain a queue in the department so that there was always someone waiting. This led to patients waiting for a long time, before and after their X-ray. The process map identified all the stages and delays, and helped the team suggest areas for improvement.

In Case 6.1 above, the team may have suggested that the wards try to write on the form a time by when the X-ray is required to help prioritisation, or times when the patient might be unavailable. It might be agreed that the X-ray department could call for more portering help if there was more than one patient waiting. These changes could be tried in PDSA cycles. PDSA cycles are rapid change cycles, so that a momentum for improvement is established in a team. If the change achieves an improvement, it can be made permanent. If it does not, then it can be amended or another suggestion tried.

PDSA cycles will help to develop a culture where everyone has a responsibility for changing the service, and where changes can be tried out. If a change does not result in an improvement, effective learning can still be achieved. However, there are some changes that could be made, where a failure would not be acceptable, particularly relating to patient safety. Introducing a new treatment or procedure, for example, is likely to have a clear procedure within a Trust's governance framework. So although there are efforts being made to empower clinicians who deliver services to make changes, these changes have to be made within the context of the organisation and its governance arrangements.

A **PDSA** (plan–do–study–act) cycle is a rapid way of trying and evaluating a small change in a work process to see if the change leads to an improvement.

PART 3: EXPLORING MANAGEMENT AND LEADERSHIP

To conclude this chapter on management and leadership we discuss a number of issues that provide some critical perspectives. First, we will consider some views about whether the NHS has too many managers, which seems to be a popular view among many members of the public and health professionals. We will also briefly consider some more substantive critiques.

The relationship between managers and health care professionals

In 2007, the NHS Confederation, which represents NHS organisations, published a report entitled *Management in the NHS: The facts* (NHS Confederation 2007). This addressed key issues such as why the NHS needs managers, and what they do, noting that they 'often find themselves criticised and derided for being faceless bureaucrats or pointless pen-pushers' (NHS Confederation 2007, p. 2). The NHS Confederation pointed out that 'the traditional image of NHS managers – perpetuated by TV programmes such as *Casualty* and *Holby City* – is of men in sharp grey suits, who are not really interested in patients' (NHS Confederation 2007, p. 6). The reality is that 59 per cent of managers and senior managers in the NHS are female, and over 50 per cent have a clinical background. Only 2.7 per cent of the NHS workforce are managers, compared with 15 per cent of the UK workforce as a whole. Management costs were around 5 per cent of total NHS expenditure in 2000, falling to 4 per cent in 2005. In addition, as we have discussed in this chapter and others, the NHS is going through major changes, which have to be managed. These figures were updated by the NHS Confederation (2015) when they noted that between 2009 and 2013 there had been a decline of almost 20 per cent in the number of health service managers, following the reforms of the NHS discussed in Chapter 5.

Evidence such as this might give an objective view, but figures on this scale are difficult to relate to in practice. There are some difficulties in defining exactly what a manager is – would you, for example, count a Ward Sister or Charge Nurse as a manager? The views of many NHS staff may be formed more by their experience of management, rather than statistical evidence.

There has been a considerable amount of practical interest in the relationship between managers and health professionals. One reason that tensions remain between the clinical professions and managers is the changing way that health care is delivered, with greater emphasis on uniformity in clinical processes, with care and treatment being increasingly 'systematised' (as opposed to being based on individual decisions of clinicians), and increased efficiency becoming more important (Degeling *et al.* 2003). Degeling *et al.*

171

I. Snelling, C. Havard and D. Pontin

TABLE 6.6 Attitudes on modernisation

Elements of health services modernisation	Mcedical clinicians	Mcedical managers	General managers	Nurse managers	Nurse clinicians
Recognise connections between clinical decisions and resources	Oppose	Support	Equivocal	Support	Oppose
Transparent accountability	Oppose	Support	Support	Support	Oppose
Systematisation	Oppose	Oppose	Support	Support	Equivocal
Multi-disciplinary team	Oppose	Oppose	Equivocal	Support	Support

(2003) offer some international evidence on attitudes to various aspects of modernisation. Table 6.6 shows how medical clinicians and managers, nurse clinicians and managers, and general managers view key issues in health service reform. Although this research is now quite dated, it remains widely cited, and remains a useful framework to consider attitudes.

Interestingly, nurse managers were the only group supporting all four elements, and Degeling *et al.* (2009) go on to argue that managers and doctors should engage more directly with nursing and allied health colleagues. This paper suggests that nurses as managers and clinicians have a particular perspective, outside the much-discussed divide between management and medicine.

Evidence-based management

The rise in the evidence-based health care movement has provided the inspiration for calls for managers to use similar processes of using evidence in their decision-making. There are clear differences in evidence-based clinical practice and evidence-based management, particularly in the availability of evidence. Difficulties in applying evidence to management practice are widely acknowledged and relate to issues that include differing cultures, the strength (or lack) of the research base and the nature of decision-making. A lack of a clearly defined body of knowledge in health care management has led to a view that to attempt to apply the principles of evidence-based clinical practice to management is simply misconceived. Instead a call has been made to examine the 'craft' of management, which draws on the work of Schön (1983) on the 'reflective practitioner' to create a more critical and 'evidence aware' approach (Hewison 2004). The debate about evidence-based management raises some questions about the status of the 'profession' of management, how its practitioners should be educated, and how they should relate to health care professionals who have an increasing reliance on an explicit evidence base.

Unexamined assumptions that support established interests

There has been considerable growth in research about management in the health service in recent years. Learmonth (2005) reviewed the literature relating to a number of key issues and concluded that much management research 'takes commonsense managerial imperatives as simply a natural part of the way that the world is, assumptions used to construct particular worlds' (Learmonth 2005, p. 110). In other words, there is insufficient examination in much management research of basic assumptions; they give 'a version of the world [that], while appearing neutral, tacitly supports elite interests' (Learmonth 2005, p. 93). These assumptions might include the inevitability of legitimate power in organisations, or the importance of management techniques.

An example of this is given in McDonald (2004), in a study of an initiative in a PCT to 'empower' staff, which is a theme of recent service improvement initiatives, as discussed earlier. She suggests that the 'empowerment' of staff may be seen as a different way of exercising control, through moulding identities acceptable to the organisation, to value staff who are 'loyal, positive, and embrace change' (McDonald 2004, p. 946).

This serves to reinforce a point made in the chapter. Management is not a science, which gives you the right answers in a specific context. Understanding management and leadership requires sustained critical reflection on your experience, with the help of a range of models, theories and concepts. As this last section has attempted to show, there are some fundamental debates about the status of management, its role in the NHS and its relationship with the health care professions.

CONCLUSION

In this chapter, we have asked you to think about management and leadership not only as part of your working environment, but also as important activities that you will undertake from the very beginning of your career. Theories and concepts in management and leadership do not contain truths that can tell you, for example, what management behaviour will make a team successful, or what is the 'correct' way to assess risk. But they do give you ideas that you can use to help reflect on your experiences and to develop your understanding of your work environment and how you develop your own role and behaviour.

The importance of clinical professionals being leaders was emphasised in the Francis report (Francis 2013). Further improvements in the NHS, particularly in the quality and safety of services, will not happen unless staff at all levels are prepared to take on responsibility not only for their own professional actions, but also as leaders. In your career you may also wish to follow a management route. In either case, we hope that this chapter has given you some useful ideas to consider.

SUGGESTED FURTHER READING

Barr, J. and Dowding, L. (2012) *Leadership in Health Care* (2nd edn). London: Sage.
Gopee, N. and Galloway, J. (2013) *Leadership and Management in Health Care* (2nd edn). London: Sage.
Iles, V. (2005) *Really Managing Health Care* (2nd edn). Maidenhead: Open University Press.
Sullivan, E. J. and Garland, G. (2013) *Practical Leadership and Management in Health Care for Nurses and Allied Health Professionals* (2nd edn). Harlow: Pearson.
Thomas, J. (2013) *A Nurse's Survival Guide to Leadership and Management on the Ward* (2nd edn). London: Churchill Livingstone.

REFERENCES

Aiken, L. H., Sermeus, W., Van den Heede, K., Sloane, D. M., Busse, R., McKee, M., Bruyneel, L. *et al.* (2012) Patient safety, satisfaction, and quality of hospital care: cross sectional surveys of nurses and patients in 12 countries in Europe and the United States. *British Medical Journal*, **344**, doi: 10.1136/bmj.e1717

Belbin, R. M. (1993) *Team Roles at Work*. Oxford: Butterworth-Heinemann.

Croft, C., Currie, G. and Lockett, A. (2015) Broken 'two-way windows'? An exploration of professional hybrids. *Public Administration* **93** (2), 380–394.

Davies, H. T. O. and Mannion, R. (2013) Will prescriptions for cultural change improve the NHS? *British Medical Journal*, **346**, f1305.

Degeling, P., Maxwell, S., Kennedy, J. and Coyle, B. (2003) Medicine, management, and modernisation: a 'danse macabre'? *British Medical Journal* **326**, 649–652.

DH (Department of Health) (1998) *A First Class Service: Quality in the NHS*. London: DH.

DH (2000) *An Organisation with a Memory*. London: DH.

Francis, R. (2010) *Independent Inquiry into Care Provided by Mid-Staffordshire NHS Foundation Trust January 2005–March 2009*. London: Stationery Office.

Francis, R. (2013) *Report of the Mid-Staffordshire NHS Foundation Trust Public Inquiry*. London: Stationery Office.

HSE (Health and Safety Executive) (2009) *How to Tackle Work-Related Stress: A guide for employers on making the Management Standards work*. HSE.

HSE (2015) *What is Stress?* www.hse.gov.uk/stress/furtheradvice/whatisstress.htm (accessed 5 January 2015).

Healthcare Commission (2009) *Investigation into Mid-Staffordshire NHS Foundation Trust*. London: Healthcare Commission.

Hewison, A. (2004) Evidence-based management in the NHS: is it possible? *Journal of Health Organisation and Management* **18** (5), 336–348.

Hochschild, A. R. (2012) *The Managed Heart: Commercialization of human feeling* (2012 edn). Berkeley, CA: University of California Press.

Iles, V. (2005) *Really Managing Health Care* (2nd edn). Maidenhead: Open University Press.

Katzenbach, J. R. and Smith, D. K. (1993) *The Wisdom of Teams: Creating the high-performance organisation*. Boston, MA: Harvard Business School Press.

Kennedy, I. (2001) *Learning from Bristol: The report of the public inquiry into children's heart surgery at the Bristol Royal Infirmary 1984–1995*. CM 5207 London: The Stationery Office.

Kenny, C. (2008) *The Best Practice: How the new quality movement is transforming medicine*. New York: Public Affairs.

Keogh, B. (2013) *Review into the Quality of Care and Treatment Provided by 14 Hospital Trusts in England: Overview report*. London: NHS England.

Langley, G., Nolan, K., Nolan, T., Norman, C. and Provost, L. (1996) *The Improvement Guide: A practical approach to enhancing organisational performance*. New York: Jossey-Bass.

Learmonth, M. (2005) Making health services management research critical: a review and a suggestion. *Sociology of Health and Illness* **25** (1), 93–119.

Lyubovnikova, J., West, M. A., Dawson, J. F. and Carter, M. R. (2015) 24-Karat or fool's gold? Consequences of real team and co-acting group membership in health care organizations. *European Journal of Work and Organizational Psychology* **24** (6), 929–950.

McDonald, R. (2004) Individual identity and organisational control: empowerment and modernisation in a primary care trust. *Sociology of Health and Illness* **26** (7), 925–950.

Mackay, C. J., Cousins, R., Kelly, P. J., Lee, S. and McCaig, R. H. (2004) Management standards and work-related stress in the UK: policy background and science. *Work and Stress* **18** (2), 91–112.

Martin, G. P. and Waring, J. (2013) Leading from the middle: constrained realities of clinical leadership in healthcare organisations. *Health* **17**, 358–374.

Monitor and Trust Development Agency (2015). *Price Caps for Agency Staff: Rules*. www.gov.uk/ government/uploads/system/uploads/attachment_data/file/484834/price_caps_for_agency_staff _rules_final_rev11dec.pdf (accessed 7 February 2016).

National Patient Safety Agency (NPSA) (2008) *A Risk Matrix for Risk Managers*. London: NPSA (www.npsa.nhs.uk).

National Reporting and Learning System (NRLS) (2015). *Patient Safety Data*. www.nrls.npsa. nhs.uk/patient-safety-data/ (accessed 7 February 2016).

NHS Confederation (2007) *Management in the NHS: The facts*. London: NHS Confederation.

NHS Confederation (2015) *NHS Managers: Busting the myths*. London: NHS Confederation.

NHS England (2015) *Root Cause Analysis (RCA) Investigation*. London: NHS England. www.nrls.npsa.nhs.uk/resources/collections/root-cause-analysis/ (accessed 7 February 2016).

NHS Institute for Innovation and Improvement (2010) Improving health care quality at scale and pace. Lessons from The Productive Ward: Releasing time to care programme. http://eprints. soton.ac.uk/344686/ (accessed 7 February 2016).

NHS Leadership Academy (2013). *The Healthcare Leadership Model*. www.leadershipacademy.nhs.uk/ resources/healthcare-leadership-model/ (accessed 7 February 2016).

NMC (Nursing and Midwifery Council) (2015) *The Code: Professional standards of practice and behaviour for nurses and midwives*. London: NMC.

Pearce, C. (2006) Ten steps to effective delegation. *Nursing Management* **13** (8), 9.

Perry. J., Bell, F., Shaw, T., Fitzpatrick, B. and Sampson, E. L. (2014) The use of PDSA methodology to evaluate and optimise an inner city memory clinic: a quality improvement project. *BMC Geriatrics* **2014** (14), 4.

Reason, J. (1997) *Managing the Risks of Organisational Accidents*. Aldershot: Ashgate.

Rost, J. (1993) Leadership development in the new millennium. *Journal of Leadership and Organizational Studies* **1** (1), 91–110.

Sawbridge, Y. and Hewison, A. (2011). *Time to Care? Responding to concerns about poor nursing care*. Policy paper 12. Health Services Management Centre, University of Birmingham.

Sawbridge, Y. and Hewison, A, (2013). Thinking about the emotional labour of nursing: supporting nurses to care. *Journal of Health Organization and Management* **27** (1), 127–133.

Schön, D. (1983) *The Reflective Practitioner*. New York: Basic Books.

Smith, J. (2002) *The Shipman Enquiry: First report*. London: The Stationery Office.

Storey, J. and Holti, R. (2013) *Towards a New Model of Leadership for the NHS*. NHS Leadership Academy. www.leadershipacademy.nhs.uk/wp-content/uploads/2013/05/Towards-a-New-Model-of-Leadership-2013.pdf

Trebble, T. M., Hansi, N., Hydes, T., Smith, M. A. and Baker, M. (2010) Process mapping the patient journey through health care: an introduction. *British Medical Journal* **341**, c4078.

Tuckman, B. (1965) Developmental sequence in small groups. *Psychological Bulletin* **63** (6), 384–399.

Wanless, D., Appleby, J., Harrison, A. and Patel, D. (2007) *Our Future Health Secured? A review of NHS funding and performance*. London: King's Fund.

West, M. A., Topakas, A. and Dawson, J. (2014) Climate and culture for health care performance. In *The Oxford Handbook of Organizational Climate and Culture*. Barbera, K. and Schneider, B. (eds). Oxford: Oxford University Press, pp. 335–359.

West, M. A., Dawson, J. F., Admasachew, L. and Topakas, A. (2011). *NHS Staff Management and Health Service Quality: Results from the NHS Staff Survey and related data*. London: Department of Health.

Wong, C. A., Cummings, G. G. and Ducharme, L. (2013) The relationship between nursing leadership and patient outcomes: a systematic review update. *Journal of Nursing Management* **21**, 709–724.

7

INTERPROFESSIONAL WORKING

Katherine Pollard, Julie Bugler and Sally Hayes

LEARNING OUTCOMES

After reading and reflecting on this chapter, you should be able to:

- identify why interprofessional working is important;
- acknowledge your responsibilities and obligations as a registered nurse in relation to interprofessional working;
- outline different types of interprofessional working within nurse practice environments;
- identify evidence to support interprofessional working;
- outline the history of interprofessional working in UK health and social care services;
- discuss the different forms interprofessional working can take;
- identify factors that enhance or inhibit interprofessional working.

INTRODUCTION

Interprofessional working/collaborative practice is seen to be an essential aspect of the delivery of health and social care in general and nursing care in particular. In this chapter we aim to present a comprehensive overview of the issues you need to consider in order to acquire the necessary understanding and skills to engage in effective interprofessional working.

The chapter is divided into three parts. In Part 1, we provide an outline of interprofessional working explaining in general terms why it is important, what it looks like, and what sorts of skills and attitudes are needed to make interprofessional working effective.

In Part 2, we further explain the importance for nurses of interprofessional working before looking at how professions in the UK and other countries have interacted in the past. We also investigate specific features of interprofessional working more closely, and examine some of the barriers to effective interprofessional working. Part 2 concludes with an outline of the current evidence base for interprofessional working.

In Part 3, we explore interprofessional working in nursing practice in more depth, and discuss the skills that nurses need to ensure successful interprofessional working. Issues of relationships and communication affecting collaboration are highlighted, as well as nurses' involvement in leadership and co-ordination between different groups of professionals, care sectors and agencies. The chapter concludes with a consideration of the role of the nurse in effective interprofessional collaboration.

PART 1: OUTLINING INTERPROFESSIONAL WORKING

Case 7.1

Mr Blake was admitted to hospital 3 weeks ago after a failed discharge home 3 days earlier. This is his fourth admission in as many months with decompensated heart failure. Mr Blake wants to return home. Involved in the discharge planning arrangements are an occupational therapist, social worker, discharge nurse, senior staff nurse in charge of the ward that day, a medical consultant and a junior doctor. They meet to discuss and jointly work out a plan of care, which involves, among other things, making some modifications to Mr Blake's home and arranging tele-health and a care package before he is discharged. Mr Blake's preferences and opinions about his discharge are sought and considered by the discharge team, who will liaise with the general practitioner (GP) and the community nursing team, including a community heart failure specialist nurse. Mr Blake has no children. His next of kin is his niece Sally, who lives 40 miles away.

Case 7.2

Tom is 15 years old, with a moderate learning disability and severe anxiety. He is an only child living with his mother, Louise, who is struggling after a recent separation from Tom's father. Tom attends a mainstream school and receives one-to-one support, but wants to move schools to gain more life skills and become more independent with cooking, budgeting, travelling and making friends. He has very few friends, but has a girlfriend, Ella, who he sees at school; they send each other text messages, which concerns Louise, as they are sometimes sexual in content. Tom suffers from chronic constipation and has faecal leakage, mainly at night. He is prescribed a powerful laxative, but the treatment regime causes both Tom and Louise considerable distress. Recently they have started arguing a lot and she has approached his social worker, Ravi, for help with the general situation. Ravi has referred Tom to the Specialist Services for Children with Learning Disabilities for help with medication, education regarding constipation and guidance around growing up and making friends and relationships. Following the referral, Louise is contacted by Claire, a community learning disabilities nurse from the services, to arrange a meeting for an initial assessment.

K. Pollard, J. Bugler and S. Hayes

Why interprofessional working?

Nurses rarely work in isolation. Typically, as illustrated in the cases of Mr Blake (Case 7.1) and of Tom (Case 7.2), patients will find practitioners from more than one professional group, and sometimes from more than one organisation or agency, involved in the delivery of their care. Although the range of professionals and practitioners will vary, it is unusual to find health care situations where nurses are not involved. Thus it is a fact of professional life that nurses must work with others in the delivery of care. This recognition is the starting point for effective **interprofessional working** and it is no accident that in both acute and community care settings, nurses are often ideally placed to take on responsibility for co-ordinating processes and procedures involving other professionals and practitioners.

What is interprofessional working?

Interprofessional working is understood as a particular way of working with others. The essential feature of interprofessional working is collaboration; hence the use of such terms as collaborative working or **collaborative practice**, which involves both professionals and non-professionals in the provision of care. Thus interprofessional working is more than merely having contact with other professionals involved in the care of a given individual. It requires the recognition that no one professional or practitioner can meet all the needs of any one client. This being so, nurses need to develop the skills and attitudes that foster collaborative ways of working in order to minimise the fragmentation of care that **patients** might otherwise experience.

What skills and attitudes are needed for effective interprofessional working?

A number of barriers to effective interprofessional working have been identified and some of these will be detailed and explored later in the chapter. For now it is enough to say that a commitment to interprofessional working necessarily involves attempting to overcome obstacles to collaborative practice. Effective interprofessional working does not just happen; it requires an active contribution from each member of the interprofessional team as well as an environment that provides the opportunity for all members to participate in discussion and decision-making.

To engage with interprofessional working it is necessary for individuals to have, among other things:

- a knowledge and understanding of the roles and responsibilities of other care providers;
- a willingness to identify personal strengths and weaknesses together with a willingness to accept the need for personal and professional development;
- a willingness to trust, respect and value the contributions of all involved in the delivery of care; and
- well-developed communication skills.

PART 2: EXPLAINING INTERPROFESSIONAL WORKING

Why interprofessional working is important for nurses

Interprofessional working is seen as a way of minimising the fragmentation of services that often accompanies the delivery of health care when two or more professional groups are involved (and arguably, there is always more than one professional group involved in the care of any one particular service user).

There are obvious dangers inherent in a system in which different professional groups organise themselves in different ways and specialise in particular aspects of care delivery. The most common dangers are the failure to collaborate and the failure to communicate. Sometimes these problems lead directly to tragic outcomes, as reported in the inquiries into a number of high-profile cases (see, for example, Francis 2013, Laming 2003, 2009). One of the key consequences of these inquiries has been the recognition that no profession or agency has a monopoly on care. Interprofessional working, with an emphasis on collaborative working and effective communication, is seen to be one way of preventing failures of care such as those explored by Laming (2003, 2009) and Francis (2013).

The ideal of interprofessional working is that different professionals work together in an attempt to reduce the fragmentation of care as experienced by service users. For example, accurate assessment of a service user's condition or situation is important for the subsequent delivery of appropriate care. The common information available from a single systematic and structured assessment ought to be able to serve as a basis for subsequent profession-specific assessments without the need for a patient to respond to the same questions from three or four different professionals. Yet traditionally professional groups have perceived a need for profession-specific assessment processes. Arguably **the best interests of the patient** trying to rest in a hospital bed are not served by a succession of visits from, for example, a nurse, a phlebotomist, a pharmacist, another nurse, an occupational therapist and a social worker, as well as a ward round of doctors all within the space of a single morning. Attempts to reduce this sort of fragmentation are not new and the ideas of seamless care, integrated care pathways and a unified, co-ordinated assessment process are consistent with and, in some cases, pre-date the move towards interprofessional working. These processes all require professionals to orientate their work in terms of patient benefit rather than on the basis of professional identity and/or boundaries. A key report on the future direction of the National Health Service (DH 2008) highlighted shared accountability as an important principle underpinning the roles and obligations of all health care practitioners.

How have professions in the UK interacted in the past?

In the UK the work of health and social care practitioners is highly institutionalised. Acts of Parliament have established professional and statutory bodies for the registration and regulation of different professional groups: the Nursing and Midwifery Council (NMC) for nurses, midwives and health visitors; the General Medical Council (GMC) for doctors; and the Health and Care Professions Council (HCPC) for social workers and allied health professionals (including, among others, radiographers, physiotherapists and occupational therapists). Although similar arrangements exist in most developed industrialised countries, this is by no means a global phenomenon. In some developing

The best interests of the patient: the crux of interprofessional working is that it focuses on patient-centred care delivery and puts the interests of the patient ahead of the interests of any given professional.

K. Pollard, J. Bugler and S. Hayes

countries, such as Haiti, there is no organised health or social care system (St Boniface Haiti Foundation 2015).

Even in the UK, the institutionalisation of health care is relatively recent. Health care has been organised and regulated for little over one hundred years, while the organisation and regulation of social care has been even more recent (Vatcher and Jones 2014). Across the health and social care spectrum, different professions have different histories with different social trajectories. The most powerful of the professions has been, and arguably remains, medicine. The delivery of health care was controlled and directed predominantly by medical professionals during the whole of the twentieth century. Where health and social care practice intersected, the medical profession often retained primacy (Hudson 2002). Medical professionals directed the practice of other health professions even more closely, often controlling their establishment and regulation from the outset (Witz 1992). Although nursing skills have been exercised by individuals for centuries, nursing as a distinct profession was only recognised at the end of the nineteenth century; national regulation of nursing (albeit featuring medical control) was only established in the UK in 1923 (Dingwall et al. 1988).

The two major developments affecting the organisation of health care in the UK during the twentieth century were the creation in 1948 of the National Health Service (NHS) and of the World Health Organization (WHO). Before World War II (1939–1945), health and social care in the UK was provided by a patchwork of civic bodies, charitable institutions and individual professionals in private practice. Collaboration between these various entities occurred only on an ad hoc basis, dependent largely on individual inclination and ability. Recognition that the needs of the population could not be met by such a piecemeal approach resulted in the establishment of the NHS, and the implementation during the 1940s of legislation concerning education and social care for vulnerable groups, including children (Gladstone 1995). However, communication and collaboration between different professions continued to occur in a disjointed manner, often dominated by medical priorities, and dependent on individual initiative and inclination, rather than on systematic processes (Pollard et al. 2014).

In the 1990s UK governments and health and social care professionals started to address these issues in a systematic fashion. However, this period also saw the rise of not-for-profit organisations such as social enterprises, whose involvement in the provision of health care services has been advocated by successive governments (Addicott 2011). During this time, private companies were encouraged to invest in the health care 'market' in the UK (Pollock 2009). In other changes, some health care services have been allocated to different agencies in the public sector; for example, health visiting and other public health services are now the responsibility of local authorities, rather than of the NHS (Stephenson and Wiggins 2014). All these developments have resulted in a landscape where service provision is once again fragmented, so that it becomes increasingly important for health care professionals to be aware of their obligations concerning interprofessional collaboration, as well as knowing how to communicate effectively across a range of different organisations (Francis 2013).

Professional interactions beyond the UK

In the wider social context, collaboration between epidemiologists from different European countries has been occurring since the 1920s initially through the League of Nations Health Organisation. The main concern of this body was public health and the incidence

180

and control of communicable diseases across Europe (League of Nations Health Organisation 1931). The scope of the organisation expanded after World War II, culminating in the establishment of the WHO, whose aim is that all people everywhere should attain the highest possible level of health. Health is defined in WHO's Constitution as 'a state of complete physical, mental and social well-being and not merely the absence of disease or infirmity' (WHO 2015). WHO continues its influential role today, and provides a forum through which health professionals from all over the world are able to share knowledge, opinions and perspectives. In addition, governments of both developed and many developing nations aim to implement WHO recommendations.

A closer look at interprofessional working

Case 7.2 (continued)

After the initial assessment, a meeting was called so that all the professionals involved could collaborate to ensure that consistency of care for Tom would be achieved. These included Claire (learning disabilities nurse) and a psychologist from the Specialist Services for Children with Learning Disabilities, Ravi (Tom's social worker), a speech and language therapist, a teacher, and a practitioner from a national charity that provides support and advice about continence for children. Tom and Louise attended the meeting and participated in making decisions. The meeting was held at Tom's school because he felt most comfortable there and didn't want to miss any lessons. Tom chose to come for only part of the meeting during his lunch break. Claire chaired the meeting and ensured everyone contributed their thoughts. Ravi took the minutes. Louise was surprised at how many different services were involved and was able to get a clearer picture of who could support her. The professionals worked together to decide who would be best to do joint work and who best to do individual work.

Interprofessional working is one of those things that most people agree is a good idea but about which there are multiple understandings. For some, interprofessional working is just a new name for the way nurses have always operated. Looking at the number of different professionals involved in care services for Mr Blake (Case 7.1) and for Tom (Case 7.2) it is easy to imagine a nurse saying something like: 'we have always worked with other professional groups so interprofessional working is nothing new'. While it is possible that this claim may have some basis in truth, there is a good chance that what she or he thinks of as interprofessional working is merely a matter of regular contact with other professionals such as doctors, physiotherapists, social workers and so on.

Effective interprofessional working is more than merely having contact with individuals from other professional groups. Nurses often claim to have different perspectives from those of doctors, and interprofessional working assumes nurses can and should make a valuable and valid contribution to patient care. Interprofessional working requires that individuals within an interprofessional team regard each other with mutual respect (Sommerfeldt 2013). A fundamental aspect of collaboration is the recognition that each member has an important contribution to make in meeting the needs of an individual patient or client.

K. Pollard, J. Bugler and S. Hayes

Participation and collaboration

While it is true that during their working day nurses often have contact with other professionals, the current emphasis on interprofessional working suggests that the relationship between nurses and other health care professionals may not always be effective.

Case 7.1 (continued)

In handover the nurse in charge of Mr Blake's care explains to the staff nurse taking over that the team would like a referral to the community heart failure specialist nurse-led service. She also mentions that, having noticed Mr Blake coughing a lot in the mornings, she has left a sample pot with him in order to collect a fresh sputum sample. The doctor has reviewed him and is concerned that he has a chest infection but does not want to prescribe antibiotics. Mr Blake does not want to take any new medication until the hospital has tested a sample. Unfortunately Mr Blake is transferred to another medical ward that afternoon in order to 'free up' beds for the weekend; the pot is forgotten, and the information is not handed over to the staff.

This simple failure of forgetting about the sample pot can easily happen in a busy hospital environment, but the consequences for a patient can be serious. You may have come across similar examples of poor communication leading to missed opportunities for collaboration resulting in fragmentation of care.

Activity 7.1

Think about health care settings you have been in and try to identify the sorts of working between different professionals that took place. Make a note of all the professionals or non-professionals involved.

As you will probably have identified from Activity 7.1, working practices between professional groups can be undertaken in different ways. The essence of interprofessional working, as it is currently understood, is *participation and collaboration*. There are a number of terms used to describe interprofessional working and they are sometimes used as if they are interchangeable. However, these terms can reflect a range of different understandings about the nature of interprofessional working. Although it is true that interprofessional working can take many forms, and can be described using a variety of terms, what is often referred to as *interprofessional* working might be better described as *multiprofessional* working.

Common terms in use are: *interprofessional, multiprofessional, interdisciplinary, multi-disciplinary, interagency* and *multi-agency*. As a **general rule** the prefix *inter* implies that all individuals engaged in the process will actively contribute to it, as demonstrated at the meeting held to discuss Tom's care (Case 7.2); by contrast, where the prefix *multi* is used, there is no such implication. *Interprofessional* working implies that communication and

182

decision-making concerning care delivery will involve representatives from each profession, discipline or agency concerned: '[Nurses] must know when and how to communicate with and refer to other professionals and agencies . . . promoting shared decision-making, to deliver positive outcomes and to co-ordinate smooth, effective transition within and between services and agencies' (NMC 2010, p. 21). A *multiprofessional* meeting may mean that individuals from a range of different disciplines are in attendance, but that not all of them will take an active part. It should also be noted that the term *interdisciplinary* usually refers to collaboration between different disciplines (for example, archaeology and psychology) or to initiatives that promote the sharing of resources and knowledge between different disciplines or professions. The term *interprofessional* refers specifically to situations where individual health or social care professions contribute their own professional perspective to an overall plan or activity (D'Amour and Oandasan 2005, Parse 2015, Payne 2000).

In the context of interprofessional health care practice the term *team* is also in common use but is interpreted in different ways. Teams can vary and can range from close-knit groupings of individuals who work alongside one another on a regular basis, to loose networks of individuals from different agencies and services, who collaborate only when a particular situation demands it. Decision-making processes can vary considerably between different types of teams, and may even differ within a single team. A key feature of successful interprofessional working is that all those involved agree about what sort of collaboration is envisaged, and in particular, what sort of communication and decision-making processes are to be established (D'Amour and Oandasan 2005, Payne 2000).

Interprofessional working does not exclude contributions from non-professional carers

Although the term *interprofessional working* implies collaboration between qualified professionals, a more flexible interpretation is often needed. In most health and social care settings, the **contribution of support workers**, such as health care assistants and home carers, as well as administrative staff, is an integral part of care provision. Some professions have established a tradition of **involving service users** in the planning and delivery of care, for example social care and mental health services (DH 1994, Social Care Institute for Excellence (SCIE) 2001). More recently in the UK, the NHS Act 2006 and the Health and Social Care Act 2012 have stipulated that all health and social care professionals can and should involve service users and/or carers actively in the planning and delivery of care (DH 2012). Service user involvement is illustrated within the two cases used in this chapter.

The concept of the 'expert' is very powerful among both health and social care professionals and the wider public, and there remains a widespread assumption that an integral aspect of the professional role is to make decisions regarding the course of action service users should follow, sometimes without engaging them in a consultation process. Some professionals still regard this as normal practice; however, organisations' mandatory obligation to obtain and act on patient feedback about the care they receive is slowly changing culture in this respect (www.nhs.uk/NHSEngland/). Awareness of the rights of the individual service user has spread among professions, and it is now widely accepted that the service user voice should be heard in the process of service provision (Donskoy and Pollard 2014). So it is generally understood that the term *interprofessional working* implies collaboration between qualified professionals, support workers, administrative

The contribution of support workers to interprofessional working is both invaluable and indispensable – for example, home care assistants, health care assistants and administrative staff.

Involving service users in decisions about their care is an integral and mandatory aspect of interprofessional care.

183

K. Pollard, J. Bugler and S. Hayes

Effective
interprofessional
working demands
that individual
practitioners
transcend **their own
point of view** in
order to appreciate
the views of other
individuals involved.

staff, service users and/or carers, in various combinations. For these reasons and because it more accurately describes the kind of working envisaged, there are some who use *collaborative practice*, *collaborative working* or *partnership working* in preference to the term *interprofessional working*.

Case 7.2 (continued)

Tom and Louise are active members of a local participation group, where their activities include helping to recruit new health and social care staff; they have learned interviewing skills from Barnardo's staff. They also take part in training new staff about ways to include participation within day-to-day work. They have been consulted on other new services and have given opinions on service leaflets, letters and policies. Tom and Louise have taken part in films made to educate a wide range of practitioners, which have been shown in the local NHS Trust to help others understand the importance of participation and service user involvement. They have also been to local universities to contribute to teaching sessions for students studying learning disabilities nursing and social work.

As can be seen from Case 7.2, service users' and carers' contributions to collaborative practice can take many forms, and can extend to involvement in education and training for a range of health and social care practitioners.

What gets in the way of effective interprofessional working?

When asked whether interprofessional collaboration is a good idea, most health or social care professionals are likely to answer in the affirmative. However, getting individuals to work well together can be problematic. Possible barriers to effective interprofessional collaboration include:

- different professional priorities and boundaries;
- lack of understanding of others' roles and obligations;
- communication mechanisms;
- poor interpersonal skills.

(see Day 2013, Keeping 2014)

Different professional priorities and boundaries

When considering the needs of service users, individual professionals are likely to prioritise their own professional perspectives. For example, and broadly speaking, social workers are likely to focus on issues of social support, medical staff will probably remain primarily interested in physical symptoms or disease progression, and occupational therapists will be concerned with the provision of an environment conducive to promoting a person's ability to perform daily activities. In some circumstances the values of different professional groups may be at odds with one another: for example, there may be significant disagreements about issues such as the extent of service user representation or consultation in decision-making. In some contexts, it may not be possible for some professionals to get **their own point of view** taken as seriously by colleagues either as they would wish or

184

as they would consider appropriate. A key aspect for nurses working interprofessionally is to ensure that other professionals appreciate and understand the nursing contribution to interprofessional care (Sommerfeldt 2013).

Activity 7.2

Think about all the professions involved in arranging Mr Blake's discharge (Case 7.1) and care for Tom (Case 7.2). How important do you think it is that consideration is given to each of the different professional perspectives?

Despite differing perspectives, there is often significant overlap between different professionals' spheres of practice, and this can lead to conflict as professionals react to protect what they consider to be 'their territory' (see, for example, Booth and Hewison 2002). However, such issues of territoriality are often a result of habit and accompanying assumptions about who is capable of carrying out a specific task. Once all those involved become accustomed to different ways of working, there is evidence to suggest that time and exposure can result in role overlap becoming a routine and unremarkable element of practice; nurse prescribing is a case in point (Blanchflower et al. 2013, Moller and Begg 2005, Parr 2011).

Lack of understanding of others' roles and obligations

Of course, all professional perspectives are important, and should be borne in mind: however, it is sometimes difficult for individual professionals to appreciate the concerns of other professional groups, particularly where knowledge of the roles and values of those other professions is limited (Aguilar et al. 2014).

Case 7.2 (continued)

Claire (the learning disabilities nurse) visits Tom at home regularly and supports both him and Louise with many of their concerns, but particularly with those around Tom's constipation. Claire liaises effectively with the paediatrician, and on one occasion arranges and delivers a repeat prescription for Tom's laxative to him. Tom sees his GP soon afterwards about an unrelated condition and is asked about his constipation. Louise explains that Claire has organised a prescription for him. The GP is concerned, as she is unaware that community nurses can obtain prescriptions for their patients directly from medical specialists and asks why the nurse visits Tom at home and whether she wears a uniform. Louise relates this incident to Claire, who contacts the GP to explain her role and also sends her a leaflet about the Specialist Services for Children with Learning Disabilities.

While the likelihood is that most professionals have some idea of what their colleagues do, they may over- or underestimate the scope and extent of their spheres of practice and professional responsibility, as demonstrated in Case 7.2 above. In these circumstances, it becomes particularly important that nurses share pertinent details about their role with

185

K. Pollard, J. Bugler and S. Hayes

Where communication mechanisms between different professions, care sectors and agencies are not **streamlined**, professionals need to be particularly vigilant about making sure that relevant information is shared with everyone who needs it.

other professionals (Sommerfeldt 2013). Thus, it is equally important for nurses to find out about their professional colleagues' role and sphere of practice in order to prevent misunderstanding and inappropriate action and to ensure patients receive optimum care.

Activity 7.3

Find out how much you really know about the roles and responsibilities of other health and social care professionals by selecting and reading a chapter from *Interprofessional Working in Health and Social Care* by Thomas et al. (2014) (see suggested further reading).

After reading the chapter try to identify:

1   the differences between the role and responsibilities of nurses and those of whichever other professional group you chose to read about; and
2   any areas of overlap that might lead to conflicts or duplication of effort.

Egalitarian approaches to planning and delivering care can be hampered by hierarchical structures, which always operate within the context of a power imbalance (Keeping 2014, McNeil *et al.* 2013). In the past there were many health care settings where occupational hierarchy determined who was authorised to make decisions. Traditionally, the medical profession dominated this hierarchy, while other professions jostled for position on the lower rungs (Witz 1992). However, this situation has changed significantly since the turn of the twenty-first century. Although the medical profession still enjoys higher status than many other health care professions, non-medical professionals, including nurses, do make decisions about patient care without medical input, and are often in a position to influence medical decision-making (Traynor 2013, Williamson *et al.* 2010).

For nursing, in particular, the drive for professional autonomy coupled with the extension of the nursing role and development of specialist and senior managerial nursing posts has resulted in the profession gaining higher status and an acceptance of nurses' legitimate involvement in decision-making. An expectation that nurses now work in collaborative teams in many health care settings has reinforced the perception that nurses are 'professionals in their own right', with concomitant accountability for decisions that they make and care that they deliver (Miers 2010, Traynor 2013, Williamson *et al.* 2010).

Communication mechanisms

There is a considerable variety of mechanisms available for communication between different professionals in different health and social care settings. In some areas of practice, regular meetings are held, attended by all professionals involved in care delivery; in other areas, communication may be haphazard and ad hoc, reliant upon individuals being in the right place at the right time.

In many acute areas information is relayed between professionals in written form. While the written record may be **streamlined** and well-organised with each professional writing in a single set of notes for individual service users, it is still common to find information about clients held in a number of different types of records: for example, nurses may write

186

in one set of notes while medical staff write in another; and other professionals may or may not write in either. Since professionals will tend to read only the set of notes in which they write this can result in individual professionals not having all the information necessary to meet the needs of the service user; and of course, this problem will be compounded where individuals neglect to write pertinent information anywhere at all.

Case 7.1 (continued)

When chatting to a nurse caring for him on the new ward, Mr Blake makes it known that on his last discharge his GP had not been contacted by the hospital. On checking the discharge summary, the nurse discovers that, while it had been typed, it was not actually sent to the GP practice. This alerts the nurse to the necessity of checking that details about Mr Blake's current discharge will be sent to the community-based services.

Many professionals rely on the telephone and/or electronic communications for conveying information, so it is crucial that messages are relayed appropriately. Community practitioners spend a great deal of time away from their office base, and often rely on answerphone messages or e-mails. When these messages are not coherent or do not contain sufficient detail, important information can be missed. When contacting patients directly by means of mobile phones, it is important that professionals remember that patients may not have enough credit to listen to a voicemail message, but can receive text messages for free.

In all health care organisations in the UK, electronic storage of patient/service user information is commonplace (Whitewood-Moores 2011); furthermore, the health status of some patients is monitored remotely through the use of tele-health techniques (British Computer Society 2012). In community settings, patient information is increasingly being recorded on handheld electronic devices (Community Practitioner 2014). However, communication between computer systems in different sectors and organisations is often difficult, if not impossible (Giordano *et al.* 2011, *Lancet* 2011); issues of data protection, following the requirements of the UK Data Protection Act 1998, can also make sharing electronic information problematic. E-mails between the NHS and Social Services may need to be encrypted in order to remain confidential. It is important that nurses and other health care professionals are aware of pertinent aspects of the electronic systems they and their collaborators use, and ensure that effective communication is not compromised as a result of technical limitations or idiosyncrasies.

Ineffective interpersonal skills

An examination of the factors listed above supports the conclusion that effective collaboration is fundamentally dependent on both the willingness and the ability of individuals to communicate effectively with others. If any member of an interprofessional working group is not committed to the principles of collaboration problems may ensue, particularly if the member in question holds a relatively powerful position in the organisation. Ineffective interpersonal skills on the part of any member can lead to misunderstandings and unanticipated reactions, which may have knock-on effects on the way care is provided. Language itself can be divisive: most professions ascribe meanings to words that may be understood differently by members of other professions and, similarly,

The ability to listen is an essential skill for effective interprofessional working.

professionals frequently use acronyms or jargon when they speak. Hence interprofessional collaboration can be hampered by a lack of awareness of profession-specific meanings for a word and by the unintelligibility of professional acronyms. In addition, some professionals tend to colonise service users when, for example, speaking about 'my patient' or 'my client'. If this is interpreted as one profession claiming exclusive responsibility for the well-being of a service user, other colleagues may become alienated from the process of collaboration (Keeping 2014).

Of course, expressing oneself is only one component of communication. If professionals are unwilling or unaware of the need **to listen** to what colleagues are saying, or to give due consideration to individuals' priorities, then it is unlikely that they are going to be able to work well together (McNeil *et al.* 2013) (see Chapter 14 for more information on communication and interpersonal skills).

The evidence base for interprofessional working

In the UK, health professionals are obliged to provide evidence-based care and evidence often takes the form of guidelines, in particular those issued by the National Institute for Health and Clinical Excellence (NICE) targeting specific areas of practice. In 2000, the Health Development Agency (HDA) was established to develop the evidence base for care delivery and to help implement that evidence in practice with the stated aims of improving health and reducing health inequalities. A key strategy for the HDA was to work with organisations such as Local Government Associations, which represented local authorities at a national level. In 2005, the functions of the HDA were transferred to NICE. While there is no NICE guideline focusing specifically on interprofessional issues, relevant principles are embedded in a range of guidance, for example, the necessity to 'ensure clear and timely exchange of patient information' between all those involved in someone's care, especially at the point of transfer from one setting/environment to another (NICE 2012).

Support for interprofessional working comes from an assumption that working collaboratively will reduce the fragmentation of care delivery through closer teamworking among professionals. Yet the idea of interprofessional working is not without its critics, and it has been found that where interprofessional working is ineffectively implemented, it can impede teamwork (McNeil *et al.* 2013). Nevertheless, inquiries into high-profile cases identify, among other things, failure of communication between different professionals involved in care as a significant feature contributing to negative patient outcomes (Laming 2003, 2009, Francis 2013). This suggests that service users will benefit from better co-ordination of care and better communication between the professions, as well as from the targeted allocation of resources across different services and agencies. However, despite an increasing focus on interprofessional practice in health care settings since 2000, the evidence base to support this assumption is still not well developed (Brandt *et al.* 2014).

One of the reasons for the paucity of evidence concerning the effect of interprofessional collaboration on service user outcomes is that it is a difficult topic to research. Processes that involve communication and joint working between different groups are complex and varied, and involve a number of interdependent factors: these include the effect of individual personalities, differing professional perspectives, the way systems are set up, how decisions are made, and how or whether actions follow those decisions. Other factors that affect care outcomes include service users' conditions or requirements, as well as relevant psycho-social factors such as individuals' social support systems. Because of these and other issues it is almost impossible to isolate and assess the effect of any single factor contributing to this amalgam of conditions and influences.

These difficulties notwithstanding, some researchers have attempted to contribute to **the evidence base** supporting interprofessional collaboration. Problems conducting research into interprofessional issues can be minimised if settings are chosen where staff turnover is relatively low; where most of the professionals involved in delivering care are located in the same place; and where systems and processes for staff interaction are clearly articulated and understood. Projects that have attempted to assess the link between interprofessional collaboration and outcomes for service users tend to be conducted within dedicated settings where small teams of professionals provide care for specific service users. For example, in studies of care for renal patients on dialysis (Dixon *et al.* 2011), the intensive care unit (Randall Curtis *et al.* 2012), fast-track hip surgery (Pape *et al.* 2013) and maternity care (Nijagal *et al.* 2015), researchers have been able to demonstrate a positive impact of interprofessional collaboration on service user outcomes.

> Carefully planned research can help to build **the evidence base** supporting interprofessional working in health and social care.

RESEARCH FOCUS 7.1

Pape *et al.* (2013) report results from a study examining the influence of daily interprofessional meetings on patients' length of stay following fast-track hip surgery in a Danish hospital. Fast-track hip surgery aims to optimise pain management and enable early mobilisation, so as to diminish the length of stay in hospital. A daily interprofessional meeting was introduced for all staff involved in patient care: surgeons, nurses, occupational therapists and physiotherapists. A checklist was used to discuss problems and to identify optimal care strategies. Joint decisions were made about which health care profession should take responsibility for specific procedures and tasks. A case control study compared hospital length of stay in 75 patients who received surgery and aftercare before the introduction of the daily interprofessional meeting, with that in 88 patients treated after its introduction. Length of stay in the latter group diminished significantly.

There have also been attempts to widen the evidence base supporting interprofessional collaboration. While the emphasis on specific service users has remained, some researchers have shown effective interprofessional working makes a positive contribution to outcomes where care is delivered in more diverse settings, with less clearly defined processes (e.g., Strandmark *et al.* 2013). Other studies, exploring the views of both service users and staff, have found higher levels of satisfaction (a 'soft' outcome in terms of service delivery) in settings where effective communication and co-ordination of care between professionals has been established (Birkeland *et al.* 2013, Dufour *et al.* 2014).

The evidence base has been extended further by reviews examining results from collections of small studies. This can result in a reinforcement of the idea that there is insufficient evidence to support the effectiveness of interprofessional collaboration in a particular area (Britton and Russell 2006). However, some of these reviews have helped to show that good working relationships and integrated practice do contribute to improved service user outcomes (Cameron 2005, Colter Smith 2015, Courtenay *et al.* 2013, Martin *et al.* 2010).

RESEARCH FOCUS 7.2

Birkeland *et al.* (2013) conducted a mixed-methods study to explore the way Swedish interprofessional paediatric cardiology teams work together. Thirty teams completed questionnaires about the organisation of work, relevant tasks and the attitudes of staff involved. Focus groups were held with 29 team members from a range of professions to explore in depth individuals' experiences and opinions about interprofessional working. The questionnaire results revealed positive attitudes to interprofessional collaboration, particularly where a nurse took the team co-ordinator role. The focus group data indicated that all the professionals involved considered interprofessional working to be essential in order to deliver a good service to children in their care. The respondents commonly stressed the need for adequate time to develop relationships and skills within their teams, to optimise the quality of the service offered.

RESEARCH FOCUS 7.3

Martin *et al.* (2010) conducted a literature search in PubMed, CINAHL and Cochrane Library in order to review the evidence base concerning the influence on patient outcomes of interprofessional collaboration between doctors and nurses. Two researchers independently found 14 randomised controlled trials (RCTs) for review. Most of the studies compared outcomes within older patients who had received either collaborative care or usual care. The RCTs compared outcomes involving a range of interventions of varying length, including promotion of community-based services and care co-ordination. Clinical and functional outcomes were commonly measured, as well as social and patient-reported outcomes. Results were mixed across the sample; however, 13 of the RCTs reported at least one improved outcome, which was statistically significant following the interprofessional intervention.

Although it can be argued that much research in the field has not produced results that can be thought of as 'hard science', there is a logic in the assumption that improving interprofessional communication and practice to enhance the quality of care will lead to improved outcomes for service users, a view supported by health care professionals (Pollard *et al.* 2012). Most available research findings agree with this logic.

PART 3: EXPLORING INTERPROFESSIONAL WORKING

The main rationale for improving interprofessional collaboration is the belief that it will enhance service user outcomes and experience (Pollard *et al.* 2014) so it is crucial to consider factors influencing interprofessional collaboration in terms of the effect on service delivery. It is rare that poor outcomes in health and social services are caused by a single event; it is much more usual to see a cascade of occurrences involving poor relationships, poor communication, poor leadership and/or poor co-ordination (Laming 2009, Francis 2013).

Activity 7.4

Make a list of all the professionals involved in the care of Mr Blake (Case 7.1) and Tom (Case 7.2). In each case give reasons for who you think should be responsible for ensuring relevant information is passed between the various professionals at different points in time.

One of the things that doing Activity 7.4 should help to illustrate is the complexity of relationships between different professional groups. Although effective communication is a necessary requirement, effective interprofessional working is also dependent on clear understandings about leadership and co-ordination of care.

What does interprofessional working in nursing practice look like?

Nurses contribute to many different types of interprofessional working in a variety of settings. In the acute sector, nurses interact closely and systematically with a range of other health and social care professionals, support workers, administrative staff and service users, particularly in specialist areas such as stroke rehabilitation, neurology and intensive care. Collaborative episodes involving nurses may be more sporadic in other acute settings (such as within general medical wards) but the effectiveness of collaboration in these environments is equally important.

Case 7.1 (continued)

Over the weekend a number of health care professionals have looked after Mr Blake and have noticed his cough appears to be worsening. His oxygen levels have remained stable but his respiratory rate has increased, he feels weak and looks less well. A health care assistant on duty, who cared for him the day before, reports her concerns to a staff nurse who asks a doctor to review Mr Blake once more. The staff nurse also asks a physiotherapist to assess Mr Blake and to support him with some breathing exercises.

As Mr Blake's case demonstrates, nurses' ability to engage in effective interprofessional collaboration may be particularly significant precisely when it is infrequent and/or irregular.

The widespread increase of community-based care at the turn of the twenty-first century resulted in new patterns of caregiving. However, as a result of major changes in the UK political landscape over the last decade, different ways of working have moved in and out of fashion. For example, there was a trend towards establishing integrated health and social care teams, such as those whose function was to deliver complete packages of care to service users with learning disabilities (Walker *et al.* 2003). These teams were managed by social services, and typically employed, among others, psychiatrists, psychologists, physiotherapists, occupational therapists, learning disabilities nurses and social workers. Many of these teams were, however, discontinued as services were radically

Mutually agreed **decision-making processes** are crucial for successful interprofessional working.

restructured. It is interesting to note that the idea of 'integrated care', the purpose of which is to provide more streamlined care in a more efficient fashion particularly to older people and those with long-term conditions, is enjoying a resurgence (see, for example, www.nottinghamcity.nhs.uk). However, whatever the formal structure of care delivery, nurses involved in community-based care must liaise and often co-ordinate care with a range of different practitioners: these may include all those mentioned as belonging to the integrated team above, as well as support workers in care homes, general practitioners, other medical professionals, allied health professionals such as dietitians and a variety of different nursing groups employed by both acute and community health service providers.

Whatever settings nurses work in, both cases in this chapter illustrate how complex service users' needs may be. It is therefore crucial that all professionals involved collaborate effectively to provide appropriate person-centred care.

Activity 7.5

Consider the need for nurses caring for Mr Blake (Case 7.1) and for Tom (Case 7.2) to co-ordinate services and liaise with other professionals. What characteristics and competencies do you think the nurses involved need to possess?

What do nurses need to do to ensure successful interprofessional working?

Most of the obstacles outlined in Part 2 of this chapter can be overcome if professionals are willing to engage in activities that promote mutual understanding and respect. Although organisational barriers to collaboration may be difficult to change, individuals can enhance collaboration by ensuring that they have an understanding of their colleagues' professional roles, as well as an understanding of the scope and limits of their own professional practice. An appreciation and acceptance of the differences between various professional perspectives and values is essential, as is the appropriate involvement of all interested parties, including service users. A key feature of effective interprofessional collaboration is the development and implementation of **decision-making processes** that are acceptable to all those concerned. It should be obvious that effective communication skills, combined with attitudes that encompass trust, respect and the valuing of contributions from all parties, play a pivotal role in determining the quality of interprofessional interaction and collaboration (Keeping 2014).

An important starting point for nurses engaged in interprofessional collaboration is an awareness of the different perspectives, priorities and values of other professional groups. Nurses need to have confidence in the value of the nursing contribution, as well as respect for other professionals' points of view: both components are needed if one professional perspective is not to be eclipsed by another.

Traditionally nurses have been subservient to doctors, and this history is reflected in some of the structures within which nurses practise today (Dingwall *et al.* 1988). You may not be in a position to affect some of the wider factors militating against effective collaboration, for example, the professional hierarchy in the NHS. However, by equipping yourself with appropriate skills, you can influence the way in which you work together with your colleagues. For example, learning how and when to use negotiation skills and assertiveness techniques can be useful in preventing inappropriate decisions being made that may result in service users not receiving the most suitable care. A major benefit of developing such skills is that they can help you to avoid difficult interpersonal situations arising from an overly compliant or confrontational stance. Thus it would seem appropriate for nurses to take advantage of the many and varied techniques for developing effective communication skills.

Support may not always be forthcoming for junior nursing staff to contribute constructively to interprofessional interaction. Nursing in the UK has developed from a model drawing on the structures of both the armed forces and domestic service and the hierarchical nature of both remains in evidence (Dingwall *et al.* 1988). It has been found that while senior nurses often communicate and collaborate effectively with colleagues from other professions, nurses in more junior positions are not always included in these processes. In many instances, this situation may simply be a result of habit, rather than any conscious attempt to exclude junior staff from interprofessional interactions. The role of the nurse continues to develop and there is now an expectation that all nurses will embrace professional values, particularly those related to autonomous thinking (Traynor 2013). If junior staff display appropriate communication skills they will, in many cases, be able to establish themselves as full members of the team.

Nurses are in key positions in many areas, often being well placed to have a clear overview of a service user's requirements (Sellman *et al.* 2014). It is therefore essential that nurses engage effectively in interprofessional collaboration, so that these requirements can be clearly stated and considered by colleagues from appropriate disciplines (Sommerfeldt 2013). The antidote to barriers to the nursing contribution resides in individual nurses developing:

- attitudes of confidence in their own perspective and abilities;
- trust and respect for their colleagues from other disciplines; and
- appropriate communication skills, which enable them to facilitate decision-making in the best interests of service users.

Relationships and communication affecting collaboration

Case 7.1 (continued)

Sally, Mr Blake's niece, arrives later that day. She notices the deterioration in her uncle, and raises her concerns with the staff nurse looking after him. Mr Blake tells his niece he is going home in the next few days when a package of care is organised. Sally is concerned about how he will cope alone at home and asks to see the medical team and social worker the next day to discuss the plan. She is disappointed that they have not approached her before, but the staff nurse explains Mr Blake has capacity and has asked that she not be bothered by the team, and therefore refused permission for them to contact her.

Relationships between patients and carers

Professionals need to remember that relatives or other carers may play a significant role in interprofessional working. Relationships among family members and/or family friends can have a powerful influence on collaboration with and between professionals. Relatives and carers often feel they need to act on behalf of their relatives/friends, just as Sally did in seeking to 'champion' her uncle's need for care. However, professionals must recognise that relatives and carers, even if they think they are acting in the individual's best interests, do not always have the latter's needs as a priority (Donskoy and Pollard 2014). Being aware of differing agendas between the relative/carer and the service user is vital.

While relatives may often want to be involved and informed about a loved one's care, health and social care staff have an obligation to prioritise the service user's privacy above relations' concerns. The Mental Capacity Act 2005 and associated policies (DH 2010) stipulate that all individuals who have capacity must be consulted and involved in decisions about their care; in particular, the principle applies to individuals with mental health difficulties and learning disabilities, as well as those who have suffered neurological trauma (Donskoy and Pollard 2014). This issue always needs to be taken into account when deciding on an appropriate course of action within collaborative practice. Health and social care professionals should never routinely discuss a patient's care with relatives or carers without the express permission of the patient.

Relationships between the professionals involved in patient care

Interprofessional teams are often made up of diverse groups of practitioners and even those who work in the same setting may see one another infrequently. In addition, modern professional roles continue to change and develop; there is no guarantee that a member of one profession will be aware of changes in the scope or role of another, as demonstrated in Case 7.2 by the concern shown by the GP on learning that Claire had obtained a prescription from the paediatrician for Tom. This is particularly so in the case of doctors and nurses, who have a long history of hierarchical relationships; unless they receive explicit information to the contrary, many doctors are not aware of the practical implications of nurses' increasing autonomy (Dingwall *et al.* 1988, Traynor 2013, Williamson *et al.* 2010).

Individuals who need to collaborate occasionally are often based in different buildings or services with infrequent contact, particularly where formal channels of communication have not been established. Such lack of contact can contribute to a poor grasp of colleagues' roles and responsibilities and to ignorance concerning some details of an individual service user's care, thus compounding problems with interprofessional collaboration and communication.

It is important that nurses develop negotiation skills so they can practise to their full capacity. They need to demonstrate this capacity in order to gain the trust of professional colleagues, patients and carers, some of whom may not be conversant with recent developments in the nursing role, and who may therefore lack confidence in nurses' clinical skills and knowledge.

The interface between the acute and primary sectors

Another crucial component for improving care delivery is the establishment of effective, functioning systems and relationships between the acute and primary sectors. Although both are staffed and run by health and/or social care professionals, the nature of the environment, the professional role and the relationships with service users vary considerably (Sellman *et al.* 2014). Many professionals working in the community will have worked in hospitals at some time during their career; however, because of a greater emphasis on community provision of care, it is no longer unusual to find newly qualified practitioners employed in community posts. Hospital-based staff may never have had any experience of community practice. In particular, nurses working on hospital wards and those working in the community may hold different priorities, expectations and experiences concerning the nature of the nursing role (Sellman *et al.* 2014). Just as it is important for professionals from different disciplines to understand each other's roles, so too it is important that practitioners from the same profession, but based in different environments, understand the implications for co-ordination of care delivery when service users move between different facilities.

This situation becomes more complex when health and social care practitioners working collaboratively are employed by a combination of NHS organisations and non-NHS organisations in the public, private and/or voluntary sectors. It is crucial for effective collaboration that everyone involved understands and appreciates the varying organisational demands and priorities influencing workers' capacity to act, as well as the differences in professional obligations and cultural norms (Francis 2013, McNeil *et al.* 2013).

Nurses' involvement in leadership and co-ordination

Issues of co-ordination and leadership within an interprofessional team are important (Laming 2009). A common cause of ineffective interprofessional working is a lack of clarity regarding roles and responsibilities within the team. A decision about who is best suited to take on the lead role is vital as this person is ultimately accountable for the plan of care. In addition, for the service user and/or carer it provides a single point of contact. Clear guidelines need to exist for ensuring that one named member of the team takes the lead in co-ordinating care.

In many cases, nurses are particularly well placed to co-ordinate care, and to take on leadership in their professional roles (Sellman *et al.* 2014). There is increasing expectation that they will do so, although nurse leaders do not yet always receive sufficient interprofessional support and recognition in practice to enable them to function to their full capacity (Franks 2014). However, evidence is starting to appear that demonstrates the benefits of nurse leadership in multiprofessional settings (Birkeland *et al.* 2013, Clarke 2014, Lloyd *et al.* 2015) and formal initiatives have been established to promote leadership skills among nurses as well as among other health care professionals (www.leadershipacademy.nhs.uk/).

Leadership in the community

Case 7.1 (continued)

Sally meets with the medical team and the social worker the next day. She expresses her concerns about her uncle's discharge home. The team explain they have sent all the relevant details to his GP and have also arranged for tele-health monitoring. In addition, they have contacted the community heart failure specialist nurse, who will be visiting him within two days of discharge. Mr Blake knows the community heart failure specialist nurse, as she visited him soon after he went home following his previous admission. However, on that occasion, the GP felt that her input was not required, so she was not able to continue offering him care.

Every individual has to share **responsibility** for team tasks if interprofessional working is to succeed.

Appropriate **leadership and co-ordination** are essential components contributing to good interprofessional working.

General practitioners have traditionally been considered gatekeepers in providing medical care in the community, although increasingly, specialist nurses working in collaboration with general practitioners are taking more of a lead role (Sellman *et al.* 2014). However, where there is an overlap in practice, as demonstrated in the case of the GP and the community heart failure specialist nurse in Case 7.1, negotiation may be required to establish who has **responsibility** for providing care in particular circumstances.

Case 7.2 (continued)

Louise is still anxious about Tom's relationship with his girlfriend, Ella, and worries that they may be becoming sexually active. She discusses her concerns with Claire, saying that she has no idea how to handle this situation. She finds it very difficult to consider Tom as an adult, particularly in this area. Claire gives her information about services that can help educate and support young people with learning disabilities with regard to sexual and relationship issues. Claire also gets permission from Louise to share her concerns with Ravi (Tom's social worker), so that he can also support both her and Tom with this situation.

As can be seen in Case 7.2, leadership can involve a variety of different activities and responsibilities. The professional who co-ordinates care and support for a service user not only needs to liaise directly with other practitioners involved as appropriate, but must also be aware of the range of existing services, some provided by the voluntary sector, which may be able to offer citizens assistance with specific issues. It is also important that the lead professional knows how service users and/or carers can access such services.

Activity 7.6

Who do you think is the most appropriate professional in the community to take the lead role in providing care to Mr Blake or to Tom? Why? If you were the district nurse caring for Mr Blake, or the community learning disabilities nurse caring for Tom, what steps might you take to ensure that an appropriate system for co-ordinating care between all the relevant professionals was in place?

The cases of Mr Blake and Tom illustrate the need for professionals (including, and perhaps particularly, nurses) to be aware of a number of key factors concerning **leadership and co-ordination** if they are to promote effective care delivery for service users. These factors include:

- The need for clear guidelines for leading and co-ordinating a team successfully.
- The need for all involved to know and agree about who should be the overall co-ordinator of care.
- The need to ensure clear lines of communication about who is responsible for which particular aspects of care.
- The need to ensure no one professional's input is being ignored or overlooked.

- The need to recognise that different practitioners based in different environments may have different priorities, expectations and experiences of their role, even when they belong to the same profession.
- The need for practitioners based in different environments to understand the implications for co-ordination of care delivery when service users move between them.

It would be unrealistic to assume that all professionals will equip themselves with the requisite skills and knowledge to promote effective interprofessional collaboration so that service users receive the care they need. However, in most health care settings, nurses are well placed to take on co-ordination if not leadership roles within interprofessional teams (Birkeland *et al.* 2013, Sellman *et al.* 2014). If nurses take it upon themselves to develop appropriate skills and to practise as part of an integrated interprofessional team, then they can make a real difference to the way that care is co-ordinated and delivered on the ground.

CONCLUSION

This chapter has attempted to illustrate the importance of interprofessional working together with some of the factors that can hinder or help in the development of effective interprofessional care. By reading this chapter we hope that you will have come to recognise that you can influence the quality of care given to patients, clients, service users and citizens and that you can contribute to effective interprofessional working by following a relatively simple course of action that includes:

- involving service users in plans of care;
- consulting service users about their circumstances and in particular finding out which other professionals are involved in their care;
- making sure that you understand the nature and scope of colleagues' professional roles;
- ensuring all professionals involved with service users remain informed about issues affecting care;
- taking care that communication between different individuals, both professional and non-professional, is both effective and reliable;
- providing sufficient detail to colleagues about the nursing role, particularly in areas where assumptions may be operating, for example, the limits to the scope of nursing practice.

This may seem to imply that nurses must single-handedly take on the responsibility for improving interprofessional collaboration. This is not so; but if nurses are to fulfil their professional obligations to their patients, then they must lead the way and demonstrate an awareness of and capacity for effective interprofessional working.

SUGGESTED FURTHER READING

Day, J. (2013) *Interprofessional Working: An essential guide for health- and social-care professionals.* Andover: Cengage Learning.

Thomas, J., Pollard, K. and Sellman, D. (eds) (2014) *Interprofessional Working in Health and Social Care: Professional perspectives.* (2nd edn). Basingstoke: Palgrave Macmillan.

REFERENCES

Addicott, R. (2011) *Social Enterprise in Healthcare: Promoting organisational autonomy and staff engagement.* London: King's Fund.

Aguilar, A., Supans, I., Scutter, S. and King, S. (2014) Exploring how Australian occupational therapists and physiotherapists understand each other's professional values: implications for interprofessional education and practice. *Journal of Interprofessional Care* 28 (1), 15–22.

Birkeland, A.-L., Hägglöf, B., Dahlgren, L. and Rydberg, A. (2013) Interprofessional teamwork in Swedish pediatric cardiology: a national exploratory study. *Journal of Interprofessional Care* 27, 320–325.

Blanchflower, J., Greene, L. and Thorp, C. (2013) Breaking down the barriers to nurse prescribing. *Nurse Prescribing* 11 (1), 44–47.

Booth, J. and Hewison, A. (2002) Role overlap between occupational therapy and physiotherapy during in-patient stroke rehabilitation: an exploratory study. *Journal of Interprofessional Care* 16 (1), 31–40.

Brandt, B., Lutfiyya, M. N., King, J. A. and Chioreso, C. (2014) A scoping review of interprofessional collaborative practice and education using the lens of the Triple Aim. *Journal of Interprofessional Care* 28 (5), 393–399.

British Computer Society (2012) *Health Informatics: Improving patient care.* E-book. British Computer Society.

Britton, A. and Russell, R. (2006) Multidisciplinary team interventions for delirium in patients with chronic cognitive impairment. *Cochrane Library Database* (1), (CD000353).

Cameron, D. (2005) Co-ordinated multidisciplinary rehabilitation after hip fracture. *Disability and Rehabilitation* 27 (18/19), 1081–1090.

Clarke, U. (2014) Nurse leadership in sustaining programmes of change. *British Journal of Nursing* 23 (4), 219–224.

Colter Smith, D. (2015) Midwife–physician collaboration: a conceptual framework for interprofessional collaborative practice. *Journal of Midwifery & Women's Health* 60 (2), 128–139.

Community Practitioner (2014) Scottish community nurses get tech savvy. *Community Practitioner: The Journal of the Community Practitioners' & Health Visitors' Association* 87 (3), 6.

Courtenay, M., Nancarrow, S. and Dawson, D. (2013) Interprofessional teamwork in the trauma setting: a scoping review. *Human Resources for Health* 11 (57). doi: 10.1186/1478-4491-11-57

D'amour, D. and Oandasan, I. (2005) Interprofessionality as the field of interprofessional practice and interprofessional education: an emerging concept. *Journal of Interprofessional Care* 19 (s1), 8–20.

Day, J. (2013) *Interprofessional Working: An essential guide for health- and social-care professionals.* Andover: Cengage Learning.

DH (Department of Health) (1994) *Working in Partnership: A collaborative approach to care. Report of the Mental Health Nursing Review Team.* London: HMSO.

DH (2008) *NHS High Quality Care for All: NHS next stage review final report.* Chair, Lord Darzi. CM 7432. London: The Stationery Office.

DH (2010) The Mental Capacity Act 2005. www.legislation.gov.uk (accessed 28 May 2016).

DH (2012) Liberating the NHS: No decision about me, without me. Government Response. www.gov.uk/(accessed 24 January 2016).

Dingwall, R., Rafferty, A. M. and Webster, C. (1988) *An Introduction to the Social History of Nursing.* London: Routledge.

Dixon, J., Borden, P., Kaneko, T. M. and Schoolwerth, A. C. (2011) Multidisciplinary CKD care enhances outcomes at dialysis initiation. *Nephrology Nursing Journal* 38 (2), 165–71.

Donskoy, A.-L. and Pollard, K. (2014) Interprofessional working with service users and carers. In *Interprofessional Working in Health and Social Care: Professional perspectives* (2nd edn). Thomas, J., Pollard, K. and Sellman, D. (eds). Basingstoke: Palgrave Macmillan, pp. 35–46.

Dufour, S. P., Brown, J. and Lucy, S. D. (2014) Integrating physiotherapists within primary health care teams: perspectives of family physicians and nurse practitioners. *Journal of Interprofessional Care* 28 (5), 460–465.

Francis, R. (2013) *Report of the Mid-Staffordshire NHS Foundation Trust Public Inquiry*. London: The Stationery Office.

Franks, H. (2014) The contribution of nurse consultants in England to the public health leadership agenda. *Journal of Clinical Nursing* 23 (23–24), 3434–3448.

Giordano, R., Clark, M., with Goodwin, N. (2011) *Perspectives on telehealth and telecare: Learning from the 12 Whole System Demonstrator Action Network (WSDAN) sites*. WSDAN briefing paper. London: King's Fund.

Gladstone, D. (1995) Individual welfare: locating care in the mixed economy. Introducing the personal social services. In *British Social Welfare: Past, present and future*. Gladstone, D. (ed.). London: UCL Press, pp. 161–170.

Hudson, B. (2002) Interprofessionality in health and social care: the Achilles' heel of partnership? *Journal of Interprofessional Care* 16 (1), 7–17.

Keeping, C. (2014) the processes required for effective interprofessional working. In *Interprofessional Working in Health and Social Care: Professional perspectives* (2nd edn). Thomas, J., Pollard, K. and Sellman, D. (eds). Basingstoke: Palgrave Macmillan, pp. 22–34.

Laming, Lord (2003) *Inquiry into the Death of Victoria Climbié*. London: The Stationery Office.

Laming, Lord (2009) *The Protection of Children in England: A Progress Report*. Norwich: The Stationery Office.

Lancet (2011) The NHS IT nightmare. *Lancet* 378 (9791), 542.

League of Nations Health Organisation (1931) *League of Nations Health Organisation*. Geneva: WHO Information Section.

Lloyd, A., Clegg, G. and Crouch, R. (2015) Dynamic nurse leadership in high-pressure situations. *Emergency Nurse: Journal of the RCN Accident and Emergency Nursing Association* 23 (3), 24–25.

McNeil, K.A., Mitchell, R.J. and Parker, V. (2013) Interprofessional practice and professional identity threat. *Health Sociology Review* 22 (3), 291–307.

Martin, J. S., Ummenhofer, W., Manser, T. and Spring, R. (2010) Interprofessional collaboration among nurses and physicians: making a difference in patient outcome. *Swiss Medical Weekly* 140 w130632. doi: 10.4414/smw.2010.13062

Miers, M. (2010) Professional boundaries and interprofessional working. In *Understanding Interprofessional Working in Health and Social Care: Theory and Practice*. Pollard, K.C., Thomas, J., and Miers, M. (eds). Basingstoke: Palgrave Macmillan, pp. 105–120.

Moller, P. and Begg, E. (2005) Independent nurse prescribing in New Zealand. *New Zealand Medical Journal* 118 (1225), 1724.

NICE (National Institute for Health and Care Excellence) (2012) Patient experience in adult NHS services. http://pathways.nice.org.uk (accessed 29 May 2016).

Nijagal, M. A., Kupperman, M., Nakagawa, S. N. and Cheng, Y. (2015) Two practice models in one labor and delivery unit: association with cesarean delivery rates. *American Journal of Obstetrics and Gynecology* 212 (4), 491.e1–491. e8.

NMC (Nursing and Midwifery Council) (2010) *Standards for Pre-Registration Nursing Education*. London: NMC. www.nmc.org.uk/standards/(accessed 24 January 2016).

Pape, B., Thiessen, P. S., Jakobsen, F. and Hansen, T. B. (2013) Interprofessional collaboration may pay off: introducing a collaborative approach in an orthopaedic ward. *Journal of Interprofessional Care* 27 (6), 496–500.

Parr, C. (2011) A strategy for nurse prescribing. *Nurse Prescribing* 9 (7), 318–320.

Parse, R. R. (2015) Interdisciplinary and interprofessional: what are the differneces? *Nursing Science Quarterly* 28 (1), 5–6.

Payne, M. (2000) *Teamwork in Multiprofessional Care*. Basingstoke: Macmillan.

Pollard, K., Miers, M. and Rickaby, C. (2012) 'Oh why didn't I take more notice?' Professionals' views and perceptions of their pre-qualifying interprofessional learning as preparation for interprofessional working in practice. *Journal of Interprofessional Care* **26** (5), 355–361.

Pollard, K., Sellman, D. and Senior, B. (2014) The need for interprofessional working. In *Interprofessional Working in Health and Social Care: Professional perspectives* (2nd edn). Thomas, J., Pollard, K. and Sellman, D. (eds). Basingstoke: Palgrave Macmillan, pp. 9–21.

Pollock, A. M. (2009) *NHS plc: The privatization of our health care (New updated edition)*. London: Verso Books.

Randall Curtis, J., Ciechanowski, P. S., Downey, L., Gold, J., Nielsen, E. L., Shannon, S. E., Treece, P. D., Young, J. P. and Engelberg, R. A. (2012) Development and evaluation of an interprofessional communication intervention to improve family outcomes in the ICU. *Contemporary Clinical Trials* **33** (6), 1245–1254.

St Boniface Haiti Foundation (2015) *St Boniface Haiti Foundation: Never Let Go of Hope* www.haitihealth.org (accessed 24 January 2016).

SCIE (Social Care Institute for Excellence) (2001) About SCIE. www.scie.org.uk (accessed 24 January 2016).

Sellman, D., Godsell, M. and Townley, M. (2014) Nursing. In *Interprofessional Working in Health and Social Care: Professional perspectives*. (2nd edn). Thomas, J., Pollard, K. and Sellman, D. (eds). Basingstoke: Palgrave Macmillan, pp. 100–116.

Sommerfeldt, S. (2013) Articulating nursing in an interprofessional world. *Nurse Education in Practice* **13** (6), 519–523.

Stephenson, J. and Wiggins, K. (2014) Councils to have legal obligation to run their health visitor services. Nursing Times.net. www.nursingtimes.net/(accessed 24 January 2016).

Strandmark, K. M., Bengt, A. and Hjalmarson, H. V. (2013) Developing interprofessional collaboration: a case of secondary prevention for patients with osteoporosis. *Journal of Interprofessional Care* **27** (2), 161–170.

Traynor, M. (2013) *Nursing in Context: Policy, politics, profession*. Basingstoke: Palgrave Macmillan.

Vatcher, A. and Jones, K. (2014) Social work. In *Interprofessional Working in Health and Social Care: Professional perspectives*. (2nd edn). Thomas, J., Pollard, K. and Sellman, D. (eds). Basingstoke: Palgrave Macmillan, pp. 174–185.

Walker, T., Stead, J. and Read, S. G. (2003) Caseload management in community learning disability teams: influences on decision-making. *Journal of Learning* **7** (4), 297–321.

Whitewood-Moores, Z. (2011) A single NHS language: SNOMED. *British Journal of Health Care Assistants* **5** (11), 565.

WHO (World Health Organization) (2015) *About WHO*. www.who.int/about/en/ (accessed 24 January 2016).

Williamson, G. R., Jenkinson, T. and Proctor-Childs, T. (2010) *Contexts of Contemporary Nursing*. (2nd edn) Exeter: Learning Matters Ltd.

Witz, A. (1992) *Professions and Patriarchy*. London: Routledge.

8

EVIDENCE-BASED PRACTICE

Mark Broom, Elaine Mahoney and Derek Sellman

LEARNING OUTCOMES

After reading and reflecting on this chapter, you should be able to:

- identify the range and scope of evidence;
- have an awareness of hierarchies of evidence;
- acknowledge the relevance of evidence to nursing practice;
- outline some of the difficulties in using evidence in practice.

INTRODUCTION

There is a great deal written about evidence-based practice and the phrase has come to mean different things to different people. Some suggest that the wholesale adoption of evidence-based practice in nursing is a bad idea, while others believe it should underpin everything we do. Whatever the reality, evidence-based practice is now considered essential for safe and effective nursing practice. In this chapter we offer some information that we hope will be useful to you in your attempt to practise from an evidence base.

The chapter is divided into three parts and structured around four phases of evidence-based practice:

- reviewing practice;
- finding evidence;
- appraising evidence; and
- changing practice.

In Part 1, we offer some general ideas about evidence. We note that not all evidence is of equal value, that the evidence of our senses can be wrong and we outline the reasons nurses need to be able to appraise evidence in whatever form it appears.

M. Broom, E. Mahoney and D. Sellman

As well as **'evidence-based practice'** you are likely to come across terms such as evidence-based medicine', 'research-based practice', 'evidence-based health care' and 'evidence-based nursing'. Sometimes these terms are used interchangeably, yet they each mean slightly different things: to use them interchangeably is to confuse medicine with nursing and to confuse evidence with research. For reasons that should become clear as you read this chapter we prefer the term 'evidence-based practice'.

In Part 2, we say more about the nature of evidence and begin to offer some ideas around the notion and importance of reliability. We offer some examples of how we all use evidence in our everyday lives and non-nursing situations and we outline some important sources of evidence with a few tips on searching the literature. The focus is on reviewing practice and finding evidence.

In Part 3, we explore ideas around recognising the value of different forms of evidence before engaging with some issues of critical appraisal. The focus is on reviewing evidence with a few suggestions about implementing change where that proves to be appropriate.

PART 1: OUTLINING EVIDENCE-BASED PRACTICE

Case 8.1

It is Alan's first day as a student nurse on Charterhouse Ward. He is surprised to find the 'underarm lift' being used routinely by staff on the ward. When he asks why this discredited lift is still being used when the evidence points to its potential to cause harm to both patients and staff, Kathy, his mentor, says it is because of: pressure of time; busyness of the ward; lack of training in effective use of equipment and so on. Finally Kathy admits that the underarm lift should not be used but says 'it is just what we do here'.

Of course, it does not happen like this in all practice areas but in asking the seemingly innocent question 'why do it that way?' Alan has uncovered the complex nature of the relationship between evidence and practice. Even in cases where the evidence is uncontroversial (such as in relation to the underarm lift) there is no guarantee that nurses will base their practice on that evidence. There are many possible reasons for this and some of these will be explored later in this chapter.

Why evidence-based practice?

That practice should be based on evidence seems so self-evident that it is hard to understand why anyone would disagree. Yet the continued emphasis on the need for nurses to base their practice on evidence suggests not only that some current nursing practice is not evidence-based but also that the idea of **evidence-based practice** is not as straightforward as it might appear.

We all make use of evidence every day. We use the evidence of our senses to see, hear, smell, taste and feel the things around us. Under normal circumstances we can rely on the evidence of our senses. When we wish to cross a road we interpret the evidence that comes from our eyes to determine the distance and speed of approaching cars. We turn our head to see who is running when we hear the rapid fall of footsteps behind us and we discard the milk that smells bad rather than use it in our coffee. Such everyday decisions are made on the basis of evidence. In these examples the evidence comes from our senses and our senses usually serve us well. Generally speaking we know the evidence of our senses to be reliable although we also know that it can sometimes be unreliable. Some of the things our senses tell us are real we know to be illusory: for example, we know that railway lines do not converge in the distance despite the evidence of our eyes and similarly

202

we know that a straight stick does not magically become crooked when partly immersed in a pond.

We already know there is evidence that we can rely on and evidence about which we should be wary. To ignore the evidence about an approaching car when we cross the road would be foolish indeed but it would be equally foolish to walk on railway lines believing that trains cannot travel on tracks that converge. In both situations we make a judgment about the evidence before deciding what action to take. In other words, the evidence does not speak for itself. Rather we make an assessment about which evidence we should pay attention to and which evidence we should ignore. In making such a judgment we demonstrate that not only do we already know not all evidence to be of equal value, but also that we have the ability to appraise evidence; that is, to make judgments about the relative value of different pieces of evidence.

You appraise evidence daily in relation to all sorts of decisions you make and actions you take. The effectiveness of these decisions has been learned over time, you have skills that assist you to accept or discard evidence that influences a choice that you have acted upon. To appraise evidence for nursing effectively requires you to learn a new skill set for making judgments about the value of different pieces of evidence. In other words, if you are going to be able to make effective choices you need some guiding principles that will identify evidence you should pay attention to or be wary of as you go about your everyday nursing practice. Just as you have previously learned what you know about the dangers of approaching cars and walking on train tracks, so you can learn how to distinguish between weak and strong evidence for nursing practice.

Simply put, evidence-based practice requires nothing more than:

- reviewing your practice;
- finding evidence;
- appraising the evidence; and
- changing practice where appropriate.

Of course, it is not quite that simple, as each of these activities requires specific knowledge, skills and confidence. Reviewing practice requires some form of reflection; finding evidence requires search and retrieval skills; appraising evidence requires knowledge of the criteria against which judgments are made; and changing practice requires, among other things, effective interpersonal skills as well as leadership and management skills.

Nevertheless, Alan has set the ball rolling for evidence-based practice and he and Kathy, his mentor, are about to embark on a steep learning curve in order to discover best manual handling practice and to try to implement it on Charterhouse Ward.

PART 2: EXPLAINING EVIDENCE-BASED PRACTICE

Why evidence-based practice is important for nurses

The adoption of evidence-based practice for nursing follows the development of evidence-based medicine that recognised the importance of the need for a systematic appraisal of the evidence on which clinical decisions are made. Evidence-based nursing is seen as attractive because it offers an alternative to the 'sister knows best' or 'this is the way it

RESEARCH FOCUS 8.1

Without rejecting the potential value of the saline bath, Walsh and Ford found that a specific concentration of salt would be required to achieve any therapeutic effect yet routine practice was merely to pour an unspecified amount of table salt into a bath. Thus the possibility of therapeutic action became a matter of chance depending on how much salt any particular nurse put into the bath water on any particular occasion. If a saline bath is to have a beneficial effect then those responsible for preparing it should at the very least be able to know how to get the correct concentration.

is done on this ward' approach to the delivery of nursing care. This approach, which had been so pervasive for so long, came in for criticism particularly during the 1980s and was given voice in the book *Nursing Rituals* (Walsh and Ford 1989) in which everyday routine nursing practices (such as pre-operative fasting, the use of saline baths, and the taking of temperature) were scrutinised against the available evidence. What Walsh and Ford found was a dominance of ritual over rational action. Clinicians are well advised to pause to ask why they are doing an activity and what evidence underpins it. What may be understood as good practice at the point of qualification as a nurse may quickly become redundant in the light of developments in technology and knowledge.

The use of evidence for professional practice

The use of evidence is common among professional groups. For example, we all know that the police need to gather sufficient evidence of wrongdoing before a person can be charged with a crime. We also know that both the prosecution and the defence will use evidence in court in the attempt to persuade a jury of the guilt or innocence of the accused. We like to think that any evidence used during criminal proceedings is sufficiently accurate to ensure the defendant gets a fair trial. If we subsequently find that the evidence used to convict someone turns out to be faulty, or was used in such a way as to give a false impression of guilt or innocence, then we immediately recognise that something has gone wrong. When this happens we know that recompense is required: the trial will be abandoned; the prisoner found guilty as a result of false evidence will be released and so on.

Generally speaking, we like to think that only the guilty go to prison and we like to think that the evidence on which they are found guilty is definitely true. Yet, as noted in Chapter 4, even in law evidence does not have to be conclusive. In criminal law, the role of evidence is to 'prove' something beyond reasonable doubt, whereas in civil proceedings all that is required is that evidence leads to a conclusion on the balance of probability. In other words, even in an area that we often imagine requires straightforward and well-defined standards of evidence, the evidence can be (and often is) contradictory, contestable, and open to interpretation.

In this respect nursing is no different. The evidence that nurses use to guide their practice can also be (and often is) contradictory, contestable, and open to interpretation; it can also be less or more reliable and generally stems from research in some way. The safe and competent nurse is the one who, among other things, is able to distinguish between reliable and unreliable evidence; and who can identify contradictions in evidence, understand why some evidence is contestable, and recognise that in some cases different interpretation of the same evidence is possible. Thus while sometimes the evidence for nursing practice is comprehensive and uncontroversial (such as the evidence in relation to the prohibition on the underarm lift) it may be more common to find the evidence either inconclusive or weak. Thus in order to appraise evidence for practice a nurse may need to act not only for the defence as well as for the prosecution, but also as judge and jury.

In court it is the job of both the prosecution and defence lawyers to convince the jury of:

1   the strength of the evidence supporting their case; and
2   the weakness of the evidence of their opponent.

The questioning and cross-examination of witnesses is designed to test the strength of the evidence on which the jury is asked to make a decision and the role of the judge is to ensure that only relevant and appropriate questions are asked. It is in asking and answering questions that the strengths and weaknesses of the evidence are exposed.

Similarly there is a need to ask relevant and appropriate questions of the evidence on which nursing practice is based or proposed. **Critiquing frameworks** are merely systematic ways of asking relevant and appropriate questions so that judgments can be made about the strength of the research process that underpins the evidence.

Thus a critiquing framework is a tool to aid in the appraisal of evidence. We need to know the strength of different pieces of evidence in order to base nursing decisions and actions on the strongest evidence available: where strong evidence exists it would be foolish to rely on weak evidence. We do not walk on train tracks because the evidence of our eyes (in this instance) is weaker than other, stronger evidence telling us that train tracks do not converge.

It might be helpful to think about this in terms of the use of evidence in court. The strongest evidence is that which leaves the jury in no doubt about the guilt or innocence of the accused. If there remains room for doubt, then the next strongest evidence is that which is 'beyond reasonable doubt'. Where there is still reasonable doubt, then the next level of evidence is that which leads to a conclusion on the 'balance of probability'. So we have three levels of evidence:

1   evidence about which there is no doubt;
2   evidence that leads to a conclusion 'beyond reasonable doubt'; and
3   evidence that leads to a conclusion based on the 'balance of probability'.

On this account, 'balance of probability' evidence is the weakest type. Yet in the practice of nursing this is the most likely form of evidence to be readily available. This goes some way to explaining why so much emphasis is placed on the **hierarchy of evidence** and helps to explain why 'beyond reasonable doubt' evidence is given such high value.

The ability to successfully analyse or critique research requires knowledge and understanding of the research process and method. **Critiquing frameworks** are tools comprising a series of focused questions that help to determine the usefulness of research in practice. Later in this chapter you will encounter a variety of different critiquing approaches.

The ability to rank or categorise evidence assists the practitioner when making decisions about the quality of a research article. **Hierarchies of evidence** are systematic and robust tools used when classifying the reliability of research articles.

Activity 8.1

Imagine you are planning to buy a brand new car. Have a go at making a list of questions you might use to help you choose which car to buy.

When decisions are influenced by our own experience or personal interpretation of that experience then it is deemed to be **subjective**. In contrast, objective decisions are said to be undistorted by factors of this type making them easier to quantify and reproduce by others when similar decisions are required.

With such an expensive item it is likely you will spend time browsing through manufacturers' glossy brochures and, perhaps, reading one or two motoring journals. This will provide you with a range of information (or evidence). Some of this information will be in the form of 'hard' evidence (e.g., statistics on fuel economy or CO_2 emissions) and some will be of the more 'soft' variety (e.g., descriptions of comfort, design or style).

The hard information will include statistics such as the number of miles travelled for each litre of petrol, figures for carbon dioxide emissions and the passenger safety record. Having information of this type allows you to make judgments about, for example, the relative environmental impact of the cars on your shortlist. However, if each manufacturer is using a different test to calculate carbon dioxide emissions then some cars may appear to be more environmentally friendly than others. This is similar to assuming foods advertised as low fat are healthy options (this is not necessarily true as noted in Chapter 15). It is only possible to make direct comparisons when the figures from all manufacturers are based on standard tests. Thus figures on fuel economy for different cars can only be meaningfully compared if manufacturers adopt standardised testing, and this is exactly what manufacturers are required to do in the UK. So if you think fuel economy is important then you can make a direct comparison between different cars because manufacturers produce data for fuel consumption based on a standard urban cycle.

The type of hard evidence illustrated above can be relied upon precisely because it allows direct comparisons to be made. To return to the law analogy, it represents 'beyond reasonable doubt' type of evidence. Using this kind of evidence you can say with some confidence that, for example, car X performs best in terms of fuel economy, carbon dioxide emissions and passenger safety and that on these grounds it would be the best car to buy. However, you may not choose to buy car X for all sorts of other reasons, some of which are more rational than others, and most of which will be derived from evidence that is difficult to quantify (soft evidence).

Although often crucial, soft evidence cannot be compared in the same way as hard evidence. There is no point in buying the car with the best environmental record if when you sit in the driving seat your feet do not reach the pedals. So you need to try it out. You need some first-hand information on things such as comfort, all-round visibility and ease of manoeuvrability. It will not matter how persuasive the hard evidence is if you find car X uncomfortable to drive, or if you find you cannot see out of the rear window. In fact, this evidence is not soft at all, but neither is it quantifiable in the way fuel economy is. Nevertheless, it is evidence that is no less important to you than the hard evidence.

There is yet more soft information (or evidence) that may influence your choice. You may have a bias against a particular manufacturer as you may have heard people say things like 'you wouldn't see me dead driving one of those'. You may have what advertisers call 'brand loyalty' based on positive previous experience of a manufacturer; or you may have a preference for a particular colour or shape. This information is much more **subjective**, and may well involve your emotions. As such, it is less reliable and may lead you to neglect or ignore relevant evidence. For example, you may simply not consider any car from one manufacturer because they once had a reputation of producing cars that rust; or because a distant uncle had no end of trouble with one in the 1970s and no one in the family has ever bought one since.

Activity 8.2

Look again at the criteria you made earlier (Activity 8.1). Try to work out which items on your list relate to hard evidence and which equate with soft evidence.

Chances are that your list will contain some hard and some soft types of considerations and both influence our choices. If we choose a car purely on soft types of evidence we may be swayed by factors that relate to our feelings or preferences alone; we might choose a car that comes in our favourite colour only to find later that it is much more expensive to run, or that the nearest service centre is 50 miles away. If we choose purely on the rational grounds of hard evidence we would try to consider each make and model on its merits. We would try not to let our feelings (either negative or positive) get in the way of making the best decision. We would rely on current rather than past evidence. We would look for the most recent evidence to see if the 'rust bucket' reputation is still deserved; and we would recognise the possibility that our uncle's experience might not have been as bad as family mythology makes out (he may just have been particularly unlucky).

In using hard evidence as a starting point we not only increase the choices available to us, we also reduce the influence of unreliable evidence on our decision-making. In this sense, at least, evidence-based practice is an attempt to reduce the influence of unreliable evidence on nursing decisions.

The choices nurses make in relation to the delivery of care are subject to the same pressures, biases and irrational feelings that we all share when making other life choices. The difference is that while it is acceptable to allow these things to influence our choice of car (because that is a personal choice) it is not acceptable to allow them to dominate choices in relation to nursing care. This is because nursing decisions need to be related to the needs of patients rather than to our own preferences. So while some of the different types of information and evidence illustrated in the buying a car example will be appropriate to decision-making in nursing, other types will be unhelpful and possibly harmful. As a registered nurse, it is important to be able to distinguish between the two. Table 8.1 illustrates the similarities in evidence used when buying a car and when making choices for nursing practice.

TABLE 8.1 Comparison of types of evidence used in buying a car or providing nursing care

Buying a car	Providing evidence-based care
Seeking up-to-date advice from the literature by exploring motoring magazines and brochures	Looking for best practice in academic and professional journals
Analysis of performance data	Analysis of statistics and results
Discussion with friends and family	Peer discussion on best practice
Your attitude, the feel and the drivability of the car	Feelings and the lived experience presented by qualitative research
Past experience of driving and car ownership	Established nursing practice/how it has always been done

Reviewing practice

Reviewing practice is a precursor for evidence-based practice. Reviewing practice requires thinking about nursing. This may range from merely wondering if there might be a better way of doing something to undertaking a full-blown structured reflection following a critical incident and using one or other of the established models of reflection (see Chapter 17 for more information on the process of reflection).

If we give Alan (Case 8.1) the benefit of the doubt we can say that he was merely asking an innocent question because he has received conflicting information about nursing. His tutors (who are not there with him in practice) point him to the evidence about the dangers of the underarm lift, while the nurses with whom he is working use it all the time. Alan merely wants to know who is right so that he can become a safe practitioner. He finds it hard to imagine that the nurses on Charterhouse Ward would knowingly put themselves and the patients at risk of harm so he thinks they must know something he does not and tries to find out what this something is by asking his mentor.

If we also give Kathy (Alan's mentor and the ward sister) the benefit of the doubt and assume she is not deliberately trying to put the nursing staff or the patients at risk of harm, then we might say that she has to ensure everything gets done within the available time. Hence Kathy has a bigger picture in mind as she allows the practice to continue. She knows the underarm lift is not good practice but since she became ward manager she has had a number of more demanding pressures to deal with and anyway, no one has been injured as far as she can tell. Hence she has just let poor practice continue. However, now Alan has raised the issue she realises it is time to do something about it. In this sense then, and despite being a first-year student nurse, Alan has made a difference; he has acted (albeit unintentionally) as an agent of change.

Finding evidence

Case 8.1 (continued)

Most of the patients on Charterhouse Ward need help with mobility. Having been prompted to action by Alan, Kathy now wants to learn more about best practice in manual handling. As a first step she will need to find the evidence.

Kathy goes in search of the Trust policy on manual handling. She is disappointed with what she finds. While it contains some useful information about the need to undertake mobility assessments on individual patients and has some references, it is undated and provides only a few specific recommendations for good practice, although it does reinforce the message that the underarm lift is about as far away from good practice as it is possible to get. Thus Kathy's search for evidence is far from over, and she decides to enlist the help of Alan with his new-found knowledge gained from the university about evidence-based practice. Unfortunately, Alan has only just begun to learn about searching the literature so they agree to work together to see what they can find.

Finding evidence is a crucial step in evidence-based practice. This much should be obvious, but it needs to be the right sort of evidence; and finding the most appropriate evidence for any particular aspect of nursing practice can be a daunting prospect. While the Internet has undoubtedly made searching for information relatively easy, finding reliable evidence means you need to know something about sources of information, and how authoritative those sources are. Using search engines and online encyclopaedias will certainly help you to access a huge amount of information but that in itself can create difficulties. When there is so much information, it can be difficult to choose between articles; when there is so much information you need some form of **search strategy**.

Computer literacy

It is reasonable to suggest that most entering nurse education have been through schools or colleges that have embraced the online learning environment. Whether an individual watches television, shops or seeks to book a holiday, the skills utilised in these online endeavours are applicable to searching for clinical evidence. Searching through large bound bibliographies sitting in a library is a thing of the past, but this does not mean all health care practitioners have the skills to navigate around the electronic databases or effectively utilise the World Wide Web in the pursuit of information. Without the necessary skills the very tools that should liberate can frustrate the health care practitioner.

Information overload

With so much information available in a variety of differing media, it is easy to become overwhelmed when searching a topic. The ability to filter good from poor evidence is essential to remain focused and to ensure you capture the essence of the problem under investigation. Results from using an Internet search engine will give you an indication of the depth of evidence available but it can also present a challenge in determining the credibility of sources. Effective search patterns utilising databases such as CINAHL and MEDLINE help to focus a search, making the process manageable. The results from this type of search will generally yield credible sources based on research.

Effective searching

Being able to develop and use search patterns and transfer these from one database to another allows efficient use of search time and means a greater likelihood of finding the information you need. Having these skills and knowing what different databases have to offer makes searching the literature easier and less time-consuming. It does take time and effort to learn, and you may make some frustrating mistakes along the way but help is at hand through a number of helpful resources. Libraries and librarians are particularly helpful when learning how to search the literature. Most education institutions and/or libraries have individuals available to help you learn about and explore these valuable tools.

Sources of evidence

There is a staggering array of health care information available to practitioners. As well as local policies and procedures, information is available from books, journals, colleagues, electronic databases and indexes, the Internet, professional organisations, Governments and clinical guidelines. Of course, each source has its advantages and disadvantages with some based on research while others are based on perceived best practice.

A little time spent planning your **search strategy** results in a more realistic outcome and in less frustration from a practitioner's perspective. The use of key words, time range, limits on language, type of article (e.g. original research, literature review or full text) will help give focus to your search. Spending time learning how to use databases and search engines effectively will be rewarded in the future in less time spent exploring search results that do not match your original criteria. Thus finding the right sort of information requires an element of computer literacy, avoiding information overload and searching effectively.

Local policies and procedures

Local policies and procedures are usually readily available and sometimes take the form of clinical guidelines (see below). However, they can quickly become out of date unless there is a conscious effort to keep them under review in the light of new and emerging evidence. Spend time looking for the review date, the credibility of the authors and investigate the source of evidence that underpins the recommendations.

Books

Books are perhaps the most easily accessible form of information and many now contain a substantial evidence base. However, information in books can quickly become out of date. In subject areas in which new knowledge is emerging rapidly a book, which may take around 6–9 months to reach the shelves once the manuscript has been delivered, may be almost out of date on publication. Nevertheless, not everything in books becomes out of date so quickly so it is helpful to recognise which information within a book is likely to need updating and which is likely to remain current. For example, Piaget's theory of cognitive development is unlikely to change from old to new editions of general introductory textbooks on psychology, although research evidence supporting or disputing his theory may not appear in older editions so ensuring you are working from the most recent edition is important. It appears a common trend with a number of publishers to produce a companion website with each newly published book giving the author an opportunity to make amendments to the original text and add new evidence as it enters the public domain.

Journals

Journal articles have the advantage of being more current than books because the turnaround time between acceptance and publication can be much shorter. Generally journals are the first publication choice for researchers and those producing evidence-based opinion papers. Not all journals have equal standing: while double blind peer review is standard for some, others publish case studies and opinion papers following less stringent external review. Alongside a hierarchy of evidence you are also able to rate the journal's impact, influence or prestige. Using highly ranked journals minimises the risk of citing poor evidence but the content of the paper should still be critiqued because the fact of publication does not guarantee quality research.

Colleagues

You can always rely on your colleagues having an opinion. However, you cannot rely on the accuracy or validity of their opinion. There is a tendency for students to assume that qualified nurses have up-to-date and comprehensive knowledge on a huge range of topics and issues. The reflective nursing student asks such questions such as 'why is it done this way?' If the received answer has no evidence-based justification then you are in danger of following the 'sister knows best' school of justification. If however, your answer is on the lines of: 'because my mentor has shown me the current evidence from a reliable source that recommends this way of doing it as best practice', then there is a good chance you are using evidence-based practice.

Electronic databases and indexes

Electronic databases and indexes allow you to search and cross-reference journals using keywords, author details or journal title. While each database or index can be searched individually it is increasingly common to make use of 'portals', such as Ovid or FindIT that allow you to search a number of different databases using an easy to use interface. Some of the more commonly used (and perhaps most generally useful) electronic databases are MEDLINE, CINAHL, PubMed, EMBASE, Midwifery and Infant Care, Alt Health Watch and the Cochrane Collection. Each database has a unique slant on the literature it represents so searching a number of databases gives the best possible search result.

The Internet

The Internet has made it possible for more individuals than ever to access information and to learn in new and exciting ways. The power of the Internet to transform the educational experience is awe-inspiring, but it can also be a frustrating and time-consuming pastime, particularly if you are unfamiliar with or unaware of the tools that can make it easier. One of the most efficient ways of retrieving information from the Internet is to use a **'search engine'**. Search engines trawl the Internet in different ways so it is worth trying different search engines to maximise your results. Commonly used search engines include: Google (www.google.co.uk); Yahoo (http://uk.yahoo.com); and Alta Vista (http://uk.altavista.com/web/default). This list is by no means comprehensive: it is merely a starting point and you are encouraged to try out other search engines although all Internet browsers will allow you to search the Internet.

Professional organisations

Professional organisations provide an important source of evidence and information ranging from professional guidance or legislative change through to archives of relevant journals. Useful information and differing perspectives can be gained by searching the websites of professional organisations. For example, the Nursing Midwifery Council website (www.nmc-uk.org) gives a nursing perspective on nurse prescribing whereas the Royal Pharmaceutical Society of Great Britain website (www.rpsgb.org.uk) offers a similar strategic message but with a somewhat different professional slant. However, it should not be assumed that a strong evidence base exists for all documents produced by professional organisations and users are guided towards appropriate appraisal of information from these sources.

Policies and reports

There have been a myriad of reports produced on a wide range of topic areas from international, national and local perspectives. Intranets that search local Trust databases are a useful first step to find polices on all manner of themes specific to your locality. Reports and publications as well as health statistics are easily obtained from the Department of Health website (www.dh.gov.uk). A regional perspective on health care can also be found by accessing the relevant web pages for each UK region.

A **search engine** is an automated software program that trawls the Internet collecting and cataloguing data from web pages. This is presented to the user as an indexed list ranked in order of the best match to your search parameters. Search engines complete this task astonishingly quickly.

211

M. Broom, E. Mahoney and D. Sellman

The terms primary and secondary evidence are used regularly in the literature. Primary evidence is original and you are reading the authors' report directly as it was written. **Secondary sources** of evidence may be gathered when reading a report or document where the author refers to another author's research. Unless you then refer to the primary source you are unable to determine whether context and meaning have been altered when applied to the secondary source. As such, primary evidence is considered more reliable than secondary evidence.

Evidence that stems from experimental designs such as **randomised controlled trials** (RCTs) provides an effective way of determining the cause–effect relationship between intervention and outcome (Parahoo 2014). If well designed, RCTs can form the scientific basis of high-quality change. If flawed or poorly designed, incorrect inferences may result in inappropriate care practices being adopted.

Clinical guidelines

Clinical guidelines are a useful source of information for the busy practitioner and may be of local, regional or national origin. They represent **secondary sources** of evidence in which a critical appraisal of the primary evidence is linked to other aspects of evidence-based practice (patient preference, professional expertise and available resources) in order to make recommendations for practice.

Clinical guidelines generated by respected national bodies tend to carry greater authority, for example, those from the National Institute of Health and Clinical Excellence (NICE) are held in particularly high esteem, but as a nurse you still need to be convinced that such guidelines are appropriate for your client group and practice area.

With so much easily available information and so much new information being published it would be unreasonable to think that a nurse can keep up to date with all the evidence relevant to their area of specialty. As such the practitioner is faced with the challenge of attempting to discriminate between good and poor evidence. Reviewing the literature is both a time-consuming and a skilled activity and most practitioners have neither the time nor the inclination to undertake a comprehensive appraisal of the literature. Nevertheless, there is a need to understand why appraisal is necessary and to have an idea of the process if nursing practice is to be based on the current best evidence available. This level of engagement with evidence has been described as being 'research aware' or 'research literate' (Moule 2015) and it is to appraisal that we now turn in Part 3 of this chapter.

PART 3: EXPLORING EVIDENCE-BASED PRACTICE

Appraising the evidence

Hewitt-Taylor (2013) reminds us that many nursing actions appear to be based upon tradition, habit or on the unsubstantiated preferences of influential health care professionals. It is possible that in some instances traditional practice is perfectly safe and may even be best practice, but it is difficult for a nurse to justify such practice without evidence supporting its effectiveness. Some nursing practices have changed little in 20 or more years, others have changed in light of evidence demonstrating beneficial patient outcomes, but one of the expectations of evidence-based practice is that nurses should continue to review practice in order to introduce change to practice where the evidence suggests this is necessary.

Whatever form the evidence takes it is necessary to make a judgment about its value or worth. This is to say that there is a need to find out whether or not a particular piece of evidence can or should be used to inform practice.

The appraisal process starts with an identification of the category to which a piece of evidence belongs. Merely determining whether it is research evidence or non-research evidence is to make a judgment about its value. Research evidence is generally considered to be more reliable than non-research evidence. Thus in any hierarchy of evidence **randomised controlled trials** (RCTs) will be placed higher than clinical expertise or professional opinion (see Figure 8.1). For those seeking hard evidence that offers 'beyond reasonable doubt' type conclusions, the RCT sets the standard to which other forms of evidence aspire. Some consider studies that do not meet the RCT standard to have little part to play in evidence-based practice.

212

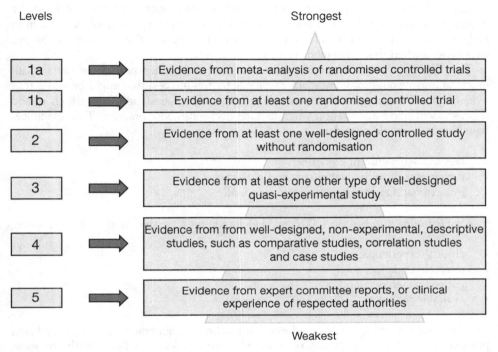

Levels   Strongest

1a	Evidence from meta-analysis of randomised controlled trials
1b	Evidence from at least one randomised controlled trial
2	Evidence from at least one well-designed controlled study without randomisation
3	Evidence from at least one other type of well-designed quasi-experimental study
4	Evidence from from well-designed, non-experimental, descriptive studies, such as comparative studies, correlation studies and case studies
5	Evidence from expert committee reports, or clinical experience of respected authorities

Weakest

FIGURE 8.1
Hierarchy of evidence

Source: Flemming and Fenton (2002, p. 114).

A **systematic review** will critically summarise the literature using a process of quality assessment and appraisal of material. Studies that are unsound are rejected leaving the reader with a concise, reliable account to work from (Boland, Cherry and Dickson 2014).

Meta-analysis is a technique for quantitatively combining the results from multiple studies. A meta-analysis of RCTs would produce evidence that would be considered even more valid and reliable than that from a single RCT.

Gerrish and Lathlean (2015) define **quantitative research** as a systematic process of getting quantifiable information presented numerically and analysed through the use of statistics.

Hierarchies of evidence

Hierarchies of evidence take different forms. The hierarchy of evidence reproduced in Figure 8.1 is used by Flemming and Fenton (2002) and takes a familiar form. In this hierarchy the strongest form of evidence is at the top in the form of meta-analyses (level 1a in the diagram) closely followed by what they call 'Evidence from at least one RCT' (Flemming and Fenton 2002, p. 114). This would include single RCT studies as well as **systematic reviews**.

In this hierarchy it is evidence from levels 1a and 1b that meets the 'beyond reasonable doubt' standard. All the other levels from 2 down to 5 provide evidence that might meet the 'balance of probability' standard. Flemming and Fenton note that 'As you move down the hierarchy the chances of reaching reliable, accurate and unbiased answers decrease' (2002, p. 113) but they reject the idea that only the evidence of RCTs should be used in clinical decision-making. While RCTs, systematic reviews and **meta-analyses** provide the strongest evidence, this type of research can only answer those types of questions where direct comparisons between interventions and outcomes can be made.

Thus if you want to know the most effective way of transferring an immobile patient from bed to chair, level 1a and 1b studies can provide the answer but only within a set of detailed parameters. For example, well-designed level 1-type studies can tell you the quickest or the most efficient method because these things can be measured, counted and quantified (hence they are **quantitative research**) but such studies will struggle to provide meaningful data on patient comfort or preference, or information about which equipment staff find easier to use.

Just as the most fuel-efficient car is unsuitable if you cannot reach the pedals, so the equipment needed for the most efficient method of transferring immobile patients from bed to chair will be unsuitable if patients cannot tolerate the level of discomfort experienced when that equipment is used.

Thus RCTs, systematic reviews and meta-analyses cannot provide answers to all practical nursing questions. For many nursing activities the best that might be said is that evidence from these types of studies will provide a firm foundation from which to add other evidence and information when making decisions about practice. Thus evidence-based practice should consider:

- best available current evidence;
- preferences of individual clients and patients;
- expertise and experience of the professional.

For Flemming and Fenton (2002, p. 114) it requires a combination of the following:

- clinical experience;
- research evidence;
- patient preference; and
- available resources.

This last point is an often-neglected item on the list of requirements for evidence-based practice. Even if the equipment recommended from level 1 studies is both the most effective and the most comfortable, it may not be available but this does not necessarily represent a failure of evidence-based practice.

Evidence categorisation

Being able to rank or categorise evidence assists the health care practitioner in the pursuit of reliable evidence for guiding practice. Since the 1970s, a growing number of organisations have been involved in classifying and reviewing evidence for the benefit of health care practitioners. If nurses are to have confidence in the recommendations of systematic reviews and clinical guidelines then there must be a systematic and robust approach (Grade Working Group 2004). The system used in the development of guidance for many clinical and public health interventions involves the hierarchy used by the Scottish Intercollegiate Guidelines Network (SIGN) and reproduced by the National Institute for Health and Clinical Excellence (NICE) to explore the review and grading of evidence (see Table 8.2).

As noted earlier, a hierarchy of evidence provides an indication of the relative confidence you can place in a particular piece of evidence. In the SIGN hierarchy evidence at levels 1^{++} and 2^{++} is deemed to be research of the highest quality and it is papers meeting the criteria of such studies that are used in generating a systematic review. This provides the best chance of producing reliable evidence of effectiveness.

Evidence at both levels 1^- and 2^- and levels 3 and 4 involves the use of research approaches that are variations of the scientific experiment or studies that do not use an experimental approach. Such approaches have limitations and, as a result, findings from these studies are placed lower down the hierarchy. Thus the chance of producing reliable results of effectiveness is lower than that obtained using higher-level studies.

TABLE 8.2 The Scottish Intercollegiate Guidelines Network hierarchy

1^{++}	High-quality meta-analyses, systematic reviews of RCTs, or RCTs with a very low risk of bias
1^{+}	Well-conducted meta-analyses, systematic reviews of RCTs, or RCTs with a low risk of bias
1^{-}	Meta-analyses, systematic reviews of RCTs, or RCTs with a high risk of bias
2^{++}	High-quality systematic reviews of case-control or cohort studies.
	High-quality case-control or cohort studies with a low risk of confounding, bias or chance and a high probability that the relationship is causal
2^{+}	Well-conducted case-control or cohort studies with a low risk of confounding, bias or chance and a moderate probability that the relationship is causal
2^{-}	Case-control or cohort studies with a high risk of confounding, bias or chance and a significant risk that the relationship is not causal
3	Non-analytic studies (for example, case reports, case series)
4	Expert opinion, formal consensus

Source: SIGN (2004).

Qualitative research may be any type of research that produces findings not arrived at by statistical procedures or any means of quantification (Parahoo, 2014). This is an all-embracing term that attempts to understand human behaviour and a rationale for that behaviour.

Qualitative research findings are not included in this hierarchy. This is not to say that qualitative research has no value or that it is unreliable; it is merely to recognise that it does not offer evidence of effectiveness in the way that quantitative research evidence does. Qualitative research does have a contribution to make to evidence-based practice, although not everyone agrees on the value of that contribution. Qualitative research methods are used to study events or experiences in their natural setting, attempting to make sense of poorly understood areas of care. In some cases a better understanding of a situation that emerges from a qualitative study may identify a particular phenomenon amenable to research using quantitative approaches.

It is now accepted in some circles that both quantitative and qualitative research have a part to play in evidence-based nursing practice. For example, an RCT is a frequently utilised approach when exploring the efficacy of drugs, while qualitative approaches will help us understand the experiences of clients undergoing particular treatments. Throughout your professional career you are likely to read reports that have utilised both quantitative and qualitative research approaches.

In the SIGN hierarchy, expert committee reports, professional opinion and clinical expertise represent the least reliable forms of evidence in terms of effectiveness. However, sometimes this is the only type of evidence available in which case it cannot be dismissed out of hand, but it still needs to be viewed with a critical eye. The message here is that whatever form of evidence is being used, there is a need to appraise its value in terms of its application to any particular nursing action.

The recommendation table that accompanies the SIGN hierarchy (Table 8.3) provides an indication about the level of evidence you are using to provide care in any particular situation.

Deciding how the literature you are examining compares to the level of evidence in Table 8.3 will give a reasonable idea of the strength and rigour of the design and of the evidence base for your practice. However, you need to remember that evidence in any

TABLE 8.3 Level of evidence table

A	At least one meta-analysis, systematic review, or RCT rated as 1^{++}, and directly applicable to the target population; or a systemic review or RCT or a body of evidence consisting principally of studies rated as 1^+, directly applicable to the target population, and demonstrating overall consistency of results
B	A body of evidence including studies rated as 2^{++}, directly applicable to the target population, and demonstrating overall consistency of results; or extrapolated evidence rated as 1^{++} or 1^+
C	A body of evidence including studies rated as 2^+, directly applicable to the target population, and demonstrating overall consistency of results; or extrapolated evidence rated as 2^{++}
2^{++}	Evidence levels 3 or 4; or extrapolated evidence rated as 2^+

Source: SIGN (2004)

category will not necessarily meet the standards of reliability set for that form of evidence: hence the need for critical appraisal.

Critical appraisal

Journals provide an excellent source of recent research papers, although as we pointed out earlier, not everything that gets published is of high quality. Using the skills of critical appraisal will help you to make a judgment about the value of a particular piece of evidence. Regardless of the form of evidence under review, the process of critical appraisal is broadly similar. Undertaking a critical appraisal is a bit like being a detective. The purpose is to sift the weak from the strong evidence.

Just like prosecution and defence lawyers in a trial, effective critical appraisal relies on asking the right sort of probing questions. There are a number of critiquing frameworks designed for this purpose: that is, to ask specific and probing questions of evidence to help you make a judgment about its quality. For example, LoBiondo-Wood and Haber (2013) provide a framework for evaluating qualitative research and a separate one for evaluating quantitative research. Similarly, there are frameworks specifically designed to appraise systematic reviews and clinical guidelines. While the questions in one framework will be different from the questions in another and will be different again for appraising, for example, clinical guidelines and RCTs, the basic premise in each will be the same. In all instances a framework will seek answers to questions designed to assess whether the accepted standards of the particular type of evidence have been met. If those standards have been met then there is a greater chance that the evidence is reliable. Critical Appraisal Skills Programme (CASP 2013) suggest that when appraising evidence we need to decide three things:

- Is the study valid?
- What are the results?
- Are the results useful?

Effective critical appraisal is something that you can learn. Just as you have learned not to trust your eyes when faced with railway tracks and just as you have learned not to be deceived by the appearance of a partly submerged stick, so you can learn what to look out for when reviewing evidence.

The chances are that at some point during your pre-registration nurse education programme you will be asked to make an appraisal of some evidence. It is likely that you will be expected to appraise evidence using a critiquing framework and you may wonder why you are being asked to do this. Well, the answer is that in order to be an autonomous and accountable practitioner you need to be able to make an independent judgment about the evidence you use to guide your practice. It is no more acceptable to use clinical guidelines (or any other form of evidence) uncritically than it is to practise on the basis of the discredited 'sister knows best' model that evidence-based practice is trying to replace. Being able to do a bit of critical appraisal means you may be able to avoid basing your actions on unreliable evidence that can be worse than not using evidence at all (CASP 2013). The more critical appraisals you do, the easier it becomes, and the more likely critiquing will become a normal part of your reading technique.

Case 8.1 (continued)

If we return to the situation on Charterhouse Ward you will remember that Kathy acquired a copy of a local guideline on manual handling: because this document makes recommendations for practice it can be classed as a clinical guideline. Alan remembers that one of the lecturers mentioned something about an appraisal tool for clinical guidelines and he eventually tracks it down. It comes as part of the CASP package and he and Kathy attempt to use it to appraise the clinical guidelines on manual handling.

The CASP package is an open learning source (CASP 2013) specifically designed for health care professionals. It contains a framework for appraising RCTs, qualitative research, systematic reviews, cohort studies and case-control studies. It follows a checklist approach that is easy to follow and well worth a view.

Activity 8.3

Have a look at Kathy and Alan's answers to the questions of an appraisal framework (Table 8.4). Do you think Kathy and Alan are going to be able to trust the results of this piece of evidence?

TABLE 8.4 Examples of answers to questions in the CASP framework for appraising clinical guidelines

Responsibility for guideline	Yes	No	Not sure
Is the agency responsible for the development of the guidelines clearly identified?			✓
Was external funding or other support received for developing the guideline?	✓		
If external funding or support was received, is there evidence that the potential biases of the funding body(ies) were taken into account?		✓	

In this example (Table 8.4) the author of the guideline is clearly stated. Although she is unknown to Kathy, the author had previously been employed by the hospital some years earlier in the role of nurse development manager. So while the author was identified, there is no statement about who was responsible for the development. If the answer to two additional questions about who has responsibility for reviewing and updating the guideline and when this should be done are equally unclear then the signs are that this guideline may be out of date, especially if no date of publication is given.

Similarly, the support of a company that manufactures lifting and handling equipment is acknowledged, but there is no mention of any steps taken to make sure that support did not influence or bias the results.

In this case both Kathy and Alan are surprised (even a little shocked) to find that it appears that the guideline represents unreliable evidence for practice. They have no way of knowing how recent (or old) it is; they have no way of knowing if it has been recently reviewed and updated and they have no way of knowing if the equipment recommended was influenced by the financial support given by the manufacturer.

As Polit and Beck (2013) suggest, regardless of the framework used, a critiquing tool should take into consideration the following aspects of the evidence (whatever form that evidence takes):

- the credibility and accuracy of the results;
- the meaning of the results;
- the importance of the results;
- the extent to which the results can be generalised or have the potential for use in other contexts;
- the implications for practice, theory or research.

To even think about making a change in practice on the basis of evidence that has not been subject to some form of appraisal is to fail to understand your own professional accountability. It may be tempting to encourage change on the basis of one piece of research evidence but the only professional approach is to have some idea of the validity of that piece of evidence: thus some form of critical appraisal is a necessary skill for effective nursing practice.

When reading research papers, sections on method, sample selection and data collection may be difficult and uninspiring. Yet it is important not to ignore these sections and read them alongside the introduction, discussion and conclusion. A critical read of all sections of the paper is the only way to be sure that a full critical appraisal has been undertaken. Questions on the lines of the following are common in critiquing frameworks and provide information for making a judgment about the value of a piece of research evidence.

1   Is the chosen methodology the most effective for the topic area?
2   Is there sufficient sample for the chosen method?
3   Is the data collection tool available for scrutiny and does the author give sufficient information to judge issues of reliability and validity?
4   Is sufficient data published to allow scrutiny of the figures for accuracy?
5   Does the researcher answer their research statement, question or hypothesis?
6   Do the author's discussion and conclusions stem from the data collected?

218

By looking for answers to questions of this type you will be analysing and reviewing the literature rather than merely reading uncritically. Critical appraisal is about coming to a balanced review of a research paper (or other form of evidence) while looking for both positive and negative aspects. It should not be just an account of all that is wrong with the paper. As Hibbard (2004) states: 'Critiquing research is a very high order cognitive skill. It requires knowledge of the conceptual, methodological and ethical components of research' (p. 37).

The more often you try appraising evidence using a critiquing framework the more analytical and natural the critiquing process will become. As a result of this process you will become a more informed practitioner whose care is based on evidence. Think back to your first clinical experience, sitting in the Charge Nurse's office and receiving a handover report. Remember how complex and bewildering it all seemed then, yet now you know what is going on (most of the time) and you may even be involved in giving handover. Understanding the research process and becoming comfortable with critical appraisal is a very similar learning experience.

Changing practice

In purely practical terms, making a change to existing or established practice is perhaps the most difficult phase of evidence-based practice. A willingness to change is a fundamental requirement; if you are not prepared to change the way you do things there is little point in either reviewing practice or finding and appraising the evidence. The point of engaging with these activities is to try to find out whether or not existing practice is supported by current best evidence. If you are unwilling to make changes to your practice in the light of evidence suggesting that change is needed then the purpose of evidence-based practice is undermined.

Case 8.1 (continued)

Both Alan and Kathy have already demonstrated they are willing to make changes to practice. As ward manager Kathy has tried to implement other changes with varying degrees of success. In this respect she has, at least, some experience; enough to know that there is nothing easy about making and sustaining changes to practice. Alan on the other hand, finds it difficult to understand why people are reluctant to change, particularly when there is so much evidence to show a need for that change.

Managing change is far from straightforward. On the face of it, it is reasonable to expect people to want to change practice when the evidence is sufficiently compelling. If only it were so simple! The reality is that people do not always behave in reasonable ways and not everyone is willing to change the way they do things. While some people embrace change, others will resist it; some people are more easily convinced of the need for change than others; some will only change once they recognise the inevitability of it and even then may resist in subtle and not so subtle ways. Yet others may be too willing to change, or seek change merely for the sake of change. In other words, change is dependent on people, and managing change is a skilled and complex activity. The skilled change agent can draw from a range of different change management theories and you can find more information about these theories in Chapter 6 of this book.

RESEARCH FOCUS 8.2

On being willing to change

Sellman (2003) claims open-mindedness as a prerequisite for evidence-based practice on the grounds that the two failures of open-mindedness (closed-mindedness and credulousness) help explain the tendency of nurses (and other health and social care practitioners) to adopt the comfort of ritual and routine. For Sellman being open-minded requires a capacity to recognise the possibility that one's current beliefs and/or practices might be incorrect, together with a willingness to change those beliefs and/or practices in the light of compelling evidence.

On this account closed-mindedness (an unwillingness to acknowledge the possibility that one might hold an erroneous belief) and credulousness (a tendency to adopt a belief in the absence of supporting evidence) are both person-located barriers to evidence-based practice.

As Sellman (2015) later notes, nurses tend to be drawn to evidence that supports rather than challenges their strongly held beliefs. Thus the closed-minded person is unlikely to engage with evidence that indicates they should revise their current practices – so a nurse who believes there to be nothing wrong with using the underarm lift and thinks on the lines of: 'well, I've been using it for 35 years and it hasn't done me any harm' is not going to be convinced easily of the need to change their practice.

Similarly, Sellman notes that the credulous nurse is someone who might, for example, accept uncritically and act on a call from an eminent professional who merely expresses an opinion that nurses should no longer be involved in the manual handling of patients.

There are, of course, different levels of change, each requiring a different level of engagement with other people in a range of positions in the hierarchy of the organisation. These include a change that needs to be addressed immediately and takes planning, or a change that can be immediately implemented. It could involve a new practice protocol that needs to be developed as a result of new evidence or a change that needs addressing by the organisation as a whole.

It should be apparent that you would need to use a different approach for each level of change. Changes that involve only yourself should be easy to implement while those that affect whole organisations will require engaging with different individuals and negotiating through bureaucratic processes. It is, after all, likely to be easier to effect change in a small team of nurses than to introduce change to practice across a large organisation. Nevertheless, even attempts to implement change among, for example, a small team working in a single hospital ward can easily founder, especially if planning for the change is hasty or ill-conceived, or if change is being foisted on an unwilling staff.

It is relatively easy to change your own practice. For example, Alan might decide never again to take part in underarm lifting but this will have only limited effect on patient care if other members of the ward team continue the poor practice. In fact, in this situation Alan may find himself becoming unpopular and possibly isolated; and if he begins to worry this might have a negative effect on his placement assessment, then his resolve might start to slip. Such pressures are not entirely fanciful and point to the difficulty of expecting students to act as agents of change in practice areas.

However, if Kathy decides to lead by example, she will make sure everybody understands the need for change and she will work with each individual in order to demonstrate there

220

is a different way of achieving the same or better outcomes. Of course, to do this she will need to become knowledgeable about safer techniques and proficient in using specialist equipment. If she does this there is a chance that the other staff will begin to change their behaviour, at least while Kathy is present. If it happens that some others begin to adopt the better practice that Kathy is trying to introduce there is a chance that the change in practice will continue to spread among the team until those who continue to use the underarm lift are in the minority. At this point the pressure to conform will come to bear on those resisting change rather than on those implementing it. If this happens then a lasting change may have occurred but even then you will need to recognise that, if the weight of new evidence points to it, further change may be necessary. As a result it may be best to think of change as a continuous process: as evolution rather than revolution.

This is not a theory of change, neither is it offered as a recipe for change management. For this you should turn to Chapter 6. Rather it is merely an illustration of the need to plan carefully when trying to implement change, and of the need to recognise change as inevitable.

Activity 8.4

Make a list of the reasons you think the staff on Charterhouse Ward would give you if you asked them why they continue to use the underarm lift.

A time delay between the reporting of research findings and a more general recognition of the significance of those findings is common; in some cases it can be many years. It is sometimes suggested that because of this time lag, evidence for change only gradually filters into the general awareness of nurses, providing a sort of slow knowledge creep. When enough nurses recognise their practice is out of step with current evidence a suitable environment for change may have been created and change is then more likely to happen as those affected are, in theory at least, more likely to be receptive to it. Even then, resistance may occur, especially if individuals think the changes will affect them in negative ways. While a nurse may be convinced of the need to stop using the underarm lift they will not be motivated to change if the alternatives are too complicated, time-consuming or demanding. Resistance to change is often very powerful and should never be underestimated.

Activity 8.5

Having considered the rationale for using the underarm lift presented in Activity 8.4, why do you feel staff may be reluctant to embrace the research literature?

Polit and Beck (2013) provide a helpful breakdown of what they consider the four most important factors that get in the way of applying research findings to practice. Recognising these barriers can be half the battle in making it possible to look at the best ways to eliminate or minimise them. The four barriers highlighted by Polit and Beck are as follows:

Research-related barriers

In many instances research that directly addresses the practice issues faced by nurses is in its infancy, which means there may be few reports of sufficient quality on which to base practice decisions. This is one reason why it is so important to be able to understand the critical appraisal process. It is not necessarily that the pressing questions of nursing cannot be answered by high-quality and trustworthy research, but it does mean that the evidence base is just too small to make it sufficiently reliable as a guide to practice. Thus while it is still developing, nurses can make decisions on the basis of whatever evidence is available at a particular point in time. This is one reason why you need to keep up to date with evidence as it becomes available.

Nurse-related barriers

Although an improving picture overall, the research awareness of health care professionals remains inadequate. Research modules are available in most courses studied at higher education institutions but it takes more than the ability to critique to implement research findings. It is also well documented that there is a lack of motivation, resistance and reluctance to initiate change.

Organisation-related barriers

The 'culture' of an organisation can make a huge difference in the way colleagues respond to research. Some organisations actively encourage innovation and improvement. In others, the effect of established priorities and procedures can stifle innovation. With the implementation of the national Research Governance Strategy (DH 2006) research awareness has gained a higher profile throughout the NHS, and Trusts are expected to identify their research strategies. As a result a more coherent research strategy to deliver evidence for practice is emerging. This has been reinforced as nurse education became integrated into the higher education system in the UK, with an associated focus on the application of research to practice.

Barriers related to the nursing profession (and barriers between professions)

It is useful to think about two categories of professional barriers:

1 *Barriers between health care professionals and researchers.* Researchers and health care professionals do not always see things in the same way and the priorities of each can sometimes conflict. In addition, researchers and practitioners do not always trust each other. Research by its very nature attempts to control or focus in on predefined problems. This is seen as alien to many practitioners who view the care of their clients from a holistic perspective.

2 *Barriers between different health care professions.* It is not uncommon for a single piece of research to have implications for members of different health care professions. Again, the track record here is not always a good one, although progress is certainly being made.

Authors categorise the barriers to the implementation of evidence in different ways, but the characteristics Polit and Beck (2013) outline have been identified consistently over time and similar barriers are evident in many professional groups. Although a little old now, an interesting and comparatively brief literature review on the topic of getting research into practice (Tordoff 1998) highlights barriers under four similar headings of:

1   problems with the research itself;
2   individual resistance to implementation;
3   organisational factors; and
4   cultural issues.

Reviewing practice in relation to current evidence takes place in an environment where many other factors influence the decisions we make. Muir Gray (2001) suggests there are three factors that influence the assimilation or otherwise of evidence into everyday health care and these factors are represented by interlinking circles in Figure 8.2. Muir Gray

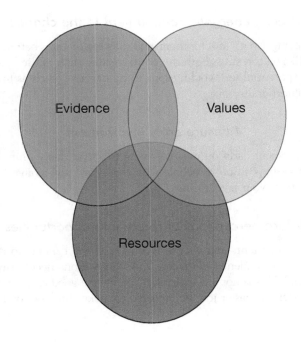

FIGURE 8.2
The influences of values, resources and evidence on actual decisions

Source: Adapted from Muir Gray (2001).

argues that the quality or otherwise of the evidence is only one factor in the complex activity of decision-making. Values and resources have a significant influence on decisions made regardless of the weight or quality of evidence supporting change. Proposals for changes that have significant resource implications are likely to be modified in an effort to keep costs down to that which the organisation can afford, while those proposed changes that appear inconsistent with the strongly held values of nurses are likely to be resisted, subverted or even ignored altogether. Muir Gray claims that the influence of values and resources on actual decisions made is greater than the influence of evidence, regardless of the quality of that evidence.

In *Managing Change and Making it Stick* (1987 pp. 33–34) a classic text of its time, Plant suggests six key activities for maximising commitment to change, designed to help others to accept and come to terms with the change, to maximise their commitment to it and to lower their resistance to it.

1 Help individuals or groups face up to change

This involves helping people to accept the need for change. In particular, you need to work with those who are positive so that you harness the power of the supporters. You also need to decide what you can do that will let the more hesitant people come round in their own time.

2 Communicate like you have never communicated before

Make sure that everyone knows everything that is relevant to them and do not assume they will find out through the grapevine. Rumour and misinformation flourish where real information is missing, and trust can be weakened as a result.

3 Gain energetic commitment to the change

This means identifying 'what's in it for them' and showing that it is better, and less painful, than standing still. You can stress both the positive sides, such as the benefits to patients or clients and the potential for avoiding something negative, such as unnecessary costs, wasted time and effort and so on.

4 Ensure early involvement

One unit of energy spent early on avoids having to spend many units later, when you may have the active opposition of people who otherwise might have been with you if they had been party to your level of insight.

5 Turn perceptions of threat into opportunities

Stress the benefits to patients and clients and also sell the benefits to the practitioners themselves. There is a tendency to assume that innovations necessarily bring additional work with them. This is not always true. If you have a good case for arguing that the result will be a better *and* easier job, be prepared to make this case loud and clear.

6 Avoid over-organising

Planning is not a one-off process. Protocols and guidance may need to be revised in the light of experience; if you are asking other people to be flexible, you need to show flexibility yourself when it is needed.

CONCLUSION

The point of evidence-based nursing practice is to ensure practice is based on best available evidence and that any changes made have benefit to those in receipt of nursing care. Making a decision to change, or wanting changes to be implemented, is only one part of this. There always needs to be some way of finding out if a change has produced a beneficial outcome. This is the essence of evaluation. Just as there are significant barriers to overcome in implementing changes in practice so there are some difficult aspects of trying to measure the benefit of changes made. In a way, evaluation is a necessary part of reviewing practice in a reflective way. Merely asking the types of questions reflective practitioners routinely ask (e.g., Why do it this way? Is there a better way to do it?) is to be engaged in evaluation of practice, and if this leads to another round of finding the evidence and subjecting it to critical appraisal with a willingness to change if the evidence is sufficiently compelling then one can say that evaluation is taking place. In this way evidence-based practice is one way to guard against a slide towards poor practice.

By reading this chapter we hope that you have begun to understand the importance and relevance of evidence-based practice for nursing. We also hope that the information contained in these pages will help you to think about and review practice so that you can play your part in influencing nursing practice in positive and beneficial ways.

SUGGESTED FURTHER READING

Boland, A., Cherry, M. G. and Dickson, R. (2014) *Doing a Systematic Review: A student's guide*. Los Angeles, CA: Sage.

Gerrish, K. and Lathlean, A. (eds) (2015) *The Research Process in Nursing* (7th edn). Oxford: Blackwell.

Lipscomb, M. (ed.) (2016) *Exploring Evidence-Based Practice: Debates and challenges in nursing*. London: Routledge.

Websites

Care Quality Commission: www.cqc.org.uk
Department of Health: www.dh.gov.uk
National Institute of Health & Clinical Excellence: www.nice.org.uk
Northern Ireland Assembly: www.niassembly.gov.uk/
Scottish Executive: www.scotland.gov.uk/Topics/Health
Welsh Assembly Government (Health): http://new.wales.gov.uk/topics/health/

REFERENCES

Boland, A., Cherry, M. G. and Dickson, R. (2014) *Doing a Systematic Review: A student's guide*. Los Angeles, CA: Sage.

CASP (Critical Appraisal Skills Programme) (2013) *Making Sense of the Evidence*. www.casp-uk.net/ (accessed 5 October 2015).

DH (Department of Health) (2006) *Best Research for Best Health: A new national health research strategy*. www.dh.gov.uk (accessed 22 January 2016).

Flemming, K. and Fenton, M. (2002) Making sense of research evidence to inform decision making. In *Clinical Decision Making and Judgement in Nursing*, Thompson, C. and Dowding, D. (eds). Edinburgh: Churchill Livingstone, pp. 109–129.

Gerrish, K. and Lathlean, A. (eds) (2015). *The Research Process in Nursing* (7th edn), Oxford: Blackwell.

Grade Working Group (2004) Grading quality of evidence and strength of recommendations. *British Medical Journal* **328** (7454), 1490–1498.

Hewitt-Taylor, J. (2013) *Understanding and Managing Change in Healthcare: A step-by-step guide*. Basingstoke: Palgrave Macmillan.

Hibbard, C. (2004) Accessing sources of knowledge. In *Research into Practice: Essential skills for reading and applying research in nursing and health care* (2nd edn), Crookes, P. A. and Davies, S. (eds). Edinburgh: Bailliere Tindall, pp. 23–28.

LoBiondo-Wood, G. and Haber, J. (2013) *Nursing Research: Methods, critical appraisal, and utilization* (8th edn). St Louis, MO: Mosby.

Moule, P. (2015) *Making Sense of Research in Nursing, Health and Social Care* (5th edn). London: Sage.

Muir Gray, J. A. (2001) *Evidence-Based Health Care: How to make health policy and management decisions*. Edinburgh: Churchill Livingstone.

Parahoo, K. (2014) *Nursing Research: Principles, process and issues* (3rd edn). London: Palgrave Macmillan.

Plant, R. (1987) *Managing Change and Making it Stick*. London: Fontana.

Polit, D. F. and Beck, C. T. (2013) *Essentials of Nursing Research: Appraising evidence for practice* (8th edn). Philadelphia, PA: Lippincott Williams & Wilkins.

Sellman, D. (2003) Open-mindedness: a virtue for professional practice. *Nursing Philosophy* **4** (1), 17–24.

Sellman, D. (2015) Ethical competence and evidence based practice. In *Exploring Evidence-based Practice: Debates and challenges in nursing*, Lipscomb, M. (ed.). London: Routledge, pp. 195–203.

SIGN (Scottish Intercollegiate Guidelines Network) (2004) *SIGN 50. A Guideline Developer's Handbook*. Edinburgh: SIGN.

Tordoff, C. (1998) From research to practice: a review of the literature. *Nursing Standard*, **12** (25), 34–37.

Walsh, M. and Ford, P. (eds) (1989) *Nursing Rituals: Research and rational actions*. Oxford: Butterworth Heinemann.

9

ASSESSMENT

Derek Sellman, Stephen Evans and Jackie Younker

LEARNING OUTCOMES

After reading and reflecting on this chapter, you should be able to:

- explain the importance of assessment for nursing practice;
- describe the skills needed for effective assessment;
- consider the usefulness of assessment tools;
- discuss the relationship between systematic assessment and safe care.

INTRODUCTION

As Barrett *et al.* (2012) note 'Assessment . . . is as much about finding out what the patient can do as it is about what they cannot do' (p. 22). In this chapter 'finding out' is emphasised as the foundation of nursing care. Without finding out appropriate information about patients and clients it is difficult to determine suitable nursing care. Being systematic in assessment ensures the gathering of information necessary to deliver safe and effective care. Thus, assessment is an integral part of becoming a nurse in each of the four fields of nursing in the UK.

The chapter is divided into three parts. In Part 1, we offer information about assessment, emphasising the importance of effective patient assessment.

In Part 2, we explain general aspects of the skills of observing, measuring and interviewing: all necessary for effective assessment. We also offer examples using specific assessment tools to illustrate the general and transferable principles of assessment tools in general.

In Part 3, we detail some aspects of the head-to-toe physical assessment and begin to outline the nature of assessment beyond the physical realm.

PART 1: OUTLINING ASSESSMENT

Case 9.1

> Maureen is a first-year student nurse. Today is the end of her first week on her second placement: a busy ward at the local hospital. She is having difficulty making sense of much of what she sees going on around her and she is beginning to worry that she will never manage to prioritise her workload as her mentor (Alia) does so effortlessly. By way of an example, when they enter a bay of patients, Alia seems to notice many things that Maureen doesn't, and Maureen recognises that she is in danger of missing important aspects of patient care unless she can begin to see the things obvious to Alia.

Activity 9.1

Imagine you are friends with Maureen (Case 9.1) and she has asked you for advice. Write down some suggestions that might help Maureen to find a way of seeing those things that appear obvious to Alia.

The importance of patient assessment cannot be overstated. Every time you approach a patient you will be making some type of assessment. This may be as simple as noticing a patient looks better today than yesterday; or thinking they look uncomfortable, or worried, or happy and so on; or it may involve purposeful, deliberate and systematic collection of information. Using only the former you may struggle to obtain accurate or relevant information, particularly if you do not check out your assumptions against an external source. For example, if you change a patient's position because she looks uncomfortable without checking that she *actually* is uncomfortable, then you may cause rather than relieve discomfort. Being systematic means you are less likely to miss information important for making patient care decisions.

Maureen needs to start making her observations count: she needs to become attentive to the nursing environment in order to discriminate between relevant and irrelevant information regarding patients, their treatments and their care. Becoming appropriately selective is something Alia has learned and which has now become 'second nature' to the extent that she sometimes finds difficulty understanding why things that are obvious to her are not obvious to others. Of course it has not always been so, just like Maureen, Alia started out as a novice. Benner (1984) describes novice nurses as reliant on checklists; a reliance that diminishes with experience in the move towards expert performance.

Assessment precedes action. At the mundane level we assess how much toothpaste we need *before* brushing our teeth; how much shampoo is in the bottle *before* washing our hair; and how much cheese to slice *before* making cheese on toast. Poor assessments in these examples matters little, for the effects of too little or too much toothpaste, shampoo or cheese will, under normal circumstances affect individuals without significant effect on others.

Assessment is something we learn, and we can learn it well or poorly. We learn to assess the speed of oncoming traffic *before* crossing the road (we did not always have this skill); we learn to assess how long it will take to get to the airport *before* we leave to catch a plane (we may have learned to allow extra time to account for unexpected delays); and we assess how much debt we can afford *before* taking out a mortgage (we may have learned to balance income with expenditure). Getting these types of assessments wrong can have more harmful consequences for us and others. If we get hit by a car when we step into the road because our assessment of its speed was inaccurate, the effects may be felt by many including the driver and passengers, and (potentially) the emergency and hospital services. Missing a flight may ruin a holiday for our friends, and if we failed to account for the total costs of home ownership we may end up causing considerable hardship to our families.

Assessment in professional life may have more profound consequences. Ineffective assessment has the potential to cause serious harm to patients. The nurse who undertakes an ineffective assessment of routine observations (temperature, pulse, respirations and blood pressure) of a postoperative patient may fail to notice a significant change in that patient's condition that could result in a delay in recognising and/or preventing serious postoperative complications.

Assessment in nursing stretches beyond the physical, recognising that patients and clients have other needs (e.g., psychological, social and spiritual). However, this chapter concentrates primarily on physical aspects of assessment, although other domains are incorporated, because the tools for physical assessment are well established and largely uncontroversial compared with assessment tools for non-physical domains. Indeed, while most nurses acknowledge the interdependence of the physical, psychological, social and spiritual, it is not clear that nurses are sufficiently skilled to undertake assessment in all four domains.

To summarise, we have identified four important aspects of assessment:

1 Assessment precedes action.
2 Effective assessment skills can be learnt.
3 Ineffective assessment can have harmful consequences.
4 Comprehensive assessment necessarily involves more than physical assessment.

To act without undertaking assessment; not to learn the skills of effective assessment; and/or to practise ineffective assessment is to fail in one essential aspect of becoming a safe and competent registered nurse. As a novice, Maureen will need to spend time and expend effort in moving from novice to becoming safe and competent. There is no doubt that a checklist approach helps the novice to learn to be thorough and systematic, which is an important element of reducing the potential for harm to patients of ineffective assessment.

PART 2: EXPLAINING ASSESSMENT

Case 9.1 (continued)

Despite her concern that she does not notice all the things Alia (her mentor) notices, Maureen does have some skill in observation, measurement and interviewing. She brought these everyday skills with her; now she is beginning to develop these skills as part of her learning. That Maureen knows she needs to further develop these

D. Sellman, S. Evans and J. Younker

skills shows that she is recognising some of the things she will need to learn if she is to become a safe and effective practitioner.

Effective assessment requires a systematic approach to the collection of data using a variety of sources as appropriate in any given situation. In everyday life our assessments are based on familiarity and assumptions that usually suffice. However, in our professional lives the need to be systematic in assessment is crucial in order to ensure nursing actions are based on accurate and relevant information. The systematic gathering of information, together with a recognition that patients' health status will change (and therefore require ongoing assessment) can help nurses to be sure they are delivering care that relates to patient need.

Assessment and the nursing process

Assessment is the first step in the **nursing process**, which enables nurses to recognise each patient as an individual whose situation is unique, despite having presenting signs and symptoms common among particular patient populations. Without effective assessment not only are the experiences of individual patients likely to be subsumed within a category (surgical, cardiac, etc.) but also the care provided is likely to address collective rather than individual needs.

Assessment requires gathering information and this information can be either **subjective data** or **objective data**. A nursing assessment will aim to gather information about a client's health status, including biographical data, health history, health patterns, cultural, social and other norms, as well as the findings of a physical examination (Weber and Kelley 2014).

The skills of effective assessment

Observing, measuring and interviewing are essential skills for effective patient assessment. Learning to become appropriately observant requires paying attention to, and discriminating between relevant and irrelevant, information presented to the senses; learning to measure requires being accurate and consistent; learning to interview requires effective communication skills.

Observation

Our senses are bombarded with information and familiarity allows much of this information to fade into the background. It is only in unfamiliar environments that we become aware of much of this background information. During a first night away we notice the noises a building makes, the general odour of a room, the texture of sheets and so on. Yet by the second or third night much of this sensory 'noise' recedes into the background, to be noticed only when it changes unexpectedly.

This goes some way to explain why Maureen finds it difficult to know what to pay attention to when she enters a bay of patients. For Maureen, the hospital ward remains a relatively unfamiliar environment, which bombards her with sights, sounds and smells that will eventually become part of the unnoticed background of her professional environment. Unlike Maureen, Alia (Maureen's mentor) notices slight changes to the background of sensory information. Alia may detect subtleties in the sounds, sights, and smells as she enters a bay; things that Maureen has not yet learned to distinguish as significant. Alia may hear sounds in one patient's breathing that give her cause for concern where Maureen hears only breathing; may see early indications of pallor in a patient where Maureen does not; or may recognise the beginnings of an odour of infection masked to Maureen by disinfectant and other standard hospital smells.

Measurement

We are constantly measuring; measuring, for example, the time before our shift ends or the distance between the ward and the canteen. Measurements of this type can be 'rough and ready'. We have the equipment to be precise but would not normally bother and we might find it odd for others to do so unless there were good reason. In some circumstances accuracy is required. A space shuttle launch requires precise timing and an Olympic running track must have a specific length.

Interviewing

Similarly, we make everyday use of the basic skills of interviewing. To interview is merely to inquire. When we ask a friend about their favourite colour or ask a stranger for directions to the restaurant we are seeking information, and while we would not normally describe this as interviewing, that is what it is. The same skills are needed to find out things about patients. Effective interviewing skills rely on effective communication and interpersonal skills (see Chapter 14).

A comprehensive assessment of a patient requires using the skills of observation, measurement, and interview to gather data in relation to their physical, psychological, social and spiritual well-being. It is often issues related to physical well-being that bring patients into contact with the health services and thus physical assessment tends to be prioritised. There are good reasons for nurses in all fields to be familiar with physical assessment even if only to exclude physical origins of presenting symptoms. Similarly, patients under the care of nurses in all fields will have psychological, social and spiritual needs. To neglect psychological, social and/or spiritual assessment is to fail to recognise that people are more than mere physical beings. However, in the current climate of target-driven health care provision and given the time pressures under which most nurses in the UK work, it is unsurprising that many nurses find the time restrictions of their practice cause them to focus predominantly on physical aspects of care. Thus we begin with the physical assessment.

Activity 9.2 'Doing the observations'

Imagine you are a senior student charged with teaching Maureen to undertake patient observations. Do you think you know enough about the measurement, purpose and recording of patient observations to ensure that Maureen becomes safe and effective at doing the observations? Write some brief notes about the things you definitely know about doing the observations and try to identify gaps in your knowledge.

Starting the physical assessment

While most nurses will become adept at 'doing the observations' not all will develop observational skills beyond efficient task performance. Technical proficiency is merely a starting point and those who progress beyond novice will have learnt to pay attention to a range of sensory information. A systematic physical assessment begins with a general observational survey of the patient along with the measurement of their temperature, pulse, respirations, and blood pressure. The general observational survey begins at the start of the encounter between nurse and patient, and continues for the duration of the physical examination (Ball *et al.* 2015). It includes paying attention to the patient's height and weight, posture, mood and alertness, skin colour, signs of distress, grooming and personal hygiene, facial expression, as well as body and breath odours. On first encounter, Maureen may have noticed nothing more than an older woman sitting in bed, asking for a nurse. Because of her limited experience Maureen may not have realised that during the few moments it took her to generate this first impression, Alia had already begun a general survey of the patient. In those first few seconds Alia had processed a range of sensory information as part of her initial assessment of the patient's general condition.

Alia's observations will have been guided by questions such as:

- How does the patient look?
- Is she anxious, distressed, acutely ill, frail?
- Is she awake, alert and responsive to other people?
- Did she hear/notice the nurses entering the room?
- What items are on the bedside table?
- Is she interacting with visitors?
- Is she short or tall, thin or stocky?
- Are there any unusual odours?

Each of these observations helps Alia build a picture of the patient's general health and offers initial clues not only about how she might begin to shape a plan of care but

TABLE 9.1 Maureen's and Alia's initial impressions

Maureen's initial impressions	Alia's initial impressions
Maureen perceives an older woman sitting in bed surrounded by mess, asking for a nurse and rambling on a bit	Alia perceives an older woman sitting forward in bed looking anxious and short of breath. She is asking for a nurse but also calling out for her sister who is not present. On seeing Maureen and Alia she immediately asks: 'where am I and why am I here?'
	The patient looks flushed and sweaty and has removed one sleeve of her hospital gown and it looks as though she has been trying to get rid of the bed covers. The bedside locker door is open and the contents appear to have been rummaged, some appear to have fallen on the floor along with the call bell
	To Alia this indicates that the patient is restless, possibly confused and may have a raised temperature

also how best to proceed with the assessment. Table 9.1 illustrates the things that Maureen and Alia might notice from the same sensory information.

Alia's experience allows her to sift relevant information from the background and leads to her initial impression of an acutely ill patient in need of urgent attention. Her experience has enabled her to pay attention to significant information from the clutter of sensory data that confronted both Maureen and Alia as they entered the room. In her general survey, Alia had noticed important clues including the patient's colour and appearance, the apparent confusion not previously present, the call bell on the floor making it difficult to summon assistance, her position in the bed (patients experiencing shortness of breath often sit forward in the bed) and the absence of relatives or visitors. Alia captures this information in the brief moment it takes to reach the patient. For Alia, doing the observations will help to confirm her initial impressions; for Maureen, doing the observations is the staring point of assessment.

The general survey continues while doing the **observations**. The observations (temperature, pulse, respirations and blood pressure – commonly referred to as 'vital signs', 'the observations' or simply 'the obs') are a set of physiological measurements providing a basis for physical examination. Whatever the underlying disease processes, vital signs offer important objective data about a patient's condition. Thus nurses must be effective in doing the observations and noticing other indicators of patients' health and/or illness. Effective observation of patients' vital signs requires the use of effective communication skills in explaining what you plan to do and why the procedure is necessary. This is particularly important for patients who are confused, anxious, agitated, or fearful of medical procedures.

Temperature

A patient's temperature is measured against an objective scale but even before using a thermometer, Alia suspects the patient will have a raised temperature because she appears flushed and sweaty. This is confirmed by the use of touch (the patient's skin feels hot and clammy) as, using calm and measured language, Alia acknowledges the patient with a 'Hello Mrs Swinbourne' followed by a simple explanation of a need to 'take some routine observations'. Knowing there is a chance that in her distressed and possibly confused state the patient may not cooperate, Alia explains every action carefully and makes polite conversation designed to help orientate Mrs Swinbourne.

Body temperature can be measured at different sites (e.g., mouth, rectum, axillae and tympanic membrane) but as these are all peripheral sites, each reflects a slight variation from core body temperature. Thus an apparent change in temperature over time may not be a change if the measurements were made at different sites. Tympanic membrane (ear) measurement is the least invasive and most widely used. Tympanic thermometers are simple to use but can be challenging for confused, agitated or fearful patients. Fortunately, Mrs Swinbourne remained cooperative. The reading was 38.5° centigrade. This is a high temperature and suggestive of the presence of infection. It will need further investigation.

Alia pointed out to Maureen that if a patient is uncooperative or becoming distressed it may be useful to consider if other clinical signs reduce the need for a temperature measurement. For example, if there is no reason to suspect a raised temperature, if all the other observations are within the normal range, if the patient does not feel hot to the touch, or does not appear flushed then it may be appropriate to leave temperature measurement temporarily. However, if the patient is recently admitted, apparently

Observations. Temperature, pulse, respirations, and blood pressure (commonly referred to as 'vital signs', 'the observations' or simply 'the obs') are a set of physiological measurements that provide the basis for the physical examination.

233

confused and appears unwell then this may be indicative of an infection and an accurate measurement of temperature is essential.

Pulse

Another routine observation involves assessing the pulse. Sensory information from a patient's pulse contributes primarily to the assessment of cardiovascular function, although other useful information can be obtained at the same time. The standard recording is of the pulse rate, which is a measurement of the number of heartbeats (or cardiac cycles) per minute. Typically the pulse is palpated at the radial artery while counting the number of pulsations in one minute. For patients with a strong, steady and regular pulse, it is accepted practice to count the number of beats for 15 or 30 seconds and then multiply whatever number is reached by four or two respectively. However, if the pulse is weak or irregular, then the rate should be counted for a full minute. So while 'taking' a pulse involves measurement, assessment requires interpretation of a wider range of sensory information.

Variation of the pulse rate is normal and relates to the physiological need to get blood to the tissues. So an individual will have a faster pulse rate when engaged in strenuous activity than they do at rest. Maureen records Mrs Swinbourne's pulse as 100 beats per minute. This is faster than her normal 'at rest' rate recorded on her chart and may be a reflection of physiological deterioration or of her restlessness.

Tachycardia (fast heart rate) can occur with activity or movement, exercise, anxiety and stress, pain or high temperature. Bradycardia (slow heart rate) is usually a sign of heart problems and needs immediate reporting. However, some drugs lower the heart rate so it is necessary to consider a patient's history and information from the drug chart to assist in the assessment of the significance of a slow heart rate.

Normally a pulse will have a steady, regular rhythm. Some irregularities in the electrical conduction of the heart can cause the rhythm of the pulse to be irregular. A rapid, irregular heartbeat is usually a sign that the patient is unwell and needs urgent attention. The other observations (blood pressure and respirations) will provide useful additional information. Some patients with known heart disease may have an irregular heartbeat being treated with medication so being aware of a patient's medical history, medications and other findings from the general survey will assist the overall assessment. A patient's pulse is usually easy to palpate. Difficulties arise for patients with cardiovascular collapse and decreased peripheral circulation. This is also likely to be reflected in a low blood pressure and indicates the patient is critically ill.

Information that will assist in the overall assessment when a patient has either a fast or slow pulse rate will come from the answers to questions such as:

- Is this normal for this patient?
- Is the patient engaged in activity that increases heart rate?
- Are there other important clinical signs such as a change in blood pressure or an elevated temperature?
- Is the patient known to have heart disease?
- Is the patient taking drugs that affect the heart?

These and other similar questions can help in the overall assessment of the patient and will contribute to decision-making in relation to a plan of care. Of course, other sensory information is available when 'taking' a pulse. A pulse rate taken manually allows the nurse to feel the patient's skin and this can provide sensory information about skin temperature, tone, general condition and so on, all of which provides further assessment data.

Respirations

Changes in respirations can offer early indication of deterioration in a patient's health status. Often regarded a poor relation in the observations, the value of accurate measurement of respiratory rate and effort can be underestimated. Respirations are counted by observing the rise and fall (one respiratory cycle) of the chest over one minute. The normal respiratory rate is about 10–20 breaths per minute. While counting the number of respiratory cycles is important, significant information can be obtained by paying attention to the pattern of a patient's breathing, as well as the nature of their respiratory effort. A patient who is struggling for breath may still have a normal respiratory rate, so this measurement is only part of the assessment of respirations. For example, a patient may have a respiratory rate of 12 breaths per minute yet have shallow chest movements and may be unable to complete a spoken sentence without gasping for breath. Clearly the care needs of this patient cannot be determined on the basis of respiratory rate alone. Factors that affect the respiratory rate include pain, raised temperature, respiratory disease, airway problems, central nervous system problems, drugs, muscle weakness and anxiety, so it is important to consider other possible causes when making an assessment of a patient's respirations.

A single measurement of respiratory rate can offer some information towards an assessment of respirations, but the trend of respiratory rate over time is of more use. For example, it would not be unusual to find a respiratory rate of 24 breaths per minute returning to, say, 12 breaths per minute in a patient who has been reassured about impending surgery; whereas a steady increase in respiratory rate over an 8-hour period from 12 breaths per minute to a consistent 24 breaths per minute would indicate a respiratory problem in need of urgent attention. This last point reinforces the importance of understanding assessment as a continuous process where measurement occurs against a background of knowledge of normal and abnormal physiological function in relation to what is normal for any given patient at any particular time.

Blood pressure

Blood pressure is the peripheral measurement of cardiovascular function. 'Taking' a patient's blood pressure has become routine but accurate assessment requires paying attention to detail and taking account of factors that might give false or inaccurate readings.

An accurate measurement of blood pressure requires the use of a **blood pressure cuff** of the correct size: one that is too narrow or too short may give a falsely high reading. The cuff is positioned on a patient's arm (about 2.5 cm above the antecubital crease over the brachial artery). The patient's arm should be free of clothing, supported, relaxed and positioned at about heart level. If these conditions are not met there is a danger of a false reading, and if the conditions vary (e.g., on a general hospital ward over a 24-hour period a patient's blood pressure may be measured by several different nurses each of whom may approximate these ideal conditions to a different extent) then there is the possibility that

Whether using a manual or automated system, the blood pressure cuff must be the correct size for the patient. The **blood pressure cuff** houses an inflatable bladder. The width of the bladder should be approximately 40 per cent of the upper arm circumference (about 12–15 cm for the average adult). The length of the bladder should be around 80 per cent of the upper arm circumference (almost long enough to encircle the arm).

D. Sellman, S. Evans and J. Younker

the pattern of readings recorded may reflect these variations rather than changes in the patient's health status. Of course, ideal conditions are not always possible as some patients may be unable or unwilling to cooperate.

A 'high' blood pressure may be 'normal' for some patients. A high reading may occur if a patient has been active, if their arm was unsupported or not relaxed, and can accompany anxiety or distress. Thus accurate assessment of blood pressure is not merely taking and recording a reading: it requires making sense of that reading in relation to other aspects of the patient's condition and environment.

Activity 9.3

Return to your responses to Activity 9.2 and make notes about what you have learned from reading the section about routine observations. Can you identify any further gaps in your knowledge base in relation to doing the observations?

Case 9.1 (continued)

Alia and Maureen perform Mrs Swinbourne's observations together. Their findings are as follows:

- Temperature: 38.5°C
- Pulse: 100 beats per minute
- Respirations: 32 breaths per minute
- Blood pressure: 110/50 mmHg

Alia knows from reading Mrs Swinbourne's notes and from the information given during handover that the patient is not taking cardiac medication and her blood pressure is normally about 140/90 mmHg. She also knows that 12 hours ago Mrs Swinbourne was sitting up in bed comfortably with a temperature of 37.5°C. Together, Maureen and Alia review the information on the patient's observations chart and note that since her admission Mrs Swinbourne's observations have been as follows:

- *Temperature.* Previously recorded within the range of 37.2°C to 37.7°C. The present reading of 38.5°C represents a change in her health status and indicates the presence of infection and a need for further investigation.
- *Pulse.* Previously recorded within the range of 72 and 80 beats per minute. The new reading of 100 beats per minute is also a change from normal and may be a function of physiological deterioration or of her apparent anxiety and restlessness.
- *Respirations.* Previously recorded within the range of 15 to 18 breaths per minute. This new measurement of 32 breaths per minute is a significant increase and together with the position she has adopted in bed indicates a breathing problem.
- *Blood pressure.* Previously recorded within the range of 135/85 to 150/90 mmHg. While this new measurement of 110/50 is within what is considered a 'normal' range, it is not normal for this patient and therefore represents a significant change in health status.

The information gathered thus far has required skills of measurement (illustrated by, for example, the use of a thermometer); the skills of interview (in asking specific questions); and the skills of observation (by, for example, using the senses to notice the texture of the patient's skin). Having completed the general survey together with the measurement of a standard set of observations, Maureen and Alia now have accurate and relevant information to contribute to their initial assessment of Mrs Swinbourne. Their findings indicate that the patient is having respiratory problems and that a more in-depth assessment of her respiratory system will be necessary.

The assessment of pain

Case 9.1 (continued)

Maureen and the drug round

While assisting on drug rounds during her first placement, Maureen noticed that closed questions such as *'do you want any pain killers?'* were routinely used by the nurses for patients with prescriptions for 'as required' pain medication. Closed questions invite brief responses such as 'yes', 'no' or 'don't know'. Closed questions offer limited use in the assessment of pain. Rather than asking, *'do you want any pain killers?'* the nurses on Maureen's second placement tend to ask, *'do you have any pain or discomfort?'* and for patients who say 'yes' the follow-up questions are more probing, such as: *'can you show me where it hurts?'*, *'is the pain in the same place as yesterday?'* or *'is it less or more painful than it was yesterday?'* Consequently, the drug round takes longer but patients' pain appears better managed with fewer complications arising from unrelieved pain (Brennan *et al.* 2007, Cousins *et al.* 2004, James 2014, Lynch 2001).

Nurses make a significant contribution to the management of pain although nurses' assessment of patients' pain is notoriously poor (Coulling 2005, Franck and Bruce 2009, Layman Young *et al.* 2006, Wøien *et al.* 2014). There are many reasons for this including suggestions that nurses tend:

- to underestimate how much pain patients have (in relation to how much pain patients report);
- to overestimate the danger of morphine addiction and respiratory depression;
- to make correlations between conditions and analgesia requirements rather than assess individual need for pain control.

It is not unusual to overhear nurses say things such as: *'he shouldn't need morphine after X days post surgery'*. In fact the patient might need morphine, although reports of severe pain from a patient under these circumstances should alert the nurse to the possibility of serious postoperative complications. Similarly, it is not unknown for nurses to continue to administer doses of morphine to cancer patients assuming their pain is associated with their cancer, when their pain might be caused by constipation: a familiar side effect of morphine. In both examples it is the failure to assess the patient's pain that has led the nurse to respond inappropriately.

Activity 9.4

List the pain assessment tools you have seen in use. Write some notes about the advantages and disadvantages of each tool you have listed.

There are a number of different tools available for the assessment of pain, but unlike tools used for collecting information about temperature, pulse, and blood pressure (e.g., different types of thermometer and sphygmomanometer) the tools used for the assessment of pain typically rely on subjective measures. It is important to address potential communication barriers when conducting pain assessment in order to achieve an objective outcome (McDonald *et al.* 2000). There are some observable behavioural and physiological indicators that can be suggestive of pain (Lynch 2001), but these indicators may be present for other reasons so cannot be relied on as sole indicators. For example, rubbing an area of the body, a general restlessness, facial grimacing, mood changes, flushing and sweating, a rise in blood pressure and/or pulse rate may all suggest but are not definitive of the presence of pain. Although for individuals unable to verbalise, such observable phenomena may be the only indicators of a patient's pain (Abdulla *et al.* 2013, RCP, BGS and BPS 2007, Zwakhelan *et al.* 2004).

A self-reporting scale is probably the most commonly used type of pain assessment tool (Kim *et al.* 2005). The essential feature of a pain scale is that it allows the patient to indicate how much pain they are experiencing in terms of a continuum ranging from no pain at one end to unbearable pain at the other; with choices along the continuum reflecting increasing levels of severity. There are different forms of pain scales (verbal, numeric and pictorial) and each has advantages and disadvantages. While some clinical areas adopt a specific scale, there will be situations where an alternative scale will be more appropriate. The point is that if a scale is to provide an effective assessment of a patient's pain then the patient must be able to understand it. Hence, a pictorial scale might be appropriate for someone with limited verbal skills or compromised cognitive function. In addition, differences in both attitudes to pain and to its meaning at the individual level make it difficult to generalise. Nevertheless, it is reported that older people tend to require a more proactive approach because of a supposed set of 'attitudes and beliefs . . . [that] may generate barriers to good pain control' (José Closs 2007, p. 12). There may be numerous reasons for this including expectations and language. Older people tend to use words like 'ache' or 'soreness' to describe pain so might say 'no' in response to the question 'Do you have pain?' Responsibility for such failures of communication and thus failures of effective pain assessment and management lies with the nurse rather than the patient.

The subjective nature of pain scales can be illustrated by a comparison with the scale for measuring blood pressure. Blood pressure is measured using a standardised and objective scale and (assuming a threshold competence in measuring blood pressure among different individuals performing the observation) variations in readings obtained will reflect actual and verifiable changes in a patient's blood pressure. There is no guesswork involved; anyone with the skill can make accurate and objective measurements of blood pressure directly comparable to blood pressure measurements of others. This is one reason why it is possible to make meaningful statements about the normal range for blood pressure in healthy individuals; or to know that a diastolic blood pressure of less than 80 mmHg will compromise kidney function. In contrast, pain can only be measured from the perspective of the person experiencing it; there can be no objective standardised numerical scale comparable to that for measuring blood pressure. This is partly because individuals have different tolerances to pain and partly because such numerical scales as exist for pain assessment rely on patients choosing a number that has no meaningful external reference point. The number chosen by a patient bears no necessary relationship either to other numbers on the scale or to numbers as chosen by other patients: on a scale of 0–10, a score of 8 for one patient bears no necessary relation to a score of 8 listed by any other patient. So it is not possible to generalise from self-reported (or even nurse-estimated) pain scores.

On the plus side, pain scales are simple to use and provide a way of capturing information about how much pain a patient has (pain intensity) and therefore help evaluate improvements (or otherwise) in pain control following analgesia. However, intensity is only one aspect of pain and thus pain scales offer only limited information towards a comprehensive assessment of an individual's pain.

One way to add to the assessment of a patient's pain is to ask them to indicate its location and to describe the pain. Location can be determined by asking a patient to mark the site of their pain on a body diagram, and the simple question 'is your pain in the same place as you indicated on this diagram?' is an easy way to ensure changes in the location of a patient's pain are quickly identified. Similarly, asking a patient to choose a word that best describes their pain can both add to the overall pain assessment and provide a common language between health care professional and patient. Mrs Swinbourne tends to describe her pain as 'aches' and 'soreness' so it would be appropriate to ask, for example: 'can you point to where it aches today?'; or 'is your soreness better or worse than it was yesterday?'

One further issue that makes the assessment of pain more difficult than, for example, measuring blood pressure, is the complicated relationship between pain and mood. An association is recognised between depression and the experience of pain although it is not clear which has the greater effect on the other: there is a suggestion that pain, particularly constant pain, can lead to depression which in turn can worsen the experience of pain. This can add a further layer of complexity because in addition to physiological aspects, there may be psychological, social and/or spiritual factors involved in the pain experienced by any one person, which means that a comprehensive pain assessment requires assessment in all four domains. The McGill Pain Questionnaire (Melzack 2005, first published in 1971) is considered one of the most reliable and sophisticated pain assessment tools. However, its comprehensiveness makes it time-consuming and unsuited to busy and pressurised clinical environments, although there is a short-form McGill Pain Questionnaire (Melzack 1987).

Nevertheless, it is useful to extract some features from the McGill pain assessment tool, especially in relation to asking the patient questions about the frequency of their pain, if it is worse at particular times of the day and whether it is related to specific activities or moods. Of course, these types of questions begin to take on aspects of the psychological, social and perhaps even spiritual assessment and while there may be appropriate assessment tools for each, it is not clear that nurses are sufficiently qualified or trained in their use.

Assessing a patient's pain is a complex activity requiring skills of interviewing, observation and measurement. In the busy practice environment the use of pain-intensity scales together with location charts should provide sufficient information to enable appropriate measures to be taken to reduce or eliminate patients' pain in the short term. However, for some patients there is a need for a comprehensive (e.g., for those with chronic or long-term pain) or an imaginative (e.g., for those with compromised cognitive capacities) pain assessment.

PART 3: EXPLORING ASSESSMENT

First impressions can be misleading. Nevertheless, our initial impressions of a patient at each encounter can offer clues about their health status. In Part 2 of the chapter we highlighted the apparent ease with which Alia was able to recognise the potential significance of some of the sensory information available when approaching a patient. Some of the things she notices may turn out to have little or no significance, but in remaining responsive to potential clues among the background of sensory information, Alia is paying attention to information that may be of importance in relation to the care of patients. Thus first or initial impressions can offer a starting point for assessment but it is only a starting point, and the assessment needs to progress in a systematic and thorough manner if it is to be effective. Just as we suggested in Part 1 that a nurse should check with the patient to see if they are as uncomfortable as they appear before making any attempt to change their position, so it is important not to be misled by the apparent significance of some tantalising clue about a particular problem being experienced by a patient. The danger of focusing assessment predominately on one aspect of a patient's health status suggested by a first impression is that it may be at the expense of other areas of needed assessment. In other words, if you prejudge your assessment of a patient you may stop looking for (or stop noticing) things that do not fit with that prejudgement and in so doing miss what might turn out to be important information. This is one reason why a systematic and thorough assessment is so important.

We have pointed out that while the systematic collection of data is essential, an effective assessment requires information gathered to be interpreted in the light of the specific circumstances of each patient. Not every patient with a blood pressure of 110/80 mmHg and a pulse rate of 110 will be critically ill: some will but this will depend on, among other things, that patient's usual blood pressure and pulse rate. It may also depend on the patient's previous level of health. A fit, healthy 32-year-old male may be able to cope physically with a change in heart rate and blood pressure following a routine operation; while an 80-year-old female with multiple health problems may become very unwell with small physiological changes in the heart rate and blood pressure after a simple procedure.

Completing the physical assessment

In Part 2 of this chapter we explored some aspects of the general survey together with observation of vital signs and noted that this initial assessment provides clues about how a more thorough assessment of a patient might proceed. A complete physical assessment requires a full head-to-toe examination but this may not be necessary if the initial assessment indicates the need for an in-depth assessment of a particular area of the body. For example, the focus of assessment for a patient identified as having shortness of breath and rapid breathing will be a detailed respiratory assessment. In this section we outline the head-to-toe approach of physical assessment.

240

Nursing in the UK is evolving. Nurses are developing the skills necessary for a variety of roles including prescribing, case management and advanced practice, and for this last, the skills of physical examination have become increasingly important (DH 2010). While it may not be necessary for all nurses to undertake head-to-toe examination, a working knowledge of it will add to the knowledge base from which effective assessment takes place.

The head-to-toe examination

Advance preparation of an environment conducive to physical examination together with having all necessary equipment readily available allows for an uninterrupted examination. The examination may take place in different locations (e.g., GP surgery, hospital ward, patient's home) but wherever it occurs consideration must be given to patient privacy, noise levels, temperature, adequate lighting, a bed or examination table for the patient, and a table or tray to hold equipment. Effective hand washing and having gloves available are further parts of preparation (Bickley and Szilagyi 2013).

It is helpful to begin the examination with familiar and less intrusive procedures such as blood pressure, pulse and respirations. This helps to reduce patient anxiety about the full examination. Throughout, it is important to explain what you are doing and why. It may also be appropriate to integrate health promotion and teaching (e.g., while examining the skin it may be appropriate to help the patient learn to look for changes to the colour, size, or shape of moles). The physical examination is generally done from the patient's right side because most examination techniques are done with the examiner's right hand. If it is necessary to change the patient's position, it is important to explain to the patient what you want them to do in clear, simple terms.

There are four basic techniques used during head-to-toe examinations: inspection, palpation, percussion and auscultation, with each adapted as appropriate for the body system being examined (Bickley and Szilagyi 2013).

Inspection

Inspection begins from the moment that you meet the patient and continues throughout the examination. It involves using the senses of vision, smell and hearing to observe and detect normal and abnormal findings. The following guidelines help with inspection:

- A comfortable room temperature – a room that is too cold or too hot may alter the patient's behaviour and skin appearance.
- Fluorescent lights may alter the skin's appearance – it is best to use natural lighting where possible.
- Completely expose the body part you are inspecting and keep the rest of the patient covered as much as possible.
- Note colour, patterns, size, location, consistency, odours, movement and sounds during the inspection.
- Compare the symmetry of body parts (e.g., eyes, ears, hands, legs).

Most inspection involves only the use of senses; however a few body systems require equipment for thorough inspection (e.g., ophthalmoscope for the eyes and otoscope for the ears).

Palpation

Palpation involves using the hands to touch the patient. Characteristics noted by palpation include:

- texture (rough, smooth);
- moisture (dry, wet);
- temperature;
- consistency (soft, hard, fluid-filled);
- mobility (movable, fixed, vibrating);
- strength of pulse;
- size;
- shape;
- degree of tenderness.

Palpation may be done with three areas of the hand, depending on the nature of the examination. The fingerpads are most often used to feel pulses and check size, texture, consistency and shape. The ulnar or palmar surface of the hand may be used to feel for vibrations. The dorsal surface of the hand is best for checking temperature. Palpation may be light, moderate or deep depending on the depth of the structure being palpated and the thickness of the tissue overlying the structure. For example, it is good practice to use light palpation to assess the abdomen followed by deeper palpation to check the location of internal organs such as the liver.

Percussion

Percussion is tapping over a body part to produce a sound wave. The sound produced helps to determine the underlying structures. Percussion has a few different assessment uses that include:

- *Determining density.* Percussion helps determine whether an underlying structure is filled with air or fluid or is a solid mass. For example, the lungs are generally filled with air and percussion should produce a resonant sound – if there is a pleural effusion, the sound will be dull, indicating a fluid-filled area.
- *Determining location, size and shape.* Percussion may be used to note changes between borders of an organ.
- *Eliciting pain.* Percussion is used to help identify inflamed underlying structures – when an inflamed area is percussed, the patient may say it feels tender, painful or sore.

Percussion is most commonly used as part of the respiratory and abdominal examination.

Auscultation

Auscultation involves using a stethoscope to listen to body sounds that are not otherwise audible. Sounds heard with the stethoscope include heart sounds, movement of blood through the cardiovascular system, bowel sounds and movement of air through the lung fields. The sounds are described by their intensity, pitch, duration and quality. The following points should be considered to help with auscultation:

- Eliminate distracting or competing noises.
- Auscultate over the patient's bare skin – listening through the clothing may obscure the body sound.
- The diaphragm (flat part) of the stethoscope can be used for high-pitched sounds such as normal heart sounds, lung sounds and bowel sounds.
- The bell of the stethoscope is used for low-pitched sounds such as abnormal heart sounds and bruits (loud sounds heard over major blood vessels such as the carotid artery or aorta).

Case 9.1 (continued)

In Part 2 of this chapter, Maureen and Alia completed their initial assessment of Mrs Swinbourne. Based on their findings of the general survey and on the significance of the measurement of temperature, pulse and respirations, Alia's hypothesis is that the patient may have a chest infection. This prompts her to undertake a more comprehensive assessment of Mrs Swinbourne's respiratory system.

Examination of the respiratory system

Here we outline in some detail the way in which the four basic techniques of inspection, palpation, percussion and auscultation help to examine and assess a patient's respiratory system.

Inspection

- *Look at the patient's overall pattern of breathing and note their respiratory rate.* Inspect the chest movement as they breathe to look for symmetry and ease of breathing.
- *Assess the colour of the face, lips and chest.* Cyanosis is a late sign of hypoxia and will make white skin appear blue-tinged. Hypoxia may also cause the lips or nails to look pale.
- *Inspect the front and back of the chest noting size, shape and symmetry.* Patients with chronic emphysema may have a characteristic barrel chest appearance.
- *Look at the client's position.* Normally breathing is relaxed with arms at the side or on the lap. Often patients with chronic obstructive pulmonary disease (COPD) will lean forward and use their arms to support their weight and lift the chest to increase breathing capacity (tripod position).
- *Inspect for use of accessory muscles.* Normally breathing uses the diaphragm and abdominal muscles. Patients with breathing problems may use the trapezius or shoulder muscles to help with inspiration.

Palpation

- Palpate the anterior and posterior thorax to assess for symmetry and general condition.
- Assess thoracic expansion. Place the hands around the chest and ask the patient to take a deep breath. Note whether both sides of the chest move symmetrically.

243

Percussion

- Percuss over the anterior and posterior lung fields. The sound should be resonant over all areas of the lungs and dull over major organs (heart, liver, spleen).

Auscultation

- Ask the patient to breathe deeply through the mouth. With the diaphragm of the stethoscope, listen to the anterior and posterior lung fields, starting at the apex and moving to the base. It is important to listen from side to side to make comparisons, while listening through a full inspiration and expiration cycle at each point. Normal breath sounds are described as:
  - *vesicular* – heard over most of the lung fields, soft and clear, low pitch, expiration sound is short;
  - *bronchovesicular* – heard over main bronchus and upper right posterior lung field area, medium pitch, expiration equals inspiration;
  - *bronchial* – heard over the trachea, high pitch, expiration sound is loud and longer than other areas.
- Breath sounds may be difficult to hear or absent. Fluid or secretions in the lungs or airway will change the sound (e.g., crackles or rhonchi). Narrowing of the airway will also affect lung sounds (wheeze).

Case 9.1 (continued)

Alia's findings:

- Mrs Swinbourne appears short of breath; she is not using accessory muscles; she is sitting forward in bed (which may indicate anxiety or a breathing problem); she also has a non-productive cough that is worse when she lies supine.
- There is symmetry between the anterior and posterior thorax. Both sides of the chest move when the patient takes a deep breath, however, the breaths are shallow and it is difficult for her to breathe deeply.
- Percussion reveals dullness over both bases.
- Crackles heard at both bases of the lungs that do not clear with coughing. The breath sounds are also diminished in both bases.

Alia now has information that has been collected using a systematic approach. This information allows Alia to make an informed assessment of Mrs Swinbourne's well-being and to begin to shape an appropriate plan of care. The assessment includes findings from the history, basic observations, the general survey and the more thorough assessment of the respiratory system. All these findings support Alia's initial impression of an acutely ill woman in need of urgent care, but now Alia has data drawn from the systematic assessment to communicate to other professionals (such as other nurses, doctors and physiotherapists) involved in the patient's care. This thorough assessment led to a well-planned package of care and Mrs Swinbourne's speedy recovery led to a focus on arrangements for transfer home.

Assessment for transfer

Arrangements for the transfer of a patient from hospital to home or to a different care facility (often referred to as 'discharge planning') requires a comprehensive assessment of a patient's capacities for self-care. Ideally, the assessment for transfer begins on admission and continues during a patient's hospital stay. All patient assessment relies on the same set of core skills; observing, measuring and interviewing. In assessment for transfer the focus shifts from assessment a client's nursing needs to the assessment of the client's capacities for self-care. In many instances this will necessitate the involvement of professionals from different disciplines.

Case 9.1 (continued)

Prior to Mrs Swinbourne's transfer home Maureen has been working with several other professionals in an attempt to ensure that the discharge arrangements are suitable. Maureen and Alia had met with Mrs Swinbourne and the Intermediate Care Team (a community-based team comprising a nurse, a care manager, a physiotherapist and an occupational therapist who work alongside Mrs Swinbourne's GP). The team advised Mrs Swinbourne that they would continue to provide medical care and rehabilitation once the hospital-based team determined that she was well enough to return home. During the meeting Mrs Swinbourne told everyone that prior to this hospital admission she had managed very well at home. She says she needs no assistance with personal care, can cook a hot meal every day at lunchtime, and can shop for her own groceries at the small local supermarket, who deliver to her door. The care manager reported that Mrs Swinbourne received home help once a week for two hours to do the heavy housework, such as vacuuming and laundry. Mrs Swinbourne stated that she thought the home help was unnecessary and complained that they 'always put things back in the wrong place'.

The care manager advised the meeting that before her admission to hospital, Mrs Swinbourne had been living alone in a second-floor, local authority-owned flat. Despite her 82 years, she had until recently been working as a volunteer in the hospital's gift shop. Prior to this admission she had little contact with the health services. A neighbour had called an ambulance when she found Mrs Swinbourne sitting at the bottom of the stairs inside their block of flats, unable to respond and looking pale. The neighbour had reportedly advised the paramedics that she had been concerned about Mrs Swinbourne for some time. In the meeting it was decided that Maureen would accompany Mrs Swinbourne on a pre-discharge home visit, to be met there by Melissa (the Intermediate Care Team nurse) and Raina (the occupational therapist).

The Intermediate Care Team service is based on government policy and intended to ease the transition from hospital to home for older people, as well as to reduce the likelihood of re-admission and to allow timely discharge (DH 2008). Of course, nursing and other care and rehabilitation processes continue once a patient is deemed suitable for transfer home (or to another care setting). This continuity of care will be essential to ensure the problems that Mrs Swinbourne was facing prior to her hospital admission, both in terms of her health and other aspects of her home life, do not reach such an acute level that she needs to be re-admitted to hospital. Partnership-based Intermediate Care Teams have been developed in most localities across the UK to bridge the gap between hospital care and community-based health and social care services.

The focus on the physical aspect of the nursing assessment in the earlier parts of this chapter reflects the patient journey as the priority for most hospital patients is to improve their physical health so that they are well enough to return home. Generally speaking, the acute hospital environment, with its emphasis on minimising the duration of patient stay, is not particularly conducive to systematic evaluation of a person's psychological, social and spiritual well-being. This is in part because in being removed from familiar surroundings an individual may feel socially and spiritually detached. Clearly, the acute health reason for the initial hospital admission must take priority and once this had been addressed, other non-physical or less urgent physical health and environmental factors can be assessed. As noted in Part 2 of this chapter, to entirely neglect these matters from the nursing assessment is to fail to realise that people are more than mere physical beings. To continue to do so up to the point of transfer is likely to endanger the patient and substantially increase the risk of re-admission to hospital. It is the meeting with the Intermediate Care Team that begins to systematically take account of these other issues, which can help Maureen to assess how safe Mrs Swinbourne will be when she returns home; as well as what further nursing and other supports will be required to ensure that she can remain at home.

The things that Maureen has observed

The first thing that Maureen may have observed from the meeting with the Intermediate Care Team is that Mrs Swinbourne is an independently minded lady. She believes she can manage personal activities of daily living, such as self-care and feeding and that she does not require the services she previously received to help with domestic activities of daily living. This may contradict Maureen's own observations of how Mrs Swinbourne has been coping with her self-care while in hospital, as well as the data provided by the care manager on the home help provided for Mrs Swinbourne prior to her admission. It indicates to Maureen that Mrs Swinbourne may lack insight into her current physical health problems and their impact on what she can do for herself. It illustrates that Maureen needs to continue to assess Mrs Swinbourne's ability to self-care while on the ward, and perhaps refer her to a hospital occupational therapist who can work with Mrs Swinbourne on some activities of daily living (e.g., cooking simple meals) until her discharge.

As the emphasis of care moves away from primarily physical concerns towards non-health factors that could be obstacles to a successful and sustainable discharge home for Mrs Swinbourne, so the assessment methods change. Assessment now will rely less on the interpretation of objective, measured data, such as vital signs, and more on subjective data from the nurse's personal observation of the patient's behaviours, from the reports of others members of the multidisciplinary team, and from reports of the patient, carers and other people within their social circle.

Maureen will have noted that the neighbour had been concerned about Mrs Swinbourne before the event that led to her admission. This may lead Maureen to obtain more information from the neighbour if she sees her visiting Mrs Swinbourne on the ward. Thus the process of assessment (gathering information, interpreting it and acting upon it) is a cycle that continues throughout each patient episode. All the information gathered by Maureen can be used to feed into Melissa's assessment for an individualised community care plan for Mrs Swinbourne.

Case 9.1 (continued)

On the day of the visit, Maureen accompanies Mrs Swinbourne to her home by hospital transport to meet Melissa (the nurse) and Raina (the occupational therapist) from the Intermediate Care Team. When they arrive, they find Mrs Swinbourne's flat in a dishevelled state, with clothing lying on the floor together with dozens of chocolate wrappers. In her kitchen there are several opened bags of frozen food that have been spilt and left to go mouldy, with the freezer door left open. Mrs Swinbourne offers her visitors a cup of tea, but initially is unable to find the switch on her kettle. She finds two cups in a cupboard, which Maureen notices are not clean. Mrs Swinbourne misses the cups and spills hot water from the kettle. On the worktop there are several open bottles of pills and Maureen notices that most have passed their expiry date.

Maureen's earlier concerns regarding Mrs Swinbourne's ability to cope at home seem to have been confirmed by her observations during this visit. Assessment through observation of how a person behaves, or appears to be behaving in their own home environment is crucial for successful and sustainable community living for people with complex health problems. Maureen's interpretation of what she has observed during her visit to Mrs Swinbourne's flat could include the following:

* Mrs Swinbourne may have been unable to keep her home tidy prior to admission.
* Mrs Swinbourne's diet and nutritional intake may have been poor prior to admission.
* Mrs Swinbourne may have a visual or cognitive impairment causing her not to see the kettle switch or the dirty cups (although the kettle should be familiar to her).
* Mrs Swinbourne may have a visual-perceptual deficit, impaired upper limb strength and/or impaired mobility causing her to spill the hot water when attempting to pour it into the cups.
* Mrs Swinbourne may not have been able to manage her own medication prior to her admission.

This list is not exhaustive and the only way that all possibilities to explain the patient's behaviour can be explored and the reasons for her behaviour identified, in order to determine whether discharge home is feasible, is through a systematic assessment by practitioners from appropriate professional groups.

On return to the hospital and after talking things through with Raina, Maureen begins to realise that the priorities she has as a nurse (with emphasis on the physical) are not shared by occupational therapists. This became clear as Raina explained that the distinctions that Maureen (and other nurses) tend to make between physical, social, psychological and spiritual assessment (while understandable in the acute stages of a patient's illness) are less important for other professional groups such as occupational therapists who tend not to compartmentalise medical and health issues as separate from other factors that contribute to (or inhibit) a person's well-being.

247

Case 9.1 (continued)

On the day before transfer home, Maureen notices Mrs Swinbourne leaving the ward bathroom and walking with her wheeled walking frame, as she usually does, back towards her bed. However, on this occasion Mrs Swinbourne passes by her bed and makes her way out of the ward. Maureen follows and asks if she is looking for something, to which Mrs Swinbourne replies that she is trying to find her spectacles because one of the doctors had taken them from her. Maureen suggests that she may have left them by her bedside or in the bathroom and that she will help look for them. Maureen accompanies Mrs Swinbourne back to the bed, but they cannot find her spectacles there; Maureen helps Mrs Swinbourne to sit comfortably by her bed and then proceeds to the ward bathroom where she finds the spectacles on the floor. She notices the washbasin taps have been left running and water is spilling over into large puddles on the floor.

Later that day, Mrs Swinbourne is visited by Charlotte, one of the hospital social workers. Charlotte chats to Mrs Swinbourne for about half an hour, after which she writes something in the medical notes and promptly leaves the ward without speaking to anyone else. Maureen looks at the medical notes and sees that Charlotte has written that, other than reinstating pre-admission home help, no services are required to be put in place for Mrs Swinbourne's discharge tomorrow.

Maureen is distressed by this cursory assessment of Mrs Swinbourne by the social worker and with her new-found understanding about the complexities involved in comprehensive assessment recognises how important it is for all professionals involved in the care of a patient such as Mrs Swinbourne to communicate with each other and work together constructively. In effect, Maureen now realises the importance not only of developing effective skills of assessment but also of interprofessional working (see Chapter 7).

CONCLUSION

It is not possible in a chapter of this length to cover all aspects of patient assessment: as a result we have focused on the skills needed for effective assessment regardless of which aspect of a patient is being assessed. While the physical domain predominates we are at pains to point out that this is meant to be illustrative: that is, we take it that the skills of observation, measurement and interviewing detailed in this chapter can be put to use in the assessment of any domain of patient experience. Thus these skills are transferable.

We would like to make three final points before leaving the reader to find the best way to make use of the learning that will have occurred as a result of reading this chapter.

1   Effective assessment lies at the heart of safe and effective nursing practice, wherever and whenever that practice takes places.
2   There are many different assessment tools available that can assist in the pursuit of effective assessment but these tools should not be mistaken as replacements for the need for careful observation, measurement and interviewing. Even with the most valid and reliable assessment tools there remains a need for professional judgement and discretion in interpreting the information gathered from using such tools.

3   A focus on assessment in the physical domain is a necessary component of all the assessments that nurses undertake, and the need for effectiveness in physical assessment will remain whatever other domain is being assessed.

We hope that by reading this chapter you have gained a deep understanding of the importance of effective assessment and of the relationship between systematic assessment and safe and effective care.

SUGGESTED FURTHER READING

Baid, H. (2006) The process of conducting a physical assessment: a nursing perspective. *British Journal of Nursing* **15** (13), 710–714.

Barker, P. J. (1997) *Assessment in Psychiatric and Mental Health Nursing: In search of the whole person.* Cheltenham, UK: Stanley Thomas.

Weber, J. R., and Kelly, J. H. (2014) *Health Assessment in Nursing* (5th edn). Philadelphia, PA: Wolters Kluwer Health/Lippincott Williams & Wilkins.

REFERENCES

Abdulla, A., Adams, N., Bone, M., Elliott, A. M., Gaffin, J., Jones, D., Knaggs, R., Martin, D. Sampson, L. and Schofied, P. (2013) Guidance on the management of pain in older people. *Age and Ageing*, **42**, i1–i57.

Ball, J. W., Dains, J. E., Flynn, J. A., Solomon, B. S. and Stewart, R. W. (2015) *Seidel's Guide to Physical Examination* (8th edn). St Louis, MO: Elsevier Mosby.

Barrett, D., Wilson, B. and Woollands, A. (2012) *Care Planning: A guide for nurses* (2nd edn) Harlow: Pearson Education.

Benner, P. (1984) *From Novice to Expert: Excellence and power in clinical nursing practice.* Menlo Park, CA: Addison-Wesley.

Bickley, L. S. and Szilagyi, P. G. (2013) *Bates' Guide to Physical Examination and History Taking* (11th edn). Philadelphia, PA: Wolters Kluwer Health/Lippincott Williams & Wilkins.

Brennan, F., Carr, D. B. and Cousins, M. (2007) Pain management: a fundamental right. *International Anesthesia Research Society* **105** (1), 205–221.

Coulling, S. (2005) Nurses' and doctors' knowledge of pain after surgery. *Nursing Standard* **19** (34), 41–49.

Cousins, M. J., Brennan, F. and Carr, D. B. (2004) Pain relief: a universal human right. *Pain* **112** (1–2), 1–4.

DH (Department of Health) (2008) *Older People's NSF Standards.* London: DH.

DH (2010) *Advanced Level Nursing: A position statement.* London: DH.

Franck, L. S. and Bruce, E. (2009) Putting pain assessment into practice: why is it so painful? *Pain Research & Management* **14** (1), 13–20.

James, D. N. (2014) Guidance on the provision of anaesthesia services for acute pain management. www.rcoa.ac.uk/system/files/GPAS-2014-11-ACUTEPAIN_0.pdf Accessed 20 July 2015.

José Closs, S. (2007) Assessment of pain, mood, and quality of life. In *Pain in Older People*, Crome, P., Main, C. J. and Lally, F. (eds). Oxford: Oxford University Press, pp. 11–19.

Kim, H. S., Shwartz-Barcott, D., Tracy, S. M., Fortin, J. D. and Sjostrom, B. (2005) Strategies of pain assessment used by nurses on surgical units. *Pain Management Nursing* **6** (1), 3–9.

Layman Young, J., Horton, F. M. and Davidhizar, R. (2006) Nursing attitudes and beliefs in pain assessment and management. *Journal of Advanced Nursing* **53** (4), 412–421.

Lynch, M. (2001) Pain as the fifth vital sign. *Journal of Intravenous Nursing* **24** (2), 85–94.

McDonald, D. D., McNulty, J., Erickson, K. and Weiskopf, C. (2000) Communicating pain and pain management needs after surgery. *Applied Nursing Research* **13** (2), 70–75.

Melzack, R. (1987) The short-form McGill Pain Questionnaire. *Pain* **30** (2), 191–197.

Melzack, R. (2005) The McGill Pain Questionnaire: from description to measurement. *Anesthesiology* **103** (1), 199–202 (first published in *Anesthesiology* in 1971).

RCP, BGS and BPS (Royal College of Physicians, British Geriatrics Society and British Pain Society) (2007) *The Assessment of Pain in Older People: National guidelines. Concise guidance to good practice series, No 8*. London: RCP.

Weber, J. and Kelley, J. (2014) *Health Assessment in Nursing* (5th edn). Philadelphia, PA: Lippincott Williams & Wilkins.

Wøien, H., Værøy, H., Geir, A. and Bjørk, I. T. (2014) Improving the systematic approach to pain and sedation management in the ICU by using assessment tools. *Journal of Clinical Nursing* **23** (11–12), 1552–1561.

Zwakhelan, S. M. G., Katinka, K. A., Hamers, J. P. H. and Huijer Abu-Saad, H. (2004) Pain assessment in intellectually disabled people: non-verbal indicators. *Journal of Advanced Nursing* **45** (3), 236–245.

10

SOCIOLOGICAL CONCEPTS FOR NURSING

Margaret Miers

LEARNING OUTCOMES

After reading and reflecting on this chapter, you should be able to:

- recognise and describe the influence of social factors on a) own identity, biography, values and beliefs, and on b) nursing as a profession;
- identify key sociological concepts and approaches relevant to the understanding of health, illness, disability and professional practice;
- consider factors that inhibit promotion of health for all groups of inclusion, exclusion and discrimination;
- consider impact and sources of power in professional–client relationships.

INTRODUCTION

What is sociology and why does it matter?

A simple definition of **sociology** is the study of society. In Latin, the word 'socius' means 'companion', which suggests that sociology is the study of companionship, or, more broadly, social relations. Social relations can be informal, individual and unstructured, or formal, collective and organised. Sociology studies them all, as well as the two-way relationship between the individual and the collective, and the processes through which individuals and society are (knowingly or unknowingly) connected. Nursing involves many important social connections between individuals, social relations between nurses and patients, and among nurses and other members of care teams; and nursing, as a professional activity, involves a contract with society as a whole.

This chapter will help illuminate ways in which knowledge of sociology may help nurses achieve competences by

A simple definition of **sociology** is the study of society.

251

C. Wright Mills, in a book first published in 1959, identified the **sociological imagination**, an ability to link everyday individual concerns to wider social phenomena, as an essential tool of sociology.

- encouraging reflection on self and on the role and power of health professions;
- explaining approaches and concepts relevant to understanding health, illness and disability;
- describing patterns of inequality in health and care;
- exploring experiences of health, illness and health care.

Society continues to change, thus sociology remains an evolving discipline – the relevance of information in this chapter will change as the world and the health service change. The enduring contribution of sociology is through the cognitive skills it fosters. Most important is scepticism, a mode of thought that questions what is taken for granted in order to identify and question underlying assumptions and patterns of behaviour. C. Wright Mills, in a book first published in 1959, identified the **sociological imagination**, an ability to link everyday individual concerns to wider social phenomena, as an essential tool of sociology. He described this as a capacity that 'enables its possessor to understand the larger historical scene in terms of its meaning for the inner life and the external career of a variety of individuals' (Mills 1970, p. 11). Mills identified tools of the sociological imagination as an ability to distinguish between 'the personal troubles of the milieu' and 'the public issues of social structure' (1970, p. 14), and to recognise links between private troubles and public issues.

It is sociology's questioning and searching approach that helps unravel the nature and influence of culture, relations of power and processes of inclusion and exclusion. Such key skills are nurtured through a reflexive approach that prompts analysis of our own social position and behaviour, particularly in a professional role. Self-awareness is a prerequisite for supportive and enabling patient-focused care.

Sociology is often denigrated as being no more than common sense and sociology may not appear as a separate course of study within the nursing curriculum. One explicit advantage of recognising the scope and interests of sociology as a distinct discipline is that familiarity with social science literature and research helps develop analytical skills, through conceptual analysis and through understanding the relevance of social research. Research focus 10.1 introduces important studies and surveys that explore the relationship between social factors and health. Extracts from Erving Goffman's work in Box 10.1 exemplify sociological analysis.

The chapter is divided into three parts: Part 1 provides an outline of sociology; Part 2 reviews the relevance of sociology to health care; and Part 3 explores the relevance of sociology in nursing.

PART 1: OUTLINING SOCIOLOGICAL ASPECTS OF NURSING

Case 10.1

Mrs Johnson has been admitted to Accident and Emergency (A & E) after suffering a transient ischaemic attack at home. She is 82 years old and has begun to experience symptoms of possible dementia. She is accompanied by her husband and daughter. As Mrs Johnson appears confused and disorientated, Mr Johnson is very careful to explain that although his wife's full name is Jessica Vera Johnson, she has always been known as 'V': she has never been known by the name 'Jessica'. Mr Johnson is also very careful to provide accurate information about the tablets

Mrs Johnson takes and the timing of her medication.

Following examination in A & E, two nurses wheeled Mrs Johnson to a ward. Now 7 o'clock, Mr Johnson asks if his wife could be given her teatime medication. One nurse responded 'Too late. You should have been here at 4 o'clock'.

Mrs Johnson's daughter, Mary Butler, visited her mother the following morning. She was dismayed to discover that her mother had not received her medication until 11 o'clock at night. Initially she was perplexed to find staff talking to her about a patient they called 'Jesse'. She eventually realised that staff were talking about her mother, but were using an abbreviation of her first name, a name she had never used. Mary was relieved that her father, who was deaf, did not realise this. She explained her mother was known as 'V'.

Mrs Johnson was discharged after two days on the ward. Mr Johnson was pleased to have his wife home, but very worried about her confused state.

Activity 10.1

Note down your thoughts about staff response to Mrs Johnson and her family. Reflect on nursing activities and hospital routines that a) support and b) inhibit individualised care.

Durkheim (1893) and Marx developed theories and concepts that helped explain the **structure** of society.

Durkheim used an organic analogy that viewed society as an organism, identifying ways in which forms of organisation and social relations brought unity to a social group. His work on the structure of society and forms of consensus influenced the development of **functionalism**.

The development of sociology

Sociology emerged as a discipline in the nineteenth and early twentieth centuries during a time of considerable social change. The industrial revolution had led to new ways of manufacturing and distributing goods, and to new systems of financing and controlling production. Capitalism emerged as a dominant form of economic activity in the Western world and the rise and decline of Western colonialism shaped global relationships. During the twentieth century, diverse political philosophies such as liberalism, socialism, communism and fascism led to contrasting forms of political organisation based on democratic or totalitarian structures. The growth of bureaucracies aimed to make administration more rational and efficient and the growth of medical and scientific knowledge challenged religious dominance. The 'modern' world of industrialised and urbanised countries was very different from earlier traditional rural societies.

For much of the twentieth century, sociology took on the task of exploring and explaining the complexity of this modern world. The founders of sociology generally used a scientific approach, developing the use of social surveys to gain valuable data showing the influence of factors such as social class, age, race and gender on opportunities and experience, including health, disability and disease (see Research focus 10.1). Key writers such as Emile Durkheim, Karl Marx and Max Weber (seen as the founding fathers of sociology) developed theories and concepts that revealed different ways of understanding and explaining the social world. These different approaches, briefly summarised in Table 10.1, stimulated critical thinking about the relationship between the individual and society. Sociology remains a discipline that encourages debate. Durkheim (1893) and Marx developed theories and concepts that helped explain the **structure** of society: **Durkheim** used an organic analogy that viewed society as an organism, identifying ways

Marx's critique of capitalist society illuminated the importance of **conflict** in social change and the centrality of economic power in structuring social systems and relations.

Weber (1930, 1968) emphasised the importance of **social action** and its meaning for individuals.

Social interactionism and a linked development, social constructionism, have had a profound influence on sociology's understanding of the experience of health, illness and disability.

in which forms of organisation and social relations brought unity to a social group. His work on the structure of society and forms of consensus influenced the development of **functionalism**, (by Robert Merton (1949) and Talcott Parsons (1951)). In contrast, **Marx**'s critique of capitalist society illuminated the importance of **conflict** in social change and the centrality of economic power in structuring social systems and relations.

Not all social theorists were primarily concerned with overall explanations for the structure of society. Weber (1930, 1968) emphasised the importance of **social action** and its meaning for individuals as well as the importance of ideas (such as the Protestant ethic) and processes (such as rationalisation, which he saw as a mix of bureaucratic organisation and the development of scientific thought). Weber's emphasis on social action led to further theoretical developments focused on interaction, notably Mead's (1927) notion of symbolic interactionism, significantly developed by Goffman (1968a, b). **Social interactionism** and a linked development, social constructionism, have had a profound influence on sociology's understanding of the experience of health, illness and disability.

TABLE 10.1 Some sociological theories

Functionalism	Conflict theories	Social action	Postmodernism
Society is seen as a system, made up of social institutions (such as the family, the economy, the political system) and social roles	Karl Marx is the major conflict theorist	Society is maintained and shaped through individual interactions. It is our capacity to assign meaning to and understand and control symbols that makes interaction possible	Postmodern theorists argue that modernist theorists misled the world about the certainty of knowledge
Society works in a way similar to a biological organism	Societies are divided by classes that are determined by the relationship to the means of production (such as land and factories)		Knowledge is relative, standpoints are plural and diverse
Social institutions carry out activities that are beneficial (functional) for society as a whole. For example, the family and education system support social values that maintain cohesion	In capitalism the interests of the dominant bourgeoisie and subordinate proletariat are opposed and class conflict is inevitable	Symbols used in social construction are learned and communicated through interaction. Hence the term symbolic interactionism	Culture has become more important and cultural relations are no longer determined by economic status and structures. In a postmodern world we produce and consume cultural images
Order and equilibrium are based on consensus	Marxists see class position as a prime source of individual identity. Other conflict theorists paid more attention to the importance of political and cultural spheres in shaping interests that divide society		Culture is contestable and fragmented, leading to diverse, fluid and multiple identities

---

RESEARCH FOCUS 10.1

Longitudinal studies

Social surveys have provided significant information about the relationship between social factors such as social class, education, employment status and life experience including health status. Our understanding of social determinants of health has been enhanced through a series of longitudinal cohort studies that have followed individuals over their life course and have been able to illuminate the effect of life circumstances on health and well-being. These, as well as national panel surveys and census data, provide datasets that monitor social conditions and behaviour. The first cohort study, the National Survey of Health and Development (NSHD), was established in 1946 as a result of an investigation into maternity services. The study was based on interviews (by health visitors) with all mothers who gave birth in one week in March 1946. Although it had not been intended to study the babies, funding has been found to follow them throughout their lives. The key studies are listed below:

National Survey of Health and Development (NSHD) established in 1946, ongoing www.nshd.mrc.ac.uk/

National Child Development Study (NCDS) established 1958 www.cls.ioe.ac.uk/ncds
A study of individuals born 3–9 March 1958 in England, Scotland and Wales with information collected at 11, 16, 23, 33, 42, 46, 50, 55

1970 British Birth Cohort Study (BCS70) www.cls.ioe.ac.uk/bcs70
Individuals born in 1970 with information collected at birth, 5, 10, 16, 26, 30, 34, 38, 42

Office for National Statistics (ONS) Longitudinal Study www.statistics.gov.uk
A study based on a 1 per cent sample of those enumerated in England and Wales census, begun in 1971

Health Survey for England www.natcen.ac.uk/series/health-survey-for-england
An annual survey instituted in 1991 to monitor trends in the nation's health

Millenium Cohort Study (MCS) www.ioe.ac.uk/mcs
Longitudinal study of 15,000 UK babies born over a year from 1 September 2000. Information at 9 months, 3, 5, 7, 11

Whitehall Studies www.ucl.ac.uk/whitehalllI Longitudinal studies of British civil servants, led by Professor Sir Michael Marmot, to determine factors that affect health.

In the late twentieth century sociologists began to question the founding theorists' explanations. Feminist writers argued that mainstream sociological theory was *malestream* theory (Abbott and Wallace 1990), rooted in patriarchal relationships in which men have power. Feminists have argued that knowledge is gendered. Men and women have different experiences and construct their knowledge through different standpoints. Modernist explanations have also been questioned because of significant global change. In the United Kingdom and other Western societies labour intensive industries such as mining and ship building declined. Manufacturing has relocated to (for example) China, India and Indonesia. Western economies became reliant on the retail and service sectors.

255

Margaret Miers

From the late twentieth century onwards, national economies have become increasingly affected by the global economy and the arrival of the digital age. Individuals in the West are now more important as consumers than as producers. Fashion and leisure have become more important in people's lives. The growth of information technology and the Internet changed the distribution of knowledge, changing the role of many established groups. In health care, for example, the roles and power of professionals have altered alongside the growing importance of the patient as an active consumer rather than a passive recipient of health care. Writers have variously described the late twentieth century onwards as late modernity (Giddens 1991), liquid modernity (Bauman 2000) or postmodernity (Featherstone 1991, Fox 1993, Lyotard 1984).

In the twenty-first century the social structure appears more fluid and uncertain, bringing opportunities for diverse experiences and to forge multiple identities, but there are also risks and insecurities, particularly at times of economic recession. Postmodernism (see Table 10.1) brings a recognition that to make sense of the changing world it is important to understand the subjective experience of individuals in a consumerist society where appearance, body shape, music, leisure (culture) are possibly as important to individual identity as position in the social structure. Sociology has therefore become concerned with links between identity, biography and social worlds (real and virtual). Different sociological approaches can be further explored through considering their different views on the development of identities – our sense of who we are.

Personal and professional identity: who are we?

Activity 10.2

Think about how you would describe yourself. If working with other students, take time to introduce yourself to someone who does not know you and ask them to introduce themselves to you. In addition, look at personal pages on the Internet and at profiles on social media. How are individuals presenting themselves? What characteristics do they identify as important? Do they tell a 'story' about their life? What, and who, influences our sense of who we are?

Different sociologists have emphasised different approaches to understanding identities. Humans are social beings who learn to be group members through a process known as socialisation. Through socialisation they learn the culture of the group – that is the knowledge, values, norms, roles and expectations that shape social life. **Structural functionalists** have viewed **socialisation** as a process of role learning. Social roles such as teacher or nurse have prescribed sets of obligations and expectations that provide templates of how to behave. Individuals learn to conform to role expectations through external pressures involving rewards and punishments as well as internalisation, a process encouraged through role taking and observation of role models. Wrong (1961), however, criticised such a view of human development as being an 'oversocialised conception of man'.

Whereas functionalists emphasised a process of conformity through learning roles associated with social statuses, **symbolic interactionism** sees identities as constructed

256

through a process of interaction and negotiation in which responses of others are crucial to the creation of meaning. Children and adults constantly interpret and assign meaning to the actions and reactions of each other. Interaction is fostered through meanings assigned to symbols and it is through use of symbols that individuals interpret, reflect upon and develop patterns of behaviour that constitute culture. A doctor wearing a white coat and carrying medical instruments is using symbols that indicate expertise and professional status. (Professionals wearing 'normal' clothes often do so to avoid creating a barrier between themselves and clients.) It is through interactions with others that children become aware of themselves as separate individuals, acquiring a sense of personal identity and social identity. Social identities derive from being a type of individual such as boy or girl, son/daughter, older brother, younger sister. Social identities can encompass, inter alia, ethnicity, religion, nationality, locality, occupation, gender, sexuality, leisure activity. They differ from personal identities associated with individual characteristics such as honesty, recklessness, optimism, but nevertheless clusters of personal characteristics may be perceived as linked to particular social roles or groups, thus ensuring that social identities become fundamental to individual lives.

The interactionist approach to understanding identity is most vividly portrayed in the work of Erving Goffman who saw social interaction as performance whereby actors control information made available to others and interpret and attempt to control others' responses. Two of Goffman's books have particular relevance for health care. In *Asylums*, Goffman records his analysis and observations of the experience of hospitalised mental patients. He notes the changing sense of self as an individual experiences the power relations of the hospital. Staff construct an image of the person as sick and resist attempts to construct the individual as normal. Admission processes (see Box 10.1) strip patients of their former identity and as patients submit to staff expectations they come to accept the staff definition of the situation and their identity as an ill person.

Goffman's *Stigma* has also influenced our understanding of society's treatment of individuals perceived as different. Disability results from stigmatisation of impairments (see Box 10.1). Understanding interaction helps us understand how responses to social difference can constrain and undermine the identity of a person with impairments. Goffman stressed that stigma was not a fixed entity but a relational concept. One attribute may be normal in one context but discreditable in another. The colour of one's skin has led to different treatments in different societies at different times. Race, religion, gender, sexuality, age, physical and mental impairments, for example, have all been attributes that have led to widespread discrimination, and at times still do. The strength of symbolic interactionism is the close attention given to the impact of social action on individuals' own perceptions of themselves. The impact of racial discrimination on self-perception is illustrated, for example, by a statement by James Hood, a civil rights campaigner in the USA who, in 1963, challenged Alabama University's policy of admitting white students only. Despite this challenge Hood has noted that, 'at the time I believed we were inferior to white folks. That's what I was taught growing up in Alabama'. Hood insisted civil rights were 'not rights for black people but rights for all peoples. Equality, the freedom to become someone' (*The Times* 2013).

The interactionist approach to understanding identity, however, has been widely challenged for ignoring structural inequalities that underpin negative judgments made about attributes such as gender and race. The impact of social structure may be better explained by structural functionalist and conflict approaches. Marx saw an individual's economic position, that is, class position, as central to a sense of identity. Furthermore,

257

BOX 10.1

Asylums

The recruit comes into the establishment with a conception of himself made possible by certain stable social arrangements in his home world. Upon entrance, he is immediately stripped of the support provided by these arrangements.

(Goffman 1968a, p. 24)

[C]ertain roles are lost to him by virtue of the barrier that separates him from the outside world. The process of entrance typically brings together other kinds of loss and mortification as well. We very generally find staff employing what are called admission procedures, such as taking a life history, photographing, weighing, fingerprinting, assigning numbers, searching, listing personal possessions for storage, undressing, bathing, disinfecting, haircutting, issuing institutional clothing, instructing as to rules, and assigning to quarters.

(Goffman 1968a, pp. 25–26)

Stigma

The Greeks . . . originated the term **stigma** to refer to bodily signs designed to expose something unusual and bad about the moral status of the signifier. The signs were cut or burnt into the body and advertised that the bearer was a slave, a criminal or a traitor – a blemished person.

(Goffman 1968b, p. 11)

Society establishes the means of categorising persons and the complement of attributes felt to be ordinary and natural for members of each of these categories . . .

. . . When a stranger comes into our presence, then, first appearances are likely to enable us to anticipate his category and his attributes, his 'social identity' . . .

. . . evidence can arise of his possessing an attribute that makes him different from others in the category of persons available for him to be, and of a less desirable kind . . . He is thus reduced in our minds from a whole and usual person to a tainted, discounted one. Such an attribute is a stigma.

(Goffman 1968b, p. 12)

[Stigma can lead to] varieties of discrimination, through which we effectively, if often unthinkingly, reduce his life chances.

(Goffman 1968b, p. 15)

subjective awareness of class position (class consciousness) was central to the development of a social class into a political force able to play a historic role in the development of a society. Marx and Engels (1848) thought that, in a capitalist society, the proletariat would move towards becoming a 'class for itself' (a class aware of, and pursuing, its own interests). The trade union movement and the Labour Party developed through working class awareness of shared interests and sense of solidarity. By the 1990s, however, the relationship between class structure and position and cultural beliefs and practices had become increasingly complex. Beck (1992) argued that the ability to manage one's life in a 'risk' society had become more important than class position.

Identity in a postmodern society

Giddens (1991) has argued that in the late twentieth century rapid change meant that individuals could select and discard identities that attain or lose meaning. Identity has become a reflexive project of the self. Nevertheless, the need to maintain 'ontological security', that is, a sense of confidence in self-identity, means that identity work involves seeking coherence among constructed personal and social identities. Reflexivity is a key skill. Bauman (1995) argued that whereas the challenge had hitherto been to build a solid and stable identity, in the contemporary postmodern world the lack of clear stable pathways for individuals to follow means that maintaining a range of choices as to what kind of person to be is important. Flexibility is key and the growth of the Internet and the possibilities of virtual communities, without boundaries of space and time, present opportunities for creation and recreation of identities and adoption of multiple identities.

Activity 10.3

Look back at Case 10.1 and think about the experience of Mrs Johnson in the light of ideas about identity.

Do hospital staff support Mrs Johnson's sense of identity? Consider the relevance of Goffman's work in relation to hospitalisation.

Barriers to the 'freedom to become someone': processes of separation and exclusion

Despite societal changes that may offer individuals freedom to choose a lifestyle, there is still concern, particularly during a prolonged period of recession, that structures and processes inhibit individual 'freedom to become someone'. Sociologists see the history of capitalism and colonialism as important in understanding the endurance of patterns that separated social groups and led to social exclusion. Barriers to opportunities have emerged through assumptions about social groups that promote discrimination on the basis of factors such as gender, race, sexuality, age, different abilities, sexuality and socio-economic background. The continuing legacy of world history, including Western colonialism can be seen in current relations between countries and religions, political tensions around immigration and concerns about religious intolerance and terrorist activity.

Separating identities: gender in industrial capitalism

Gender inequalities have been influenced by a history of a growing separation of work and home during industrialisation that led to increased separation between the spheres of men and women. Such separation led to cultural emphasis on and construction of gender differences. Women were seen as passive, caring and emotional whereas men were seen as strong, active and rational. Biological differences were seen as determining men's and women's behaviour and historical differences in men's and women's opportunities and social status were therefore seen as 'natural'. The impact of such thinking on nursing has been profound. Garmarnikow (1978) suggested the doctor–nurse relationship paralleled the relationship between Victorian husband and wife. Nurses, like women, were seen as naturally subordinate, responsible for others and naturally caring. The fact that, in the 1950s, boys became doctors and girls nurses led to cultural images of nurses as sex objects, a prevalent but contrasting image to that of the cultural view of nurses as angels. Patriarchy reinforced this thinking about women and their attributes, yet in turn this sexism led to a growth in feminism and women's challenge to excluding and discriminatory practices. Although women now participate in many areas of life on an equal basis in the UK, concern remains about the low numbers of men in nursing and the low proportion of women in senior positions in politics, law and business. Recent revelations about sexual abuse perpetrated by public figures have revealed the prevalence of views of women as sex objects in the 1960s and 1970s.

Separating sexualities

The two sex/gender emphases on male/female differences also reinforced the categories of sexuality acknowledged by society. Adrienne Rich (1980) argued that in the nineteenth century 'compulsory heterosexuality' became a vehicle of patriarchy, supporting a view of women as sexually passive and, as Connell (1987) has argued, to a 'hegemonic masculinity' – a view of masculinity as heterosexual, dominant and powerful. Homosexuality became pathologised and medicalised and male homosexual subcultures emerged, providing members with mutual support to resist negative judgments about their identity. Although attitudes to different sexual preferences have changed considerably over recent decades, homosexuality remains unacceptable in some cultures.

Separating races

In the sixteenth century the word 'race' referred to diverse populations in Europe. It was only after European colonial expansion into the Pacific, Africa and the Americas that the word was used to refer to physical characteristics and differences. Developments in scientific understanding of evolution and genetics led to an idea that racial traits were fixed. The Nazis in Germany in the 1930s and 1940s emphasised the idea of racial superiority. The subsequent defeat of political racism after World War II led to debate about the nature of human biological variations and the notion of discrete racial characteristics became discredited. Race is now understood as a social construct used in everyday discourse to reflect people's perceptions. In sociology it is a term used to reflect the ways people have racialised their relations with each other through racist discourse, that is, a set of ideas and arguments that reflect historical patterns of dominance and subordination unified around ideas about the inferiority/superiority of different groups. Such racist discourse supports racism, structures and patterns of behaviour that disadvantage and discriminate against groups

groups and individuals. The Macpherson Report (1999) used the term 'institutionalised racism' to describe processes that can disadvantage certain ethnic groups when a diffuse racialisation of ethnic difference is inherent in routines and practices (such as recruitment and promotion policies) as well as through overt prejudice. Macpherson was reporting on institutionalised racism in the Metropolitan Police following identified inadequacies in the police response to the murder of a young black man, Stephen Lawrence, in 1993. As a result of the Macpherson Report, the Race Relations Act was extended to the whole of the public sector, leading to the introduction of equal opportunities and race awareness training throughout public and many private organisations. The case in 1998 of David Bennett who died when restrained by five nurses identified similar difficulties within mental health services (DH 2005).

Conflict theorists saw racism as deriving from capitalism and colonialism and from slavery, systems of economic domination and exploitation. Throughout the world segregation and discrimination have, at times, restricted opportunities for particular ethnic groups and affected individual identities.

Identity and social class

The impact of class position on social identity remains an issue for debate despite the declining relevance of Marxist thought and changing economic activity such as the decline of mining and manufacturing in the UK. Bourdieu's influential work inextricably linking economic and social/cultural worlds has sustained an interest in the relationship between culture and other resources. Bourdieu emphasises the dynamic structuring of practice, that is, the way our practice is shaped by dynamic processes. His explanatory terms are 'field', 'habitus' and capital. 'Fields' are 'structured spaces of positions' (Bourdieu 1993, p. 27) in which individuals act or 'play the game'. Interested individuals in the field are skilful and competence in the field is crucial to gain the rewards accessible within the field. A health care setting, for example, a hospital ward, is an example of a 'field'. 'Habitus' is a 'structuring structure' (Bourdieu 1986, p. 170) that is both social positions and a set of perceptions and understandings. Individuals' habitus are socially acquired and it is their habitus that affects their ability to operate successfully in fields. Bourdieu sees fields as interrelated, fluid and changeable. As individuals move between fields they become aware of differences in stakes and practices in different fields, supporting reflexivity about their own practice and position. Bourdieu identifies types of 'capital' that contribute to an individual's habitus: economic, cultural, social. All can play an empowering role in an individual's life. Cultural capital comprises types of cultural advantage that can lead to economic gains, most notably educational qualifications, but also including what Bourdieu (1997) calls 'long-lasting dispositions of mind and body'. Social capital includes social networks and sociability. Cultural capital can bring the skills necessary for building social networks (social capital), which in turn can bring advantages not just in terms of wealth but in terms of health and well-being. Our identities, therefore, are framed and supported by our habitus and our types of capital, and affect our movement within and across fields.

Whereas Bourdieu's ideas can help explain fluidity in social structure and the complexity of factors that shape our identity, they do not deny the enduring power of dominant groups and the entrenched processes of social exclusion that limit individual opportunities. Bourdieu's work also emphasises the importance of culture. Culture is studied through ethnography, a research approach largely involving observation and listening to participants in social groups and settings. Ethnography is also used to study institutions through close consideration of texts and talk. Institutional ethnography examines how people are organised to accomplish daily activities, looking at connections between relations, seeking the ruling relations that co-ordinate knowledge and activities (Rankin and Campbell 2009, Smith 2005).

Activity 10.4

Look again at Case 10.1. Consider the hospital as a 'field' and the role of the drug round in shaping the field as a 'structured space of positions'. Consider Mr Johnson's attempts to influence his wife's care and why he is unsuccessful.

Professional identity

For many individuals the job they do is an important part of their identity. Professions are occupations that have been assigned particular status and rewards in return for skilled work contributing to the well-being of society. Functionalist explanations for professions' role identified key attributes of a profession: a body of knowledge transmitted through prolonged education and training; motivation for public service rather than private gain; adherence to a code of ethics; regulation by a professional body. In return for these attributes, professions gained prestige and financial reward. Functionalist approaches were criticised for being a justification for a privileged position rather than an explanation. Freidson (1970) was the first of many to clarify the importance of power and control in preserving professional status. Control over position in the labour market (by restricting the supply of workers qualified to take on professional roles and restricting access to areas of work) is important. Parkin (1979) identified control over education and training as a strategy of occupational closure, restricting access to opportunities that ultimately lead to professional rewards. Witz (1992) described the process of seeking professional status as a 'professionalising project' and argued that nursing used dual closure strategies (exclusion and usurpation) in the fight to become an independent profession. In arguing, in the early twentieth century, for state registration, a uni-portal system of entry and centralised control over education and training, nurses were arguing for a system that could exclude nurses trained in different ways (as the practice of local control through individual hospitals allowed). It can be argued that nurses' professionalising project is continuing. Professional boundaries are fluid and as nurses take on more of doctor's tasks, gain higher academic qualifications to support more autonomous work, they may be 'usurping' some medical work. At the same time health care assistants and assistant practitioners take on activities that can be seen as usurping nurses' work. Nurses retain control over the title 'nurse' but may not be able to retain control over care activities.

Illich (1977) and Zola (1975), from a conflict perspective, saw the medical profession as all powerful, serving self-interest not the interests of society, a criticism that can be applied to all professions. Feminist writers such as Witz have argued that professions are patriarchal structures through their dominance by men, a historical dominance supported by women's lack of access to universities. Celia Davies (1995) has argued that the notion of profession celebrates a masculine view of expertise in which individual mastery of skills and knowledge base are valued. She argued for a new model of professionalism emphasising the importance of reflective practice and the engaged, embodied collaboration with colleagues and clients.

The Code (NMC 2015) published by the Nursing and Midwifery Council supports such a model of professionalism in emphasising the importance of teamwork.

Activity 10.5

Note down your reasons for choosing nursing and reflect on people and factors that influenced your choice.

If working with other students, discuss your pathways to becoming a nurse. Read Research focus 10.2 and consider whether the research findings reflect your experience. How important were altruistic motives, professional rewards, long-standing motivation, client orientation and personal interest/abilities in your choice of profession?

What factors do you think influence society's views of nursing?

RESEARCH FOCUS 10.2

Miers *et al.* (2007) explored the career motivation of students entering a range of non-medical health professions in one faculty in England in 2001–2002. Data were collected through an open-ended question about motivation (What was your main reason for deciding to join your chosen profession?) on a questionnaire completed at entry and at qualification. The professions included in the study were: radiotherapy, diagnostic imaging, physiotherapy, occupational therapy, midwifery, adult nursing, children's nursing, mental health nursing and learning disabilities nursing. Some 821 students answered the question on entry and 560 on qualification. On entry and across all professions, the desire to work with people with an altruistic/helping orientation was identified as the main reason for joining the professional programme. Personal interest and/or a perception that personal attributes would suit the role was the second most popular reason, followed by professional rewards and values (including remuneration, status, job security and opportunities to develop knowledge and skills). Further reasons given were prior experience, commitment to client group and long-standing motivation.

On qualification, a significantly lower percentage of students cited altruism or professional rewards as motivating factors. Nursing students reported altruistic motives less frequently than students from other non-medical professions on entry and on qualification. This may be due to children's nursing, mental health and learning disabilities nursing as well as midwifery showing a strong commitment to the client group.

There were few differences between men and women in reasons for choosing a profession although women described a long-standing motivation (e.g., 'I have always wanted to be a nurse') more often than men. Although all age groups ranked altruism high on entry, only 46.78 per cent of young adults aged 21–30 years, compared with 62.64 per cent of students under 21 and 59.26 per cent of 31–40 year olds expressed service-oriented reasons for entering health care. Those aged 21–30 years old (born 1971–1980) were the group least likely to claim altruistic orientation to health care, perhaps because of a realistic view of the demands of health work or because they are testing opportunities and are uncertain about their commitment to the profession. Although adult and children's nursing entrants reported a long-standing motivation to nurse, mental health and learning disabilities nurses did not, suggesting a stereotypical image of hospital-based nursing attracts recruits at an early age.

Iatrogenesis is illness caused by medicine and medical practice.

Social iatrogenesis is where **medicalisation** leads to more and more aspects of life becoming subject to the scrutiny and control of health professionals.

The study shows that nursing is not the only choice for those with a service/altruistic orientation and although nursing remains unique in its capacity to foster early commitment, graduate programmes in other non-medical professions are strong competitors for possible nursing recruits. Responses suggested a significant decline in expectations of professional rewards between entry and qualification.

PART 2: EXPLAINING SOCIOLOGICAL ASPECTS OF NURSING

Approaches to understanding health, disease and the experience of care

Different sociological approaches and concepts have shaped the discipline's contribution to understanding health and disease.

Biomedicine

Sociologists, as well as exploring how social contexts shape experience of health, illness and disability, have commented on the prevalence, dominance and impact of the bio-medical model of health. The influence of the bio-medical model increased rapidly during the nineteenth and twentieth centuries. Its underlying assumptions include:

- Disease is a deviation of normal biological functioning.
- Diseases have specific causes.
- The body is seen as a machine, to be restored to full functioning through treatment.
- The health of society is largely dependent on medical knowledge and medical services.

Bio-medical dominance was consolidated through the growth of hospitals in the nineteenth and twentieth centuries as well as through laboratory-based developments in medicines and in understanding of disease processes. Such dominance, however, is not without its critics and arguments against the importance of the bio-medical model are many, notably the view that public health reforms (including clean water supplies, sanitation and improved nutrition) have contributed more to the health of the nation than medicine (McKeown 1976).

Medicalisation

A much more radical critique of modern medicine, however, came from Ivan Illich (1977) who argued medical practice caused harm as well as improved health. He argued society was experiencing an epidemic of **iatrogenesis**, that is, illness caused by medicine and medical practice. He identified types of iatrogenesis; medical (or clinical) iatrogenesis, when treatment itself causes harm (e.g., through side effects of drug treatments); social iatrogenesis whereby **medicalisation** leads to more and more aspects of life becoming subject to the scrutiny and control of health professionals leading to experiences such as pregnancy, childbirth, grieving and unhappiness becoming medicalised; cultural iatrogenesis whereby individuals cease to accept personal responsibility for health and become unwitting passive consumers of medical dominance.

Discourse and surveillance: Foucault

Michel Foucault's writings have also furthered our understanding of the power of medicine, particularly through exploring the ways in which the development of medical practice from the late eighteenth century onwards has allowed modern states to exercise powers of surveillance over populations. He identified how new institutions such as hospitals and prisons developed ways of controlling and disciplining individual bodies. The bio-medical model of illness established doctors as possessing expert knowledge about bodies and centralising medical practice in hospitals led to what Foucault called the medical or clinical 'gaze', a way of seeing and defining the sick as dysfunctional bodies entailing investigation and clinical intervention (Foucault 1976). Scientific practice necessitated an objective, detached approach to 'cases' and 'symptoms'. Foucault argued health care became part of a 'disciplinary society', characterised by state surveillance over individuals. Prisons exemplified surveillance particularly through the design of Pentonville whereby staff can see into all areas of the prison and inmates are subjected to 'panoptic' surveillance (Foucault 1977). However, for Foucault, physical surveillance was not as important as the way in which knowledge and power are inextricably linked through 'discourse'. Discourses are sets of common assumptions that frame the way we see the world, what counts as knowledge and as normal practice. Discourses 'create' reality. Hence knowledge cannot be treated on its own terms but as an expression of power relations. Power is everywhere, through all social relations and communications – through discourse. Nevertheless, for Foucault, the ubiquity of power always prompts resistance – 'where there is power, there is resistance' (Foucault 1979, p. 95).

Foucault's view of power is significantly different from approaches to power adopted by early sociologists, who focused on identifying the social structures (such as economic class position) and the groups (such as political elites) that had the power to promote their own interests over others. He challenged the view that power is only exercised in particular circumstances, for example, through decision-making. For Foucault power is everywhere, inherent in language and in the process of interaction between individuals.

Models of disability

Disability theorists and activists have also strongly criticised the medical model. The medical model of disability focused on impairment. If a medical 'cure' was not possible, the afflicted individual was expected to adjust to the environment and the management goal was to prepare an individual to adapt through rehabilitation. Disability was seen as a personal tragedy; wider social issues about the exclusion of disabled people from aspects of social life, including employment were ignored. In the 1960s and 1970s writers influenced by conflict theories and inspired by disability activists explored the development of the medical model of disability in the context of historical change. As Oliver and Barnes (2012) explain,

> the creation of the disabled individual occurred at a particular historical point, namely the coming of industrial society. The collective labour of agrarian society gave way to the individualised wage labour of the factory, fundamentally changing all other social relationships as well. From this point on people with functional limitations became a problem for government because often they were not able to operate the new machinery.
>
> (p. 16)

Margaret Miers

Since the 1980s there has been widespread acceptance of a **social model** of disability that recognises that it is the way society is organised that disables those with physical and mental impairments.

The sick role

Not all social theories concerning health and illness are, however, critical of biomedicine and medical dominance. Talcott Parsons (1951), a structural functionalist, saw illness as disruptive to the normal functioning of society. He argued that the deviant behaviour that might result from ill health can be controlled if individuals conform to the expectations of what he identified as the **sick role**. These expectations are to seek medical help and to become a 'patient', wanting to get well. In return, patients are allowed to give up normal responsibilities and are not seen as being responsible for their illness. The sick role is a temporary role, legitimated by the medical profession. Individuals who do not appear to want to get well will be seen as malingerers and those who do not accept medical advice will be seen as deviant. Understandably there have been many criticisms of Parsons' sick role concept. Whereas it may describe societal response to acute illness it does not 'fit' the experience of chronic illness. The sick role encourages patient passivity and dependence and is an unhelpful model for health care in the many settings where services are provided for healthy individuals, for example, maternity care, reproductive health, screening services. Nevertheless, it is a model of care that aligns with a model of professional power and patient compliance.

Illness experience

Interactionism offered an alternative approach to understanding health and illness behaviour. Whereas from a functionalist perspective professional–patient encounters were seen as shaped by conformity to expectations of patient compliance and professional control, interactionism illuminated the importance of negotiation, whereby the significance and meaning of experiences and behaviour could be re-shaped. Early research into illness behaviour demonstrated that individuals took time to perceive themselves as possibly requiring professional help. Social interaction as well as bodily changes played a role in the process of becoming ill. The experience of chronic illness (long-term conditions) involved a long-term process of changing views of normality (see Research focus 10.3). Bury (1982) used the term **biographical disruption** to describe the way in which long-term conditions can challenge an individual's sense of self and self-worth, altering a person's life situation and relationships. One reason why a person's self-identity can be disrupted through the onset of long-term disease is the meaning attributed to the limitations (such as changes in mobility) that may be experienced. Some limitations, for example paralysis following stroke, may be stigmatised by society, or indeed by the individual, bringing fears about negative labelling and a diminished view of self alongside fears about managing the uncertainty of a long-term condition. Coming to terms with such changes in health takes time and, as Banner et al. (2012) identify, renegotiation of normality. Williams (1984) has argued that individuals use narrative to explain their experience within their own biography, leading to a 'narrative reconstruction' of events in order to reduce the threat to everyday meanings in everyday life.

RESEARCH FOCUS 10.3

Illness experience: women's experience of cardiac surgery

Banner *et al.* (2012) explored the experience of women diagnosed with coronary heart disease and undergoing coronary artery bypass graft surgery through semi-structured interviews with 30 women. Women from two urban teaching hospitals in England and Wales were interviewed pre-operatively and 6 weeks and 6 months post-operatively. A grounded theory approach was used to analyse the data. The core category of normality embraced all stages of the illness experience. During a period of symptom recognition and translation participants sought to preserve normality but as symptoms and limitations increased women experienced disrupted normality. Hospital admission led to relinquished normality and sleeping difficulties, pain, wound healing problems and impaired mobility all led to anxiety during early recovery. Nevertheless during the recovery period participants 'renegotiated normality'. Cardiac rehabilitation programmes were pivotal in assisting women to evaluate their situation positively.

Throughout all stages of the illness experience, women engaged in an ongoing dialogue between the private and public aspects of their experience. A public–private dialogue involving public sharing of private perceptions and responses eased the process of renegotiating normality. Establishing boundaries around activities that enabled women to preserve their domestic role was crucial. The study offers insights into women's illness experience that can assist in developing gender-sensitive preventative and management interventions to support recovery from cardiac surgery.

Illness as deviance: labelling and mental illness

Interactionism has also contributed significant insights into the understanding of mental health services, particularly through labelling theory. Becker (1963) argued that once a deviant label is assigned, the social reaction to the behaviour can make it harder for an individual to behave differently, or for their behaviour to be interpreted differently. For example, if an individual uses illegal drugs, the fact that the drugs can only be obtained through participating in drug subcultures, which may involve exposure to further illegal behaviour means the individual gains more opportunities for deviance and experiences expectations to continue drug taking. Similarly, Szasz (1970) argued that people call others 'mad' when they do not accept their behaviour as normal. If behaviour is defined as indicating mental illness, subsequent reactions from others including drug treatments and hospitalisation may in itself prompt behaviour seen as conforming to the 'mad' label.

In order to resist such labelling, mental health user groups have argued for a greater emphasis on social approaches to mental health, including non-medicalised community provision and support as well as attention to the links between mental health issues and social exclusion.

The 'expert patient': new models

The transition to a post-modern society in which health information is freely available through media and Internet sources has led to challenges to some established ideas about dependency on medical knowledge. Individuals are seen as consumers, and services now recognise the importance of the patient voice. Fox (1993) has argued that modernist views of health and illness are framed through a discourse whereby identities as 'healthy' or 'sick' are inscribed on bodies, as Foucault explained. Fox seeks a post-modern understanding whereby health is a possibility shaped through resistance to discourse and through individual narratives that create subjectivities, meaning and experience. In Fox's understanding, care practices in organised health care have become controlling (termed 'care-as-discipline'). Nevertheless, following Foucault's analysis of resistance to power, Fox argues that resistance to care-as-discipline is possible through individual practices between carer and cared-for; a 'gift of care' is possible (Fox 1995).

It could be argued that the development of self-management and expert-patient programmes in the NHS and the emphasis on user involvement are examples of significant change in professional–client relationships recognising the importance of patients' knowledge of the impact of disease and the value of sharing experience and stories. However Bury (2010) explored these initiatives in the context of changes in NHS management practices and concluded that although self-management may appear to empower individuals by deflecting power away from the medical profession, the programmes are part of cost control and can serve to curtail expectations about what might be possible in a resource-constrained health service. Research into user involvement shows the difficulties service users experience trying to shape agendas and change discourse. Nevertheless, personal budgets may offer some individuals the chance to gain more control.

Case 10.2

Power

This summary is based on Mitchell's story: Personal health budgets.

For a full account of the case study see UCL Institute of Health Equity webpage www.instituteofhealthequity.org/projects/mitchells-story-personal-health-budgets

Mitchell is a teenager with complex health needs. In 2001 he suffered a medical crisis requiring prolonged hospitalisation. After a year he was discharged home with a home care package to support his need (he has a gastrostomy, tracheostomy and is on long-term ventilation). His mother describes the frustration and hopelessness felt by Mitchell and his family at this time. Although support staff enabled Mitchell to remain with his family, the lack of control over who fulfils that role was a challenge. Hospital policies and procedures dictated practice. For example, staff were prevented from using aromatherapy oils to massage Mitchell at home because of the risk to other 'patients'. 'The service was central to decision making rather than the needs of the children and families'. Mitchell's family applied for more control of his care package through seeking permission to take on responsibility for a personal health budget. This process took 4 years during which time the family were supported by advocates and utilised a third party domiciliary care agency to act as holder of Mitchell's indicative budget. Mitchell's mother noted she had found 'professional power had often made us anxious; knowing an individual can influence the fabric of your life can be very stressful'. Working with their trusted advocates during the process was a tremendous help as 'they did not take responsibility for us but encouraged us to find and exercise our own power and resources'.

After the change to the individual budget some staff continued to support Mitchell. Staff had felt constrained by an inflexible service and one noted 'the thing that stands out is that Mitchell has more freedom to do what he wants to do'.

Activity 10.6

Consider Mitchell's story in the light of Foucault's and Illich's arguments about the power of biomedicine and Fox's views about care-as-discipline. Note how hospital discourses influence home-based care. Consider Mitchell's mother's experience of professional power and note down reasons why health professionals fail to provide personalised care.

Reflect on instances when you have felt constrained or frustrated by the care you provide and consider reasons for your dissatisfaction.

Social determinants of health

Sociologists have contributed to a deepening understanding of social determinants of health over recent decades. Longitudinal studies and panel surveys (see Research focus 10.1) as well as national and international studies of mortality and comparable morbidity data have all identified inequalities in health and a consistent gradient in health across socio-economic groupings. Throughout the developed world research has identified that the poorest people have the highest mortality rates and mortality rates for those in middle incomes are between those at the bottom and the top. Gender, ethnicity and geographical location also all show influences in health. Heart disease, for example, is unequally distributed across regions in the UK. Death rates from coronary heart disease are highest in Scotland and the north of England, lowest in southern England.

A 2012 Royal College of Nursing Policy Briefing identified the social determinants of health as housing, education, financial security, the built environment and acknowledges the World Health Organization's view that economics, social policies and politics are overriding factors that affect these determinants (RCN 2012). Government statistics illustrate health inequalities that cannot be explained by biological or individual factors, for example, unskilled workers are twice as likely to die from cancer as professionals.

Evidence relating to the social determinants of health has been summarised by a series of Committee and Enquiry reports, notably the WHO Global Commission on the Social Determinants of Health Report (WHO 2008), the Scottish Government's ministerial task force report (SG 2008) and the Marmot Review in 2010. Social scientists contribute to discussions about possible explanations for variations in health and to discussions about strategies to work towards health equity. Possible explanations include material circumstances (income, housing, working environment), social selection, involving people with good health moving into well-paid employment and those in poor health being liable to move down the employment ladder, and cultural and behavioural factors. Smoking, exercise, diet, uptake of preventative services and help-seeking behaviour can all affect health. The complexity of influential factors is now widely accepted and models of layers of influence are used as a way of understanding social determinants of health.

269

Key contemporary debates

Income inequality

Although it is clear that inequalities in income are linked to inequalities in health there is debate about whether it is the absolute lack of resources to keep warm, eat healthily, afford a secure home, or whether it is the *relative* lack of income that has a negative effect on health. At a population level, absolute income theory has been supported by a strong relationship between gross domestic national product (GDP) and life expectancy. At an individual level, an accumulation of negative material factors in early life can damage health across a life course. For example foetal development, birth weight and educational attainment can all be affected by material factors and have a long-term effect on health.

Evidence for the relative income hypothesis comes from global comparisons of population data that show that among developed nations, the richest countries in terms of GDP do not necessarily have the highest life expectancy. A 2006 review of 170 studies of income inequality and health showed that life expectancy, infant mortality, low birth weight and self-rated health have repeatedly been shown to be worse in more unequal societies (Wilkinson and Pickett 2006). The website of the Equality Trust www.equalitytrust.org.uk provides resources supporting this view, including graphs showing a relationship between inequality and levels of obesity and experience of mental illness. The explanation for inequality leading to poor health is that living in an unequal society is stressful, due to status differences and status competition. Chronic stress affects the cardiovascular and immune systems.

Work, stress and health

The results of the Whitehall studies of civil servants (see Research focus 10.1) have strongly supported the importance of this psycho-social pathway. These studies showed a social gradient in morbidity for a range of diseases: heart disease, some cancers, depression, suicide, chronic lung disease, gastrointestinal disease, back pain and general feelings of ill health. Someone in the middle of the hierarchy had poorer health than those above them and better health than those below. Smoking, lack of physical activity, obesity all showed a social gradient, as did cholesterol levels and blood pressure. Explanations offered for these gradients among civil servants focused on stress at work, particularly the combination of high demands and low control. In the Whitehall studies control is measured by degree of authority over decisions and use of skills, including the opportunity for skill development. High-grade jobs have high demands but high levels of control: the lower the grade of employment, the less control. This demand–control model of work stress has been developed further to include the impact of social support. *The Whitehall II Study* showed that working with supportive colleagues and managers improves mental health and reduces sickness absence and that social support outside work had health benefits. Other relevant findings included the impact of an imbalance between high effort and low reward, which increased illness rates, as did job insecurity and poorly managed organisational change (Ferrie 2004).

PART 3: EXPLORING SOCIOLOGICAL ASPECTS OF NURSING

Nursing and patients

Nursing involves important social relationships, notably with individual patients and clients. The Francis Report on the failures at Stafford Hospital showed deficiencies in physical care but it is the distress felt by patients and carers concerning the perceived failure of staff to treat hospitalised patients with dignity and respect that has attracted widespread attention (Mid-Staffordshire NHS Foundation Trust 2013). How can sociology help explain the lack of individualised care within hospital settings?

Consider the different approaches mentioned in Part 1 of this chapter. Interactionism focused on the micro level of society – individual actions and reactions. Goffman's insights into the working of asylums and on the impact of stigmas on individual identity can help us think more carefully about the experience of hospitalisation from the point of view of the actors involved. Admission to hospital involves separation from normal daily life, losing opportunities to make individual decisions, including when to take one's own tablets, or when to eat meals. Whereas patients may feel vulnerable and belittled by this experience, for staff, the hospital is a familiar environment in which they are in control. Hospital routines, such as drug rounds, are activities shaped by medicalisation and by professional and managerial power. The drug round may be an efficient and safe way of providing medicines but it is also a symbol of professional and institutional power over vulnerable individuals. Foucault's work can alert us to the ubiquity of power and its links to knowledge.

Early nursing research indicated that until the 1970s and the development of the nursing process, nurses' work was largely seen as completion of tasks, procedures, physical care and ward management rather than caring relationships. Menzies (1960) in her study of a hospital nursing service argued that the task list system of organising work served as a protection against nurses experiencing potential distress and anxiety deriving from patients' suffering. Ritual task performance led to depersonalisation and categorisation for both nurse and patient. Such a work system served as a social defence system against anxiety, yet it also contributed to staff stress levels and minimised satisfaction. In a study of interpersonal relationships in general wards, Stockwell (1972) found that nurses most enjoyed caring for patients who communicated readily, knew nurses' names, were able to laugh and joke and cooperated with helping to get well. Unpopular patients were those who grumbled, did not enjoy being in hospital, appeared to suffer more than nurses believed appropriate and suffered from conditions nurses viewed as not the responsibility of their ward. Nurses sanctioned unpopular behaviour by ignoring patients, forgetting requests, enforcing rules and using sarcasm. Overall, nurses did not see conversations with patients as legitimate work. Despite developments in nurse education and the philosophy of nursing, these early studies are worth reconsidering in the light of criticisms of care and alongside critiques of bio-medical models of care. Nurses have, for many decades, worked in systems that have not prioritised individualised care.

Sociologists have examined the difficulties of caring work through analyses of emotional labour, that is the management of one's own and others' feelings. The term 'labour' clarifies that emotion work has exchange value and, outside of the home, becomes a commodity, with a price (Hochschild 1983). James (1992) and Smith (1992) saw emotion management as devalued in society because 'emotion' is held in contrast to 'rational' and because emotions belong in the home. The consequent devaluing of care remains a central problem in care services.

Nurses in health care services

Developing caring and therapeutic relationships is now seen as central to nurses' work. Nevertheless nurses' relationships with patients and clients are shaped by the organisations and societies in which they work. Nurses are not immune from discriminating and excluding practices prevalent within the wider world, nor are they always able to maintain their capacity for care in all organisational settings. Bridges *et al.* (2012), in a review of ethnographic studies of acute nurses' relationships with patients, found that whereas the organisation of work in critical care settings supported therapeutic relationships, nurses on general wards reported moral distress due to unsatisfactory care. Distress led nurses to withdraw from emotional engagement. Ethnographic work on hospital systems in Canada has shown how information systems used to drive efficient bed use can affect nurses' use of their professional knowledge. Rankin and Campbell (2009) found that electronic monitoring of care pathways allows hospital performance in relation to length of stay and bed utilisation to be compared, leading to greater efficiency pressures. Although nurses identified troubling issues concerning patient readiness for discharge, the care pathways and bed utilisation electronic programmes worked as technologies of surveillance and control, constraining nurses' use of professional discretion in caring for individuals.

Studies of nurses at work have reported negative aspects of nursing as a profession. Nursing teams have historically been hierarchically organised, emphasising obedience and conformity. Nurses' roles have been subordinate to medical dominance. Roberts, in 1983, saw nurses' passive behaviour as a sign of being an oppressed group that accepted a dominant view of themselves as inferior. Feelings of oppression and frustration can lead to aggressive behaviour towards subordinates, reinforcing submissive behaviour among junior staff. The perpetuation of a bullying and silencing culture within the NHS has become a national concern within the UK, with the development of an open and honest reporting culture being seen as a necessity for service improvement (Francis 2015).

There has been a strong body of sociological work considering nurses' relationships with colleagues through an analysis of the division of labour and changing professional boundaries. Whereas research in some settings has found evidence of conflict between nurses and other occupational groups (Timmons and Tanner 2004), in other settings, analysis of the micro politics has adopted an interactionist, 'negotiated order' perspective, emphasising the situated nature of work demarcation, with individual doctors and nurses adopting variable practices (Allen 1997). The changing expectations of clients, changing professional roles and changing management systems bring risk and uncertainty for individual nurses, but different sociological theories and concepts can bring different perspectives to challenging situations. Social research may help identify practices that constrain nursing care, but also observe the way individuals create space for supportive care.

CONCLUSION

Sociology offers nurses conceptual tools and ways of thinking that can help nurses reflect on their own personal, social and professional identity and recognise the importance of processes and pressures that shape, support and disrupt our sense of who we are and what we do. Despite the imperatives of following care pathways and procedures that are directed as much by management systems as by professional knowledge and judgment, nurses have a patient-focused role and coordinating responsibilities that bring unique opportunities for individualised care. Recognising the inherent dehumanising dangers in care systems and the reality of health inequalities is a prerequisite for supporting an individual and providing care. Understanding ways in which nursing is influenced by professional and organisational cultures may also help face the challenge of being a nurse.

SUGGESTED FURTHER READING

Sociology textbooks

Fulcher, J. and Scott, J. (2011) *Sociology* (4th edn). Oxford: Oxford University Press.
Giddens, A. (2009) *Sociology* (6th edn). Cambridge: Polity Press.

Sociology and health care texts

Nettleton, S. (2013) *The Sociology of Health and Illness* (3rd edn). Cambridge: Polity Press.
Taylor, S. and Field, D. (2007) *Sociology of Health and Health Care* (4th edn). Oxford: Wiley-Blackwell.

Sociology and nursing texts

Denny, E. and Earle, S. (eds). (2005) *The Sociology of Long Term Conditions and Nursing Practice*. Basingstoke: Palgrave Macmillan.
Denny, E. and Earle, S. (eds). (2009) *Sociology for Nurses* (2nd ed). Cambridge: Polity Press.
Goodman, B. and Ley, T. (2012) *Psychology and Sociology in Nursing*. Sage: Learning Matters.
Miers, M. (ed.). (2003) *Class, Inequalities and Nursing Practice*. Basingstoke: Palgrave Macmillan.
Porter, S. (1998) *Social Theory and Nursing Practice*. Basingstoke: Macmillan.
Wilkinson, G. and Miers, M. (eds). (1999) *Power and Nursing Practice*. Basingstoke: Macmillan.

Journals

Social Science and Medicine
Sociology of Health and Illness

REFERENCES

Abbott, P. and Wallace, C. (1990) *An Introduction to Sociology: Feminist perspectives*. London: Routledge.
Allen, D. (1997) The nursing–medical boundary: a negotiated order? *Sociology of Health and Illness* **19** (4), 498–520.
Banner, D., Miers, M., Clarke, B. and Albarran, J. (2012) Women's experiences of undergoing coronary artery bypass graft surgery. *Journal of Advanced Nursing* **68** (4), 919–930.
Bauman, Z. (1995) *Life in Fragments: Essays in postmodern morality*. Oxford: Basil Blackwell.
Bauman, Z. (2000) *Liquid Modernity*. Cambridge: Polity Press
Beck, U. (1992) *Risk Society: Towards a new modernity*. London: Sage.

Becker, H. (1963) *Outsiders: Studies in the sociology of deviance*. Chicago, IL: The Free Press.

Bourdieu, P. (1986) *Distinction*. London: Sage.

Bourdieu, P. (1993) *Sociology in Question*. London: Sage.

Bourdieu, P. (1997) The forms of capital. In *Education, Culture, Society, Economy*. Halsey, A. H., Lauder, H., Brown, P. and Wells A. S. (eds). Oxford: Oxford University Press, pp. 46–59.

Bury, M. (1982) Chronic illness as biographical disruption. *Sociology of Health and Illness* **4** (2), 167–182.

Bury, M. (2010) Chronic illness, self-management and the rhetoric of empowerment. In *New Directions in the Sociology of Chronic and Disabling Conditions: Assaults on the life world*. Scambler, G. and Scambler, S. (eds). London: Palgrave Macmillan, pp. 161–180.

Bridges, J., Nicholson, C., Maben, J., Pope, C., Flatley, M., Wilkinson, C., Meyer, J. and Tziggli, M. (2012) Capacity for care: meta ethnography of acute care nurses' experiences of the nurse–patient relationship. *Journal of Advanced Nursing* **69** (4), 760–772.

Connell, R. W. (1987) *Gender and Power*. Cambridge: Polity Press.

Davies, C. (1995) *Gender and the Professional Predicament in Nursing*. Buckingham, UK: Open University Press.

DH (Department of Health) (2005) *Delivering Race Equality: An action plan for improving services inside and outside mental health care and the government's response to the independent inquiry into the death of David Bennett*. London: DH.

Durkheim, E. (1893) *The Division of Labour in Society*. London: Macmillan 1984.

Featherstone, M. (1991) *Consumer Culture and Postmodernism*. London: Sage.

Ferrie, J. E. (ed.). (2004) *Work Stress and Health: The Whitehall II Study*. London, Council of Civil Service Unions/Cabinet Office.

Foucault, M. (1976) *The Birth of the Clinic: An archaeology of medical perception*. London: Tavistock.

Foucault, M. (1977) *Discipline and Punish: The birth of the prison*. New York: Pantheon.

Foucault, M. (1979) *The History of Sexuality, Volume I: An introduction*. London: Allen Lane.

Fox, N. J. (1993) *Postmodernism, Sociology and Health*. Buckingham, UK: Open University Press.

Fox, N. J. (1995) Postmodern perspectives on care: the vigil and the gift. *Critical Social Policy* **44/45**, 107–125.

Francis, R. (2015) *Freedom to Speak Up: An independent review into creating an open and honest reporting culture in the NHS*. www.webarchive.nationalarchives.gov.uk (accessed 29 May 2016).

Freidson, E. (1970) *Profession of Medicine*. Chicago, IL: University of Chicago Press.

Garmarnikow, E. (1978) Sexual division of labour: The case of nursing. In *Feminism and Materialism*. Kuhn, A. and Wolpe, A.-M. (eds). London: Routledge & Kegan Paul, pp. 96–123.

Giddens, A. (1991) *Modernity and Self Identity*. Cambridge: Polity Press.

Goffman, E. (1968a) *Asylums*. Harmondsworth: Penguin Books.

Goffman, E. (1968b) *Stigma: Notes on the management of spoiled identity*. Harmondsworth: Penguin Books.

Hochschild, A. (1983) *The Managed Heart: Commercialisation of human feeling*. Berkeley, CA: University of California Press.

Illich, I. (1977) *Limits to Medicine: Medical nemesis: The expropriation of health*. London: Routledge.

James, N. (1992) Care = organisation + physical labour + emotional labour. *Sociology of Health and Illness* **14** (4), 488–509

Lyotard, J. F. (1984) *The Postmodern Condition: A report on knowledge*. Manchester: Manchester University Press.

McKeown, T. (1976) *The Modern Rise of Population*. London: Edward Arnold.

Macpherson, W. (1999) *The Stephen Lawrence Inquiry*. Cmnd 4262–I. London: The Stationery Office.

Marmot Review (2010) *Fair Society Healthy Lives: Strategic review of health inequalities in England post-2010*. London: Institute of Health Equity, University College: London. www.ucl.ac.uk/marmotreview (accessed 19 January 2016).

Marx, K. and Engels, F. (1848) *The Communist Manifesto*. Harmondsworth: Penguin 1967.

Mead, G. H. (1927) *Mind, Self and Society*. Chicago, IL: Chicago University Press.

Menzies, I. E. P. (1960) A case-study in the functioning of social systems as a defense against anxiety. *Human Relations* **13** (2), 95–121.

Merton. R. K. (1949) *Social Theory and Social Structure*. New York: Harper & Row.

Mid-Staffordshire NHS Foundation Trust Public Inquiry (2013) *Report of the Mid-Staffordshire NHS Foundation Trust Public Inquiry*. London: The Stationery Office.

Miers, M. E., Rickaby, C. E. and Pollard, K. C. (2007) Career choices in health care: is nursing a special case? A content analysis of survey data. *International Journal of Nursing Studies* **44**, 1196–1209.

Mills, C. W. (1970) [1959] *The Sociological Imagination*. Harmondsworth: Penguin Books.

NMC (Nursing and Midwifery Council) (2015) *The Code: Professional standards of practice and behaviour for nurses and midwives*. London: NMC.

Oliver, M. and Barnes, C. (2012) *The New Politics of Disablement*. (2nd edn). Basingstoke: Palgrave.

Parkin, F. (1979) *Marxism and Class Theory: A bourgeois critique*. London: Tavistock.

Parsons, T. (1951) *The Social System*. New York: Free Press.

Rankin, J. M. and Campbell, M. (2009) Institutional ethnography (IE), nursing work and hospital reform: IE's cautionary analysis. *Forum: Qualitative Social Research* **10** (2), Art 8. www.qualitative-research.net/index.php/fqs/article/view/1258/2720 (accessed 19 January 2016).

Roberts, S. J. (1983) Oppressed group behaviour: implications for nursing. *Advances in Nursing Science* 5 (4), 21–30.

RCN (Royal College of Nursing) (2012) *Health Inequalities and the Social Determinants of Health*. London: Royal College of Nursing.

Rich, A. (1980) Compulsory heterosexuality and lesbian existence. *Signs* **5** (4), 631–660.

SG (Scottish Government) (2008) *Equally Well: Report of the ministerial task force on health inequalities*. Edinburgh: Scottish Government.

Smith, D. E. (2005) *Institutional Ethnography: A sociology for people*. Toronto: AltaMira Press.

Smith, P. (1992) *The Emotional Labour of Nursing*. Basingstoke: Macmillan.

Stockwell, F. (1972) *The Unpopular Patient: The Study of Nursing Care Project Reports, Series 1, No. 2*. London: Royal College of Nursing.

Szasz, T. (1970) *The Manufacture of Madness*. New York: Harper Row.

Timmons, S. and Tanner, J. (2004) A disputed occupational boundary: operating theatre nurses and operating department practitioners. *Sociology of Health and Illness* **26** (5), 645–666.

The Times (2013) Obituary: James Hood. 21 January.

Weber, M. (1930) *The Protestant Ethic and the Spirit of Capitalism*. London: George Allen & Unwin (and subsequent editions)

Weber, M. (1968) *Economy and Society*. eds G. Roth and C. Wittich. Berkeley, CA and Los Angeles, CA: University of Chicago Press.

WHO (World Health Organization) (2008) *Closing the Gap in a Generation: Health equity through action on the social determinants of health: final report of the Commission on Social Determinants of Health*. Geneva: World Health Organization.

Wilkinson, R. G. and Pickett, K. E. (2006) Income inequality and population health: a review and explanation of the evidence. *Social Science and Medicine* **62** (7), 1768–1784.

Williams, G. (1984) The genesis of chronic illness: narrative reconstruction. *Sociology of Health and Illness* **6** (2), 175–200.

Witz, A. (1992) *Professions and Patriarchy*. London: Routledge.

Wrong, D. (1961) The oversocialised conception of man in modern sociology. *American Sociological Review* **26** (2), 183–193.

Zola, I. (1975) In the name of health and illness: on some practical consequences of medical influence. *Social Science and Medicine* **9**, 83–87.

11

PSYCHOLOGICAL CONCEPTS FOR NURSING

Daniel Farrelly and Paul Snelling

LEARNING OUTCOMES

After reading and reflecting on this chapter you should be able to:

*   understand the importance of psychology for nursing care;
*   recognise and describe the influence of a range of key psychological concepts on individual behaviour;
*   consider how these factors affect life choices and patient care.

INTRODUCTION

What is psychology and why does it matter?

Broadly speaking, **psychology** is concerned with the study of brains and behaviour.

This question is of course of immediate interest to nurses who care for patients with primary disorders of mood or behaviour, but there is now conclusive evidence of the link between physical and mental health. This means that in acute illness or planned surgery, nurses can aid both physical and mental well-being by caring for patients in a way that understands and takes account of the links between mind and body. There is growing awareness of the way that psychological processes have a significant and yet unconscious influence on the way we all live our lives, and a deeper understanding of these will lead to more insight and greater control for both nurses and patients. The subject area of **psychology** is vast and cannot be covered in a single chapter, so the aim of this chapter is to highlight the fascination and value of some different aspects of psychology to nursing practice, helpfully showing the full benefit of being 'psychologically literate'. The chapter is divided into three parts. In Part 1, psychology is defined, and the link between physical and psychological health is introduced. In Part 2, a range of psychological concepts will be discussed, and their implications for nursing care introduced. In Part 3, the developing concept of evolutionary psychology is discussed.

PART 1: OUTLINING PSYCHOLOGICAL CONCEPTS FOR NURSING

Case 11.1

Since childhood, Johannes has always been an anxious person, and he says that part of his response to anxiety is that he tends to eat comfort food and drink alcohol every night. He understands that this isn't good for him and he has put on some weight as a result. Now he just feels worse because of his weight and doesn't want to go out or do anything at all. He says that all his family are overweight but this doesn't make him feel any better; and he says that people, including some health care professionals, are just looking at him and disapproving.

The word 'psychology' is Greek in origin, coming from 'psych' meaning 'of the mind and soul', and 'logia', meaning 'the study (of)'. As such psychology incorporates many different aspects of human nature, offering depth to our understanding of it. Traditionally, psychology has been separated into different areas of interest, which include the following:

- *Biological psychology* – the biological basis of behaviour, includes the nervous system, hormones, the brain, neurotransmitters, genetics and evolution.
- *Social psychology* – includes personal and intimate relationships, all aspects of social interactions, and group behaviour.
- *Cognitive psychology* – includes how memory works, language, perception, decision-making and how we learn.
- *Developmental psychology* – includes all aspects of psychology that relate to child and infant development, such as language, morality, and empathy.
- *Individual differences* – relates to the variation of psychology traits between individuals, including personality and intelligence, and how to measure these.

However, one aspect that is important to note when describing psychology is to also describe what psychology is *not*. It is inevitable that a subject that explores our thoughts, behaviours, and feelings should be of interest to us all, and our introspective and reflective nature often leads to misconceptions and misunderstandings about psychology that unfortunately become widely accepted by non-psychologists. Examples of this are that humans only use 10 per cent of their brains, or that dreams have hidden, symbolic meanings. Yet research in psychology points to actual findings that can be more interesting than such myths, and more about these will be presented in Parts 2 and 3. Also of relevance here are the types of topics that psychology covers. Particularly in medical and caring professions, the term psychology is often viewed synonymously with mental health, therapy and/or counselling. No doubt these are important and deserving of attention in nursing education and textbooks, but there are many other areas in psychology that can enrich the knowledge and ability of nurses in all fields. The link between psychological and physical health is very well known. Illness that is initially physical is known to cause psychological symptoms, and primary psychological symptoms such as anxiety are associated with a range of physical effects. For many of us, even short periods of acute anxiety, such as waiting for a flight, speaking in front of class, or a job interview, result in familiar physical sensations: dry mouth perhaps, a racing heart, sometimes even a tremor or nausea. The practice of holistic care often refers to the term

277

Heritability
is an estimate of how much of a particular characteristic is due to genetics as opposed to any environmental effects.

biopsychosocial care indicating the interconnectedness of different aspects of health and care into a single model.

A good example is the nursing care of people who have irritable bowel syndrome (IBS). Tanaka *et al.* (2011) demonstrate the complexity of the link between psychological and physical factors in IBS; long-standing abdominal pain, like many other sorts of pains causes anxiety and in turn anxiety via the autonomic nervous system causes an exacerbation of pain. Anxiety, therefore, can be considered both as a cause and a consequence of the physical symptoms of IBS (Smith 2010). Similarly the psychological impact of a life-changing cancer diagnosis will result, for many, in a range of psychological symptoms including distress, depression and anxiety, which can be assessed and treated as necessary. In many cases this requires specialist input (Holland and Alisi 2010). Treating anxiety with drugs and/or other specialised psychological techniques may help gastric symptoms and the distress of a cancer diagnosis, but there is clearly a need for closer understanding of the link between physical and psychological health in all settings. Having a minor procedure as day case surgery involves some stress and anxiety, and as well as this being unpleasant in itself, stress and pain are known to delay wound healing (Woo 2012). Nurses giving reassurance, detailed information facilitating choice as far as possible, and maintaining a calm environment can help reduce stress (Mitchell 2007). Caring in this holistic way may cause some difficulty in an environment that is very busy as these interventions take time and close attention, but acknowledgement of the genuine stressors and their effect on health is necessary. As with many things in nursing, relatively minor interventions can make a big difference.

PART 2: EXPLAINING PSYCHOLOGICAL CONCEPTS FOR NURSING

In this section a number of aspects of psychology will be introduced. The research base from the discipline of psychology will demonstrate how the field has developed, and the implications for nursing practice in each area will be introduced.

Biological psychology

Behavioural genetics

To understand the origin of different psychological traits and how these can impact on an individual's health, scientists estimate the amount that an individual's genes contribute to it. This contribution can be between 0 (no genetic contribution at all) to 1 (entirely due to genetics), and is known as the **heritability** of a trait. Behavioural genetics is an area of psychology that seeks to find out what the heritability is for different traits. Most traits are controlled by many different genes and therefore we cannot say if a certain gene is present based on just observing the trait unlike, say, eye colour, which is controlled by just one gene. Take height, for example, where there is a strong but not perfect correlation between an individual's height and that of their parents. This suggests that there is a genetic component, but also that there are environmental influences, for example, diet and development. Calculating an estimate for heritability enables us to separate genetic from environmental causes.

Heritability can be calculated from twin studies. This is because of the different types of twins and the amount of genes they share. Monozygotic (MZ) twins are identical (they grow from the same egg) and share 100 per cent of their genes, whereas dizygotic (DZ) twins are equivalent to full siblings (they grow from different eggs) and share approximately 50 per cent of their genes. Behavioural geneticists assume that all twins have had a shared upbringing, including things such as diet, home life, relationships with parents and schooling. Apart from this, twins will have a non-shared environment that includes all life events that happened to each twin separately and uniquely, such as illnesses or accidents. Therefore, how similar a particular trait is between two twin siblings (known as the concordance rates) will be due to a combination of this shared upbringing and also their shared genetics. Now, because there is a difference in how many genes are shared between MZ and DZ twins, we can use this to calculate heritability. Box 11.1 has an example.

There are, however, problems associated with estimating heritability. First it makes the assumption that the shared environments of both MZ and DZ twins are the same, but this may not always be the case. In particular we could perhaps assume that DZ twins would have less of a shared environment, due to the fact that they will be less similar than MZ twins from a very early age. This may be due to physical differences, or differences in personality, for example there may be a 'shy one' who will be treated differently and respond to different cues, and often gender differences. Furthermore there will even be differences between the upbringing of MZ twins; they will have different names, and one will always be the 'older one' even if it is just by seconds! In the above example even MZ twins who have a shared upbringing and identical genetics still do not have perfect concordance rates with 0.13 of concordance unexplained suggesting that the non-shared environment can have a significant influence.

However, despite these problems, behavioural genetics has made a great contribution to our understanding of the origin and development of different traits. It has been used to help our understanding of different psychiatric disorders such as schizophrenia, bipolar disorder and depression. It has also been relevant in our understanding of complex psychological conditions such as autism. In almost all cases heritability is difficult to calculate and is the result of the interaction and activation of a large number of different genes. However, they show that heritability is greater than 0, which points to a partial genetic basis of these, and a great deal of other traits in psychology. This will of course include other behaviours relating to health and well-being, such as responses to stress, dietary and exercise behaviour and addiction. Knowledge of this is important, as this is something that patients and their families want to know about, and ask for more

---

BOX 11.1 **The size of brain structures**

In a study by Geschwind *et al.* (2002), the total volumes of cerebral hemispheres were measured in a sample of both MZ and DZ twins. The concordance rate for MZ was 0.87 whereas it was 0.56 for DZ, making a difference between them of 0.31. As their shared upbringing is assumed to be identical between MZ and DZ, the remaining 0.31 difference must be due to the difference in the shared genetics between the two types of twins. As concordance is greater with MZ and they share twice as many genes as DZ twins do, doubling this value (Falconer's estimate of heritability) gives the final estimate size of the genetic component (the heritability) of the size of brain structures as 0.62.

information on, sometimes out of curiosity but other times out of fear. Being able to speak comfortably and with knowledge as a nurse will be of great value, as it can help allay their fears or guide them to look for the right information and ask the right questions.

Obesity, genetics and stigma

In 2008, the American *Journal of Clinical Nutrition* published a large UK study, which recruited over 5000 sets of twins aged between the ages of eight and eleven (Wardle *et al.* 2008). The study aimed 'to quantify genetic and environmental influences on BMI (body mass index) and central adiposity in children growing up during a time of dramatic rises in paediatric obesity' (Wardle *et al.* 2008, p. 398), finding that heritability for both BMI and waist circumference was, at 77 per cent, substantial. The editors of the journal commended the study, noting that it confirmed the genetic influence of obesity that had been known for two decades.

Publication was widely discussed on the television news (BBC 2008) and in the print media. Reported in *The Times*, the study's principal author was quoted as saying 'This study shows that it is wrong to place all the blame for a child's excessive weight gain on the parents' (Henderson 2008). The complexities of genetic influence are recognised in detailed academic analyses (Holm 2008), but more popular discussions, even those in broadsheet newspapers, can readily reduce the issue to a crude 'nature–nurture' dichotomy. Under the title 'Face it, fatty, your genes are innocent', a comment article in the *Sunday Times* included:

> I hate to blithely dismiss a whole swathe of scientific findings but I don't believe a word of this. Fat gene, my foot. Funny how it seems to manifest itself only in the prosperous, cake-guzzling, carb-and-sugar-laden West. Where are the obese Sudanese toddlers? The porky Ethiopians? [. . .] You can choose to make sacrifices or choose to be lazy and remain fat – and if you choose to be lazy and remain fat, then fair enough, but accept that it's your own doing and take responsibility for it. [. . .] Above all, we need to get to grips with the fact that fatness is a personal choice, one that can't be blamed on anybody or anything other than our own greedy behaviour.
>
> (Knight 2008)

Comments like this can been seen throughout the press and also on social media and contribute to an environment where obesity is stigmatised (Puhl and Heuer 2009). Some find the social unacceptability of obesity to be a good thing, regarding it is an encouragement for behaviour change (Callahan 2013). This view seems to assume, like India Knight, that obesity is a matter of personal choice. Experimental research by Major *et al.* (2014) (see Research focus 11.1) suggests that for some, this perceived motivational force of stigma not only does not work, but actually increases obesity. Though professional ethics of nurses and other health professionals require a non-judgemental attitude to patients, numerous studies (for example Brown 2006, Swift *et al.* 2013) have shown that this is not the case for many. In the UK survey on trainee health professionals by Swift *et al.* (2013) student nurses were less judgemental than other professionals, as were those who understood that weight control was not solely under personal control; and Nicholls *et al.* (2015) found that student nurses did recognise and implement person-centred care of obese people. These studies are reassuring and reinforce that caring for people who are

---

RESEARCH FOCUS 11.1

More perhaps so than nursing research, psychological research is often experimental in nature, and often doesn't reveal full details to participants during the experiment. Major *et al*. (2014) conducted an experiment that hypothesised that exposure to weight-stigmatising news reports would increase calorie consumption. The researchers recruited 93 female university students, in return for course credit or $10. All had previously assessed their own weight, which was significantly correlated to their measured weight. After randomisation, half were asked to read an article, ostensibly from the *New York Times*, entitled 'Lose weight or lose your job'. The other half were asked to read a highly similar article entitled 'Quit smoking or lose your job'. The articles described reasons why employers were reluctant to hire people who are obese or who smoke. Then both groups were asked to do the same things – talk about the employment policies for 5 minutes, followed by a break while they waited to complete a questionnaire. They were unobserved during the break, and told to help themselves to snacks. But the participants did not know that the snacks had been pre-weighed so the researchers knew exactly what each subject had consumed. They were told that the articles were not genuine and had been written for the experiment *after* they had completed the questionnaire, but were not told that the study was about weight or eating. A great deal of data was obtained. Of the women who perceived themselves as overweight, those reading the weight article consumed significantly more calories than those who read the smoking article, but there was no difference between the groups of women who did not think that they were overweight. Other findings of the study included that self-perceived overweight women felt significantly less capable of controlling their food after reading the weight-stigmatising article than the smoking-stigmatising article. The study was relatively small and used young women as subjects, so the authors caution against wide generalisation, and suggest areas of further research. But the tentative implication is that weight stigmatisation, including public health policies, can actually make things worse.

---

trying to lose weight requires an understanding of the psychology of what has contributed to their condition as well as a non-judgemental approach.

The role of hormones in behaviour – testosterone and oxytocin

When people hear '**testosterone**', they often immediately think of the public perception that this **hormone** has. It is often viewed negatively, often paired with '-crazed' or '-fuelled' and linked to aggressive and/or violent acts, particularly in males. How much of this is true? Indeed, the presence of testosterone is linked to competitive behaviour, aggression and dominance, as would be expected. But this is not the full story, as a study by Eisenegger *et al*. (2009) showed. In this study, participants were given either testosterone or a **placebo** and then asked to play a simple game that measured cooperative behaviour. They found that rather than being aggressive or competitive, participants given testosterone were actually more cooperative than those who received a placebo. This is against what might be expected, as the authors found when they interviewed the participants afterwards. Those who were less cooperative *believed* they had received testosterone. According to the authors this is because testosterone is a hormone whose role it is to encourage individuals to achieve higher status. In most cases this can be through increased aggressive or dominant behaviour as it is in other animals but in

Hormones
are chemicals that occur naturally in the body. They are mainly released from different parts of the endocrine system including glands, such as the pituitary gland, into the bloodstream to affect an organism's moods, behaviour and development.

Testosterone
is a particular form of hormone known as androgens, which plays a role in the development of sexual characteristics in males.

281

Daniel Farrelly and Paul Snelling

A **placebo** is an inert substance that has no medical effect and can be administered to patients. If the patient *believes* that the substance has an effect, then it will have a positive influence on their health (i.e. the placebo effect).

some cases, as in the study by Eisenegger *et al.*, it can be through being cooperative and helping others.

With this further insight into this hormone, how testosterone changes over a man's lifetime can clearly be understood. This is more relevant to men as testosterone is an androgen, which is in higher levels in men than women, for good reason. Males of (almost) all animal species need to compete more to be chosen by females as sexual partners, and humans are no exception. This is due to the greater investment that mothers put into caring for offspring, meaning they need to be 'choosier' (Trivers 1972). Therefore, from puberty onwards men have a dramatic increase in testosterone in their bodies. This causes a number of different changes to young men's bodies, such as increasing growth of facial and genital hair, deepening of the voice and changes in body shape. It also causes some important behavioural changes, such as increasing competitive behaviour so that individuals can increase their status and thus be a more desirable partner. Such behaviour, and levels of testosterone, is highest when men are young, as this is where mating effort is highest. This is reflected in the fact that men's productivity in different cultural displays such as art, music, science, and even crime is highest at a younger age, as these are used in modern days to signal one's status (Kanazawa 2000, 2003; Miller 2000). However, such productivity declines as men get older, as do their levels of testosterone. Similarly, men's testosterone levels also drop when they become married, and further still when they have children (Gray *et al.* 2002). This makes sense as married men and fathers have no further need to compete for status and it is better for them to instead direct their time and effort to caring for and supporting their partner and offspring.

Similarly, oxytocin has become a very well-known but also misunderstood hormone that affects many health outcomes. It is often portrayed to the public as the 'love hormone' due to its role in promoting social relationships in different contexts, including between mother and newborn child, friendships and also romantic relationships. However, and as with testosterone, this over-simplifies the role oxytocin has and how it actually affects our behaviour. Oxytocin is secreted from the pituitary gland, and as a protein hormone it can act rapidly. It has an important role in female reproduction, such as in childbirth. It stimulates cervical dilation before birth and also stimulates contractions of the uterus during the later stages of labour such that injections of oxytocin are also used to induce or accelerate labour. It is also important in breastfeeding as it causes the 'letdown reflex', where stimulation of the nipple from sucking by the infant leads to nerve impulses in the brain causing oxytocin to be created and released. Oxytocin then causes mammary glands to contract and thereby release milk to the infant. This same reflex can be caused by hearing an infant crying (a reliable cue that it is feeding time), including infants other than their own which may cause embarrassment in public!

Beyond this, oxytocin has an interesting role in the formation of relationships and bonding. In prairie voles, who unusually for mammals form monogamous relationships as humans do, making them an ideal species to research to understanding social relationships, oxytocin performs a key role in the bonding between mother and pups (van Leengoed *et al.* 1987) and also in males' partner choice (Bales and Carter 2003). In humans, we can see in more detail how oxytocin affects our behaviour towards others. Kosfeld *et al.* (2005) investigated trust, an important factor in forming social attachment. In their study, participants played a game in which they can win more money if they trust others to help and the others then return this trust. Prior to the game participants received either oxytocin or a placebo but they were unaware which. The experimenters wanted to see how oxytocin influenced trusting behaviour and they found that participants who received

282

oxytocin were more trusting, which suggests its role in social bonding may be due to increased willingness to trust others. Furthermore, oxytocin can cause people to maintain trust with others, even after they have betrayed their trust previously (Baumgartner *et al.* 2008). However, oxytocin affects social interactions in many other related ways. It also makes us more willing to rate strangers as more trustworthy and attractive (Theodoridou *et al.* 2009), increases fixation on eyes when interacting with others (Guastella *et al.* 2008) and makes us better at judging emotions from eyes (Domes *et al.* 2007).

Therefore, it is clear that the public perception of testosterone and oxytocin does not really reflect what psychological research has revealed. Both have a complex but important role to play. Testosterone is particularly important in men across their lifetimes, and perhaps does not deserve the negative view it currently has. However, the action of testosterone on people's health, either directly or through the effects it has on behaviour, can lead to negative health outcomes such as depression, stress and heart disease. Similarly, oxytocin is more nuanced than the 'love' hormone, and goes beyond its known role in female reproduction to affect the formation of social relationships in many different ways. This can be relevant to health outcomes as poor relationships can adversely influence well-being, and can also play a role in conditions relating to this, such as autism (Bartz *et al.* 2010). It is important for health care professionals to have a greater awareness and understanding of these hormones and others such as cortisol, adrenaline and oestrogen. By gaining knowledge of what they actually do (and why), effective interventions, recognition of possible effects and engaging with public understanding can then be part of a nurse's means to help increase well-being.

Finally, as with many other areas of psychology, hormones have a key role to play in an individual's risk of obesity. A section of the brain known as the hypothalamus is part of the endocrine system, and controls the release of hormones into an individual's bloodstream that can regulate their appetite. It responds to the levels of different gut hormones such as leptin as an indicator of fat reserves. Problems with this link between leptin levels and the hypothalamus can cause individuals to over-eat, particularly food high in calories, as they still 'feel' hungry.

Social psychology

Obedience, conformity and social influence

One of the most infamous findings in twentieth-century psychology is Stanley Milgram's work on obedience. This research happened shortly after the trial of Nazi war criminal Adolf Eichmann, and this would prove an important motivation for Milgram. At his trial, Eichmann denied any active involvement in the Holocaust, but instead insisted that he was merely following the orders of his superiors, the so-called 'Nuremberg defence'. Could this be true, could individuals conform to commit cruel acts on others just from being asked to?

This is what Milgram explored, in a series of studies. The most commonly cited version of his experiment (Milgram 1974) has two participants; one real and one 'stooge' who appears to be a real participant but is actually part of the experiment. One becomes the 'learner' who was asked to recall a series of words (this was always the stooge), and the other (the real participant) becomes the 'teacher' who will test the learner. The teacher is told that they must administer an electric shock of increasing size to the learner whenever they get a word wrong. The participant does not know that the electric shock is not real, and the learner received no such punishment. Importantly, the teacher is told that the experimenter assumes all responsibility, and that they should continue until the experiment ends.

Surprisingly, Milgram found that participants would be obedient to the experimenter, even at extreme levels. In many cases, participants would administer up to what they believed were 450 volts, with labels such as 'Danger: severe shock' on the dial, and would continue even when hearing screams from the learner next door. Often participants would question whether they should continue, but were greeted with just the same response each time from the experimenter, 'the experiment must go on', and would then continue to administer the shocks. Follow-up studies revealed more about the nature of conformity. Victim remoteness (learner and teacher being in separate rooms), authority-figure legitimacy (such as wearing a white coat), and diffusion of responsibility (the experimenter taking sole responsibility) all led to increased levels of obedience.

The relevance of this to nursing is demonstrated the more realistic hospital-based study of obedience by Hofling (1966). Hofling used a stooge (a 'Dr Smith') to phone 22 real nurses on separate occasions while they were on night shifts at a hospital. 'Dr Smith' asked each nurse if they had the drug astroten (a fake drug, which was actually just a sugar pill) in stock. When they checked and found that they did, 'Dr Smith' then asked the nurses to administer 20mg of the drug to a patient called 'Mr Jones' who was also a stooge. However it clearly stated on the box that the maximum dose for this drug was 10mg. Finally, 'Dr Smith' stated that he was short on time and would sign any authorisation form when he next came to see 'Mr Jones'. Alarmingly, Hofling found that 21 of the 22 nurses obeyed the orders of the doctor. In contrast, out of another 22 nurses who were interviewed about such scenarios, 21 of those said they would not comply with the doctor's orders. It is to be hoped that these findings would not be repeated today.

Clearly this reveals how unconscious social influences affect our behaviour, even when we believe that they would not. Nurses face tough situations every day, and often have to take immediate action in response, but as this study and many real-life, often tragic examples show, it is important to be aware of how different social influences may adversely affect our behaviour. As part of working teams of health professionals, nurses often defer responsibility to others while retaining personal accountability for what they do, but knowledge of the social psychological effects of obedience can help in terms of asking the right questions at times. For example, are physical but unreliable cues of obedience like the attire and appearance of other medical professionals influencing me? Does the lack of responsibility I perceive make me more obedient when perhaps I should speak up? Does my own belief that I will not blindly obey others (as the latter nurses in Hofling's study clearly had) mean that I can justify it when it does occur? Obviously such reflection is difficult at times, but can also clearly have vital benefits.

Social influence can also be seen in how we conform to the beliefs and behaviours of others. Asch (1956) asked groups of participants which of three lines displayed on a screen were the same length as an additional line, even though it was very clear that only one of the three lines was the same as the other. In Asch's study however, only one participant was real, with all the others acting as stooges, who deliberately stated that another of the three lines was the same as the other, though this was clearly incorrect. Instead of going with their own (accurate) perception, the real participants, when asked to select a line after each other group member had selected a different one, often agreed with the rest of the group. Why did people do this? Possibly because of a fear of rejection and potential embarrassment (if *everyone else* believes it, maybe *I* am the one who's wrong?), and from a desire to be part of a group. Interestingly, this **conformity** reduced dramatically if there was another dissenting individual in the group who also disagreed with the other group members and selected the correct line. This is similar to minority influence, whereby the influence of a consistent minority within a group can influence others in the majority to conform to their beliefs (Moscovici *et al.* 1969). Interestingly, there are cross-cultural differences in levels of conformity. *Collectivist* cultures including many from Asia and the Middle East place more emphasis on the interdependence of the individual as part of the larger group or community including their society and/or family. Individuals from such cultures show higher levels of compliance with their group in replications of Asch's experiment than those from individualistic cultures, such as Western cultures, where individuals are more independent (Bond and Smith 1996).

Nurses and nursing students can be affected by conformity in two different ways. First as a wielder of power over their patients they should be aware that some (though not all) will relinquish control to others and meekly obey instructions (Henderson 2003). In another sense, nurses themselves may simply become obedient not only to doctors as in Hofling's study, but also to a general 'culture' within a ward or organisation. In an interview study, Levett-Jones and Lathlean (2009) found that some students were more willing to comply with various nursing practices, including poor practice, rather than confront them as this would increase their chance of acceptance within the ward team. It is easy to see how such attitudes can lead to the instances of poor care that have been reported recently, highlighting the importance of health care professionals being aware of how obedience can restrict their own and patients' decisions.

Altruism and empathy

It is undeniable that humans will help, support and care for each other. This is common across the world, and happens regularly enough for us to be able to conclude that helping others is a central facet of our nature. However, to view altruistic behaviour as natural is actually quite problematic. When Charles Darwin (1859) wrote *On the Origin of Species*, which presented his theory of evolution by natural selection, he described the existence of **altruism** in different species as puzzling. This was because he perceived that natural selection, whereby individual organisms engage in behaviours that increase their own survival and reproduction, would mean that behaviours where individuals helped others at costs to themselves would not be *adaptive*, that is they would in fact be detrimental to the altruist's survival and/or reproduction. With this in mind, how then can we explain why individuals will often incur great costs to themselves to help other individuals, often who they will never meet? When we understand the motivations and desires of altruists in different contexts, can we put this to good use to promote care and compassion for others, an important force that can permeate throughout nursing and health care in general?

One of the earliest theories as to why we help others is that we do so because of kin selection. In simple terms, this is the fact that we are more likely to help people we are related to than others, and can be understood from an evolutionary perspective. As Darwin noted, we engage in behaviours that aid our survival, so that our genes are successfully passed into the next generation. However, we share a lot of our genes with relatives, so if we help relatives survive then our genes will also be successfully passed on even though they are in another organism. William Hamilton (1964) originally explained this mathematically to explain altruism to kin in different organisms. He expressed this

Conformity
is the tendency of an individual to allow their opinions, behavior or actions to be influenced by those of others.

Altruism
refers to any act where an individual engages in a helping behaviour that incurs a cost to them yet benefits another.

in a formula, known as *Hamilton's rule*, which is $rB>C$, where r is the relatedness between two individuals, B is the benefit to the recipient of the act, and C is the cost to the actor of performing the act. So, the bigger the value of r (in other words, when two individuals are more closely genetically related), the more likely they are to help each other. Relatedness can be expressed as the (approximate) percentage of genes two individuals share. As such, it is known that our relatedness (r) with our siblings, parents and offspring is 50 per cent, whereas it is 25 per cent with our uncles/aunts, nephews/nieces, and grandparents/grandchildren, and 12.5 per cent with our first cousins and so on. Therefore it is no wonder that we see the greatest levels of help and compassion between members of one's immediate family, less so than with more distant relatives, but still more than with non-relatives.

Other theories explain how altruistic acts occur between non-relatives. One such theory is that of reciprocal altruism (Trivers 1971). According to this theory, individuals will cooperate with others who they are not related to, because the individual they help will return the favour to them in the future. In simplest terms, it's a case of 'you scratch my back, I'll scratch yours'. According to Trivers, there are three conditions that must be met in order for reciprocal altruism to occur. First, the cost of performing the altruistic act must be less than the benefit that is received from such acts; second, species in which it occurs must regularly interact socially so that the opportunity for reciprocation arises; and finally such species must also have the necessary cognitive abilities (e.g. memory, perception) to remember the interactions between individuals. As a result of this, it is perhaps unsurprising that we find reciprocal altruism occurring in intelligent social species like humans and also other primates such as chimpanzees and baboons.

However, this still cannot account for why individuals will perform altruistic acts for individuals who they are not related to or cannot return the favour in the future. This is important because such acts are common and include the vast majority of charitable acts such as donating blood, helping out at a homeless shelter and giving money to charities such as Cancer Research or the RSPCA. It seems, though, that these acts can be explained as they benefit the altruist in terms of enhancing their reputation to others, not necessarily the recipient of the altruistic act. When that information is broadcast to others it shows that they would be a reliable cooperative partner in the future, and they will be viewed more favourably should they need help themselves from others. In other words, it is viewed as being indirect reciprocity, where the reciprocation for an altruistic act can come from someone other than the recipient (Nowak and Sigmund 1998). Altruistic acts can also be viewed as costly signals, that is they are costly to produce and so altruists must themselves be of high quality in order to produce them (Gintis *et al.* 2001). As a result, altruists benefit from displaying their quality to others, which perhaps explains why charitable acts such as red noses, poppies, or named hospital wings are often displayed clearly. So who are these costly altruistic acts aimed at? One possibility is it is potential romantic partners, as being altruistic is viewed as desirable in long-term partners as it can signal the individual will be a good partner and parent (Farrelly 2011).

The above explanations of altruism are examples of ultimate causes of behaviours. In other words, they explain why a behaviour occurs in an adaptive sense, that is how it aids survival and/or reproduction. However, more obvious explanations of why we help others are examples of proximate causes, and include the fact that helping others improves one's mood. The negative state relief model (Cialdini *et al.* 1982) views helping behaviour as a tactic used to alleviate temporary low mood as part of mood management. These two levels of causes of altruistic behaviour are not mutually exclusive, and both can act to explain why such behaviours occur. The empathy–altruism hypothesis (Batson *et al.* 1991) is a similar proximate cause of helping behaviour that is relevant here. According to this hypothesis, people are motivated to help when they experience an empathic concern for another individual. As such, this concern causes a high emotional arousal that motivates the person to engage in an altruistic act to help them, which in turn leads to a drop in arousal. This is something that many charities are fully aware of, as is evident by the emotive content of the advertisements and leaflets they produce – they know that this will cause high levels of empathic concern in viewers, who will be motivated to donate to the charity in response.

A perhaps simplistic view of nursing (Smith 1995, ten Hoeve *et al.* 2014) is of a profession dedicated to the selfless care of others, and this can be seen in official documentation including the 6Cs, which lists includes compassion, which involves an emotional response to suffering. In the public eye at least, this view can be supported by views of nursing as a feminine vocation undervaluing the professional status of nurses and nursing. Unfortunately for the idea of professional nursing, high profile failures of care, stoked by a media sceptical of graduate preparation (Gillette 2012, 2014) can reinforce the wide normative view that nursing should return to a simpler account. In an innovative analysis, Carol Haigh (2010), a professor of nursing, has attempted to place nursing altruism into a biological evolutionary framework, and on this account the altruism of nurses is primarily concerned with ensuring the survival of the meme of nursing. Haigh concludes that a re-examination of altruism as a motivating factor for nurses and nursing is overdue, and should be undertaken using more than traditional frameworks. On an individual level, an understanding of the psychology of altruism can lead to greater insights about our own motivation and approach to nursing care.

Cognitive psychology

Our biases and heuristics

Case 11.1 continued

Johannes will undoubtedly be required to make choices about many things, and as part of his attempt to lose weight he may be required to make choices based on some sort of calculation, of calories, or of risks. He is the first to admit that he finds these considerations and calculations difficult.

Without doubt, we are an extremely intelligent species; the most intelligent species that has ever lived (so far and on earth) by quite some distance. However, this does not mean that our understanding and decision-making is perfect. In fact, when we look at human cognition in detail we see that it has many flaws, and as in Johannes' case, this can be quite dangerous. The medical diagnosis problem is an example:

If a test to detect a disease whose prevalence is 1/1000 has a false positive rate of 5 per cent, what is the chance that a person found to have a positive result actually has the disease, assuming that you know nothing about the person's symptoms or signs?

(Casscells *et al.* 1978, p. 999)

A **bias** is a preference for one choice over others, even when such preferences are not logically correct (e.g. people's tendency to choose 'heads' over 'tails' in coin flips)

287

This problem was given to members of Harvard Medical School who had knowledge and understanding of disease prevalence and test success rates. However, only 18 per cent of them got the right answer (the correct answer is 2 per cent). Almost half of them gave the answer as 95 per cent, which ignores the base rate information about false positives. Why do we have problems understanding this, including supposed experts? Cosmides and Tooby (1996) believe it is because of how the information is presented to participants. To test this, they replaced information about probabilities in the original medical problem with frequency information:

> 1 out of every 1,000 Americans has disease X. A test has been developed to detect when a person has disease X. Every time the test is given to a person who has the disease, the test comes out positive. But sometimes the test also comes out positive when it is given to a person who is completely healthy. Specifically, out of every 1,000 people who are perfectly healthy, 50 of them test positive for the disease.
>
> Imagine that we have assembled a random sample of 1,000 Americans. They were selected by lottery. Those who conducted the lottery had no information about the health status of any of these people. Given the information above, on average, How many people who test positive for the disease will actually have the disease? _____ out of _____

(Cosmides and Tooby 1996, p. 24)

This time, 76 per cent of participants got the right answer. Cosmides and Tooby believe that this shows that we have a better ability to reason when we are presented with frequency information than probabilistic information. However they also found that performance improved to 92 per cent correct when the same information (apart from a change in prevalence from 1/1,000 to 1/100) was presented *visually*, with the following information and a picture of 100 squares below it (see Figure 11.1).

So why do we struggle so much with problems in some forms and do better in others? Does this show that our cognitive abilities are flawed and riddled with errors? Well, not exactly. Our mental abilities are probably being judged too harshly, as many standard tests of our thinking attempt to detect ability on too narrow a focus. Instead, we can understand our cognitive abilities better if we understand the sort of problems our brains are adapted to solve.

Our ancestors would have had to make decisions based on what they observed, and where there was uncertainty such decisions would have to be made according to what regularities they had observed. For example, how often rainfall followed thunder or how often illness followed being bitten by a particular snake. This is sometimes referred to as the ecological structure of the environment that our ancestors lived in. In response to this, they developed ecological rationality, cognitive mechanisms that respond to the ecological structure of their environment to solve problems reliably. Therefore, our problem-solving abilities are adapted to respond well to problems framed in terms of ones we faced in our evolutionary history, but poorly to artificial, abstract or novel ones. This is an issue if we try to measure and understand human cognition using the latter type of problems, an example of which is the original version of the medical diagnosis problem above. Our world is full of arbitrary problems that are based on logic, but this does not necessarily match what our minds have adapted to solve.

FIGURE 11.1
Visual representation of the medical diagnosis problem

Source: adapted from Cosmides and Tooby 1996, p. 34.

"The 100 squares pictured below represent this random sample of 100 Americans. Each square represents one person. Using these squares, we would like you to depict the information given above. To indicate that a person actually has the disease, circle the square representing that person. To indicate that a person has tested positive for the disease, fill in the square representing that person. Given the information above, on average,

(1) Circle the number of people who will have the disease.

(2) Fill in squares to represent the people who will test positive for the disease.

(3) How many people who test positive for the disease will actually have the disease? ___ out of ___".

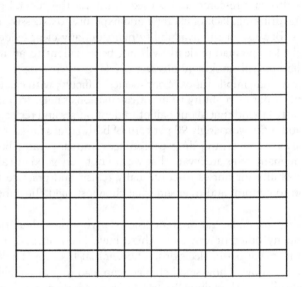

In the example of the original medical diagnosis problem above, participants are asked to make judgements based on information about the probability of a single event having a particular disease. This is logically correct, but does not match how we interpret the world. Another example would be informing a couple trying to conceive that they have a 35 per cent chance of becoming pregnant in the next 12 months. When there are only two possibilities (pregnant/not pregnant), our brains struggle to make sense of a probability of 35 per cent. We are used to reasoning and problem solving about frequencies. These are observable and concrete, such as knowing that after visiting a location 10 times that 7 of those times led to food being found. Therefore, by having brains that are designed to solve problems based on information about frequencies than about percentages, it is no surprise that the latter forms of the medical diagnosis problem above led to better reasoning and more people getting the correct response.

Not all of our reasoning is based on information about frequencies of events, but it is more likely when information can change over an individual's lifetime. Also, events that

A **heuristic** is a cognitive process whereby shortcuts or algorithms are used to make decisions.

are more personal or immediate to an individual (*local* sampling) will have more weight than general sampling, as these would have been more relevant and important. For example, the frequency of close group and family members who contract a disease is a good source of information about one's own likelihood of also contracting the disease. However, in the modern day we have access to lots of similar information that may appear local but actually is not. For example, the reporting of the global spread of bird flu in the national news may trigger our brains to believe that the threat is more local then it actually is. This is an example of the availability **heuristic** (Carroll 1978), where people base their understanding of events occurring on vividness and emotional impact rather than on their actual probability. As well as leading individuals to over-estimate the impact of vivid events such as diseases, plane crashes or shark attacks, it can also lead to misunderstanding of information presented in terms of populations. This is prevalent in medical and health care research and is used to inform the general public about the dangers of smoking, drinking, lack of exercise and exposure to excessive sunlight, among many other things. Because of the availability heuristic, any clear evidence of smoking being strongly linked to premature death will not be as salient to an individual whose 90-year-old grandfather still smokes 40 cigarettes a day!

There are many nursing implications of our species' difficulty with calculations, starting with an assessment of our own ability to make calculations safely. In a large UK survey, McMullan *et al.* (2010) found that about half of student nurses and registered nurses failed a numeracy test, and more worryingly 90 per cent of both groups failed a drug calculation test, with calculations concerning drug percentages and drip rates being particularly problematic. While many of us are aware that we are not very good at calculations, there is a special responsibility for nurses to continually revisit and practice the calculations we are called upon to perform and to ensure that the most rigid checking procedures are maintained.

People's inability to make rational decisions involving calculations have been demonstrated in many different ways, but these have been utilised in subtle ways to encourage people to make better decisions. The seminal book by Thaler and Sunstein (2008) entitled *Nudge* showed how small changes can lead to positive behaviour change. People can be 'nudged' towards making 'better' decisions for themselves in areas as diverse as food choice, pension contribution and organ donation. This is known as 'libertarian paternalism': libertarian because even though it might be argued that people's choices are being manipulated, no one is actually being forced to make any choices. Others see our inability to make rational choices as justification for more coercive paternalism, for example, the phasing out of cigarette smoking (Conly 2013).

A systematic review of studies investigating communication with patients about evidence showed that probabilities are best represented as event rates (natural frequencies) in relevant groups of people, better than words, or summarised as effect measures such as relative risk reduction (Trevena *et al.* 2006). Health promotion advice doesn't always follow this evidence-based approach. For example, the recently revised alcohol advice simply concentrates on guidance on how many units should be consumed in a week and the consequences for exceeding this are not easy to find on the www.drinkaware.co.uk website. When they are found the risks of drinking more than the minimum advice are expressed in relative rather than absolute terms, for example: 'Men are 1.8 to 2.5 times as likely to get cancer of the mouth, neck and throat, and women are 1.2 to 1.7 times as likely' (Drinkaware 2016). This information is impossible to use to make a decision about how much alcohol an individual chooses to drink unless it can be interpreted in the light of the prevalence of diseases stated, and this is not available. There is a suspicion, therefore, that the information is not being presented to allow people to make informed choices, but rather to concentrate effort on following the guidelines (Snelling 2014). This is a dilemma for nursing practice because two fundamental aims of the profession appear to conflict. Seeking to promote health suggests that we should present information in a way that encourages certain behaviours, perhaps 'nudging' people into following them, whereas seeking to promote choice requires that information is presented in a way to increase understanding of risk, and this may result in people choosing to accept risks that are consistent with their understanding of their preferred 'good' life, but against health advice.

> **Emotional intelligence** is the capacity to perceive emotions, assimilate emotion-related feelings, understand the information of those emotions and manage them.

Activity 11.1

Imagine that you are on placement in a general practitioner surgery seeing a patient who explains that he really likes his evenings in the pub with his friends, even though it means he is drinking double the recommended amount of alcohol. He asks you to explain what the extra risk to his health is in a way that he can understand. How would you approach this?

Individual differences

Emotional intelligence, labour and resilience

Emotional intelligence (EI) first became popular in the 1990s, when Daniel Goleman (1995) published his book *Emotional Intelligence*. Since then it has become a major area of research and application within psychology and is of great importance to nursing and health care in general. It is also an area of debate and consideration within the scientific community and has achieved a great deal of public interest recently. The need to reliably and consistently define EI often plays a key role in the debates. Currently no definition has widespread or unanimous acceptance, which is problematic as this can lead to the concept of EI being misunderstood. However, a simple and commonly used definition from Mayer *et al.* (1999) describes EI as being 'involved in the capacity to perceive emotions, assimilate emotion-related feelings, understand the information of those emotions, and manage them' (p. 1).

Although different definitions exist, there is some agreement about what makes up EI. To summarise, EI can be thought of as being made up of the following:

- *perceiving emotions*, which includes reading the emotions of others;
- *understanding emotions*, which includes an awareness of one's own emotional state;
- *managing emotions*, which includes the regulation and control of emotions; and
- *using emotions*, which is utilising different emotional states to perform certain tasks.

Resilience is an individual's ability to adapt to stressful situations or crises.

Of further interest is whether EI is best viewed as an ability, much like IQ, or whether it is actually a personality trait, like extraversion or conscientiousness. Academic debate continues about this, particularly in regard to how EI can best be measured. Can we test for it like an ability, even though there are no right or wrong answers about emotional problems? Or can we test for it like a personality test, with self-report items that may lead to biased or inaccurate responses?

In spite of all this debate, however, we should not lose sight of the fact that EI has been shown to be linked to many positive life outcomes. These include academic success (Barchard 2003), performance in business (Zeidner et al. 2004), health outcomes (Gohm et al. 2005), and leadership (George 2000). The link between EI and emotional labour is particularly relevant and careers such as nursing are clearly very high in the latter. Emotional labour was first introduced in the 1980s, in response to the perhaps traditional belief that the workplace should be a rational place with no role for emotions. Clearly this is not true of many jobs, where part of what employees earn their wage for is managing their emotions to improve outcomes, often in difficult and trying situations. Emotional labour is increasingly being seen as an important aspect of many different jobs. This is possibly due to recent growth of the service sector, with increased level of interaction with customers. It is also due to the inevitable increase in levels of social interactions in most jobs, with more need for teamworking and dealing with complex organisational structures, such as those in the NHS. Examples of careers high in emotional labour include air traffic controllers who need to deal with high anxiety and stressful situations to respond calmly and correctly, call centre workers who need to continue in a positive and happy mood after receiving abusive and angry calls from some customers, and of course nurses (Sawbridge and Hewison 2013).

Emotional intelligence has clear benefits, and individuals high in EI perform better in careers high in emotional labour. This is because of the successful coping strategies they can use in emotionally demanding situations. Specifically, individuals high in EI display more 'deep acting' coping, which includes a modification of one's own inner feelings and emotional state. They also display less 'surface acting' coping, which includes a modification of one's own language or facial expressions. A 'deep acting' coping strategy is more successful and appropriate, and helps individuals with high EI to cope better and avoid 'burnout', which is common in careers with high levels of emotional labour. A further examination between EI and coping strategies was conducted by Petrides et al. (2007). They found that people high in EI tend to use adaptive coping strategies such as rational coping (take action to change things) and detached coping (just take nothing personally). People low in EI, however, tend to use maladaptive coping strategies such as emotional coping (feel worthless and unimportant) and avoidance coping (feel that time will sort things out).

This suggests that emotional **resilience**, the ability to adapt to stressful situations or crises, will be a great trait in careers high in emotional labour. In other words, individuals with high EI and successful coping strategies will be better able to 'roll with the punches' that high emotional labour often provides. There are recognisable traits that emotionally resilient people have, which include emotional awareness, support, perseverance, a sense of perspective, an internal locus of control, that is in other words, the ability to attribute life events to being under one's own control, a sense of humour, optimism, and an ability to handle troubling emotions.

Activity 11.2

Think about colleagues you know who are either student or registered nurses – how many of these traits do you recognise in these individuals? Also think about those who you think will be or already are very successful in this career: do they have clearly greater levels of any of these traits?

Considering the benefits of having high EI, an important question is whether it is possible to increase or develop your own EI. This is not straightforward, particularly as we have seen there is still no consensus of what EI actually consists of. There have been many attempts to improve individuals' EI, but there are some issues with earlier attempts, which tended to concentrate on particular groups (school children, managers, individuals with emotional disorders); only concentrated on some aspects of EI or traits only related to EI; and results were often based on just short-term, subjective views on whether EI had developed. More recent attempts to increase people's EI scores have been more comprehensive. For example in the study by Nelis *et al.* (2009), the EI levels of a group of young adults were measured at the start of a training programme. In sessions across 4 weeks, they were taught the theory behind emotions and EI, and given guidance and advice about applying emotional skills to everyday life. The programme included short lectures, tasks, role play scenarios, and participants were asked to keep a diary where they could record their emotional experiences over this period. At the end of the 4 weeks, their EI levels were measured again, but importantly this was re-measured 6 months later. The researchers found that not only had EI scores increased after the programme compared to before, but that EI increases further still after 6 months. This suggests that specific attempts to train and develop EI, such as raising awareness, increasing motivation or providing successful strategies, which individuals can continue to use long after the training has finished, can have long-lasting effects. Although we are still at the early stages of discovering how we can develop and increase EI, the future is promising and with careers such as nursing where such skills can be incredibly valuable, this is good news.

A recently published integrative review into resilience in nursing students (Thomas and Revel 2016) noted that the subject is in its infancy. Nine studies were identified including just two from the UK. It found a range of definitions and concluded that resilience is important and should be fostered, but as yet there is no consensus about the value of interventions. Support of friends, family and the university are all important.

PART 3: EXPLORING PSYCHOLOGICAL CONCEPTS FOR NURSING

New directions in psychology

Evolutionary clinical psychology

Case 11.1 continued

> Johannes is morbidly obese and this is affecting his health in many different ways. He is upset about his weight, and doesn't understand why this has happened. He tries to eat healthily but fails so often and just wants to know why this happens to him?

Johannes' unhealthy behaviour may well seem peculiar as we view our current lives, but less so when we look at human life as it used to be. Our ancestors lived in very harsh environments where the vital nutrients needed for survival were sparse. These would have included sugar and other foods high in calories, as what was needed was a good source of energy. Therefore, any individual who had an innate preference for sugary and fatty foods would have a drive to seek and consume these foods, which at times of scarcity will be very beneficial in helping them survive and have offspring, who in turn would inherit that preference. However, if we fast-forward to our modern lives, we can see that cheap and processed foods with excessive sugar levels are plentiful and easily available. This is now a problem as we still have our innate desire for such foods, but this desire is now maladaptive as the over-abundance of sugary foods means that we are driven to consume far more than we actually need. In other words, our environment has changed far more quickly than our psychology can keep up with. This mismatch between our current environment and the one we evolved in can simply explain why obesity is one of the major problems that will affect the delivery of health programmes in the future.

This is just one example of how looking at health behaviours from an evolutionary perspective can help our understanding of them. Other such behaviours include why we have phobias, why we feel so much pain and why happiness is so elusive? Darwinian medicine (Nesse and Williams 1994, Williams and Nesse 1991) addresses questions such as these, recognising that psychologists have tended to view mental health problems and problematic health behaviours as maladaptive. However in Darwinian (i.e. evolutionary) terms, such behaviours in certain circumstances and at certain levels are actually beneficial, for example, anxiety or phobias may actually decrease risky behaviours that threaten our physical well-being.

Let's take depression as an example. This is usually considered to be a mood disorder, and is characterised by low mood, lack of interest in things, general fatigue, feelings of worthlessness among others. It is co-morbid with other psychological conditions such as anxiety and is a modern epidemic increasing in prevalence. Could the fact that depressive symptoms are sometimes evolutionarily in origin help explain why it is so common? Different theories suggest this, stating that depression leads individuals to accept a 'losing' strategy in social competitions to avoid further defeats (Price *et al.* 1994), or that it results from the mismatch between the modern world and the environment we evolved in (Charlton 2000). Another example is schizophrenia, which includes symptoms such as distortions of reality, uncontrolled thoughts, hallucinations and disordered emotions.

Clearly these symptoms are unhealthy and can lead to poor life outcomes, but what if these traits could be valued in certain cases? One possibility for this comes from potential links with creativity, characterised as novel and unusual thinking in different domains. Creativity can be very adaptive not only for survival through general problem solving and dealing with difficult situations, but also for mating success, where it is linked to intelligence and therefore can signal genetic quality to potential partners (Miller 2000). However, individuals with creative personality types tend to score higher on measures of schizophrenia, and individuals in creative careers, such as poets and artists tend to have higher rates of mental illness and are also more likely to have relatives with schizophrenia (Nettle 2001).

Both of these examples attempt to explain mental illnesses in evolutionary terms, by showing that in extreme forms or in extreme circumstances these adaptive behaviours can be maladaptive, leading to clinical diagnoses. However both examples are not without their critics, and such theories are certainly controversial. Furthermore, examples like this from Darwinian medicine do not attempt to dampen or question the severity with which these conditions can affect people every day. However, they may point to a new perspective that can serve health professionals well. For example, it may have implications for treatment and possibly how we can alleviate negative symptoms. Further research will help with this, and has the potential to revolutionise medical treatment for many different health outcomes.

Our early environment's effect on our health behaviour

Problem behaviours and strains on the NHS suggest that much is due to people in lower socioeconomic groups having too many children, smoking, drinking, obesity and risky behaviours, and this is a message that seems prevalent in the media. Politicians, sociologists and medical professionals among many others have attempted to address the great differences within our society when it comes to health outcomes. However one perhaps unlikely source has arisen recently, suggesting an answer from behavioural ecology, based on understanding humans the same way we understand all other species. To do so we need to look at life history theory, which is essentially how organisms allocate energy and resources to different life outcomes at different times, such as mating effort or early developmental growth. One outcome that requires a great deal of resources is investment in offspring. In these cases, organisms 'choose' the optimum time to begin allocating resources to offspring, based on the surrounding environment and the condition of the individual. A high-quality environment predicts later investment in offspring, when the parent is better placed to provide high quality support. It will also lead to a lower number of offspring as these will be of high-quality themselves and likely to survive to adulthood. Conversely, a lower-quality environment calls for earlier investment in off-spring, due to an uncertain future, which may include early mortality and increased morbidity. Similarly, low-quality environments also predict higher numbers of offspring, as poor environments can lead to decreased number of offspring reaching maturity.

The question raised, however, is does this theory also apply to humans in modern societies? Nettle *et al.* (2011) looked at the early life conditions of a large cohort of British women, to see how this might relate to the age at which they were first pregnant. They found that the socioeconomic conditions, taken as a measure of the quality of environment, did affect this. Women who, as children, lived in poor socioeconomic conditions were first pregnant at a younger age than those who lived in more affluent

295

socioeconomic positions when they were children. This also echoes the attitudes women from different socioeconomic backgrounds have towards pregnancy (Jewell *et al.* 2000). It is not just age at first pregnancy; a comparison between a neighbouring affluent and deprived area in England revealed that families in the deprived area had lower birth weights, shorter breastfeeding duration as well as lower age of first pregnancy (Nettle 2010). There was also indirect evidence that families in the deprived area had more offspring than those in the nearby affluent area. Therefore, there seems to be evidence that a poor environment leads to a 'faster' life history, characterised by early reproduction, reduced investment in children and high rates of reproduction.

It is not just early parenthood that can be explained by life history theory. Ellis *et al.* (2012) looked at the origin of risk-taking behaviour in adolescents and suggest that this is also the product of an individual's early environment. They state that harsh and unpredictable environments provide a 'weather forecast' for the future, and individuals from such environments will benefit from engaging in risky behaviour, as this will be adaptive when future conditions are also harsh. This can also be seen from a simple experiment by Griskevicius *et al.* (2011), who found that when cued about mortality, individuals from lower-quality early environments were more likely to make risky decisions for immediate gains. The opposite was true for individuals from higher-quality early environments, as being cued about mortality made them more risk averse, and they valued certain future rewards more.

Overall, these findings suggest that many of the decisions individuals make when it comes to their health are due to powerful influences of their early environment that permeate throughout their lives. Therefore, it seems no surprise that attempts by policy makers to influence health behaviours in certain groups through either incentives or punishments in later life rarely work. The same perspective too should apply to our attitudes towards certain groups who persist with what appear to be poor decisions with regard to their health. With the possibility that early life events cause such fixed effects on our later behaviour, these decisions only seem poor when viewed in the current environment. Therefore, effort should not be restricted to later life intervention, through policy or education, when the best way to encourage individuals to pursue a life history strategy that is less damaging to themselves and others is to intervene at an early age, by improving the conditions and quality of life of children in the poorer areas of our society.

CONCLUSION

The field of psychology is vast and growing and new research constantly brings new insights to human behaviour in both health and illness. The link between the brain and the body is well established and there are a number of implications for nurses in understanding this link. First, for all patients, addressing psychological needs can lead to great gains in outcome. This need not involve complex specialised techniques and real benefit is demonstrated simply by listening to people's worries and addressing them as much as you are able, and giving desired information in a way that can be understood. The psychological insights discussed in the chapter apply to all of us, but can also be more directly of use in caring for others, but perhaps the bigger influence in acknowledging these insights is a greater understanding of what might be termed the 'human condition'. The benefits of greater understanding here are likely to extend to our own lives and opinions in a range of areas, as well as more directly to our patients.

SUGGESTED FURTHER READING

Goodman, B. (2012) *Psychology and Sociology in Nursing* (2nd edn). London: Learning Matters.
Torn, A. and Greasley, P. (eds) *Psychology for Nursing*. Cambridge: Polity Press.
Upton, D. (2013) *Introducing Psychology for Nurses and Healthcare Professionals*. Oxford: Routledge.

REFERENCES

Asch, S. E. (1956). Studies of independence and conformity: a minority of one against a unanimous majority *Psychological Monographs* **70** (9), 1–70.
Bales, K. L. and Carter, C. S. (2003) Developmental exposure to oxytocin facilitates partner preferences in male prairie voles. *Behavioral Neuroscience* **117**, 854–859.
Barchard, K. A. (2003) Does emotional intelligence assist the prediction of academic success? *Educational Psychology Measures* **63**, 840–858.
Bartz, J. A., Zaki, J., Bolger, N., Hollander, E., Ludwig, N. N., Kolevzon, A., Ochsner, K. N. (2010) Oxytocin selectively improves empathic accuracy. *Psychological Science* **21**, 1426–1428.
Batson, C. D., Batson, J. G., Slingsby, J. K., Harrell, K. L., Peekna, H. M. and Todd, R. M. (1991) Empathic joy and the empathy–altruism hypothesis. *Journal of Personality and Social Psychology* **61**, 413–426.
Baumgartner, T., Heinrichs, M., Vonlanthen, A., Fischbacher, U. and Fehr, E., (2008) Oxytocin shapes the neural circuitry of trust and trust adaptation in humans. *Neuron* **58**, 639–650.
BBC (British Broadcasting Corporation) (2008) Childhood obesity is genetic. Available at: http://news.bbc.co.uk/player/nol/newsid_7230000/newsid_7231800/7231891.stm?bw=bbandm p=wmandnews=1andnol_storyid=7231891andbbcws=1 (accessed 19 February 2016).
Bond, R. and Smith, P. B. (1996) Culture and conformity: a meta-analysis of studies using Asch's (1952b, 1956) line judgment task. *Psychological Bulletin* **119**, 111.
Brown, I. (2006) Nurses' attitudes towards adult patients who are obese: literature review. *Journal of Advanced Nursing* **53** (2), 221–232.
Callahan, D. (2013) Obesity: chasing an elusive epidemic. *Hastings Center Report* **43** (1), 34–40.
Carroll, J. S. (1978) The effect of imagining an event on expectations for the event: an interpretation in terms of the availability heuristic. *Journal of Experimental Social Psychology* **14**, 88–96.
Casscells, W., Schoenberger, A. and Grayboys, T. (1978) Interpretation by physicians of clinical laboratory results. *New England Journal of Medicine* **299**, 999–1000.
Charlton, B. G. (2000) The malaise theory of depression: major depressive disorder is sickness behavior and antidepressants are analgesic. *Medical Hypotheses* **54** (1), 126–130.
Cialdini, R. B., Kenrick, D. T. and Baumann, D. J. (1982) Effects of mood on prosocial behavior in children and adults. In *The Development of Prosocial Behavior*, Eisenberg, E. (ed). New York: Academic Press, pp. 339–359.
Conly, S. (2013) *Against Autonomy: Justifying coercive paternalism*. Cambridge: Cambridge University Press.
Cosmides, L. and Tooby, J. (1996) Are humans good intuitive statisticians after all? Rethinking some conclusions from the literature on judgment under uncertainty. *Cognition* **58** (1), 1–73.
Darwin, C. (1859) *On the Origin of Species*. London: Murray.
Domes, G., Heinrichs, M., Michel, A., Berger, C. and Herpertz, S. C. (2007) Oxytocin improves 'mind-reading' in humans. *Biological Psychiatry* **6**, 731–733.
Drinkaware (2016) Your alcohol risk level www.drinkaware.co.uk/understand-your-drinking/is-your-drinking-a-problem/your-drinking-risk-level (accessed 19 February 2016).
Eisenegger, C., Naef, M., Snozzi, R., Heinrichs, M. and Fehr, E. (2009) Prejudice and truth about the effect of testosterone on human bargaining behaviour. *Nature* **463**, 356–359.

Ellis, B. J., Del Giudice, M., Dishion, T. J., Figueredo, A. J., Gray, P., Griskevicius, V., . . . and Wilson, D. S. (2012) The evolutionary basis of risky adolescent behavior: implications for science, policy, and practice. *Developmental Psychology* **48**, 598.

Farrelly, D. (2011) Cooperation as a signal of genetic or phenotypic quality in female mate choice? Evidence from preferences across the menstrual cycle. *British Journal of Psychology* **102** (3), 406–430.

George, J. M. (2000) Emotions and leadership: the role of emotional intelligence. *Human Relations* **53**, 1027–1054.

Geschwind, D. H., Miller, B. L., DeCarli, C. and Carmelli, D. (2002) Heritability of lobar brain volumes in twins supports genetic models of cerebral laterality and handedness. *Proceedings of the National Academy of Sciences* **99**, 3176–3181.

Gillett, K. (2012) A critical discourse analysis of British national newspaper representations of the academic level of nurse education: too clever for our own good? *Nursing Inquiry* **19** (4), 297–307.

Gillett, K. (2014) Nostalgic constructions of nurse education in British national newspapers. *Journal of Advanced Nursing* **70** (11), 2495–2505.

Gintis, H., Smith, E. A. and Bowles, S. (2001) Costly signaling and cooperation. *Journal of Theoretical Biology* **213**, 103–119.

Gohm, C. L., Corser, G. C. and Dalsky, D. J. (2005) Emotional intelligence under stress: useful, unnecessary, or irrelevant? *Personality and Individual Differences* **39** (6), 1017–1028.

Goleman, D. (1995) *Emotional Intelligence: Why it can matter more than IQ*. London: Bloomsbury.

Gray, P. B., Kahlenberg, S. M., Barrett, E. S., Lipson, S. F. and Ellison, P. T. (2002) Marriage and fatherhood are associated with lower testosterone in males. *Evolution and Human Behavior* **23**, 193–201.

Griskevicius, V., Tybur, J. M., Delton, A. W. and Robertson, T. E. (2011). The influence of mortality and socioeconomic status on risk and delayed rewards: a life history theory approach. *Journal of Personality and Social Psychology* **100**, 1015–1026.

Guastella, A. J., Mitchell, P. B. and Dadds, M. R. (2008). Oxytocin increases gaze to the eye region of human faces. *Biological Psychiatry* **1**, 3–5.

Haigh C. A. (2010) Reconstructing nursing altruism using a biological evolutionary framework. *Journal of Advanced Nursing* **66**, 1401–1408.

Hamilton, W. D. (1964) The genetic evolution of social behaviour. I and II. *Journal of Theoretical Biology* **7**, 1–52.

Henderson, M. (2008) Genes not poor diet blamed for most cases of childhood obesity. *The Times* 7 February 2008.

Henderson, S. (2003) Power imbalance between nurses and patients: a potential inhibitor of partnership in care. *Journal of Clinical Nursing* **12** (4), 501–508.

Holland, J. C. and Alici, Y. (2010) Management of distress in cancer patients. *Journal of Community and Supportive Oncology* **8** (1), 4–12.

Holm, S. (2008) Parental responsibility and obesity in children. *Public Health Ethics* **1** (1), 21–29.

Hofling, C. K., Brotzman, E., Dalrymple, S., Graves, N. and Bierce, C. (1966) An experimental study of nurse–physician relations. *Journal of Nervous and Mental Disease* **143**, 171–180.

Jewell, D., Tacchi, J. and Donovan, J. (2000) Teenage pregnancy: whose problem is it? *Family Practice* **17** (6), 522–528.

Kanazawa, S. (2000) Scientific discoveries as cultural displays: a further test of Miller's courtship model. *Evolution and Human Behaviour* **21**, 317–321.

Kanazawa, S. (2003) Why productivity fades with age: the crime–genius connection. *Journal of Research in Personality* **37**, 257–272.

Knight, I. (2008) Face it, fatty, your genes are innocent. *Sunday Times* 10 February 2008.

Kosfeld, M., Heinrichs, M., Zak, P. J., Fischbacher, U. and Fehr, E. (2005) Oxytocin increases trust in humans. *Nature* **435**, 673–676.

Levett-Jones, T. and Lathlean, J. (2009) 'Don't rock the boat': nursing students' experiences of conformity and compliance. *Nurse Education Today* **29** (3), 342–349.

Major, B., Hunger, J. M., Bunyan, D. P. and Miller, C. T. (2014) The ironic effects of weight stigma. *Journal of Experimental Social Psychology* **51**, 74–80.

Mayer, J. D., Caruso, D. and Salovey, P. (1999) Emotional intelligence meets traditional standards for an intelligence. *Intelligence* **27**, 267–298.

McMullan, M., Jones, R. and Lea, S. (2010) Patient safety: numerical skills and drug calculation abilities of nursing students and registered nurses. *Journal of Advanced Nursing* **66** (4), 891–899.

Milgram, S. (1974) *Obedience to Authority*. New York: Harper & Row.

Miller, G. F. (2000) *The Mating Mind: How sexual choice shaped the evolution of human nature*. London: William Heinemann.

Mitchell, M. (2007) Psychological care of patients undergoing elective surgery. *Nursing Standard* **21** (30), 48–55.

Moscovici, S., Lage, E. and Naffrechoux, M. (1969) Influence of a consistent minority on the responses of a majority in a color perception task. *Sociometry* **32** (4), 365–380.

Nelis, D., Quoidbach, J., Mikolajczak, M. and Hansenne, M. (2009) Increasing emotional intelligence: (how) is it possible? *Personality and Individual Differences* **47** (1), 36–41.

Nesse, R. M. and Williams, G. C. (1994) *Why We Get Sick: The new science of Darwinian medicine*. New York: Vintage.

Nettle, D. (2001) *Strong Imagination: Madness, creativity and human nature*. Oxford: Oxford University Press.

Nettle, D. (2010) Dying young and living fast: variation in life history across English neighborhoods. *Behavioral Ecology* **21**, 387–395.

Nettle, D., Coall, D. A. and Dickins, T. E. (2011) Early-life conditions and age at first pregnancy in British women. *Proceedings of the Royal Society of London B: Biological Sciences* **278** (1712), 1721–1727.

Nicholls, W., Pilsbury, L., Blake, M. and Devonport, T. J. (2015) The attitudes of student nurses towards obese patients: a questionnaire study exploring the association between perceived causal factors and advice giving. *Nurse Education Today* **37**, 33–37.

Nowak, M. A. and Sigmund, K. (1998) Evolution of indirect reciprocity by image scoring. *Nature* **393**, 573–577.

Petrides, K. V., Pérez-González, J. C. and Furnham, A. (2007) On the criterion and incremental validity of trait emotional intelligence. *Cognition and Emotion* **21** (1), 26–55.

Price, J., Sloman, L., Gardner, R., Gilbert, P. and Rohde, P. (1994) The social competition hypothesis of depression. *British Journal of Psychiatry* **164**, 309–315.

Puhl, R. M. and Heuer, C. A. (2009) The stigma of obesity: a review and update. *Obesity* **17** (5), 941–964.

Sawbridge, Y. and Hewison, A. (2013) Thinking about the emotional labour of nursing: supporting nurses to care. *Journal of Health Organization and Management* **27** (1), 127–133.

Smith, A. (1995) An analysis of altruism: a concept of caring. *Journal of Advanced Nursing* **22** (4), 785–790.

Smith, G. D. (2010) Psychological interventions for irritable bowel syndrome: a nursing perspective. *Gastrointestinal Nursing* **8** (9), 18–21.

Snelling, P. C. (2014) What's wrong with tombstoning and what does this tell us about responsibility for health? *Public Health Ethics* **7** (2), 144–157.

Swift, J. A., Hanlon, S., El-Redy, L., Puhl, R. M. and Glazebrook, C. (2013) Weight bias among UK trainee dieticians, doctors, nurses and nutritionists. *Journal of Human Nutrition and Dietetics* **26** (4), 395–402.

Tanaka, Y., Kanazawa, M., Fukudo, S. and Drossman, D. A. (2011) Biopsychosocial model of irritable bowel syndrome. *Journal of Neurogastroenterology and Motility* **17** (2), 131.

ten Hoeve, Y. T., Jansen, G. and Roodbol, P. (2014) The nursing profession: public image, self-concept and professional identity. A discussion paper. *Journal of Advanced Nursing* **70** (2), 295–309.

Thaler, R. and Sunstein, C. (2008) *Nudge: Improving decisions about health, wealth, and happiness*. London: Penguin Books.

Thomas, L. J. and Revell, S. H. (2016) Resilience in nursing students: an integrative review. *Nurse Education Today* **36**, 457–462.

Theodoridou, A., Rowe, A. C., Penton-Voak, I. S. and Rogers, P. J. (2009) Oxytocin and social perception: oxytocin increases perceived facial trustworthiness and attractiveness. *Hormones and Behavior* **56**, 128–132.

Trevena, L. J., Barratt, A., Butow, P. and Caldwell, P. (2006) A systematic review on communicating with patients about evidence. *Journal of Evaluation in Clinical Practice* **12** (1), 13–23.

Trivers, R. (1971) The evolution of reciprocal altruism. *Quarterly Review of Biology* **46**, 35–57.

Trivers, R. (1972) Parental investment and sexual selection: the Darwinian pivot. In *Sexual Selection and the Descent of Man*, Campbell, B. G. (ed). New Brunswick, NJ: Transaction Publishers, pp. 136–179.

van Leengoed, E., Kerker, E. and Swanson, H. H. (1987) Inhibition of postpartum maternal behaviour in the rat by injecting an oxytocin antagonist into the cerebral ventricles. *Journal of Endocrinology* **112**, 275–282.

Wardle, J., Carnell S., Haworth C. M. A. and Plomin, R. (2008) Evidence for a strong genetic influence on childhood adiposity despite the force of the obesogenic environment. *American Journal of Clinical Nutrition* **87**, 398–404.

Williams, G. W. and Nesse, R. M. (1991) The dawn of Darwinian medicine. *Quarterly Review of Biology* **66**, 1–22.

Woo, K. Y. (2012) Exploring the effects of pain and stress on wound healing. *Advances in Skin and Wound Care* **25** (1), 38–44.

Zeidner, M., Mathews, G. and Roberts, R. D. (2004) Emotional intelligence in the workplace: a critical review. *Applied Psychology: An International Review* **53**, 371–399.

12

SPIRITUAL CARE

Janice Clarke

LEARNING OUTCOMES

After reading and reflecting on this chapter you should be able to:

- understand the meaning of spirituality;
- understand how spiritual care can be incorporated into holistic patient care;
- discuss the relationship between religion and spirituality;
- discuss critiques of spirituality within health care.

INTRODUCTION

It might be thought that the idea of linking spirituality to nursing is new, but actually it's a new way of explaining some timeless aspects of nursing care. This modern way of looking at the spirituality of clients and patients has come to be seen as an essential aspect of care and central to nursing. The idea of spiritual care has grown from the recognition that many people describe themselves as being spiritual and expect this to be taken into consideration in their care. It is seen by some nurses as a way to describe an aspect of nursing care that has become lost and neglected; namely compassionately caring for the whole person as an individual, and as part of this, getting to know more about their feelings, beliefs and values, which may or may not be related to religious beliefs. It has been seen by some people as esoteric and woolly, but this chapter may be different to much of what you have read about spiritual care because it describes something practical and relevant to everything that a nurse does. Whereas often the focus is on talking, here the focus is on doing. Where often you will see spiritual care described as something additional to nursing, here you will find an approach that embeds spiritual care in everything you do.

In Part 1, Graham's case is presented and spiritual care will be outlined by describing the care that he will need. This will enable you to see a picture of what spiritual care is.

In Part 2, the underpinning ideas about what spirituality is and how it is related to nursing care are explored, in order to see why the care described in Part 1 can be described as spiritual. This section will look at why spirituality has become important to people and will describe the different ways in which spirituality is interpreted by people with a range of different beliefs. Some different ways of defining and explaining spirituality will be examined. This means looking at spiritual assessment and the role of the chaplain as well as the relationship between spirituality and religion.

Part 3 examines some of the debates and controversies that surround spirituality and spiritual care such as how spiritual well-being can be measured and whether this matters; how spiritual care differs from psychological or emotional care and from religious care; whether it matters that spirituality cannot easily be defined and whether spiritual care is something that nurses have time for.

PART 1: OUTLINING SPIRITUAL CARE

Case 12.1

Graham has been admitted to a medical ward because his tumour is causing him to vomit. He also has diarrhoea. Every night he rings the bell at least once for the nurses to change his bed. It's humiliating. He tries to stay awake as much as possible so that he doesn't 'have an accident'. He's in a side room, which he knows is for his own benefit but he feels abandoned. He thinks he's going to die but the doctors say that actually they think his chemotherapy will be effective and that he should get back to a normal life. He's 42 and divorced; he has an 8-year-old son who lives with his ex-wife Gail, who Graham rarely sees, and when he does it's a bit strained. He doesn't know what to do with him. He used to like getting out into the hills about the town and having a bit of a walk but he hasn't done that for ages. Whatever the doctors say, it all looks bleak to Graham. He's read enough to know that having a positive outlook on his illness will help him, but he can't feel positive. He feels like an old man. It's dawning on him that he hasn't accumulated that much in his life. If he died what would be left behind? Who would remember him? The nurses are efficient but he suspects they're avoiding him. He saw one nurse throw her eyes up to the ceiling when she heard his bell ring this morning. They come and go as quickly as they can. He can't really tell his Mum or his mates about the pain and the other things because he doesn't want them to feel bad. Anyway what can they do? What can anyone do?

Spiritual care

Spiritual care is new name for some very old practices. At its core, spiritual care is care that addresses the whole person, a concept that has been used in nursing for a long time but hasn't always been put into practice well, if recent criticisms are anything to go by. One of the earliest papers about spirituality or 'the other dimension' was by Piepgras (1968), arguably prompted by the realisation that the term 'spirituality' was being used more and more by members of the public as a way to describe some deeper part of a person, which makes them who they are. The spirit or spirituality of a person is a way of explaining deep inner parts of our being that are linked to our beliefs and represent our individuality, our values and our deepest needs. When we encounter a health professional who seems to appreciate this part of us and includes this appreciation in their care of us, we are more likely to feel cared for and as though we have been treated compassionately. This type of care will look and feel different. It will have the efficiency and clinical competence that all health care professionals should be delivering, but it will have an added dimension that is humane, personal and caring. This kind of care will include a questioning interest in our beliefs about life, be they religious or secular. This is holistic, person-centred care.

Graham's care

Graham has a number of spiritual needs. These are needs that if fulfilled, would help him to face his treatment and would offer hope in the future and confidence in his ability to cope (Clarke 2013). He might feel more like planning his next steps, which would make his life feel more meaningful giving him an incentive to get well and enabling him to face his treatment and its side effects with more courage and positivity. This would put him in a position for his treatment to have the best effect.

Graham's spiritual care would first consist of helping him to feel that he is a valuable and worthwhile person. This is possible by relating to Graham as though he matters and is important, so that nurses caring for Graham should behave positively about caring for him and not show signs of boredom or frustration. Drew's seminal study (1986) about what patients think care feels like showed that they know very quickly if nurses feel negative about their job. Poor care easily made them feel excluded, stupid and insignificant. Care that makes patients feel valued includes them in, rather than excludes them from, conversations.

Communicating

Simple communication skills can have profound effects. In Drew's study (1986) patients perceived that eye contact denoted care. Not allowing yourself to be interrupted when caring for Graham, or if you have to interrupt your care, making sure you go back and continue will have an effect on his sense of self-worth. Being interested in him, enquiring about his interests and his life outside the hospital would help to give him a perspective that his illness isn't all that defines him (Stein 2008). Making a point of speaking to him when there isn't any particular reason would also help Graham feel he was someone people liked and help him to feel he belongs in the world, rather than feeling as though he wouldn't be missed if he died.

Being willing to act as an advocate on his behalf, as the Nursing and Midwifery Council Code (NMC 2015) requires, representing his views to his doctors endorses Graham as a person. If a patient sees that you're willing to intervene with a person perceived to be in authority (a doctor, for example) to get the best care for them, this will increase their sense of value and self-worth. Being honest or 'authentic' is highly valued by patients and demonstrates respect, and patients value nurses who are honest enough to say 'I don't know but I'll find out' as it makes them feel as though they are in a more equal relationship with staff, which is empowering (Starr 2008). This honest, open and equal relationship feels more like accompanying a patient on their journey, an important element of spiritual care. Essential nursing skills such as taking care of a person's dignity and privacy also emphasise the value and respect you have for a patient and so helps build their self-worth.

Nurses are in a unique position to have a very positive effect on the spiritual well-being of patients because they are a constant presence in their day, involved in all their care and with patients when they are at their most exposed and vulnerable. This gives nurses opportunities for spiritual care that are not available to other health care professionals. When Graham soils his bed and feels ashamed and embarrassed by it, the way the nurse behaves can have a crucial influence on making him feel worse or better. This is expressed by this hospice worker:

> By choosing to clean him with affection, so that he can experience the fact that even when he's soiled, he's still worthy of my greatest care and attention, I have perhaps repaired his feeling of being nothing but human scrap, something rather dirty. This acknowledgment of his fundamental humanity is balm on the wound inflicted by insult.
>
> (de Hennezel 1998, p. 116)

Empowerment and dignity

If Graham could feel more relaxed about the possibility of having to ask a nurse to clean him up, he might be able to sleep better and that would help him to get well sooner and cope better. Giving Graham choices and supporting him in making decisions about, for example, what he eats, what he wears, when he has a bath or what kind of treatment he has, will help him to feel he's in control of his life and that is an empowering feeling. Someone who feels empowered is more likely to feel they can cope with adversity rather than feeling like giving up. Small things like sitting beside him to talk rather than standing over him; walking to his side to ask him if he needs any analgesia rather than shouting from the door, will also help him to feel empowered and valued, and help him to maintain his dignity (O'Lynn and Krautscheid 2011, Twigg 2000). Showing concern about Graham's lack of appetite and trying to find things that might tempt him to eat doesn't just improve his nutrition but could make him feel cared for and valued.

Touch

Touch is a particularly important part of care and is especially valued when people have wounds or conditions that are off-putting (Clarke 2013). Patients are aware when touch is purely instrumental and when it is expressive. But instrumental touch can be made to feel expressive if it is careful and unhurried, measured and accompanied by eye contact, whereas if the nurse appears to be preoccupied touch will be perceived negatively (McCabe and Timmins 2006). For instance stroking his back as you help him out of bed may be really appreciated. If you have to clean him while he's in bed because he feels particularly weak and tired, being gentle and firm would make him feel secure. Just taking the trouble to make Graham feel comfortable would enhance his spiritual well-being. Bottorff (1991) found that patients equated being made to feel comfortable with feeling connected to the world again in the midst of pain and illness.

De Hennezel describes the rhythm created by two carers moving and touching one patient in a hospice:

whenever they (*nurse's aids*) go to give whatever body assistance is required by someone who can no longer even move in bed, they are aware of how much the fact of being there for each other and of bringing the patient into this link creates a completely different kind of contact. The movements they so gently make to lift a leg and ease a patient over onto his side synchronise themselves of one accord and flow together without jolts or bumping. When one cleans a bedsore, the other embraces the enfeebled body and just stays there doing nothing but rocking it gently.

(de Hennezel 1998, p. 50)

Relationship

These kinds of relationships seemed to allow patients to be themselves with nurses and to get a different perspective on the situation helping them to feel that they are part of something bigger than themselves. Nurses who develop these quality relationships tend to enjoy their work and are less likely to suffer burnout (Leppanen-Montgomery 1991). When people are asked about spirituality they very often mention that it seems to have a lot to do with their relationships with the people around them and with anything they perceive as a higher power, energy or God. Hungelman *et al.* (1996) found that spiritual well-being seems to be a sense of 'harmonious interconnectedness'. So Graham will be helped towards a sense of spiritual peace if he has good relationships with those around him. This could mean with nurses and doctors or it could be that the nurses can help him improve his relationships with his son and ex-wife, as well as the other family members by encouraging them to visit. It might also help to talk to him about his life and his family and friends while you are carrying out care to help him explore what has gone wrong in these relationships and to decide whether there's anything he can do to make things better.

Listening and talking

Listening to patients is a big part of spiritual care. You are not expected to have a lot of answers but just to be encouraging and positive and listen while a patient thinks things through (Clarke 2013). Being interested in a patient's spiritual beliefs and trying to fulfil any particular requirements not only helps a person to stay in touch with a helping resource but also shows you care. A large part of spiritual care is about helping a patient to remember the things that give them strength and help them to cope with illness and crises. These may be things they have found helpful in the past. It could be anything from being with their family, to reconnecting with an interest or hobby. Reminding Graham about how much he used to like walking in the hills might give him a sense of hope that he could do that again. Encouraging him to look at photos or TV programmes or pictures of the kind of places he liked might give him hope in the future. He might start to think that he could even introduce his son to some of the places he liked to visit.

For many people a sense of connection and a set of resources that might add to inner strength or increase resilience might come from religion or other spiritual practices. Many people practise a religion to some degree or they believe a little and might be interested in following it up when they're ill. Spiritual care is about helping people to reconnect with the things that have given life meaning and might be a source of strength again, so it's useful to enquire about any religious leanings. If this is a part of a person's life, or has

Janice Clarke

been, it can help for them to feel that you think it's important. Giving the time and space for prayer or meditation can be really valued, as might paying attention to any particular food needs, or other things associated with religious practices. A religious person might want to talk things through with a religious specialist like the chaplain, or attend a religious service and you can help organise these kinds of activities and encourage people to take part.

No wonder Graham is feeling alone. When you've been ill and in pain for a long time, you can start to feel as though you are a burden and a bit of a bore about it. So you stop talking to your family and friends. Eventually the staff around you are the only ones you can really tell how bad you feel, so if they don't seem to want to listen you're likely to feel even worse (Stein 2008).

RESEARCH FOCUS 12.1

Tanyi *et al.* (2006) interviewed 16 women in a Midwestern US city with end stage renal failure to try to understand how they wanted nurses to address their spirituality. Using phenomenology they found that patients wanted nurses to give spiritual care by building relationships and connectedness, initiating spiritual dialogue, and mobilising spiritual resources. They said nurses did this by showing genuine caring, with patience, smiling, kindness, listening and giving information. While some patients valued also being able to talk about spiritual concerns, many didn't and for those for whom it mattered, it wasn't uppermost in their minds as a way to receive spiritual care.

Activity 12.1

Think back to a time when you have been ill and had to see a doctor or a nurse. What has made you feel better and what has made you feel worse? If you were diagnosed with cancer, how would you like people to treat you?

PART 2: EXPLAINING SPIRITUAL CARE

Why have people started to care about their spirituality?

There are many ideas as to why the term spirituality, which previously was only used by theologians, came into popular use and Heelas and Woodhead (2005) propose one of the most helpful explanations by what they call the 'subjective turn'. This means that without religion and so many of the restrictions of life that past generations grew up with, people had increasingly to look inward for more personal and individual ways of deciding what is right and wrong and which is the best way to live your life. Looking inwards meant greater focus on the inner self or how you feel inside and this inner self had to be strong to cope with all the problems of modern life. This was important because at the same time modern life was becoming increasingly complex. More freedom, the Internet, an increase in consumerism and more education means that there has been an explosion of choices and decisions compared to how it was for past generations. Added to this is the way that technology makes life faster and more instant so that people may feel insecure and stressed. We know more about other people's lives and so we have more opportunities for comparison. Mass technological systems dominate our lives but this can leave people feeling that they're not being treated as individuals. Fewer people are making the permanent commitment of marriage and easier divorce could also be said to have added to the feeling of instability and loneliness that is part of modern life. The improvements in rapid communications mean that the wars, disasters and poverty in the rest of the world are conveyed in pictures to our own living rooms and phones and this adds to the feeling that the world is a dangerous place. Better health care means that people are surviving what previously would have been life-threatening illness and we're living longer but because of that perhaps it's more likely we will experience chronic illness and dementia. In addition, fewer people experience the strong guidance that religions used to provide to signpost them through life and provide security.

All these things have led to the growing recognition that to cope with modern life, individuals need a resilient centre to provide stability in the face of instability and insecurity. In addition, people experience a desire to be treated as an individual and to be treated humanely in order to counteract the anonymity of technology. People are searching for what it is that makes them feel individual, whole and human and so this central core has become more and more important. Being aware of this core can help people to understand what matters to them in order to feel valued and this awareness seems to make us want connections with other people; it becomes particularly important at times of illness and crisis and for want of a better term, it is often called the spirit of a person.

Resilience is the capacity to withstand difficulties and crises. The ability to recover from physical, social or emotional setbacks in life.

What does spirituality mean?

To understand why it is that the care described in the previous section can be care of the spirit means exploring what spirituality is and what the related terms 'spiritual needs' and 'spiritual well-being' mean.

Spirituality

John Swinton says of spirituality:

> While the human *spirit* may be deeply mysterious, pointing as it does towards aspects of reality that are deep, unfathomable and transcendent, *spirituality* is a human activity that attempts to express these profound experiences and inner longings in terms that are meaningful for the individual.
>
> (Swinton 2001, p. 21)

There have been many attempts to define spirituality and scholars have tended to try to avoid claiming that any description or definition can be 'definitive'. This issue is explored further in the third part of this chapter. However a working definition might be that devised by Linda Ross:

> that element within the individual from which originates: meaning, purpose and fulfilment in life; a will to live; belief and faith in self, others and God and

307

Janice Clarke

Spirituality
is 'that element within the individual from which originates: meaning, purpose and fulfilment in life; a will to live; belief and faith in self, others and God and which is essential to the attainment of an optimum state of health, well-being or quality of life'. (Ross, 1997, p. 11)

Transcendence
can be interpreted in a number of ways, two of which are useful to understanding spirituality. Spirituality may be seen as being to do with beliefs about a God or energy, which is perceived as being beyond normal perception or 'transcendent'. Also being able to rise above or 'transcend' one's illness or disability and see it from a wider perspective so that you are not so affected by it could be seen as an aspect of spiritual well-being and something that spiritual care might help you to achieve.

which is essential to the attainment of an optimum state of health, well-being or quality of life

(1997, p. 11)

Spirituality and spiritual well-being are fluid ideas, which people struggle to describe and that feel personal to them. Nevertheless when asked what they think spirituality is, people answer with repeated and constant themes, for example, **transcendence**, connectedness and meaning and purpose in life (Tanyi 2002), and there is virtually no difference in concepts of spirituality now to 40 years ago.

Connection

Connection, relationship, communication and harmony are all themes that patients and nurses say are connected to spirituality in many research studies. Connection may be to parts of oneself, between people, between a person and nature, or to the universe, God or any higher power. People seem to see the quality of their connections or relationships as enhancing their spiritual well-being. The spiritual dimension is called a connecting, dynamic and unifying force, which works within a person to give a feeling of peace and harmony and helps them to relate better to other people or to a God or other spiritual entity or force. Integrating and connecting are similar concepts and one is often talked about as leading to the other so that Goddard suggests the term 'integrative energy' to describe spirituality as something that 'pervades, unites and directs all human dimensions' (1995, p. 810). Similarly, a study by Hungelmann et al. (1996) linked spirituality to connection and relationship:

> Spiritual well-being is a sense of harmonious interconnectedness between self, others/nature, and Ultimate Other, which exists throughout and beyond time and space. It is achieved through a dynamic and integrative growth process, which leads to a realisation of the ultimate purpose and meaning of life.
>
> (1996, p. 263)

Van Ness talks about spirituality as a quest for authentic relationships calling spirituality 'the quest for attaining an optimal relationship between what one truly is and everything that is' (1997, p. 5). While a concept analysis by Goldberg (1998) found terms associated with spirituality seemed to be linked to relationships. The need for relationships and attachments seems to be essential for human beings to thrive and Pattison (2010) suggests we should see it as centrally important to any understanding of spirituality. McSherry and Jamieson (2011) found that over 70 per cent of more than 4,000 nurses thought that the need for love and harmony was an important spiritual need.

Transcendence

Another aspect of spirituality is about the ability to feel connected to some energy, God or power outside yourself. During a time of illness or crisis this can become more necessary because seeing themselves as existing apart from their illness or disability and not consumed or overwhelmed by it, seems to help a person to cope with life-changing crises. Sometimes people say that they feel they *are* their illness and they don't exist apart from it. Being able to transcend your self can enable you to look at your situation and see its boundaries and its limits. This helps you to see it in perspective and to feel as though there's more to life than your illness; you rise above it. As well as transcending your own circumstances, spirituality is often expressed by the idea of connecting with a transcendent power or God who may be communicated with. This can be a strength in times of illness, change and crisis. Most people see God, however perceived, as benevolent and wanting the best for us. Speck calls spirituality 'a vital essence of our lives that often enables us to transcend our circumstances and find new meaning and purpose and can foster hope' (2005, p. 28).

Meaning

Reviews of the nursing literature usually show that for many people, spirituality has a lot to do with what gives life meaning (Martsolf and Mickley 1998, Meraviglia 1999). Research with patients, carers and staff usually finds that to have spiritual well-being you need to be leading a meaningful life (Govier 2000, Greasley et al. 2001). If life has meaning it is more fulfilling, adversity is easier to cope with, and at the end of our life we will have felt it well spent. If people know why they are doing something, it adds depth, gives it a purpose and makes it more enjoyable and easier. So that in times of sickness and trouble people may look for the meaning in what has happened and if they can't find a cause they will hope to find at least some purpose or good that has come out of the crisis. There may be no answer as to why a person has cancer and a reason for carrying on may, for many people, have to be found away from the search for a reason. Hope may be not necessarily for a cure, but for something else positive, like a good night's sleep, a day without pain, a few more months, or for your children to do well after you have died (Clarke 2013).

Many nurses have referred to Victor Frankl (1905–1997), a psychotherapist to learn more about meaning. Frankl reached his understanding of the importance of meaning in life during his experiences in a concentration camp. He believed that finding a meaning in suffering helped a person to cope with it. He believed the things that gave life meaning mattered, and just any meaning won't do (Clarke 2010). He said that meaning can be found in different ways: '(1) by creating a work or doing a deed; (2) by experiencing something or encountering someone; and (3) by the attitude we take toward unavoidable suffering' (Frankl 1984, p. 133). He said that to be fully human it was necessary to find a way to transcend your own self and look outward to the world. This suggests that spiritual well-being could come from thinking about others and being able to help them.

Frankl believed that relationships and meetings with other people can give life meaning and he thought that in the face of the worst suffering, each person has the internal spiritual freedom to choose his attitude towards it. The key is that someone doesn't have to always see themselves as being at the mercy of their circumstances. Even when the circumstances can't be changed, the way you feel about it can. As Frankl says: 'When we are no longer able to change a situation – just think of an incurable disease such as an inoperable cancer – we are challenged to change ourselves' (1984, p. 135).

Spiritual well-being

Spiritual well-being is often talked about in terms of having resources that enable coping in adversity. It is often spoken of as having an inner strength and this is a feature that has been subjected to research, which is also characterised as a personal resource that contributes to well-being and helps people to overcome challenges and adversity, and accept change as inevitable (Lundman *et al.* 2011). People with inner strength feel connected to family, friends, society and nature; they usually believe that there is a spiritual dimension to life and are able to transcend their own self. Having inner strength also seems to ensue from being able to find meaning in life despite setbacks and adversity (Lundman *et al.* 2011).

Sims and Cook (2009) see all these things as existing within a person and within communities, with relationships fundamental to the concept. This is how they sum up spirituality:

> a distinctive, potentially creative, and universal dimension of human experience arising both within the inner subjective awareness of individuals and within communities, social groups and traditions. It may be experienced as a relationship with that which is intimately 'inner' immanent and personal, within the self and others, and/or as relationship with that which is wholly 'other', transcendent and beyond the self. It is experienced as being of fundamental or ultimate importance and is thus concerned with matters of meaning and purpose in life, truth, and values.
>
> (p. 4)

Spiritual needs

If you believe that this centre or spirit is part of everyone and that it matters how strong and connected you feel, it makes sense to want to do what you can to nurture this part of you so that you can become more resilient. There is increasing evidence that helping people towards a sense of spiritual well-being will help them to cope with their illness or disability and to get more benefit from their treatment (Koenig 2012). However, nursing is not only about improving outcomes in terms of fewer days spent in hospital, but should also be about improving quality of life, and meeting spiritual needs can help to do this. Spiritual needs are the things that people say they need in order to achieve a feeling of spiritual well-being. In a qualitative meta-synthesis Hodge and Horvath (2011) found that clients most frequently mentioned meaning, purpose and hope as their spiritual needs; followed by relationship with something transcendent and spiritual practices and religious obligations. After that came the interpersonal connections with those around them followed by interactions with professional staff. This suggests that the most useful thing that nurses can do is first to help people to access or reconnect with the spiritual and religious resources that are important to them and then to make their own relationships and interactions with patients and clients spiritually enhancing by the empowering, compassionate and valuing behaviours described here.

Activity 12.2

Sit with a friend, or on your own, and ask these questions:

- Do you think of yourself as religious or spiritual in any way?
- Is there anything you do in your life that you would class as meeting a spiritual need?
- What spiritual resources or behaviours have helped you when you are ill or in a crisis in the past?

When you've considered these questions in relation to yourself also ask yourself the following:

- How did it feel to have to think about these answers?
- How would it feel to ask someone else?

Spirituality and religion: spirituality with and without God

In the 2011 census, 68 per cent of people said that they belonged to a religious group; a decline of 12 per cent on the previous census. This might make you think that Britain has become more sceptical and more rational, but actually the picture is more complicated. While there is less belief in religion a large number of people still believe in God or a higher power or force. Various surveys have persistently found this. For instance, research commissioned in 2013 by Theos (the think tank about religion and society) found in an England-wide survey that over one-third of people who never attend a religious service did believe in God or a Higher Power and nearly a quarter of atheists believe that humans have a soul (Theos 2013). It seems that people who are consistently non-religious and don't believe in God, never attend a religious service and don't believe in life after death, angels or the soul, make up only about 9 per cent of the population. The survey found that of a representative sample of adults in Great Britain while 62 per cent of Christians believed that spiritual forces have some influence on people and events in the natural world, 35 per cent of people who were not religious also believed the same thing (Theos 2013). This means that not only do nurses have to remember that many people without religious belief believe in a God of some sort and expect to have their spirituality respected but also have to remember that many people who don't believe in any kind of supernatural God or power, still perceive themselves to have a spiritual inner core that they wish to have acknowledged (Comte-Sponville 2007). However for many people, their inner core or spirit is expressed through beliefs and values that are part of a whole religious outlook. Nurses have been used to asking people about their religion but this modern concept of the person means that nurses have to get used to considering that all people have spiritual needs and many of them will not have a religion.

RESEARCH FOCUS 12.2

Ross and Austin explored the spiritual needs of patients with end stage heart failure by means of 47 semi-structured interviews with 16 end stage heart failure patients and their carers as well as in focus groups with other stakeholders. They found that the participants were struggling with spiritual concerns as well as the physical and emotional challenges of their illness. These concerns related to love, belonging, hope, coping, meaning, faith, belief and the future. As the patients' condition deteriorated the emphasis shifted from 'fighting' the illness to making the most of the time left. They said that their spiritual concerns could have been addressed by having someone to talk to, supporting their carers and by staff showing sensitivity and taking care to foster hope. These patients experienced significant spiritual needs and would have welcomed spiritual care within the palliative care package (Ross and Austin 2013).

Janice Clarke

Spiritual care
is the collection of
practices and
behaviours that are
generally seen as
aimed towards
helping someone to
find spiritual well-
being so that they
have the strength
and resilience to
cope with the crisis
they are in.

Spiritual care

Nursing has to respond to movements in society that change the needs of the people it cares for, and this contemporary idea of what a person is means that individuals are more demanding about how they want to be treated and looked after. They expect this deeper part of themselves to be cared for as well as their mind and their body and they feel that something is lacking if that doesn't happen. Most people would say they wanted to be cared for as a whole person and not just as a set of symptoms, a problem or as though they are nothing more than a biological machine; talking about their spirituality or spiritual needs is one way of expressing this. From the nurse's point of view, giving attention to the spiritual dimension of a person and of life in general has the potential to refocus the practitioner on the human aspects of care instead of only the technological or systems aspects. It is also equally relevant to practitioners as it is to patients because being able to give care in a spiritual way enhances the spiritual well-being not only of patients but also of practitioners themselves. An awareness of the spiritual dimension of life helps nurses to give spiritual care. In caring for patients with complex and challenging spiritual problems it is particularly necessary, and nurses with a strong feeling of spiritual well-being might well be able to help patients and clients with complex problems even more.

Spiritual care is the collection of practices and behaviours that are generally seen as aimed towards helping someone to find spiritual well-being so that they have the strength and resilience to cope with the crisis they are in. This often means helping them to find or use their own spiritual resources, which can help them to nurture that part of themselves, to connect to the people around them or to their notions of God, or to find their own sense of meaning in their life. Feeling valued and important as a person makes you feel confirmed and acknowledged and so adds to this sense of well-being and resilience. Therefore spiritual care can be embedded in all the caring activities that nurses undertake, from giving an injection to washing someone's hands, as long as these acts are performed with respect for the whole person: maintaining their dignity; valuing their opinion; empowering them and including them. Explained like this an understanding of spirituality and spiritual care may have the potential to put something back into nursing that many people perceive as missing (Swinton and Pattison 2010). It also has the potential to help nurses to imagine what it means to suffer and to offer a way to understand and reconnect with the people we care for as whole persons and not only as sets of needs and symptoms caught in a system that has the tendency to be less and less compassionate (Rolfe and Gardner 2014).

Spirituality has been absorbed into the nursing process so that it is often understood as being to do with specific needs that a person has and assessing their needs and planning their care accordingly. However it can also be seen as a way of being, an attitude and a desire to care for a patient in a way that could itself be seen as spiritual. While spirituality is often thought of as being exclusively concerned with talking, it is also about how physical care is performed. This is possible because a person is made up of body, mind and spirit in a way that each part interacts with the other. We know, for instance, that when we are physically hurt we feel emotionally hurt also and in the same way, how a nurse cares for you when they care for your body, can affect your mind and your spirit. The model (Figure 12.1) shows how the parts of a person are embedded in each other and constantly interacting with each other.

While spirituality is a matter of concern for all health care professions, nurses have unique opportunities to practise spiritual care that are not open to other health care

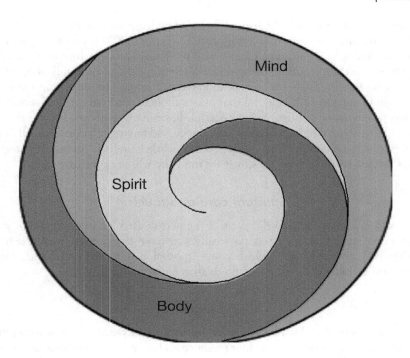

FIGURE 12.1
Integrated model
of a person
Source: Clarke
2013.

professionals because of the nurse's unique position in patients' lives. Nurses are with patients when they are at their most vulnerable and ashamed, as Graham was (Case 12.1), and nurses are uniquely able to touch and care for people when they are helping a person to wash, move and eat, in a way that other health professionals are not.

Spiritual care can help patients to find some meaning in what's happening to them, which can help them cope with their illness or disability better. Having spiritual resources can help patients to achieve better health outcomes and so it makes sense for nurses to help people find or reconnect with these resources, which may be religious. Nurses have the opportunity to help patients practise their religion and so can have an influential effect on the things that help a patient. The aim of nursing is to put patients in the best possible position for treatment to have the most positive effect, and meeting spiritual needs can help to do this.

What patients want

Reading about spiritual care is often reading about nurse-initiated discussions, but the nurses in Noble and Jones (2010) study thought that spiritual care should be guided by what patients want. The patients with cancer in Taylor and Mamier's (2005) study said that what they wanted more than talk was for the nurse to enable them to take care of their own spiritual development by providing quiet times and humour, and help them to reconnect with spiritual resources. These patients didn't particularly want to discuss spiritual concerns and they didn't want nurses encouraging them to talk by suggesting drawing or writing about spirituality. Taylor and Mamier found that patients seemed to want nurses to be a particular way rather than to overtly perform particularly spiritual tasks. For example, the patients in Conco's (1995) study described spiritual care as taking

Janice Clarke

time, being present and available, using touch and giving good nursing care. What these patients wanted most was a sense of connection. Tanyi (2002) found that patients saw spiritual care as displaying genuine caring, with patience, kindness, listening, smiling and giving information among other caring skills. While some did want to talk about it, many didn't, and those who did want to talk didn't think it was the most important thing. McSherry and Jamieson (2011) found that nurses thought spiritual care was mostly a case of helping people to have hope, being cheerful, listening to patients, having respect for privacy and dignity, giving support and reassurance and having relationships; all of which can be described as ordinary nursing care. So that while being able to talk about spiritual concerns matters in some situations, it is far from the whole of spiritual care.

Spiritual care and touch

In the model in Figure 12.1, all the parts of the person are seen as integrated – you can see that when you touch a person physically you have the potential to 'touch' them spiritually. Any physical care could become spiritual if it is performed with care and attention and genuine concern about the person being touched.

Presence

Presence is a term used to describe when you are not only physically present with someone but you have put your whole self in their presence and are giving them your full attention. When you are really present, you are making yourself completely available to another person. You can be really present with someone in a fleeting moment or in a short conversation. People can usually tell whether you are fully 'with them' or whether you're thinking of something else. Using eye contact is one way of expressing that you are fully present with someone. Another way is to pay careful attention to what they are saying.

Talking about spiritual needs

Nurses and midwives learn about patients' hopes, dreams, expectations, values, beliefs and how they live out their beliefs through getting to know them and relating to them as persons. Practitioners have to be able to create environments and relationships where patients feel free and confident to talk about personal issues when they want. To prompt a discussion about spirituality can feel daunting. Spirituality can be a difficult topic to talk about because it is so ambiguous and reactions to it vary. Some people think about it a lot and some not at all. There are a wide range of beliefs about the subject. It can help to start off with concrete and easily discussed questions and prompts and to be open to when and if the patient wants to move on to more personal beliefs. One patient in Tanyi *et al.*'s study said:

> the easiest way is just to ask, and if they [patients] are open with it, that's fine, and if they are not, well that's another sign, too, that they, you know, that they have a different way of coping with things.
>
> (2006, p. 535)

One way of starting off a conversation would be to ask a patient whether they think of themselves as spiritual or religious in any way and inviting them to explain. Then you could follow this up by asking what they use to help them in bad situations. They may tell you about anything from prayer to walking, being with their family to listening to music. Your role is then to help them to continue or reconnect with whatever spiritual resources they think may help.

A person's spirituality is deeply enmeshed in their personality and affected by their life circumstances and history. Major issues that affect spirituality are age, religious belief, illness and particularly the presence of any mental illness.

Some factors that affect a person's spiritual needs

Age and spiritual care

Case 12.2

Linda was 6 years old when she started to think about God. She was sitting looking at a butterfly in the garden and started to wonder if it knew it was a butterfly and knew it was in a garden in the afternoon. That made her think about how she came to be there, in that garden and if it was planned or an accident.

> Then I started to think about God and I suddenly realised why it mattered whether you believed in God or not. I thought of the word 'God' because I couldn't think of any other word to describe it. My parents weren't religious, we didn't go to church. But they listened to me when I said I had decided to believe in God. They just put up with it. It would have been terrible if anyone had laughed. When I went into hospital the nurse asked me if I said any prayers and I told her I said a prayer at night. She said that was very important and she'd tell the other nurses to pull my curtains round my bed after the lights went out, just for a couple of minutes if I wanted. I was glad, it made me feel better.

Children and young people are forming their identities and their spiritual needs are for security and confidence in their carers to enable them to do this effectively. Touch and the responsiveness of adults towards them has been shown to be important in this process and babies who are not touched and responded to develop insecure personalities (Autton 1989, National Scientific Council on the Developing Child 2012). Young people facing illness and disability are at risk of severe threats to their feeling of security and self-esteem, just at the time when these things are forming (Pridmore and Pridmore 2004). Spiritual care for children is therefore based around increasing and maintaining self-esteem, building trust and security, and in babies, using touch and affection. Enabling young people to make as many choices as possible is empowering and also increases self-esteem. Children have a developing sense of the spiritual from a very young age and Linda is an example of this. It should also be remembered that children may have spiritual practices they have learnt in their family such as prayer and attending services and keeping fasts. The more nurses can help children to maintain these things the stronger will be their spiritual well-being (Hay and Nye 2006). They may wonder about the meaning of life and these ponderings should be taken seriously and encouraged.

Older people are attempting to come to terms with the end of their life and need time and space to reflect. But they also still need to feel valued, respected and useful. This is the biggest problem for older people as in our society older people are often marginalised and even abused (Nygren *et al.* 2007). Again enabling choices, showing respect by being interested, including in the flow of life and conversation and caring for older bodies with as much care as younger ones, all add to the feeling of being valued and increase self-worth.

Mental health and spiritual care

Sims and Cook (2009, p. 10) explain how spirituality and religion can improve mental health. Spirituality and religion:

1 promote a positive world view;
2 help to make sense of difficult situations;
3 give purpose and meaning;
4 discourage maladaptive coping;
5 enhance social support;
6 promote 'other directedness';
7 help to release the need for control;
8 provide and encourage forgiveness;
9 encourage thankfulness;
10 provide hope.

Sims and Cook (2009) draw on Koenig's review of 1,200 studies and 400 reviews, which demonstrate that being involved in a religion seems to have positive correlations with happiness, life satisfaction, higher self-esteem, finding positive meaning, development of hope and optimism, adjusting to bereavement, having more social support and less loneliness, less depression and faster recovery when depressed, less suicide and less psychosis. It is less easy to research the effects of non-religious spirituality, as there are fewer definable ways of identifying spiritual practices and beliefs. However, the consensus in mental health care seems to be that understanding patients' beliefs and their involvement in religious and spiritual activities and encouraging and facilitating patients to continue with them, should permeate all aspects of psychiatric care (Swinton 2001, Sims and Cook 2009).

Spiritual care in helping people to recover from mental illness is concerned with helping someone to marshal their own spiritual resources, and the way you are with people with mental illness can also affect how patients recover and how they experience their illness. Relating to the whole person in the fullness of their whole being, accepting them and taking their thoughts, feelings and beliefs seriously is the starting point (Swinton 2001).

Death, dying and spiritual care

Being close to death brings a person face-to-face with the meaning of their existence and the pain of leaving loved ones behind. Death is seen as a time to review past life and people may believe that what happens to you after death will depend on how you have

---

RESEARCH FOCUS 12.3

Raffay (2014), a hospital chaplain, conducted a literature review exploring how staff and patient experience shapes our perception of spiritual care in a psychiatric setting. The following themes emerged:

1   Spiritual care may contain a religious element.
2   The work of chaplains and wider religious links were seen as important.
3   Spirituality occurs within a diverse spiritual/cultural context.
4   Training needs to be provided.
5   The relationship between service user and staff is more important in spiritual care than the tool used.
6   Staff often struggle both with the concept and with the current assessment tools that have a number of deficiencies.
7   If we are to understand spirituality and spiritual care, we need to engage with user experience.
8   It is important to understand how spirituality functions in a person's life.

---

lived your life. Consequently the time immediately before death may be seen as a time of preparation when people may want to make their peace with family or God. Some religions offer rituals of preparation and forgiveness such as anointing and blessing with oil. At the end of life, there are often important rituals associated with the moment of death, the preparation of the body after death and the timing of burial (DH 2009). Within a religious mind-set, death may not be final. There are many beliefs surrounding death and the afterlife, and many rituals and prayers have grown over the centuries to ease the transition from life to death for both the dying and those left behind.

Religious beliefs

Being religious is one way of being spiritual for many people. For a person who has religious beliefs this is an essential and core part of their life so it can't be ignored. Religions are practical and beliefs are expressed through many practical aspects of life, such as rituals, fasts, feasts, festivals and prayers. Lots of different guidance tells nurses that they should be respectful of people's beliefs, and to do that it's necessary to know a little about religions. Religions are not all the same (Prothero 2011) and it's not possible to know everything about all religions or even everything about one of them, but it is necessary to have an idea how religion might affect a person's life. More information can then be gained by asking the patient or reading about it. There is lots of information about religions on the Internet and in books. Religion may affect decisions at the start of life in respect of the type of contraception chosen, whether abortion or fertility treatment is acceptable and genetic testing (DH 2009). During treatment, religious beliefs can affect decisions about drugs because some drugs are based on alcohol, porcine products and gelatine, which may be prohibited in Islam and Judaism. Oral non-kosher medication can be problematic

Janice Clarke

Liturgy
This is the formal religious services and ritual, which exists in many religions. Today it can also be a form of prayer that a chaplain might work out with an individual to help them express thanks to a God they may not even be sure exists. A person who didn't previously think of themselves as religious may suddenly want to ask for God's help or guidance and a chaplain can help them to express their thoughts.

for Jewish people and blood products are prohibited for Jehovah's Witnesses (DH 2009). Religious beliefs may affect end of life decisions such as the amount of analgesia and sedation a person wants; whether they want their life to be prolonged, and the kind of interventions they would accept for themselves and their family. Being able to live your life as you choose according to your beliefs in itself enhances spiritual well-being and religious people should be helped to pray, worship, meditate and live, as they would at home, in an atmosphere of freedom and tolerance.

Religions should not be seen just as a social group or an interest or a prop in a person's life; they are a way of connecting with a sacred force and whether you believe this or not, you should try to respect the fact that this is how your patients see it (Clarke 2013). This is called seeing religions substantively and not just functionally. If you're going to be able to respect the beliefs of those you care for you have to take them seriously. But this doesn't mean believing in those things yourself. People will feel valued if you take an interest in their beliefs and ask questions. They will appreciate it if you help them to practise their religion in the way they live and enable them to have the privacy to pray, to meet with their priest, to attend a worship service, to continue with a fast or to celebrate a feast. At times of illness and crisis, religions can be particularly important and religious communities can be very supportive and there is a lot of evidence that religious belief helps in times of illness. So nurses should be doing everything they can to help people to continue with or reconnect with religious practices.

The role of the chaplain

Historically all health care facilities would have had access to a chaplain to help staff manage the religious concerns of their patients. However, in recent years chaplains have become more diverse in their approach and now tend to see themselves as spiritual care workers able to help patients and staff with all sorts of issues related to spirituality and not just religious issues. Chaplains aim to help people to find wholeness and inter-connection and as such their aims are the same as other health practitioners (Newitt 2010). Chaplains have a different role, different skills and different opportunities to provide spiritual care. Their specialist skills enable them to talk more easily about spirituality and as it is their main role, they are likely to have more time to focus on talking and listening. You can refer patients to chaplains, not just when they have specific religious needs but when they have spiritual needs that will need more conversation and more specialist skills than you are able to give. As **liturgy** specialists chaplains can also help people to mark transitions and events in their lives. Remember that many people have religious beliefs but they may not see themselves as part of a religion and chaplains are skilled in helping people to identify, clarify and express their beliefs without exerting any pressure to choose any particular religion or institution. They work with people to write prayers and liturgy when the traditional services of the orthodox religions don't seem right. There are often chaplains available from a variety of different religions but they are usually happy to talk to anyone, including staff. Many people today feel they need some means of thanking, worshipping, asking forgiveness of, raging against, or imploring a God who they are not sure they even believe in. So chaplains can be a source of help for everyone. The NHS publishes chaplaincy guidelines entitled 'Promoting Excellence in Pastoral, Spiritual & Religious Care' (NHS 2015).

PART 3: EXPLORING SPIRITUAL CARE

Definitions of spiritual care

Spirituality is about subjective experience that is hard to describe. It is about subtle feelings and by its very nature is nebulous and changeable. It could be said to be inherently a subversive concept because it seems to work against some trends in society such as technology, systematisation and materialistic acquisition, and similarly it resists attempts at tight definition. Definitions have the tendency to fix a single idea of a concept, which then influences research and definitions, excluding further debate. There have been many definitions of spirituality put forward by nursing academics but they have tended to be influenced by the world view and belief system of the person promoting them. They have usually not been tested on a broad enough range of participants. Consequently each definition could be rejected by some groups who feel it doesn't apply to them or represent their religion, world view or culture (Clarke 2009). Some theorists have tried to apply to spirituality the same criteria as they would any scientific concept and have called for a universal definition that can make research easier (McSherry and Draper 1998); others have argued that having a concise definition of a tricky concept like spirituality has a seductive attraction because it seems to increase understanding. Still others have argued that if definitions try to be universal and represent everyone, they become big and cumbersome and impossible to make use of in practice (Clarke 2009). Scholars have increasingly suggested that it might be better to think about descriptions of spirituality as marking out an area of thinking about which there is actually little that can easily be concretely described. Swinton and Pattison (2010), for example, say that it describes qualities or attitudes that are missing from modern health care practice. However, despite there being no universally agreed definition of spirituality, there are characteristics or family resemblances among descriptions that have remained the same over decades of research. These include the ideas of connection, transcendence and meaning discussed earlier in this chapter. A more important question about spirituality in health care is the question of what use it is and whether it can be turned to value in health care so that patients benefit from practitioners paying any attention to it. So it may be that a vague definition is fine, but it must be useful (Swinton and Pattison 2010).

One criticism of the concept of spiritual care related to the issue of definitions has been that it is indistinguishable from emotional or psychological care. Others have argued that there is a use for the term because it marks out a territory that doesn't easily fit into descriptions of emotional or psychological care (Clarke 2013). However it has to be acknowledged that there is an overlap between spiritual well-being and other forms of well-being. The type of care described in this chapter constitutes spiritual care because it aims to affect what patients perceive as their 'spirit'. Users of health services tend to agree that a part of them exists that is not only emotional or psychological but which is all these things and something more. It is also care designed to help a service user into a state of mind where they may be able to connect or reconnect with some kind of being or force or belief about such a being, if this fits with the person's mind-set, which potentially could be a help in times of crisis.

Debate about the place of spirituality in a secular society

There is a debate about whether spirituality and spiritual care is just a way to smuggle religious beliefs and biases into the way nursing is conducted. Some have thought that there wasn't any need to identify a thing called spiritual care because this was just psychological and emotional care and the reason for its introduction was to increase the profile of religion in health care. Paley (2008) has argued that it is entirely possible to reduce spirituality and spiritual care to psychological and social care and that the current way spirituality has been adopted by health care is not evidence-based or scientific. He argues with the way that in the current approach in nursing, the concept is considered universal, so that everyone must have spirituality regardless of whether they think they do or not and with the way in which spirituality has come to be associated with every aspect of human life. He also takes issue with the lack of critical analysis in discussions about what spirituality is, as have others (Clarke 2009). He has argued that the main identifying characteristic of spirituality is that it is to do with a transcendental, higher being (which may be called God) and as the health service is a secular service (no longer run by religious institutions) and the UK is a secular, post-Christian society, there is no place for spirituality in health care (Paley 2007). Therefore it should not be part of assessment systems or needs-based care planning.

Others (Ross 2008) have argued that spirituality is not wholly to do with religion and is not 'undercover' religion but that it expresses a way of being and believing that many patients and staff identify with and so it does deserve to be a part of holistic care. They have argued that it enhances nursing care and it describes an approach to care and an aspect of the person that it's not possible to describe with the tools we already have (Clarke 2013, Swinton and Pattison 2010). In other words they have argued that it cannot be reduced to psychology and sociology but that it is separate and different from these things. This is a pragmatic approach, which recognises the ubiquity of the term and seeks to find a meaningful use for it. This chapter is an example of this more pragmatic approach, because it seeks to put the idea of spirituality to the service of nursing as a means to help nurses understand why relationships with patients and acting compassionately is important. It is certainly the case, as has been mentioned earlier, that not only religious people have an interest in spirituality but that many non-religious people believe in a power or energy in the world that they may not call 'God' (Theos 2013) and they express the wish to have spiritual needs recognised even though they may consider themselves to be secular and even to be atheists (Comte-Sponville 2007). This complex picture has triggered much discussion about what it means to be secular and the relationship between spirituality and religion. The picture is not as straightforward as it appeared decades ago when people were accepted to be either religious or atheists and there wasn't a recognised place in between.

Religion and spirituality

From the earliest days of the study of spirituality in health care there has been a fear by protagonists of a secular approach to spirituality that the concept may be taken over by religious belief and religious imagery. This has resulted in a tendency to explain spirituality by differentiating it from religion and there have been strenuous efforts to maintain a distance between the two concepts (Walter 1997). However, while it is certainly true that spiritual beliefs and a spiritual outlook are not the exclusive domain of those people belonging to religions, it is a mistake to try to claim that spirituality has nothing to do with religion. The term spirituality was used exclusively by religions for generations before the modern adoption of the term and it was used to express the subjective, personal, experiential aspects of religious belief. Consequently it could be said that it is spiritual beliefs, outlooks and world views that underpin each religion. Therefore it is confusing to speak of religion and spirituality as opposites or as having nothing in common. Religions are simply one way of being spiritual in the world. If spirituality is a way to explain a human desire to connect with something sacred and transcendent and to explain how human beings are connected in the world, religions are ways in which that desire has been formalised, directed and explained over centuries of experience by particular communities of believers.

In order to differentiate spirituality and religion, theorists have had to define religion in opposition to spirituality and this has led to some mistaken assumptions about religion (Clarke 2006). Religion has been studied in depth by sociologists, psychologists, anthropologists and scholars of religious studies for decades and a number of approaches to explaining religion have been debated. Nursing scholars have not tended to refer to these debates and have defined religion very narrowly as a social, psychological or cultural phenomenon. While religion is certainly related to all these things, this is not its purpose. The purpose of religion is to connect with something sacred and this is how most religious people would see it. Therefore to be respectful to religious people it's important to try to see their religion from their point of view, which is as something immensely spiritual in their lives and not just a lifestyle choice (Clarke 2006).

A good definition of religion is this one from Berger, a sociologist:

> Religion is the human enterprise by which a sacred cosmos is established. Put differently, religion is cosmization in a sacred mode. By sacred is meant here a quality of mysterious and awesome power, other than man and yet related to him, which is believed to reside in certain objects of experience. The sacred cosmos is confronted by man as an immensely powerful reality other than himself. Yet this reality addresses itself to him and locates his life in an ultimately meaningful order.
>
> (1973, pp. 34–35)

One of the consequences of treating religion in a functionalist and reductionist way and not taking it seriously is that all religions tend to be treated as meaning the same thing when they often have very different approaches to life (Prothero 2011). Another consequence is that there is a tendency to think that religions can be broken down into lists of practices, rules and rituals. Whereas there are as many differences between people of the same religion as there are between religions and so the list approach is not very helpful. When you encounter a religious believer you need to find out how they practise their religion. Most patients would be pleased to talk about their religious practices and would be willing to explain; this shows you are interested and think it's important to know what fasts, rituals, food and hygiene rules and beliefs are important to them. It is useful to have individual information and an overall idea of why it is that someone has faith in God and why they want to follow a religion in order to understand the role it has in that person's life and how important it in their decision-making. It is also useful to be able to understand why people fast, pray or celebrate in particular ways so that you might learn how it will affect their health or management rather than to try to learn about all the details of the fast and feasts of particular religions. Taking the trouble to find out a lot about a particular religion makes sense if you work in an area where you have a lot of patients of that religion.

Janice Clarke

Activity 12.3

Members of the Muslim religion fast from food and drink from daybreak to sunset during the period of Ramadan. Lent is a time for Christian fasting. In some Christian denominations people try to give up some food that is important to them during Lent and in others, for instance, Eastern Orthodoxy, there is a strict vegan diet during Lent.

- Try to find out the reason for fasting and what believers hope to achieve.
- Find out what effect fasting can have on a person physically and emotionally and also whether there are any health benefits or health risks.
- How might your care of a Muslim diabetic patient change during Ramadan?

Why nurses find spiritual care difficult and what can be done about it

In many studies asking about experience of giving spiritual care, nurses report difficulties with understanding what spirituality is and with giving spiritual care (McSherry and Jamieson 2011, Noble and Jones 2010). McSherry has identified many of the barriers to giving spiritual care such as lack of privacy and embarrassment in talking about spiritual needs and the emotional demands and the fear this invokes. The most commonly repeated barrier cited is lack of confidence to give spiritual care because they feel poorly educated on the subject specifically in how to assess spirituality (McSherry and Jamieson 2011). When you consider that the model of giving spiritual care that most nurses recognise is one based on talking to patients, it's not surprising that lack of privacy and lack of confidence in their competence is a barrier. But realistically time and privacy are always going to be hard to provide, and education is expensive with staffing levels such that staff cannot be released for education. In addition, it seems that even when education on the subject is provided, nurses still say that they don't feel prepared. This suggests that the subject is so difficult to talk about that many nurses will feel they haven't had enough education about it no matter how much they have had. One tendency among nurses when finding talk about spirituality difficult is that they revert to talk about religion, which is more concrete. Therefore it makes sense to explore different ways of giving spiritual care, which are not so focused on having time to talk such as the way of giving spiritual care described in this chapter.

The reason for the strong focus on talking in the current approach to spiritual care may be because nurses have taken chaplains and counsellors as their role models but of course nursing is very different and based on a set of practical skills and so an approach that sees spiritual care as embedded in everything that nurses do would seem more appropriate. Some have argued for this more practical approach (Clarke 2013). Spiritual care has come to be seen as an add-on to everything else nurses do and as such it can seem like a burden and an extra responsibility when nurses are already under pressure. But seeing it as integrated into all the tasks and relationships of nursing and building on the strengths, opportunities and skills of nursing instead of emulating how other professions do it, may be a better way forward. This is the type of approach discussed in this chapter. Using the model of a person described earlier (Figure 12.1), it can be seen that a person's spirituality can be affected by how they are cared for, as much as how they are talked to. Such an approach would also have the potential of improving the quality of nursing care and nursing relationships in every situation.

However, there will always be a place for talking and finding out more about patients' spiritual needs in a more formal way. This might be termed spiritual assessment although this term has unfortunate connotations of measurement, which arguably is not appropriate. Culliford (2009) has devised a simple tool for medical students, which nurses might find helpful. There are many tools and a lot of literature about spiritual assessment (McSherry and Ross 2010), but it is still a way of talking that can seem invasive and that many nurses are not comfortable with.

CONCLUSION

This chapter has explored what spirituality, spiritual needs and spiritual care are, with a look at why these terms are even used today and why patients and nurses think they matter. An approach to spiritual care that is practical and embedded in everything a nurse does has been described because it is more suited to the way that nurses work. Some of the debates and controversies about spirituality and spiritual care have been examined. This is truly care that is spiritual and a pragmatic way of providing the benefits of spiritual care in the busy pressured health care settings that most nurses work in today.

SUGGESTED FURTHER READING

Websites

All the major religions have their own websites. For example:
Jehovah's Witnesses www.jw-org
The BBC website has lots of information about religions www.bbc.co.uk/religion/religions/islam/
Theos is a think tank that seeks to inform the debate about the place of religion in society www.theosthinktank.co.uk/

Texts

Taylor, E. J. (ed.) (2012) *Religion: A clinical guide for nurses*. New York: Springer.
 This book gives a practical overview of most religions with advice about how each set of religious beliefs affect care in circumstances such as health and well-being, illness, and death and dying.
Fowler, M. D., Reimer-Kirkjam, S., Sawatzky, R. and Taylor, E. J. (2012) *Religion, Religious Ethics, and Nursing*. New York: Springer.
 This book gives a more in-depth exploration of religion in general with an analysis of the theological and ethical beliefs of the major religions. It goes on to examine how these might affect the care patients expect and the care that nurses from that religion give.

REFERENCES

Autton, N. (1989) *Touch: An exploration*. London: Darton, Longman & Todd.
Berger, P. L. (1973) *Social Reality of Religion*. Middlesex: Penguin Books.

Bottorff, J. (1991) The lived experience of being comforted by a nurse. *Phenomenology and Pedagogy* **9**, 237–252.

Clarke, J. (2006) Religion and spirituality: a discussion paper about negativity, reductionism and differentiation in nursing texts. *International Journal of Nursing Studies* **43** (6), 775–785.

Clarke, J. (2009) A critical view of how nursing has defined spirituality. *Journal of Clinical Nursing* **18** (12), 1666–1673.

Clarke, J. (2010) Body and soul in mental health care, *Mental Health, Religion and Culture* **13** (6), 649–657.

Clarke, J. (2013) *Spiritual Care in Everyday Nursing Practice: A new approach.* Basingstoke: Palgrave Macmillan.

Comte-Sponville, A. (2007) *The Book of Atheist Spirituality.* London: Bantam Books.

Conco, D. (1995) Christian patients' views of spiritual care. *Western Journal of Nursing Research* **17** (3), 266–275.

Culliford, L. (2009) Teaching spirituality and health care to third year medical students. *The Clinical Teacher* **6** (1), 22–27.

de Hennezel, M. (1998) *Intimate Death: How the dying teach us to live.* London: Warner Books.

DH (Department of Health) (2009) *Religion or Belief: A practical guide for the NHS.* London: DH.

Drew, N. (1986) Exclusion and confirmation: a phenomenology of patients' experiences with caregivers. *Image: Journal of Nursing Scholarship* **18** (2), 39–43.

Frankl, V. (1984) *Man's Search for Meaning.* New York: Washington Square Press.

Goddard, N. C. (1995) Spirituality as integrative energy: a philosophical analysis as requisite precursor to holistic nursing practice. *Journal of Advanced Nursing* **22** (4), 808–815.

Goldberg, B. (1998) Connection: an exploration of spirituality in nursing care. *Journal of Advanced Nursing* **27** (4), 836–842.

Govier, I. (2000) Spiritual care in nursing: a systematic approach. *Nursing Standard* **14** (17), 32–36.

Greasley, P., Chiu, L. F. and Gartland, M. (2001) The concept of spiritual care in mental health nursing. *Journal of Advanced Nursing* **33** (5), 629–637.

Hay, D. and Nye, R. (2006) *The Spirit of the Child* (Revised edn). London: Jessica Kingsley.

Heelas, P. and Woodhead, L. (2005) *The Spiritual Revolution: Why religion is giving way to spirituality.* Oxford: Blackwell.

Hodge, D. R. and Horvath, V. E. (2011) Spiritual needs in health care settings: a qualitative meta-synthesis of clients' perspectives. *Social Work.* **56** (4), 306–316.

Hungelmann, J., Kenkel-Rossi, E., Klassen, L. and Stollenwerk, R. (1996) Focus on spiritual well-being: harmonious interconnectedness of mind-body-spirit. Use of the JAREL spiritual well-being scale. *Geriatric Nursing* **17** (6), 262–266.

Koenig, H. G. (2012) Religion, spirituality, and health: the research and clinical implications. *ISRN psychiatry* **2012**, Article ID 278730. doi: 10.5402/2012/278730

Leppanen-Montgomery, C. (1991) The care-giving relationship: paradoxical and transcendent aspects. *Journal of Transpersonal Psychology.* **23** (2), 91–104.

Lundman, B., Viglund, K., Alex, L., Jonsen, E., Norberg, A. Fischer, A. S., Strandberg, G. and Nygren, B. (2011) Development and psychometric properties of the Inner Strength Scale. *International Journal of Nursing Studies* **48** (10), 1266–1274.

McCabe, C. and Timmins, F. (2006) *Communication Skills for Nursing Practice.* Basingstoke: Palgrave Macmillan.

McSherry, W. and Draper, P. (1998) The debates emerging from the literature surrounding the concept of spirituality as applied to nursing. *Journal of Advanced Nursing* **27** (4), 683–691.

McSherry, W. and Ross, L. (2010) *Spiritual Assessment in Healthcare Practice.* Keswick, UK: M&K Publishing.

McSherry, W. and Jamieson, S. (2011) An online survey of nurses' perceptions of spirituality and spiritual care. *Journal of Clinical Nursing* **20** (11/12), 1757–1767.

Martsolf, D. S. and Mickley, J. R. (1998) The concept of spirituality in nursing theories: differing world-views and extent of focus. *Journal of Advanced Nursing* **27** (2), 294–303.

Meraviglia, M. G. (1999) Critical analysis of spirituality and its empirical indicators. *Journal of Holistic Nursing*, **17** (1), 18–33.

National Health Service England (2015) *NHS Chaplaincy guidelines 2015: Promoting excellence in pastoral, spiritual & religious care*. www.nhs-chaplaincy-spiritualcare.org.uk/News_and_Events/nhs_chaplaincy_guidelines_2015.pdf (accessed 15 January 2016).

National Scientific Council on the Developing Child (2012) *The Science of Neglect: The persistent absence of responsive care disrupts the developing brain: Working paper 12*. www.developingchild. harvard.edu (accessed 15 January 2016).

Newitt, M. (2010) The role and skills of a hospital chaplain: reflections based on a case study. *Practical Theology* **3** (2), 163–177.

NMC (Nursing and Midwifery Council) (2015) *The Code: Professional standards of practice and behaviour for nurses and midwives*. London: NMC.

Noble, A. and Jones, C. (2010) Getting it right: oncology nurses' understanding of spirituality. *International Journal of Palliative Nursing* **16** (11), 565–569.

Nygren, B., Norberg, A. and Lundman, B. (2007) Inner strength as disclosed in narratives of the oldest old. *Qualitative Health Research* **17** (8), 1060–1073.

O'Lynn, C. and Krautscheid, L. (2011) 'How should I touch you?': a qualitative study of attitudes on intimate touch in nursing. *American Journal of Nursing* **111** (3), 24–31.

Paley, J. (2007) Spirituality and secularisation: nursing and the sociology of religion. *Journal of Clinical Nursing* **17** (20), 175–186.

Paley, J. (2008) Spirituality and nursing: a reductionist approach. *Nursing Philosophy* **9** (1), 3–18.

Pattison, S. (2010) Spirituality and spiritual care made simple: a suggestive, normative and essentialist approach. *Practical Theology* **3** (3), 351–366.

Piepgras, R. (1968) The other dimension: spiritual health. *American Journal of Nursing* **68** (12), 2610–2613.

Pridmore, P. and Pridmore, J. (2004) Promoting the spiritual development of sick children. *International Journal of Children's Spirituality* **9** (1), 21–38.

Prothero, S. (2011) *God is Not One: The eight rival religions that run the world and why their differences matter*. New York: HarperCollins.

Raffay, J. (2014) How staff and patient experience shapes our perception of spiritual care in a psychiatric setting. *Journal of Nursing Management* **22** (7), 940–950.

Rolfe, G. and Gardner, L. (2014) The compassion deficit and what to do about it: a response to Paley. *Nursing Philosophy* **15** (4), 288–297.

Ross, L. (1997) *Nurses Perception of Health Care*. Aldershot: Avebury.

Ross, L. (2008) Commentary on Paley, J. (2008) Spirituality and secularization: nursing and the sociology of religion. *Journal of Clinical Nursing* **17** (20), 175–186.

Ross, L. and Austin, J. (2013) Spiritual needs and spiritual support preferences of people with end-stage heart failure and their carers: implications for nurse managers. *Journal of Nursing Management* **23** (1), 87–95.

Sims, A. and Cook, C. C. H. (2009) Spirituality in psychiatry. In Cook, C. C. H., Powell, A. and Sims, A. (eds) *Spirituality and Psychiatry*. London: Royal College of Psychiatrists, pp. 1–15.

Speck, P. (2005) The evidence base for spiritual care. *Nursing Management* **12** (6), 28–31.

Stein, M. (2008) *The Lonely Patient: How we experience illness*. New York: Harper Perennial.

Starr, S. S. (2008) Authenticity: a concept analysis. *Nursing Forum* **43** (2), 55–62.

Swinton, J. (2001) *Spirituality and Mental Health Care: Rediscovering a 'forgotten' dimension*. London: Jessica Kingsley.

Swinton, J. and Pattison, S. (2010) Moving beyond clarity: towards a thin, vague, and useful understanding of spirituality in nursing care. *Nursing Philosophy* **11** (4), 226–237.

Tanyi, R. (2002) Towards a clarification of the meaning of spirituality. *Journal of Advanced Nursing*. **39** (5), 500–509.

Tanyi, R. A., Stehle-Werner, J., Gentry-Recine, A. C. and Sperstad, R. A. (2006) Perceptions of incorporating spirituality into their care: a phenomenological study of female patients on hemodialysis. *Nephrology Nursing Journal* **33** (5), 532–538.

Janice Clarke

Taylor, E. J. and Mamier, I. (2005) Spiritual care nursing: what cancer patients and family caregivers want. *Journal of Advanced Nursing* **49** (3), 260–267.
Theos (2013) *The Spirit of Things Unseen: Belief in post-religious Britain*. London: Theos.
Twigg, J. (2000) *Bathing, the Body and Community Care*. London: Routledge.
Van Ness, P. H. (ed.) (1996) *Spirituality and the Secular Quest*. London: SCM Press.
Walter, T. (1997) The ideology and organisation of spiritual care: three approaches. *Palliative Medicine* **11** (1), 21–30.

13

JUDGEMENT AND DECISION-MAKING

*Pádraig MacNeela, P. Anne Scott, Gerard Clinton,
David Pontin and Derek Sellman*

LEARNING OUTCOMES

After reading and reflecting on this chapter, you should be able to:

*   identify and discuss the kinds of clinical judgements and decisions that arise in nursing practice;
*   describe the field of judgement and decision-making research;
*   identify how context influences judgement and decision-making;
*   discuss the main approaches, trends and findings of judgement and decision-making research in nursing.

INTRODUCTION

Judgement and decision-making (JDM) is part of everyday nursing. It encompasses the full range from the mundane to the complex and much of this JDM activity remains unnoticed, undocumented or based on a storehouse of knowledge increasingly reliant on personal experience. For example, many judgements and decisions are carried out repeatedly, within the familiar routines and procedures embedded in much nursing work. As a result, self-awareness regarding the searching and weighting of information for making choices is limited. When we do stop to think about how we make a judgement or a decision, the work involved is not easily captured in written form. Additionally, the judgement and decision-making process changes with experience, becoming grounded in an expanding 'library' of cases, knowledge shared with colleagues, and intuition.

Yet there is evidence to suggest that relying on intuitive judgement and customary decision-making processes is often not in the best interests of patients. For example:

*   There is growing evidence indicating that an unacceptably high number of avoidable adverse incidents are related to ineffective JDM (Thompson *et al.* 2013).

- Practising nurses tend to prioritise personal judgement over established evidence-based policies and procedures for medicine management (Haw *et al.* 2015).
- Confidence in personal judgement, often associated with experience, is no guide to the accuracy of judgements (Yang and Thompson 2010).

Consequently, much as intuition is prized by experienced practitioners and sought after by novices, there is a perceived need to reconcile professional judgement and decision-making resources with evidence-based principles to ensure nursing actions are consistent with the best interests of patients and their families. This chapter offers an introduction to some aspects of JDM theory that bear on the everyday work of nurses.

The chapter is divided into three parts. In Part 1, we make a distinction between judgement on the one hand and decision-making on the other and note how both relate to safe and effective nursing practice.

In Part 2, we describe normative, descriptive and prescriptive models of JDM as well as the influence of individual and organisational factors on approaches to decision-making.

In Part 3, we explore differences between intuitive and analytical approaches and indicate that intuition and analysis are essential components for effective JDM in everyday nursing practice.

PART 1: OUTLINING JUDGEMENT AND DECISION-MAKING

Case 13.1

Natasha is a first-year student nurse. She is surprised when her mentor (Valerie) refuses to sanction the transfer home of Mr Chin (an 84-year-old man with no further medical needs) from an acute medical unit because the family are insufficiently prepared to care for him at home. Natasha assumed that once medical staff say a patient is ready for discharge it is the nurse's job to make this happen. When Natasha asks, Valerie says that because his family are unprepared to provide the care Mr Chin needs, there is more to be lost than gained by sending this patient home. If sent home without the necessary support in place Mr Chin will likely be re-admitted within days and the family will then doubt their ability to cope. This may affect the family's willingness to take him home. Valerie explains that she plans to convince the doctor of the wisdom of delaying discharge until services are in place to help the family care for Mr Chin at home.

Nurses make numerous judgements and decisions every day; many go unnoticed, many are made from minimal information and many are made rapidly. It is not yet routine to consider JDM as a skill that can be described, reflected upon and developed. Yet, JDM is an important skill for effective nursing in increasingly pressurised environments where incomplete information and time constraints are common features of the practice landscape.

In Case 13.1 Valerie is *making a judgement* about the family's ability to manage Mr Chin's care at home and also *making a decision* about what to do. Thus Valerie is demonstrating JDM. However, she would also have demonstrated JDM had she accepted the original discharge plan; but that JDM would remain unnoticed.

Your past and current judgements and decisions will influence subsequent JDM in your professional practice. Wherever you are in the nursing programme, you will be engaged in JDM – even if you are not aware of this – and your current JDM activity will affect both the quality of the care you offer and your future time management as a registered practitioner.

During your nursing programme you are expected to develop expertise in JDM. As a first-year student it may be appropriate to rely on experienced qualified staff to prompt your JDM but as you approach qualification you will be expected to make (and justify) your independent judgements and decisions. Effective JDM is supported by theory, research and principles; and is something to be learned as part of becoming a safe and effective nurse.

The literature on JDM can be confusing. As Simmons (2010) notes, different terms are used in JDM (e.g., clinical judgement, heuristics, clinical inference, clinical reasoning, diagnostic reasoning) and not all authors differentiate between judgements and decisions. In this chapter we acknowledge **judgement** as distinct from **decision**-making.

A judgement represents a conclusion reached when a set of information cues is evaluated and integrated; whereas a decision involves choosing between alternatives. The International Council of Nursing (ICN) define judgement as: 'a clinical opinion, an estimate, or determination of professional nursing practice regarding the state of a nursing phenomenon, including the relative quality of the intensity or degree of the manifestation of the nursing phenomenon' (ICN 2002, p. 75).

The ICN definition uses terms that refer to integrating (or synthesising) different pieces of information ('opinion', 'estimate', 'determination'), highlighting that judgement involves processing information – reducing its complexity in order to summarise the meaning of different information cues. The definition refers to a 'phenomenon', meaning a feature of the patient that can be named. It could be a physiological, psychological or social phenomenon, reflecting the range and scope of professional nursing from the straightforward (e.g., body temperature) to the subjective (e.g., loneliness).

An experienced nurse integrates numerous cues when judging that a patient is experiencing a phenomenon such as anxiety. These cues range from verbal reports from a patient to indirect reports from care staff; and from visual cues to formalised assessments. To add complexity, individual pieces of information (cues) typically differ in reliability and validity.

The ICN definition highlights that qualifiers are used to report 'intensity' or 'degree' of phenomena. For example, the sliding scale of labels to describe a patient's mood. This could be constructed from informal terms (e.g., from down, low, sad and flat, through to upbeat, happy and high). Equally, formal terms could be employed (e.g., from anhedonia and blunted mood to hypomania and psychomotor agitation; and from low to medium to high risk).

It should also be noted that judgements refer to clinical and non-clinical patient states (e.g., distress, anxiety, happiness, hypotension). Moreover, although judgement tends to focus on the individual, it might equally relate to a dyad, family or community. For example, 'family capacity' could be a relevant phenomenon to assess when planning care for a patient with complex needs being transferred home.

A decision is distinct from a judgement. A decision is action-oriented, carried out to cause a change in the judged phenomenon. A decision is a choice between two or more known and available options (Hardman 2009); with a requirement of skill in assessing the suitability of one option over another and the involvement of some risk or

A **judgement** is a conclusion reached in relation to a set of information.

A **decision** involves choosing between alternatives.

329

consequence. For example, a medication decision by a nurse practitioner (NP), prompted by a judgement following consideration of cues resulting in the conclusion that the patient is experiencing the phenomenon of acute pain. The first decision (i.e., choice) taken is to prescribe pain relief medication (not to prescribe being the other option). Several associated decisions follow – the NP can make choices about the specific type of pain medication, the dosage, and the interval between doses. Some of these decisions are likely to be supported (or even determined) by a decision aid such as a medication protocol. Nevertheless, as Haw *et al.* (2015) found in a recent study the availability of national or local guidelines is no guarantee of their implementation.

Many nursing decisions are typically unnoticed, unrecorded and not supported by a formal decision aid. This does not minimise the importance of unnoticed decisions such as choices made about repositioning a patient or sitting to talk with an apparently distressed patient. Both examples follow from judgement regarding the patient's state in terms of a phenomenon (comfort and distress, respectively). Many patients are made more comfortable and many patients experience distress. The pressures of time in the practice environment means that nurses do not always intervene; but when they do, there is usually a critical level for the perception of a need that results in the decision to take action (Dalgleish *et al.* 2010). It is the nurse's judgement of the intensity of experience of a phenomenon (here, discomfort or distress) of a particular patient that triggers the decision to act.

Activity 13.1

Think about your most recent shift on placement. Take 5 minutes to jot down the types of judgements and decisions you made throughout the shift.

Don't be surprised if you found it difficult to identify the judgements and decisions you made during your most recent working shift. This is because JDM is all-pervasive within everyday nursing and it is sometimes difficult to get a clear picture of the JDM process. Some of your judgements and decisions may have been made when, for example:

- assessing patients or clients, monitoring patient condition or progress against nursing interventions;
- evaluating treatment efficacy; or
- choosing between different strategies and working with patients and families to co-ordinate their care.

You make a judgement when you think a patient looks better (or worse) today than they did yesterday. You make a judgement when you conclude that a patient is now happier or more satisfied. And you make a judgement when you feel concerned or uneasy following a conversation with a patient; and if this last judgement prompts you to ask for advice from senior staff then you have made a decision to act.

In addition to subjective and holistic judgements, there are formal judgements such as those employing tests, scales, measures or assessment tools that use objective information cues. In some practice areas, there may even be rules to guide combining cues so as to yield a verbal or numerical judgement with criteria for evaluating the judgements (e.g., low, moderate, or high risk). Of course, there different types of judgements and decisions required in each field of nursing but the formal study of JDM provides a vocabulary and set of ideas that enables effective JDM in all fields.

Nursing work involves uncertainty, and nowhere is this more apparent than in the realm of JDM as the cues or signals used to inform judgements are not without contention. One consequence of this is that making judgements and decisions means sometimes getting it wrong. There are of course many reasons for reaching inappropriate conclusions: time pressures, frequent demands and interruptions, the misreading of cues, as well as errors in combining, integrating or weighting cues (Adderley and Thompson 2015, Samuriwo and Dowding 2014). Two important and related points are:

1   *There is no necessary relationship between experience and effective JDM*. It is tempting to think that more experienced nurses will be better at JDM. However, as Yang and Thompson (2011) found, there was no difference between student and experienced nurses in terms of the accuracy of judging which patients were at risk of acute deterioration.
2   *Effective JDM is not merely a function of individual capacity*. It is easy to blame individual nurses for ineffective JDM, but this fails to account for the influence of organisations, systems and working patterns that shape our ability to make effective judgements or decisions.

PART 2: EXPLAINING JUDGEMENT AND DECISION-MAKING

Case 13.1 (continued)

Valerie has judged that there is a lack of suitable arrangements in place for Mr Chin to be transferred home and she has made a decision to influence the doctor's decision regarding the timing of Mr Chin's discharge. Valerie knows that a logical argument about the high risk of rapid re-admission will not be sufficient to convince the doctor of the need to delay Mr Chin's discharge, so she knows that she will need to decide what course of action will best achieve that aim. In order to make the best decision, it will be helpful for Valerie to have knowledge of different models of JDM.

Activity 13.2

Make notes on how Valerie might go about making a decision regarding ensuring suitable home care arrangements can be in place before Mr Chin's discharge.

Pádraig MacNeela et al.

Models of judgement and decision-making

Typically, three models of JDM processes are identified (Thompson and Dowding 2009):

1 *normative* (how a judgement or decision can best be made);
2 *descriptive* (how they are actually made); and
3 *prescriptive* (how theory can be used to improve JDM).

Normative

Normative approaches to JDM assume that people ought to make effective use of available information and choose the most efficient decision option. Rationality is key to the assumption that people wish to be logical in JDM. Central to normative models is the expected utility theory of human behaviour. This theory assumes that:

- people make decisions aware of all required information; and
- people are aware of all possible alternatives and potential outcomes.

In other words, by following the rationally determined best course of action, the **utility** of people's decision-making will be maximised; that is, they will achieve the optimum outcome (Hardman 2009).

Expected utility refers to favouring decisions with the highest expected utility. However, JDM is influenced by, among other things, environmental factors such as limitations of knowledge and levels of certainty. Thus it is important to know how people form conclusions and make choices in the face of uncertainty. Where the right answer or best decision outcome cannot be easily predicted, the risks involved in decision-making become writ large. The classic mode of research inquiry in the normative model is to ask people to evaluate trade-offs (Hardman 2009), such as asking a client to choose between alternatives on the basis of likely outcomes (e.g., choosing between medication or cognitive behaviour therapy to reduce socially unacceptable behaviour and avoid compulsory hospitalisation).

Descriptive

Descriptive models of JDM aim to show how people actually make judgements and decisions (rather than how they ought to). Underpinning descriptive models is the idea that people are not very good at using information to form conclusions or make choices. According to descriptive models, we can never be entirely rational decision-makers because we have limited **information processing** capacity (aka bounded rationality). Descriptive accounts attempt to capture how we give weight to different information cues in everyday situations where 'good enough' judgements and decisions suffice. However, in complex or time-pressured situations this good enough JDM can lead to mistakes and errors. Descriptive models typically emphasise our reliance on intuitions, beliefs and feelings over objective evidence and logical analysis, which raises the question of the accuracy of resultant judgments. In health contexts, this question becomes important if practitioners rely on intuition, beliefs and feelings rather than, for example, a simple statistical combination rule (Dowding et al. 2011).

While we are not rational decision-makers, proponents of descriptive models point out that we make intelligent use of our limited cognitive resources to make decisions by the use of **heuristics**. Heuristics are 'general rules' used in the attempt to overcome our bounded rationality. The 'stopping rule' heuristic, for example, indicates that people will stop searching for a decision once they find an option that meets their minimal acceptable criteria (Kahneman 2011) and in so doing, foreclose on the evaluation of alternatives. Nurses typically work in complex and changing environments, are often faced with incomplete information, and yet are expected to exercise JDM in situations of high-stakes outcomes. The pressure to make rapid decisions with only partial information can lead to a routine of choosing the familiar and may explain why nurses often adopt a descriptive model of decision-making. A critical question addressed in this chapter is whether this is a satisfactory option, and how the strategy can be optimised through awareness of potential pitfalls.

Prescriptive

Prescriptive models of JDM acknowledge that our use of information is rarely optimal, but recognise that ways exist to make improvements. Prescriptive models describe underlying cognitive processes that support and influence JDM (e.g., attitudes, biases and **schemas**) and suggest ways to make better use of available information (Thompson and Dowding 2009). The focus is thus on strategies used for assessing and responding to problems, on the level of mental effort required, and on the importance of accuracy to the quality of JDM.

Prescriptive models highlight factors that impinge on the quality of decision-making. According to Maule (1997) these factors include:

- time pressures;
- stress and associated emotional states (e.g., fear, anger);
- level of engagement with the problem.

In acknowledging these factors prescriptive models allow for the consideration of different strategies that will support the choice of a prescriptive action. Hardman (2009) notes that decision-making can be supported by strategies such as: decision analysis techniques and decision trees; critical incident analyses to learn from near misses and previously ineffective actions; organisational preparedness for managing critical events; and training initiatives that encourage rule-based or formal models of decision-making in the practice environment.

Judgement and decision-making in nursing practice

The literature on JDM in nursing practice is extensive (Thompson *et al.* 2013) and represents an important resource for nurses as they make everyday judgements and decisions related to setting priorities for nursing care. Here are some examples:

- *Initial assessment.* Nurses carry out initial assessments of patients to get a sense of the person's functioning, health status or abilities; or for a specific presenting problem. The initial assessment provides information to assist decision-making regarding appropriate levels of care.
- *Monitoring.* Ongoing assessment differs from initial assessment. Having established some basic patient parameters, nurses update and form evaluative judgements that

A **heuristic** is a 'general rule' strategy that circumvents the need to analyse problems through logic (Kahneman and Tversky 1973). Because of cognitive bias it cannot provide reliable forms of decision-making but its effortlessness can be valuable in situations of limited information and/or time.

Schemas are cognitive structures that represent general and specialised knowledge about objects, people or situations and the relationships between them. Intuitive or experiential nursing knowledge can be seen as a set of clinical schemas. Another form of knowledge structure is an exemplar. While a schema may suggest a general, average case, exemplars represent specific cases or instances. Nursing knowledge includes abstract knowledge, schemas and case exemplars.

TABLE 13.1 Three major types of decisions taken by nurses

Intervention choice	Choices related to choosing between different care interventions. Special attention may be given to targeting particular people. So while several patients may require skin care, the person with the highest priority for this intervention is targeted first and the best time is chosen to give the care
Communication	Choices related to the ways and means of gathering and sharing information. This may involve patients and clients, their families or carers, other members of the multi-disciplinary team and other agencies. An example here would be safeguarding vulnerable adults
Service organisation, delivery and management	Choices related to the delivery of specific services at designated times and places (e.g., deciding which staff are required to work a particular shift because of the anticipated needs of the patients/clients)

Source: adapted from Thompson *et al.* 2000.

detect stability and change. A judgement that a patient's condition is deteriorating might prompt a decision to inform appropriate others.

- *Discharge assessment.* Here the judgement about a patient's improved condition could prompt a choice between alternatives, such as recommending discharge home or transfer to a step-down facility.
- *Knowing the patient.* This requires a judgement of the patient as a whole that may range from the highly specific and clinical to the individual and holistic.
- *Risk assessment.* Judgement here aims to identify a particular vulnerability or risk (e.g., risk of infection) and a decision to act follows when a patient's state exceeds a specified threshold.
- *Concordance.* Judging how far patients and/or their families or carers have adhered to treatment or care plans (e.g., activity or dietary recommendations) or complied with medication prescriptions.

The taxonomy of decision types offered by Thompson *et al.* (Table 13.1) illustrates nurses are likely to be exposed to different levels of decision-making. Some decisions focus on activities directly related to patient care (e.g., patient positioning in acute hospital nursing or anxiety reduction in mental health nursing) while others relate to indirect interventions carried out for the benefit of patients (e.g., trying to get a patient with acute health needs admitted to a ward or place of safety). Because nurses usually work in a complex health care environment, many judgements and decisions relate to the system of health care delivery as much as to direct patient care. Nurses tend to identify with collective rather than individual decision-making (MacNeela *et al.* 2010). We argue that effective JDM is an essential component of being a competent nurse (MacNeela *et al.* 2012).

Organisational influence on JDM

There are a range of organisational features that constrain or facilitate the capacity of individual nurses to engage effectively with JDM. For example:

- Informal 'customs' and 'practices' within an organisation may differ substantially from formal communication processes.
- Seniority in organisations is associated with latitude in individual JDM.
- Different care settings present distinct types of JDM problems and resolution resources.
- Access to formal JDM aids varies between and within organisations; as do attitudes toward the use of formal aids and/or informal strategies.
- Different professional groups exhibit different cultural norms and beliefs regarding: medical or biopsychosocial models of illness; drug-based or psychosocial treatments; patient involvement in decision-making; and openness to change.
- Working relationships between different occupational groups may encourage or discourage effective JDM.

Critical social theory sometimes positions nurses as belonging to an oppressed professional group. Manias and Street (2001) argue that 'the status and development of nurses' knowledge has been largely influenced by the dominance of medical power . . . this dominance has supported the view that medicine operates from a foundation of "superior", legitimated knowledge' (p. 129). Which may be one reason why doctors are often afforded greater legitimacy than nurses in JDM. However, the 'doctor–nurse game' (Porter 1991) is one strategy that allows nurses to covertly steer medical decision-making and this may be one way Valerie can influence arrangements for Mr Chin's discharge (Case 13.1).

RESEARCH FOCUS 13.1

Manias and Street's (2001) study of critical care in Australia identified several ways in which nurses were formally excluded from decisions about patients yet still exerted influence over decision-making. Possessing knowledge that doctors needed but did not have, nurses presented information to suggest actions to doctors. This finding indicates that it is not enough to possess information, combine it well and identify appropriate decisions – it is also necessary to work effectively within systems that privilege some groups over others. Knowing how to work the system can be as important as knowing the patient. Thus documenting how informal influence exceeds formal power.

Activity 13.3

Try to identify a situation you have witnessed in which a nurse has found a way to influence the JDM of a doctor. What strategy did they use? Can you work out why the nurse felt it necessary to use a subtle approach rather than just refer to their own JDM?

Making judgements and decisions about patient care invariably occurs within systems of limited resources; where time, expense, and effective use of staff all have a bearing. This gives rise to informal and undocumented strategies for making decisions about

Pádraig MacNeela *et al.*

resources (e.g., bed management in forensic psychiatry units (Grounds *et al.* 2004)). In the USA and UK, increased visibility of the nursing contribution to JDM is seen as important in improving the standing of the profession in multi-professional teams (Buckingham and Adams 2000, Havens and Vasey 2005).

RESEARCH FOCUS 13.2

Elliott (2010) contends that nursing JDM is distinctive because of the weighting given to the thera-peutic relationship. Her grounded theory study highlighted inter-connectedness, interaction and reciprocity as influences on nursing JDM.

Gillespie *et al.* (2015) highlight the need for a balance between practice-based and evidence-based knowledge. Their multi-disciplinary study of wound care management found that practitioners give credence to both forms of knowledge, with decisions about wound care influenced by a complex mixture of patient preferences, costs and established practices. They found that practitioners oriented towards intuitive rather than evidence-based practice.

Dowding *et al.* (2011) found that an evidence-based initiative to implement an algorithm for the diagnosis of labour in midwifery required consideration of local context and circumstances and Samuriwo and Dowding (2014) noted the superior performance of pressure ulcer risk assessment tools over 'custom and practice' clinical judgement. Dowding *et al.* (2012) found prompts to assess patients for risk of pressure ulcers reduced the incidence of pressure ulcers.

PART 3: EXPLORING JUDGEMENT AND DECISION-MAKING

Intuition
is a form of knowing or understanding about something that cannot be explained by reference to facts, previous experience or the experience of others. This might be expressed sentences like 'I have a gut feeling that something is wrong with this patient'.

One of the claims of this chapter is that nursing tends towards **intuition** and heuristics in JDM rather than analysis because (at least in part) of the constraints of environment and time. Here we will begin to explore the role of intuition in JDM for nursing.

Activity 13.4

Spend some time thinking about the way you approach judgement and decision-making. Do you think others would describe you as intuitive or analytical in your judgements and decisions?

Intuitive judgements and decisions

Intuitive JDM rests on the outcome of a process of perceiving or apprehending something that triggers previous knowledge, experience or skill. This might take the form of pattern recognition (a relatively automatic categorisation of a set of cues) for example, facial grimacing and muscular tension triggers a pattern of prior knowledge that evokes the judgement that a patient is in pain. However, it takes practice and familiarity to exercise selective perception or 'see' things in this way, rather than having to think consciously. Judging that someone is anxious is of a different order to judging that they are more anxious today than they were yesterday ('descriptive judgement' and 'evaluative judgement' respectively, see Table 13.2). Both descriptive and evaluative judgements can be reached through an intuitive process using sensory evidence to prime existing knowledge, although each requires different kinds of information. The intuitive descriptive judgement above is based on an automatic recognition of cue patterns associated with anxiety, whereas the intuitive evaluative judgement requires two descriptive judgements at different times and an unconscious comparison of the two.

Intuitive type judgements serve several purposes: knowing the patient and thinking about causes of a problem (causal judgements); assessing post-intervention states (descriptive judgements); predicting rates of improvement (inferential judgements). Making a judgement of anxiety is closely linked to decision-making as recognising someone's anxiety may prompt a decision about what to do next. Natasha's mentor made a prediction that the patient would likely be re-admitted within days, having mentally simulated what would happen in the absence of adequate family support.

A consideration of intuitive judgements triggers three important issues.

1   We have a limited capacity to process information but with practice we can learn to recognise particular patterns. With limited capacity for attention and reasoning, it may be more time-efficient to trigger judgements using patterns and categories than to think deliberately about each one.
2   Fluency and flexibility in categorising environmental information is an acquired skill. Experts are able to make quick and accurate judgements based on experience and/or knowledge acquired over a long period of time and/or specific to a specialist area of practice.
3   Some tasks require rapid intuitive judgements – time pressure, stress, limited information and varied tasks may demand quick responses (Hammond 1996). Our attention is impaired by information overload, fatigue and stress from difficult or unfamiliar situations.

There is inevitably a trade-off between speed and error: the more rapid the JDM the higher the risk of error. This is perhaps a particular issue for the novice nurse with little experience of making intuitive judgements on which to draw and so is more likely to be

TABLE 13.2 Four types of judgements characteristic of nursing

Descriptive judgement	Using a label to describe a relevant state (e.g., anxious, uncomfortable, pyrexial)
Evaluative judgement	Making a comparison in relation to time, situation or other people (e.g., better/worse than yesterday, it was different last time, she is responding better than him)
Inferential judgement	Making a prediction about what may happen (e.g., I don't think she will be ready for discharge tomorrow)
Causal judgement	Stating a cause of a state (e.g., anaemia due to poor diet, erratic behaviour due to drug misuse)

Source: adapted from Lamond et al. 1996.

RESEARCH FOCUS 13.3

Novice to expert

Some nurses move from novice through intermediate levels of performance to expert with experience (Benner *et al.* 2009). This parallels Rasmussen's (1993) levels of task performance. At the highest level, task performance is skill-based (i.e., intuitive); at the intermediate and low level it is rule-based (e.g., protocol or procedure driven). Performance is knowledge-based among novices (i.e., the novice needs to think through the different options on how to approach a task). In contrast the expert nurse demonstrates skilled performance in a particular domain and it is suggested that this takes approximately 10 years or 10,000 hours to attain (Ericsson *et al.* 2007). However, experience alone does not lead to expert performance; it is the learning and development that arise from and with experience that offers a route to expert practice (and this provides one of the basic justifications for the need for nurses to engage with reflective practice – see Chapter 17). Thus higher levels of practice combined with appropriate feedback can lead to a high level of skill. Expert performance involves knowing what to do when things go wrong, as well as knowing how to make sure things go right.

---

faced with unfamiliar situations. As a result the novice will need to consciously engage with the features of unfamiliar situations in order to make judgements that will be in the intuitive realm for the expert nurse.

Heuristic thinking and situation awareness

In the previous section we suggested intuitive JDM incorporates a range of strategies. With practice it is possible to develop skill in noticing clusters and patterns of symptoms experienced by patients and clients. This is an impressive skill as health care problems rarely present in textbook fashion. According to Bargh (1994) a truly automatic judgement is one that is:

- *efficient* (requires few resources);
- *lacks intentionality* (you cannot help but see the pattern);
- *outside conscious control* (it happens and you are aware of the result);
- *outside awareness* (you are unable to say what information was used to reach the judgement).

Few judgements fulfil each criterion. Yet many judgements come close, although the accuracy of those judgements varies. This still leaves a need to account for thinking strategies and judgements that are more conscious than unconscious. We describe this mode of thought as heuristic thinking, based on the application of 'general rules' and simplified forms of analytical thinking.

Health care professionals commonly make use of only a small number of information cues when making a judgement or decision. Although more cues are usually available, the professional typically attends to between 2 and 4 cues. Despite the low number, there is no guarantee that each practitioner is paying attention to the same cues. In the case

Activity 13.5

Think about a client or patient who was leaving your placement area to return home, go to a step-down facility or transfer to a more intensive environment. Write some brief notes identifying the sequence of events and the key players involved in making judgements and decisions in relation to this patient's transfer.

of a discharge decision these information cues might include family support, the patient's wishes and their mobility status. Seeking out information on particular information cues and forming a judgement is likely to involve some conscious thinking, especially if the information cues are contradictory and hard to reconcile. While some work is involved, a heuristic of targeting a small number of cues cuts down on mental workload. To apply the idea of a 'stopping rule': if there is a very low level on any one information cue, then a default recommendation may be that discharge does not take place; if the person is under 50 years of age and wishes to go home, then the default may be to recommend discharge. Are there any stopping rules you identified in your scenario developed from Activity 13.5?

A set of general heuristics is applicable in most nursing (and non-nursing) situations (Kahneman and Tversky 1973). These deal with judgements based on:

- *similarity* (representativeness heuristic);
- *ease of recall* (availability heuristic);
- *ease of projection* (simulation heuristic);
- *an initial starting point as a guiding reference* (anchoring and adjustment heuristic).

The 'representativeness' and 'availability' heuristics rely on prior knowledge and are more automatic than conscious. The 'simulation' and the 'anchoring and adjustment' heuristics are likely to involve conscious mediation. At some level, experiential knowledge is required for each of these heuristics. As might be inferred from the earlier discussion of rationality, controversy remains attached to the question of whether heuristics benefit or interfere with clear thinking.

Early researchers on cognitive heuristics assumed a reliance on heuristics rendered JDM prone to errors and biases. For example, the availability heuristic might bring easily to mind a particular illness category when assessing a new patient because of a similar recent patient profile seen even if this exaggerates the actual probability of this illness in the population. For many heuristics researchers, a general rule is antithetical to evidence-based health care.

More recently, naturalistic decision-making (NDM) theory has gained credibility. Rather than framing experiential knowledge as a source of error, NDM highlights it as a key resource that experienced decision-makers rely on when operating in high-stakes, continually changing environments (Klein 2008). NDM assumes that prior knowledge allows us to respond adaptively to real-world situations. Typically, NDM research has been conducted with decision-makers working in highly fluid, dynamic and specialised contexts such as those found in the military, in business and in medicine; and attempts to identify how experienced practitioners make 'good enough' judgements and decisions in the face of the stress and uncertainty imposed by time pressure and incomplete

339

information. Developed from NDM, Klein (2008) captured the idea that experienced practitioners are able to use their prior knowledge to categorise new situations rapidly in his recognition-primed decision model (RPDM). Judgement here is similar to a representative heuristic, operating as a process of recognition where new instances are categorised in reference to existing knowledge. For situations that cannot be categorised this way, a more laborious, analytical judgement process ensues. RPDM is action-oriented as judgements are closely linked to decisions; the purpose of categorising being to provide appropriate action responses. Thus RPDM assumes mental reviews of possible courses of action to identify the most plausible action. Resembling the simulation heuristic, this process invokes the concept of future-oriented inferential judgement where mental simulation is considered a resource rather than a source of error.

Building on RPDM, Endsley (1995) and Durso and Sethumadhavan (2008) introduced situation awareness (SA) theory as a way to describe the degree to which we are, at any given moment, up to speed in processing and recognising the significance of information. SA refers to three separate (but linked) processes or levels, and is defined by Endsley as 'the perception of the elements in the environment in a volume of time and space, the comprehension of their meaning and the projection of their status in the near future' (1995, p. 36). This will have different meanings depending on the nursing context. The predictability and rate of change in incoming information varies from one context to another, perhaps reaching its culmination in a busy emergency department. SA fits with the applied nature of nursing where effective anticipatory or reactive responses are prioritised. For example, a patient judged to be at high risk of cardiac arrest, might prompt a decision to act because an acute deterioration in that patient's condition without immediate specialist intervention can be anticipated by projection.

Level 1 SA requires the gathering of information and a formulation of initial perceptions of the current situation. In nursing, this typically means accessing information cues relevant to a patient through sensory perception, patient self-reports and information from others. At Level 2 SA (the judgement phase) the current situation is interpreted and comprehended. An initial Level 1 SA perception of stability might require reliance on intuition to sense the patient is comfortable; if however, the Level 1 SA indicated a disconcerting or puzzling observation then Level 2 SA would become more conscious and analytical. At Level 3 SA, the process is similar to inferential judgement or simulation heuristic, anticipating future states by projection on judgements of existing situations.

Relevant to nursing as it situates judgement in complex environments, many personal influences on SA have been outlined in this chapter, including experience, prior knowledge and information processing ability. In addition to these 'person-based' influences on the capacity for making applied judgements, SA prioritises relevant task or system factors. These include the availability of decisional aids and supports, work organisation systems (e.g., autonomous versus team working, skill mix of experience and seniority), and environmental busyness (e.g., high workloads and/or long shifts promote fatigue and error arising from cognitive stress).

SA is instructive in helping understand the process from information gathering to the emergence of accurate judgements and effective projections. In addition, SA acknowledges the supports required for effective judgement as well as the risks arising from compromised awareness. SA has been applied in high-reliability industries such as aviation to understand the occurrence of human error highlighting the importance of factoring in sources of judgement failures, such as: overlooking vital information; the risk of reasoning shortcuts as a result of overfamiliarity with tasks; and the negative contribution of fatigue, time stress and interruptions. There is evidence that SA has much to offer JDM in nursing (Stubbings *et al.* 2012).

Analytical judgements and decisions

Intuitive JDM is in stark contrast to analytic JDM, which is characterised by conscious thinking and use of formal reasoning methods (Hastie and Dawes 2001). Normative models of JDM suggest how logic, utility analysis and propositional thinking should be used to yield the correct judgement or decision. This is a useful perspective, but in any given situation we are likely to lack the ability, time and information levels required to support the normative approach. Heuristic thinking strategies borrow from both analytical and perceptual methods. A heuristic is partly a conscious form of JDM, but individuals tend to make use of informal strategies, for example, peer discussion, general rules or simplified analytical strategies such as using a practice guideline or a decision tree. An analytical judgement is reached through a relatively slow, sequential consideration of information cues, as opposed to the fast and simultaneous processing of intuitive judgement (Hammond 1996).

Montgomery and colleagues (2005) assume the majority of our JDM is intuitive and heuristic and that this is expected given our limited **short-term memory** and difficulty with logical and propositional reasoning. While we often employ **probabilistic terms** they tend to be used fairly loosely. In addition, the ambiguity or time pressure associated with nursing work makes it difficult to adopt an analytic approach. As a result, our bounded rationality tends to discourage us from thinking in genuinely analytical ways precisely because of environmental and personally imposed constraints (Simon 1956).

We suggest that nursing practice has built-in conditions that encourage reliance on experiential knowledge. Nursing often requires multi-tasking in busy environments where the slowness and resource-intensiveness of analytical thinking is a disadvantage. Nursing work also requires high levels of certainty and accuracy, underscored by adverse potential consequences for patients of ineffective JDM. Nurses often try to adapt to this tension by engineering the environment: 'poor at mental calculations?' – use a calculator; 'medication errors likely?' – build in error-proof systems with checks and balances, and so on (Sharpe 2004).

One of the main trends of analytical thinking in the JDM literature is **hypothetico-deductive reasoning**. Elstein and Bordage (1988) outline four analytical stages when making a judgement or decision about patients and clients (see Table 13.3).

Most formal clinical judgements can be viewed in terms of generating hypotheses and working deductively to analyse which is most likely to be correct. To judge if a patient is under the influence of street drugs, begin by collecting information that might come from observations, colleagues, patient notes or family members. Hypotheses can be generated from the collected information, for example: the patient is using heroin, she is not using street drugs, she is using some other drug, she is using some combination of drugs and so on. In the cue interpretation stage, you consider the meaning and relevance of the information you have collected (e.g., your observation of the client's pupils). In the hypothesis evaluation stage you come to a conclusion as to which hypothesis is best supported, with different weight placed on different information cues (e.g., the presence of constricted pupils would be given a high weighting) and attempt to reconcile contradictions or inconsistencies among the information cues (e.g., the person's insistence that they have not been using street drugs as opposed to your opinion based on observation).

Short-term memory has a capacity of 7 items +/−2 (Miller 1956) and a duration of approximately 30 seconds. This limits our capacity to remember information from the environment. Working memory (Baddeley 2004) is a dynamic reading of short-term memory; representing it as the cognitive thinking and planning centre that guides your strategy in a situation, aided by attention, visualisation faculty and language-based thought. In contrast to the limitations of our conscious awareness and short-term memory, long-term memory is limitless. Declarative long-term memory is the store of verbal knowledge. Procedural long-term memory is the store of skilled knowledge. Once sufficiently well practised, task performance becomes proceduralised and increasingly automatic. Perceptual skills (such as pattern recognition) and skilled performance (in relation to a technical skill) are based on procedural memory. Episodic memory is the store for memories of specific events.

341

Pádraig MacNeela et al.

TABLE 13.3 Four analytical stages in JDM

Cue acquisition	Collecting information cues seen as relevant
Hypothesis generation	Coming up with one or more explanations that explain the patient's condition
Cue interpretation	Considering the information cues you have in light of the explanations you have generated
Hypothesis evaluation	Working out which explanation or hypothesis is correct

Source: Elstein and Bordage 1988.

Nurses do seek out relevant information as characterised by the hypothetico-deductive model. This is a skilled activity and in this instance would involve knowing what information to obtain from the family. While you might not think in terms of 'hypotheses', you may often have identified more than one explanation or possible cause for a set of symptoms or presenting features. Most information cues need to be interpreted in terms of quality and relevance to the particular situation. Sometimes individuals will think through the cause of a problem, comparing and considering the best fit with the evidence.

This four-stage model also helps us to understand how groups make judgements. A multidisciplinary team working on a clinical problem in a formal way will find the stages in the model useful as a resolution guide. However, the conditions required for a thoroughly analytical approach to JDM are seldom met. A heuristic rather than prescriptive approach is likely to be used in many cases, leading to a decision such as requesting a physiological test to confirm or refute a hypothesis. In most cases it is presumed that we use intuition and, to a lesser extent, analysis. Klein's (2008) RPDM is typical of this view. It is an example of a naturalistic decision-making theory developed to account for situations that are continually changing, which is often the case in nursing where time is of the essence in patient assessment, and where information changes rapidly requiring immediate attention and frequent updating of judgements.

Activity 13.6

Think about your most recent time in placement and try to identify a situation in which you witnessed or took part in a formal analytical JDM process.

Nursing researchers tend to focus on the hypothetico-deductive model, although it may not be the best way to describe all that nurses do in practice. We suggest that naturalistic decision-making research is needed because it focuses on complex environments where highly skilled responses are needed within short time frames in dynamic, changing situations. NDM has been used less often in the nursing literature and there is a smaller pool of work from which to draw than the hypothetico-deductive research tradition.

As noted earlier, Klein (2008) argues that people use experiential knowledge first to judge if a situation is typical, and engage in conscious, analytical approaches only if the situation or patient condition is perceived as atypical. The same person will on some occasions reach a judgement using intuition while using an analytical approach on a different occasion. Cognitive continuum theory (Hammond 1996) integrates analysis and intuition by placing each at either end of a spectrum, with numerous options in between. In keeping with the environmental sensitivity of naturalistic decision-making, situational awareness and the recognition-primed decision model, situational conditions prompt an appropriate point of intuition-analysis along the cognitive continuum for any particular occasion (Hammond 1996).

Cognitive continuum theory has enabled reconciliation between analytical and intuitive modes of information interpretation and integration (Standing 2008). Unfamiliar judgement tasks that present multiple cues, or that cannot be easily mapped onto existing 'scripts' require us to use analytic approaches. Time-pressured judgement tasks that cannot be easily reduced into component parts fit best with intuitive approaches. Ideally, judgement task conditions would direct particular cognitive strategies but in practice, pre-existing individual differences often make us gravitate towards our preferred end of the spectrum. Nevertheless, and as a general rule we should aim to suit reasoning style with judgement task for the simple reason that Thompson et al. (2013) offer: that the risk of inaccuracy or misjudgement increases in proportion to increased discrepancy between judgement task and reasoning style.

Signals and cues

To make a judgement is to (consciously or unconsciously) apprehend distinct pieces of information and bring these together. To make a decision is to determine whether the judgement made reaches the threshold for action. There is increasing evidence to support judgement analysis and signal detection theory as a means of assessing the quality and accuracy of nursing JDM.

Signal detection theory has influenced the way judgements are understood (Dalgleish 1988). This perspective explains the task as detection of whether an underlying 'signal' is present or absent in the midst of typically ambiguous or incomplete information cues that contribute to the 'noise' surrounding the signal. This applies where it is necessary to assess whether or not a critical state has been reached – for example: if a woman is in labour; if a patient is at risk of acute deterioration; or if a patient is experiencing myocardial infarction. Detecting a signal requires the ability to identify relevant signs and symptoms as well as the finely tuned calibration necessary for determining when information cues reach a critical level of 'symptomness' and thus require action or referral. Signal detection theory links judgement to decision-making; if it is judged that a particular instance exceeds a threshold for being, for example, at 'high risk', then this equates to a decision threshold prompting action.

Judgement analysis (JA) is a descriptive strategy to make transparent the weighting given to each information cue. JA is based on the lens model theory developed by Brunswik (1955). The lens model assumes that each information cue has a true information value, which is its actual relevance to an integrated judgement of multiple cues. To be capable of making the most effective judgements possible, it is necessary to know: (i) the correct weighting to apply to each cue; and (ii) the degree to which the information contained in each cue overlaps or is distinctive. Clinical algorithms and risk assessments are examples of 'gold standard' strategies that attempt to do these very things. Considering the complex and often subjective nature of patient problems and issues, there is usually some unreliability or redundancy associated with each information cue. In addition, there is no 'recipe' that specifies the weighting for each cue when integrating cues.

With experience, nurses develop a subjective sense of specific signals for particular clinical issues. For example, a nurse will tend to combine visual cues (e.g., facial features and grimacing), verbal reports and tactile cues (e.g., muscular stiffness) in an individualistic manner when judging how much pain a patient is experiencing. By under-weighting a pain cue, patient pain is underestimated and appropriate treatment options may not be put in place; while overestimating patient pain can result in unnecessary treatments and medication use. JA encourages finding ways to represent such judgements in a transparent manner open to numerical assessment. JA research allows evaluation of the 'judgement profile' of each individual, which captures typical weighting schemas for each information cue. This can in turn identify variation between individual judges and variation compared to a gold standard (if one exists) of information use patterns.

Signal detection theory also promotes the idea of the objective quality of a judgement. Each patient is or is not a 'true case' of the signal that is being assessed. In the language of signal detection theory, objective measurements of the patients to compare human judges against allows calculation rates of 'hits', 'misses', 'false alarms', and 'correct rejections'. You may have come across these four categories if you are familiar with accuracy in medical diagnosis and testing. For example: the hit rate of a general practitioner (GP) in detecting cases of streptococcal infection; the percentage of true cases of infection that the GP missed; the number of false alarms where the GP erroneously judged patients to have an infection; and the number of times the GP correctly judged that a patient was infection free.

The four numbers generated by a signal detection analysis allow us to calculate the judge's sensitivity (the degree to which true cases are detected by the judge) and specificity (how effective the judge is in ruling out non-cases of the illness or phenomenon in question). The same barometers of accuracy and effectiveness can be applied to a new biomedical test or psychometric assessment. There is often a trade-off between sensitivity and specificity. To judge all patients to have an illness would equate with perfect sensitivity, as all patients with the illness would be diagnosed. However this would display poor specificity as many patients would be diagnosed with an illness that they did not have.

The capacity to identify patients who reach a threshold for action has implications for patient welfare and for health care organisations. A nurse prescriber will seek to avoid unnecessary prescribing because of potential harmful repercussions. A nurse manager will seek to avoid unnecessary admissions in order to maximise the use of resources. Such factors support a conservative policy for triggering action, to set a very high threshold in symptom intensity before acting (high specificity). However, in both instances the nurses will also seek to avoid missing patients who require care (high sensitivity). A preceptor may lose confidence in the judgement of a novice practitioner if every instance is referred back for advice as a result of uncertainty (low specificity on the part of the novice), but will expect the novice to highlight those patients in need of care from an experienced nurse (high sensitivity).

Thus, signal detection theory provides a useful means of thinking about judgement, its links to decision-making, and the influences that apply when (consciously or not) we set a specific threshold of certainty before acting. Despite the clarity brought by JA and signal detection theory, many of the patient problems, strengths, and issues that nurses

RESEARCH FOCUS 13.4

Themes in nursing research on clinical judgement and decision-making

Judgement analysis has been used to understand health care practitioners' judgement (Brown and Rakow 2015, Hancock et al. 2012, Harries et al. 2014), and to assess nurses' judgement (Adderley and Thompson 2015, Beckstead and Stamp 2007, Yang and Thompson 2011, Yang et al. 2012).

The importance of JDM to patient well-being is demonstrated by a lack of consistency among nurses in making judgements and decisions regarding patient welfare issues such as pain, fatigue and pressure ulcers even when having access to the same information (Thompson et al. 2013). This lack of consistency could be due to levels of expertise and to the extent to which the nurse has engaged in specialised preparation.

Recalling the 'novice to expert' analogy, differences between nurses might be expected depending on length of experience. As an example, Hoffman et al. (2009) found that, compared with novices, more experienced nurses chunked information cues into different clusters. However there is mixed evidence as to whether experienced nurses are more effective in JDM than those with less experience. Several studies have shown that, for specific judgement tasks, there is no difference in effectiveness by experience (Yang and Thompson 2011). Yang and Thompson (2010) asked experienced nurses and nursing students to review 25 clinical vignettes drawn from real cases, and to identify patients at high risk of a critical event. The information cues within the vignettes included blood pressure, heart rate, respiratory rate, body temperature, and consciousness level. The relevance of nursing risk assessment in this context is self-evident as a fundamental skill of nursing practice in a critical care environment. The experienced nurses had an average of 12 years' clinical experience, including 6 years' experience in critical care. On analysing the responses, the researchers found no difference between experienced and student nurses' ability to detect which patients were actually at risk. The researchers had also asked participants to rate confidence of judgements made; experienced nurses were significantly more confident, compared with nursing students, but demonstrated no more ability to give accurate judgements.

In another recent study, Thompson and Adderley (2015) did find that specialist nurses were more effective at JDM compared with generalist nurses. They studied judgements and treatment decisions related to judging causes of leg ulceration and decisions for recommending multilayer compression therapy. The nurses reviewed over 100 clinical scenarios derived from real patient data, which were presented using text and photographs. Approximately half of these cases were signal cases (known to have a venous leg ulcer present and/or compression therapy warranted). The other half had some other kind of ulcer and/or compression therapy contraindicated. The specialist nurses were better at identifying venous leg ulcers and inappropriate treatment decisions. Yet they still exhibited individual variability and missed a significant proportion of 'true cases'. On average, they identified 75 per cent of the 'signal' cases compared with only 59 per cent of the generalist nurses. The specialists were also better at identifying more of the cases where decompression therapy should be recommended (70 per cent versus 60 per cent). Although specialists with extensive experience were more effective, even these judgements were by no means infallible.

work with are not open to the objectivity and 'knowability' demanded by these perspectives. Nurses work with many judgement tasks where there is not a known 'right answer'. Many of the judgements that nurses make, regarding comfort and discomfort, loneliness and stress and so on, may not be amenable to a gold standard for comparison.

Nevertheless, signal detection theory has been used in several recent nursing and midwifery research studies. In high fidelity clinical simulations mimicking realistic practice complexity in terms of high levels of 'noise' mixed with genuine signals, Thompson *et al.* (2012) found judgement performance to be worse than in the hypothetical scenarios more often used to assess JDM. This raises the possibility that nurses are less effective than researchers had presumed in discriminating genuine signals in noisy environments; they also found no correlation between amount of clinical experience and ability to predict detection of genuine signals. In midwifery, Cheyne *et al.* (2012) examined the decision to transfer a woman in labour to an obstetrics-led unit; a decision task frequently encountered in home delivery, rural environments and midwifery-led units. They identified considerable variation in rates of transfer between rural maternity units and obstetric units, which can be explained by having different thresholds for action in place.

CONCLUSION

In this chapter we set out to link JDM concepts and research to everyday nursing practice. We argue that being able to analyse one's JDM is valuable in providing good quality nursing care and in furthering the professional development of individual nurses. There are many options to do so, such as situation awareness, signal detection and judgement analysis. Each has been applied in other professions and environments that share similar characteristics to nursing including high-stakes outcomes and requirements for a high degree of reliability and accuracy. The relevance of these applied JDM perspectives is supported by a growing body of evidence across different nursing specialisms. The greater the degree to which individual nurses use such resources to become critically aware of the JDM process, the better the profession is positioned to argue that nursing JDM is a credible and critical resource for patient care.

We have highlighted judgement as a means for describing, tracking, explaining and predicting patient status (Lamond *et al.* 1996). We have also argued that judgement is integral to decision-making functions that, in nursing, commonly focus on intervention choices, communication options, and organisationally focused options (Thompson *et al.* 2000). Nurses support the JDM of other health professionals as well as making independent judgements and decisions. JDM is a highly purposeful activity in nursing practice carried out for the purpose of assessment, monitoring, discharge planning, risk assessment, assessing adherence to treatment and so on. Yet nursing JDM is also relational and mindful of the therapeutic relationship. One of the biggest challenges for nursing JDM is to find a balance between the acknowledgement of the value of experiential knowledge and an openness to evidence-based decision support systems.

Two of the key approaches to JDM in the literature are intuition and analysis. In most instances it is assumed that nurses use elements of both. However, in practice nurses tend towards relying on intuition because of environmental and time limitations. In this chapter we touched on the influence that organisations and groups have on JDM, as well as highlighting issues regarding JDM within the ethical domain of practice. This is to encourage nurses to consider and explore not just the cognitive processes involved in

JDM, but the practice of JDM in care environments that are marked by complex technology, interactions and working patterns. Ultimately, we argue that the cognitive, social and pragmatic factors that affect nursing work need to be articulated so that we can identify the nursing contribution to care and continue to make further improvements in care delivery.

SUGGESTED FURTHER READING

Hardman, D. (2009) *Judgement and Decision Making: Psychological perspectives*. Chichester, UK: British Psychological Society & Blackwell.

Kahneman, D. (2011) *Thinking, Fast and Slow*. London: Allen Lane.

Thompson, C. and Dowding, D. (eds) (2009) *Essential Decision Making and Clinical Judgement for Nurses*. London: Churchill Livingstone Elsevier.

REFERENCES

Adderley, U. J. and Thompson, C. (2015) Community nurses' judgement for the management of venous leg ulceration: a judgement analysis. *Journal of Nursing Studies* **52** (1), 435–354.

Baddeley, A. (2004) *Your Memory: A user's guide*. London: Carlton Books.

Bargh, J. A. (1994) The four horsemen on automaticity: awareness, intention, efficiency and control in social cognition. In *Handbook of Social Cognition, Volume 2: Application*, Wyer, R. S. and Srull, T. K. (eds). Hillsdale, NJ: Lawrence Erlbaum, pp. 1–40.

Beckstead, J. W. and Stamp, K. D. (2007) Understanding how nurse practitioners estimate patients' risk for coronary heart disease: a judgement analysis. *Journal of Advanced Nursing* **60** (4), 436–446.

Benner, P., Tanner, C. A. and Chesla, C. A. (2009) *Expertise in Nursing Practice: Caring, clinical judgement and ethics* (2nd edn). New York: Springer.

Brown, B. and Rakow, T. (2015) Understanding clinicians' use of cues when assessing the future risk of violence: a clinical judgement analysis in the psychiatric setting. *Clinical Psychology & Psychotherapy* **23** (2), 125–141.

Brunswik, E. (1955) Representative design and probabilistic theory in a functional psychology. *Psychological Review* **62** (3), 193–217.

Buckingham, C. D. and Adams, A. (2000) Classifying clinical decision-making: a unifying approach. *Journal of Advanced Nursing* **32** (4), 981–989.

Cheyne, H., Dalgleish, L., Tucker, J., Kane, F., Shetty, A., McLeod, S. and Niven, C. (2012) Risk assessment and decision making about in-labour transfer from rural maternity care: a social judgment and signal detection analysis. *Medical Informatics and Decision Making* **12**, 122.

Dalgleish, L. (1988) Decision-making in child abuse cases: applications of social judgement theory and signal detection theory. In *Human Judgement: The SJT view*, Brehmer, B. and Joyce, C. R. B. (eds). Oxford: North-Holland, pp. 317–360.

Dalgleish, L., Shanteau, J. and Park, A. (2010) Thresholds for action in judicial decisions. In *The Psychology of Judicial Decision Making*, Klein, D. E. and Mitchell, G. (eds). Oxford: Oxford University Press, pp. 165–180.

Dowding, D. W., Cheyne, H. L. and Hundley, V. (2011) Complex interventions in midwifery care: reflections on the design and evaluation of an algorithm for the diagnosis of labour. *Midwifery* **27** (5), 654–659.

Dowding, D., Turley, M. and Garrido, T. (2012) The impact of an electronic health record on nurse sensitive patient outcomes: An interrupted time series analysis. *Journal of the American Medical Informatics Association* **19** (4), 615–620.

Drach-Zahavy, A., Goldblatt, H. and Maizel, A. (2014) Between standardisation and resilience: nurses' emergent risk management strategies during handovers. *Journal of Clinical Nursing* **24** (3–4), 592–601.

Durso, F. T. and Sethumadhaven, A. (2008) Situation awareness: understanding dynamic environments. *Human Factors* **50** (3), 442–448.

Elliott, N. (2010) 'Mutual intacting': a grounded theory study of clinical judgement practice issues. *Journal of Advanced Nursing* **66** (12), 2711–2721.

Elstein, A. S. and Bordage, G. (1988) Psychology of clinical reasoning. In *Professional Judgement: A reader in clinical decision making*, Dowie, J. and Elstein, A. (eds). Cambridge: Cambridge University Press, pp. 109–129.

Endsley, M. R. (1995) Towards a theory of situation awareness in dynamic systems. *Human Factors* **37** (1), 32–64.

Ericsson, K. A., Whyte, J. and Ward, P. (2007) Expert performance in nursing: reviewing research on expertise in nursing within the framework of the expert-performance approach. *Advances in Nursing Science* **30** (1), E58–E71.

Gillespie, B. M., Chaboyer, W., St John, W., Morley, N. and Nieuwenhoven, P. (2015) Health professionals' decision-making in wound management: a grounded theory. *Journal of Advanced Nursing* **71** (6), 1238–1248.

Grounds, A., Glesthorpe, L., Howes, M., Melzer, D., Tom, B. D. M., Brugha, T., Fryers, T., Gatward, R. and Meltzer, H. (2004) Access to medium secure psychiatric care in England and Wales. 2: a qualitative study of admission decision-making. *Journal of Forensic Psychiatry and Psychology* **15** (1), 32–49.

Hammond, K. R. (1996) *Human Judgment and Social Policy: Irreducible uncertainty, inevitable error, unavoidable injustice*. Oxford: Oxford University Press.

Hancock, H. C., Mason, J. M. and Murphy, J. J. (2012) Using the method of judgement analysis to address variations in diagnostic decision making. *BMC Research Notes* **5**, 139.

Hardman, D. (2009) *Judgement and Decision Making: Psychological perspectives*. Chichester: British Psychological Society & Blackwell.

Harries, P., Yang, H., Davies, M., Gilhooly, M., Gilhooly, K. and Thompson, C. (2014) Identifying and enhancing risk thresholds in the detection of elder financial abuse: A signal detection analysis of professionals' decision-making. *BMC Medical Education* **14**, 1044.

Hastie, R. and Dawes, R. (2001) *Rational Choice in an Uncertain World: The psychology of judgment and decision-making*. Thousand Oaks, CA: Sage.

Havens, D. S. and Vasey, J. (2005) The staff nurse decisional involvement scale: report of psychometric assessments. *Nursing Research* **54** (6), 376–383.

Haw, C., Stubbs, J. and Dickens, G. (2015) Medicines management: an interview study of nurses at a secure psychiatric hospital. *Journal of Advanced Nursing* **71** (2), 281–294.

Hoffman, K. A., Aitken, L. M. and Duffield, C. (2009) A comparison of novice and expert nurses' cue collection during clinical decision-making: verbal protocol analysis. *International Journal of Nursing Studies* **46** (10), 1335–1344.

ICN (International Council of Nurses) (2002) *International Classification for Nursing Practice: Beta 2*. Geneva: International Council of Nurses.

Kahneman, D. (2011) *Thinking, Fast and Slow*. London: Allen Lane.

Kahneman, D. and Tversky, A. (1973) On the psychology of prediction. *Psychological Review* **80** (4), 237–251.

Klein, G. (2008) Naturalistic decision making. *Human Factors*, **50** (3), 456–460.

Lamond, D., Crow, R., Chase, J., Doggen, K. and Swinkels, M. (1996) Information sources used in decision-making: considerations for simulation development. *International Journal of Nursing Studies* **33** (1), 47–57.

MacNeela, P., Scott, P. A., Treacy, M., Hyde, A. and O'Mahony, R. (2012) A risk to himself: attitudes towards psychiatric patients and choice of psychosocial strategies among nurses in medical-surgical units. *Research in Nursing & Health* **35** (2), 200–213.

MacNeela, P., Clinton, G., Place, C., Scott, A., Treacy, P., Hyde, A. and Dowd, H. (2010) Psychosocial care in mental health nursing: a think aloud study. *Journal of Advanced Nursing* **66** (6), 1297–1307.

Manias, E. and Street, A. F. (2001) The interplay of knowledge and decision-making between nurses and doctors in critical care. *International Journal of Nursing Studies* **38** (2), 173–184.

Maule, J. (1997) Strategies for adapting to time pressure. In *Decision Making under Stress: Emerging themes and applications*, Flin, R., Salas, E., Strub, M. and Martin, L. (eds). Aldershot: Ashgate, pp. 271–289.

Miller, G. (1956) The magical number seven, plus or minus two: some limits on our capacity for processing information. *Psychological Review* **63** (2), 81–97.

Montgomery, H., Lipshitz, R. and Brehmer, B. (2005) *How Professionals Make Decisions*. Mahwah, NJ: Lawrence Erlbaum.

Porter, S. (1991) A participant observation study of power relations between nurses and doctors in a general hospital. *Journal of Advanced Nursing* **16** (6), 728–735.

Rasmussen, J. (1993) Deciding and doing: decision-making in natural contexts. In *Decision Making in Action: Models and methods*, Klein, G., Orasallu, J., Calderwood, R. and Zsambok, C. E. (eds). Norwood, NJ: Ablex, pp. 158–171.

Samuriwo, R. and Dowding, D. (2014) Nurses' pressure ulcer related judgements and decisions in clinical practice: A systematic review. *International Journal of Nursing Studies* **51** (12), 1667–1685.

Sharpe, V. A. (2004) *Accountability: Patient safety and policy reform*. Washington, DC: Georgetown University Press.

Simmons, B. (2010) Clinical reasoning: concept analysis. *Journal of Advanced Nursing* **66** (5), 1151–1158.

Simon, H. (1956) Rational choice and the structure of environments. *Psychological Review* **63** (2), 129–138.

Standing, M. (2008) Clinical judgement and decision-making in nursing: nine modes of practice in a revised cognitive continuum. *Journal of Advanced Nursing* **62** (1), 124–134.

Stubbings, L., Chaboyer, W. and McMurray, A. (2012) Nurses' use of situation awareness in decision-making: An integrative review. *Journal of Advanced Nursing* **68** (7), 1443–1453.

Thompson, C. and Dowding, D. (eds) (2009) *Essential Decision Making and Clinical Judgement for Nurses*. London: Churchill Livingstone Elsevier.

Thompson, C. and Adderley, U. (2015) Diagnostic and treatment decision making in community nurses faced with a patient with possible venous leg ulceration: a signal detection analysis. *International Journal of Nursing Studies* **52** (1), 325–333.

Thompson, C., McCaughan, D., Cullum, N., Sheldon, T., Thompson, D. and Mulhall, A. (2000) *Nurses' Use of Research Information in Clinical Decision-Making: A descriptive and analytical study*. London: NCC SDO.

Thompson, C., Yang, H. and Crouch, S. (2012) Clinical simulation fidelity and nurses' identification of critical event risk: a signal detection analysis. *Journal of Advanced Nursing* **68** (11), 2477–2485.

Thompson, C., Aitken, L., Doran, D. and Dowding, D. (2013) An agenda for clinical decision-making and judgement in nursing research and education. *International Journal of Nursing Studies* **50** (12), 1720–1726.

Yang, H. and Thompson, C. (2010) Nurses' risk assessment judgements: a confidence calibration study. *Journal of Advanced Nursing* **66** (12), 2751–2760.

Yang, H. and Thompson, C. (2011) The effects of clinical experience on nurses' critical event risk assessment judgements in paper based and high fidelity simulated conditions: a comparative judgement analysis. *International Journal of Nursing Studies* **48** (4), 429–437.

Yang, H., Thompson, C. and Bland, M. (2012) Effect of improving the realism of simulated clinical judgement tasks on nurses' overconfidence and underconfidence: evidence from a comparative confidence calibration analysis. *International Journal of Nursing Studies* **49** (12), 1505–1511.

14

COMMUNICATION AND INTERPERSONAL SKILLS

Victoria Lavender

LEARNING OUTCOMES

After reading and reflecting on this chapter, you should be able to:

* explain the basic components of communication;
* outline a range of communication and engagement skills that can be employed within a caring relationship with a client;
* describe the skills involved in initiating, maintaining and disengaging from the therapeutic relationship;
* discuss the importance of the development of emotional intelligence in interpersonal skills working.

INTRODUCTION

The fundamental importance of effective communication in nursing practice is acknowledged repeatedly (Egan 2014, Hargie 2011) and has long been regarded as integral to the provision of high-quality patient-focused care (Dunn 1991, Macleod Clark 1988). There is evidence that effective communication prior to and during physical procedures reduces anxiety, enhances coping and increases treatment concordance (Dickson 1999, Nichols 1993). For Faulkner the ability 'to communicate effectively . . . is at the heart of all patient care' (1998, p. 1). The nurse's competence in communicating will determine whether, and to what degree, the client's nursing needs will be appropriately assessed and met (Gallant *et al.* 2002).

Central to the healing process is the professional caring relationship (often called the therapeutic relationship) between the nurse and the client. This chapter explores some essential building blocks for creating and sustaining as well as disengaging from therapeutic relationships.

The chapter is divided into three parts. In Part 1 an outline is offered of the importance of effective communication and interpersonal skills in relation to nursing practice. This is accompanied by a brief overview of the scope of the subject area.

Part 2 provides a fuller explanation of the importance of nurses being effective in communication and interpersonal skills. A brief review of verbal and para-verbal aspects of communication is offered before explaining two aspects of building and maintaining the therapeutic relationship: (i) building and maintaining trust; and (ii) demonstrating respect, empathy and genuineness.

In Part 3, a deeper exploration of communication and interpersonal skills is provided with an emphasis on some more advanced and complex aspects of developing and maintaining a therapeutic relationship. Some information relating to barriers to and disengaging from therapeutic relationships concludes the chapter.

PART 1: OUTLINING COMMUNICATION AND INTERPERSONAL SKILLS

Case 14.1

Almira is a third-year student nurse working on a general medical ward in a small local hospital. Suzanne (Almira's mentor) is a larger than life personality who was born and brought up in the local community. Almira finds Suzanne loud and a little overbearing with her unrestrained jollity, her tendency to stand a bit too close, and her (over) use of physical contact. Almira notices that Suzanne tends to call everyone (staff and patients) 'pet' and is surprised that no one seems to mind. Almira is not sure she likes being called pet, but she does not voice her objections because it seems to be accepted as part of the ward culture and, anyway, she is intimidated by Suzanne.

The importance of developing communication skills

Stickley and Freshwater argue that 'nursing involves the formation of a meaningful relationship through the development of an effective interpersonal process' (2006, p. 13). They point out that a need for improvement remains despite emphasis placed on the importance of effective interpersonal and communication skills in nursing.

Peplau's (1991/1952) theory of nursing helped turn attention away from internal patient pathology towards therapeutic processes between nurse and patient. Peplau recognised the therapeutic opportunity for patients to understand the circumstances of their health along with the potential to make beneficial health-related changes. At the heart of the interpersonal process lies a requirement for nurses to develop effective and caring communication skills.

RESEARCH FOCUS 14.1

Mallett and Dougherty (2000) report in their study of patient satisfaction of care that the quality of nurse's communication was recorded as the least satisfying aspect. They go on to suggest that complacency or indifference to the goal of improving communication and interpersonal skills has no place in the preparation for becoming a registered nurse.

Communication and nursing

Communication can be defined as a reciprocal process of sending and receiving messages. Thoughts, feelings and information are sent as encoded messages and may be conveyed verbally via pitch, tone, inflection and speed of speech. Equally important messages are conveyed non-verbally via facial expression, eye contact, body posture, body position, movement and gestures. The receiver decodes the message to make sense of the sender's thoughts, feelings or information and generally returns messages in response to what they have understood. Consisting of a sender, a message and a receiver, this model of communication is described as linear (McQuail and Windahl 1981).

Figure 14.1 illustrates the reciprocal nature of interpersonal communication. Both sender and receiver are likely to receive simultaneous transmissions from each other requiring amendments to both coding and decoding processes. The transmission process will also be influenced by, for example, environmental factors (such as external noise levels), the degree of privacy, or the presence of others. Encoding and decoding messages is fraught with potential for misinterpretation and/or misunderstanding, and with additional barriers such as the specialised language of health care or differing attitudes, values or beliefs of the participants, this makes the communication process complex and highly individualistic.

Contemporary models of communication try to capture this complexity. In a circular transactional model, such as the one in Figure 14.2, communication is viewed as a circular process with communication as 'a reciprocal interaction in which sender and receiver influence each other as they converse' (Arnold and Underman Boggs 2016, p. 8). The emphasis here is placed on the contexts of communication within a relationship and, in contrast to the linear model, holds that feedback and validation are interdependent and dynamic elements. Feedback as the response from the receiver to the original message will affect future communication. In this model feedback is conveyed even in the absence

FIGURE 14.1
A linear model of communciation

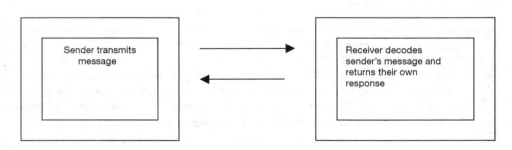

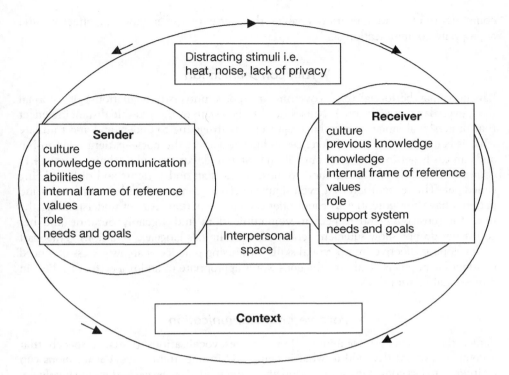

FIGURE 14.2
A circular transactional model of communication

Source: after Arnold and Underman Boggs, 2016.

of a response, and validation is understood as a form of feedback that confirms participants hold similar understandings of the message and the feedback.

Nelson-Jones (2014) categorises the basic means by which we send messages to one another as:

- *verbal messages* (via words and language);
- *para-verbal or vocal messages* (via volume, articulation, pitch, tone and speech rate);
- *non-verbal or body messages* (via facial expression, eye contact and gaze, gesture, posture, physical proximity, touch, clothing and grooming); and
- *action-taking messages* (via letters, reports and e-mails when sender and receiver are not face-to-face).

Nurses are most involved with face-to-face interactions with patients, their relatives and carers, and other health care professionals so this chapter focuses primarily on verbal, para-verbal and non-verbal communication and interpersonal skills.

PART 2: EXPLAINING COMMUNICATION AND INTERPERSONAL SKILLS

The components of communication

The complexity of the communication process requires nurses to ensure proficiency and effectiveness in clarity as senders of messages and in sensitivity of understanding as receivers. Being aware of the complexities, subtleties and dynamics of individual

Vocalisations are those parts of speech that accompany words. So volume, clarity of words, pitch, tone and rate of speech add to the meanings of spoken words and can convey messages that may or may not reflect the speaker's intention.

components of communication enables the nurse to use a range of effective and appropriate communication skills.

Verbal communication

Language may be formal (e.g., government reports, university regulations) or informal (e.g., everyday conversations). Nurses need to be aware of the possible distancing effect that professional language may have with clients struggling to understand and translate what is being said. Cultural differences in language affect the nurse–patient relationship and can easily get in the way of mutual understanding. For example, Almira (Case 14.1) comes from a different background to most of the staff and patients and dislikes being called pet. The recognition that even simple everyday conversations between nurses and patients have the potential to cause offence is an important part of understanding the need for sensitivity and respect in communication; and arguably Suzanne and her colleagues do not show sufficient sensitivity for Almira's language traditions. Thus part of developing effective interpersonal skills for nursing practice is an awareness of a need to adopt clear, precise and unambiguous words appropriate to and respectful of others in professional relationships.

Para-verbal communication

Para-verbal (or vocal) communication includes vocalisations (parts of speech that accompany words) that add to what is being said in important ways. **Vocalisations** can be interpreted as conveying information about the sender's message and include: volume, articulation, pitch, tone and speed of delivery. Each has the potential to be interpreted (or misinterpreted) by the listener regardless of the intention of the speaker.

Volume refers to loudness or softness of speech and should be appropriate to a client's hearing capacity and environmental conditions. Overly loud delivery of speech may be interpreted as conveying anger or hostility, or may simply make others feel uncomfortable (Almira wonders if some patients find Suzanne's loudness uncomfortable); undue softness may convey uncertainty, shyness or deference.

Articulation refers to clarity of words spoken and can be related to volume. For example, a nurse who mumbles will compound communication problems for someone with difficulty hearing in noisy environments (and hospital wards are often noisy environments).

Pitch refers to the height or depth of the voice and tone refers to the manner of delivery. Both can be interpreted as conveying (regardless of the intention of the speaker) the underlying thoughts, feelings and attitudes of the speaker.

The rate of speech includes the number of words spoken each minute as well as the frequency and the duration of pauses between words. A rapid speech rate may convey speaker anxiety, excitement or degree of happiness. A slow speech rate may convey ponderous thinking, pomposity or condescension.

Each para-verbal aspect of speech can obstruct clear and effective communication. When everyone understands the culturally and socially specific speech conventions, the potential for misunderstandings is minimal. So in a small, localised community with few 'outsiders', ways of communicating (including the nuances of, for example, irony, dialects and accents) will be understood by all participants. Until recently, this has been the situation on the ward where Almira is a student. Such communities are becoming rare with increasing multiculturalism and increasing diversification of language development in different communities. As populations of nurses and patients diversify so the potential for misunderstandings or offence increases. In professional life the onus is on the nurse (rather than the patient) to enable rather than hinder effective communication. So Suzanne seems to be relying on forms of communication no longer appropriate to her situation. Providing safe and effective care requires nurses to recognise responsibility for developing effective interpersonal skills as part of maintaining methods of communication that contribute to the well-being of patients, and this includes ensuring respectful communication between health and social care individuals.

Non-verbal or bodily communication

Perhaps the main vehicle for sending non-verbal messages is through facial expressions. According to Ekman *et al.* 'seven categories of emotion [mediated by facial expression] have been found . . . happiness, surprise, fear, anger, sadness, disgust/contempt and interest' (2013, p. 45)

The eyes, the eyebrows and the mouth shape are particularly effective in conveying expressed or unexpressed emotion. Eye contact both sends and collects information and helps to regulate turn-taking during conversations. Nelson-Jones (2014) suggests that during conversations, listeners look at speakers more often than speakers look at listeners (approximately 70–75 per cent for the former, 40 per cent for the latter). Speakers tend to look at listeners just before they intend to pause or stop speaking to collect feedback about the listener's reactions and to invite the listener to take a turn at speaking. However, eye contact conventions vary. Hogg and Holland (2010) note that Western under-standings of eye contact as signalling honesty is understood as rudeness or challenging in some cultures. In Arabic cultures, prolonged eye contact denotes respect, whereas in South Asian cultures it is regarded as aggressive or confrontational.

Gestures are physical movements that accompany speech and demonstrate, illustrate or emphasise particular aspects of verbal communication; sometimes replacing words, for example, nodding or shaking the head indicating agreement or disagreement respectively. Gestures too are culturally specific, so a gesture in one part of the world may mean something altogether different in another. The classic example offered by Liberman *et al.* (1975) is the hand gesture made by the thumb and first finger meeting to form a circle in the familiar 'OK' sign in many parts of the world. For Hispanic Americans, however, this signals an invitation to perform a sexual act.

Posture encompasses both the relative heights of speaker and listener and whether the body is turned toward or away from the other person. Unequal height can cause feelings of unease; for example, a nurse standing might seem to tower over a client who is lying or sitting. Turning the body or part of the body towards the other person con-veys interest. Turning the body away or crossing the arms or legs (often referred to as a closed posture) may be interpreted as lack of interest, indifference or defensiveness. An open posture with arms and legs uncrossed, relaxed and reasonably still indicates acceptance, interest and a willingness to continue communication.

Physical closeness is an important non-verbal component. Hall (1966) suggests zones of comfort in Western cultures as intimate (between 15 and 46 centimetres) for spouses, lovers, close friends and relatives; personal (46 to 122 centimetres) for acquaintances at social gatherings; social (1.22 to 3.6 metres) for people unknown to each other; and public (over 3.6 metres) for impersonal public gatherings. Some individuals do not observe these

355

Victoria Lavender

The **therapeutic relationship** is initiated, promoted, managed and sustained by the nurse for the express purpose of helping the client meet their treatment goals.

proximity zones and the zones may be different in different cultures: ignoring the social norms of any one group by positioning the body too closely may give rise to feelings of unease or even threat. This helps to explain why Almira feels uncomfortable in Suzanne's presence.

The intimacy of nursing requires nurses to be sensitive to these zones and to ensure physical proximity does not raise patient feelings of violation or distress. This can be a difficult area to negotiate as touch is such a powerful conveyor of warmth, comfort and acceptance, so an awareness of how patients might show non-verbal signs of discomfort (e.g., slight facial grimacing or physical movement away from the nurse) is important.

Activity 14.2

Face-to-face communication includes:

- *verbal components* (words and language);
- *para-verbal components* (volume, articulation, pitch, tone, rate of speech);
- *non-verbal components* (facial expression, eye contact and gaze, gestures, posture, proximity and touch, clothing and grooming).

Try to identify each of these components while you are engaged in conversation with another student. Use the questions below to help you think about how these components facilitate or hinder the communication process.

- Do you use all components in all conversations?
- In what ways do the different components interact?
- Which (if any) components dominate?
- Which (if any) components hinder communication?
- Which (if any) components enable effective communication?

The therapeutic relationship

The idea of **therapeutic relationships** between nurses and clients builds on the work of humanist psychologist Carl Rogers. The therapeutic relationship is initiated, promoted, managed and sustained by a nurse so as to help clients meet their treatment goals. It is defined as a helping relationship 'established for the benefit of the client, whereas kinship and friendship relationships are designed to meet mutual needs' (Balzer Riley 2012, p. 16). Arnold and Underman Boggs (2016) suggest that social relationships are distinguished from therapeutic ones that aim to:

- enhance well-being;
- promote recovery; and
- support self-care.

In the therapeutic relationship communication is directed towards the needs of the client although the patient is not merely a passive recipient, for inherent in the therapeutic relationship is a sense of affiliation or working in partnership. Gallant and colleagues

(2002) trace the idea of client as equal partner as consistent with contemporary emphasis on the importance of basic human rights.

Timmins (2004) and Price (2006) suggest that partnership working acknowledges and values the patient's knowledge and skills in managing their ill-health, particularly for long-term conditions. If communication is unidirectional from nurse to patient, then essential information is likely to be omitted from the assessment, planning and evaluation of client care. In the absence of partnership, giving clients information follows a pattern of 'I talk/you listen', reinforcing notions of professional dominance.

The most frequently cited benefit of partnership working is empowerment understood as enhancing the ability of a client to act in their own interest, leading to improved self-esteem and confidence (Courtney *et al.* 1996, Raeburn and Rootman 1998). Arnold and Underman Boggs (2016) describe empowerment as preparing patients to cope with difficult life situations resulting from alterations in health and well-being.

Developing and maintaining therapeutic relationships

Some of the essential skills necessary for building and maintaining a nurse–patient therapeutic relationship can be summarised as:

- building and maintaining trust;
- demonstrating respect, empathy and genuineness;
- active listening;
- listening to self and developing self-awareness;
- setting and maintaining professional boundaries.

The first two act as building blocks for the more advanced and complex skills needed for the other three. Building and maintaining trust together with demonstrating respect, empathy and genuineness will be the focus of the remainder of this part of the chapter. Active listening, listening to self and developing self-awareness, and setting and maintaining professional boundaries are considered in Part 3.

Building and maintaining trust

Trust can be defined as the firm belief in the honesty, integrity and reliability of another person. A therapeutic relationship always begins with trust (Arnold and Underman Boggs 2016). Trust is part of the psychological contract between nurse and patient. It is difficult to define but if a therapeutic relationship is to develop, the patient must be able to feel the nurse is trustworthy (Sellman 2006, 2007).

Earning a patient's trust is a lengthy process and a warm, friendly and respectful greeting is likely to start the process well. Ensuring the client's preferred form of address is used, correctly pronounced and that friends or family members are welcomed will help begin building an early rapport essential for the formation of trust. An introduction, a brief explanation of one's role in the patient's care, maintaining eye contact, an open body posture, appropriate proximity and equal height with the patient may all serve to strengthen the patient's willingness to trust the nurse.

However, these simple techniques should reflect the intentions of the nurse. If the verbal message (i.e., what the nurse is saying) does not match the nurse's facial expression, posture, or tone of voice the disparity between words and manner will create a sense of

Empathy
is the ability to 'step into' the inner world of another person in order to understand their thoughts, feelings, behaviours and meanings.

unease or even distrust. Knapp (1980) notes that we may be able to match our facial expressions and posture with what we are saying but we often fail to control the movements of our hands, legs or feet. So we can very easily 'give away' feelings of, say, anxiety, irritation or boredom, by, for example, clenching our hands, swinging our legs or tapping our feet.

Activity 14.3

Have a go at saying the sentences below to a partner or while looking in a mirror. Try to match your non-verbal and spoken messages.

- No, you're not disturbing me. It's lovely to see you, please come in.
- I feel very upset at your news, it's so sad this has happened.
- Please don't worry, it was only an old vase – I'm sure I can get another one.

Now repeat the sentences while deliberately mismatching your non-verbal behaviour with the words and the way you deliver them. For example, if the last statement is accompanied by an angry facial expression, a rigidly held posture and clenched hands, the reassuring verbal message will be lost giving the receiver the impression of the sender's anger despite the words used. Try to work out why the non-verbal message is likely to dominate and undermine the sender's verbal message.

Trust is reinforced by behaviour. The nurse who promises to pass on a message or perform a task and fails to do so without apology or explanation will quickly lose a client's trust. The Nursing and Midwifery Council (NMC) requires registered nurses to 'promote professionalism and trust' (2015, p. 15). The nurse who breaks a patient's trust damages the nurse–patient relationship, their own professional standing and the reputation of nursing.

Demonstrating respect, empathy and genuineness

Rogers (1961) claims that respect, **empathy** and genuineness are the core conditions for building and maintaining therapeutic relationships, demonstrating warmth and respect with unconditional positive regard: that is, accepting others for what they are, not on condition they behave in certain ways or exhibit particular characteristics.

Respect

Treating people with respect is fundamental to nursing. The way a nurse introduces themself to, and how a nurse addresses, a patient will convey an attitude of respect (or otherwise) to that patient. So the nurse who routinely addresses all older patients by first name or as 'pet' or 'dear' (even where that is local convention) is failing to respect those who prefer formal forms of address. The routine of asking patients how they would like to be addressed and then making that preference known to other health care professionals is one way to show respect. Valuing and acting in accord with patient preferences demonstrates respectful communication.

Being respectful entails paying close attention to what the client says, ensuring the client understands all aspects of their care, seeking permission or consent and protecting and actively promoting the client's privacy. Being respectful also includes maintaining client confidentiality, promoting choice and accepting different cultural behaviour (Lago 2006).

Case 14.2

Shirley, aged 57, has a history of mental health problems. She is currently experiencing periods of low mood, with a loss of appetite and insomnia. She tries to describe her thoughts and feelings to Marty, her named nurse. Shirley speaks hesitantly and in little more than a whisper. Marty finds it increasingly difficult to focus on what Shirley is saying and allows himself to lose concentration. His eye contact with Shirley becomes fleeting and he begins to gaze out of the window. He tries to stifle a yawn and once or twice interrupts Shirley by asking inconsequential details.

Activity 14.4

Read Case 14.2 before answering the following questions:

- How is Marty's behaviour likely to affect Shirley's expression of her thoughts and feelings?
- What might she interpret from his behaviour?
- What effect could this have upon the relationship between them?

Being respectful requires assertiveness. To be assertive involves clear and direct communication of individual needs and acknowledgement of the needs of others. When we show respect we are heeding another's right to be treated with dignity and consideration without ignoring or undermining our own needs.

Respect does not mean merely agreeing with the client's perspective, for respectful disagreement involves stating your point of view, explaining the reasons for it and acknowledging others may have a different perspective. Respect entails listening attentively, acknowledging differences and not succumbing to a need to be always right. The nurse who apologises for mistakes, misunderstandings, individual shortcomings and/or unforeseen changes to plans, demonstrates professional accountability and respect for the injured party.

Arnold and Underman Boggs describe empathy as 'the connective caring bridge between health providers and clients' (2016, p. 6). When we mentally put ourselves in the shoes of others and verbally convey what it might be like to wear those shoes, we are being empathic. Empathy aids in establishing therapeutic relationships by conveying a sense of being cared for. Balzer Riley (2012) suggests that it is not just empathy that is beneficial, but the intention of the giver and the perception of the receiver. To experience an empathic response from a nurse is to experience feelings of connectedness, of being cared for, understood and accepted. For the nurse, empathy can help establish and maintain a caring relationship with, and demonstrate respect for and acceptance of the client's internal world.

Responding empathically can be broken down into a number of steps:

1   Focusing on the speaker by filtering out distractions, paying attention to verbal and non-verbal messages, and recognising expressions of feelings.
2   Being aware of one's non-verbal responses, including facial expression, eye contact and gaze, gestures, posture, proximity and touch.
3   Being aware of one's verbal responses, choice of words, tone of voice, volume, articulation, pitch and rate of speech as well as congruence between verbal and non-verbal communication.
4   Identifying dominant feelings expressed by the speaker.
5   Verbally reflecting back the feelings you think you have heard. For example, 'It sounds as if you feel really disappointed that you won't be able to go home today as planned'.
6   Checking to see if your interpretation of the speaker's feeling is accurate. For example, 'Have I got that right?' or 'Is that how you are feeling?' Checking allows for feelings to be clarified. If your interpretation is correct the client will feel you understand them and this may further encourage them. If your interpretation is incorrect the speaker has the opportunity to clarify what they mean; 'No, it's not that I'm disappointed I'm not going home yet, it's more that I'm anxious about coping once I'm home'.

Failing to check your interpretation of the client's feelings may result in the client experiencing a sense of being told what they are feeling. Far from being understood and accepted, the client is then likely to feel alienated. Empathic responses, in reflecting back the feelings the client expresses, can serve as permission for the patient to voice what they might otherwise regard as unacceptable.

Activity 14.5

Consider the interaction between Julia, a 49-year-old patient recovering from a partial mastectomy and Lucy, a second-year nursing student.

Julia: I know I shouldn't be thinking like this. Perhaps I shouldn't even be saying this. I know I've got a lovely family. I just feel at times that I haven't got the energy to carry on. Sometimes, I just wish that I could go to sleep forever and not wake up again.

Lucy: Now cheer up, surely it's not as bad as all that!

Julia: I know you think I'm being silly.

Lucy: As you said, you have got a lovely family, very supportive. You are very lucky; you should count your blessings.

- What feelings might lie behind Julia's words?
- How might Julia feel after hearing Lucy's response?
- Is Julia likely to feel able to discuss her feelings further?
- What might lie behind Lucy's attempt to cheer Julia up?
- Try to write out a response that Lucy might give, which conveys a more empathic response to Julia's first statement.

Congruence between non-verbal and verbal communication will help to convey to the client a sense that the nurse is being genuine. The absence of genuineness is said to lead to sterile application of communication techniques (Arnold and Underman Boggs 2016). Being authentic requires the nurse to be clear about their own beliefs, attitudes, thoughts and feelings. This in turn relates to the need for assertiveness skills, self-awareness and in particular, awareness of personal limitations and some of the difficulties in managing a professional image.

Although much of current nursing literature exhorts the need for genuineness (Arnold and Underman Boggs 2016, Nelson-Jones 2014), little attention has been paid to the difficulties associated with being authentic in clinical settings. The reality of busy clinical areas often means that nurses feel they have neither the time, opportunity or energy to apply Rogerian principles of empathic understanding, respect and genuineness in their hurried and often fragmented client contact (Aiyegbusi and Norton 2013). Nelson-Jones (2014) acknowledges that inexperience or under-confidence may lead to the presentation of an inauthentic but desperately held professional façade, particularly if the client appears to question the knowledge, authority and previous experience of the professional carer. Perhaps a response that honestly acknowledges areas of inexperience, particularly in not having experienced the same emotions as the client, will be both a genuine response and one that conveys a truthful validation of the uniqueness of the client's emotional experience: a response of *I know exactly how you feel* is likely to be the point at which clients will question, albeit silently, the genuineness of the nurse.

> **Congruence** relates to the harmony or consistency in communication messages, for example, between verbal and non-verbal means.

PART 3: EXPLORING COMMUNICATION AND INTERPERSONAL SKILLS

You may have heard it said that it is unprofessional to express your personal feelings, particularly if you feel critical of the client. This suggests a need for a degree of professional detachment seemingly at odds with the requirement to be genuine within emphatic responses.

RESEARCH FOCUS 14.2

Aranda and Street (1999) explored nurses' concepts of being authentic and the need for flexibility in presenting aspects of themselves in order to respond to clients' particular needs, for example, to gain access to the details of the patient's life or seek concordance with treatments. The nurses in the study termed this being a chameleon. They expressed discomfort at changing styles of interaction with clients with its implication of being manipulative and inauthentic (even when the overall goal remained improvement of patient outcomes).

Aranda and Street propose that reconciliation of these tensions is possible through the concept of a nurse–patient relationship governed by intersubjectivity. Intersubjectivity suggests that all human relationships are co-constructed by the participants, that our reactions to others are shaped and formed by their interpretation of us. The circular transactional model of communication (Figure 14.2) illustrates the fluid nature of this process. Shifts in presentation of self are not necessarily inauthentic or manipulative; they merely represent individuals' responses to each other as each contributes to the development of the relationship.

Victoria Lavender

Advanced and complex communication skills

Active listening

Presence or attending refers to the ability of the nurse to remain physically, spiritually and emotionally attuned to the client's communication.

Many people mistakenly believe that good talkers will be good listeners. Stickley and Freshwater (2006) note there is no guarantee that a fluent conversationalist will make a good listener. Here it is useful to distinguish between hearing and listening. Hearing involves the capacity to be aware of and receive sounds. Listening involves both hearing the sounds and interpreting their meaning. According to Gordon (2000), active listening involves trying to accurately understand a speaker's messages and to demonstrate understanding by carefully chosen responses. Requiring the exercise of both receiving and sending skills, active listening is considered an essential skill in creating and maintaining the therapeutic relationship (Arnold and Underman Boggs 2016, Nelson-Jones 2014, Stickley and Freshwater 2006).

Burnard (2003) suggests that while social (or phatic) communication can aid in establishing rapport with patients, effective therapeutic communication requires the listener to move on from the phatic stage to what Wright (2006) terms 'deep listening'. For Wright, deep listening necessarily involves setting aside one's own thoughts, listening without judging and attending closely to what is being said. In this sense the effectiveness of the therapeutic conversation depends on the nurse's ability to listen and detect clues that might entail the need for sensitive responses; responses that aim to help the client explore and express their feelings. Active listening requires:

- presence or attending skills;
- asking questions;
- clarifying, restating and paraphrasing;
- using silence;
- reflecting feelings.

Presence or attending skills

Gardener (1992) identifies presence as a therapeutic gift of self and as 'the embodiment of caring in nursing' (p. 193). **Presence or attending** skills convey an unselfish interest in the client where the focus remains on the speaker. Presence refers to the ability of the nurse to remain physically, spiritually and emotionally attuned to the client's communication. Attending calls for the listener to concentrate and focus on what the speaker is saying by trying to suspend any personal thoughts or ideas in order to interpret and understand the other person's perspective.

To be effective, this intentional focus must be congruent with non-verbal messages of interest. A still and open posture, a slight lean of the upper body towards the speaker, and direct eye contact will convey the listener's focus and interest. Appropriate facial expressions such as a smile or a frown or a nodding of the head may encourage the speaker to continue. Periodically verbal encouragements such as: *go on* or *please take your time* or short vocalisations, for example, *mm* or *uh-huh* can be given. Attending skills may sound relatively straightforward, even simplistic. However, practice, concentration and a genuine desire to understand the patient are needed to ensure active listening is not 'acting' listening. Over time practice will enable these skills to be incorporated into the nurse's personal communication style and thus become both genuine and subtle.

362

Asking questions

Asking questions enables the nurse to find out about the patient. **Open questions** are useful in eliciting clients' thoughts or feelings. Perhaps the most common exception to this is the everyday *how are you?* which, although an open question, is commonly understood as a greeting rather than an enquiry: thus tends to be met with a *fine* or an *OK*-type response. However, it can be easily adapted to become a more open question, as it would be, for example, in the enquiry *how do you feel about having surgery tomorrow?* If the invitation to expand is rebuffed by a simple *OK thanks*, it is appropriate to remember that therapeutic questioning is not interrogation. Therapeutic questioning requires a sensitive and accurate reading of the verbal and non-verbal messages from the client and a willingness to adopt flexible communication strategies based on responses received.

Closed questions are appropriate when information is needed quickly or in a structured format. Examples of closed questions might be *when did you have your last insulin injection?* or *does the pain get worse on exertion?* A variation of the open question is the focused question, which is useful when seeking specific information about a particular subject or issue, for example, *can you tell me more about the pain in your shoulder?* or *can you describe your pain?*

Circular questions (Arnold and Underman Boggs 2016) focus on the interpersonal context in which an illness occurs and are designed to identify family relationships as well as the impact illness might have on individual family members. Questions of this kind can help illuminate the patient within the contexts of family or others involved in their care. An example might be, *who in your family is likely to be most affected by your father's illness?* or *how is your younger sister coping with your mother's diagnosis?*

Open questions are those that require more than a mere *yes, no* or similar response.

Closed questions are those that require no more that a mere *yes, no* or similar response.

Activity 14.6

Can you identify which of the following are open questions, which are closed questions, and which are circular questions?

- How do you feel about being discharged from hospital?
- Have you lost weight recently?
- Do you feel overwhelmed by all your visitors?
- How will your partner manage the house and the business without you?
- Do you have any pain?
- Can you tell me if your child lost consciousness?
- What do you feel is the best course of treatment for you right now?
- Can you squeeze my hand?
- Ten milligrams a day – is that your normal dose?
- How will your father view his son's refusal to visit?
- How do you feel about having a different community nurse?

While most of these questions clearly fall in one or other category, others incorporate elements of more than one type. For example, the question, *do you feel overwhelmed by all your visitors?* can be answered as both an open and a closed question. You might find it useful to discuss your ideas about which are open, closed or circular questions with other students.

Clarifying, restating and paraphrasing

Seeking clarification is sometimes necessary if the nurse is to understand the client's message. Using a neutral tone to ask the client to elaborate or explain helps ensure that they do not feel they have to justify or defend their thoughts and feelings. A simple question that asks for clarification, such as, *can you explain that to me?* demonstrates interest in the client, checks the accuracy of interpretation and allows the client to feel heard.

Restating is the repetition of a small section of the sender's message, often in the form of a query, using the sender's own words. This allows the sender to hear for themselves what they have said and provides the opportunity for them to clarify, amend or be more specific. For example, a client might say: *since my heart attack I just can't get on with the things I want to do. I feel I'm no use to anyone any more.* In restating the fragment . . . *no use to anyone?* as an enquiry, the nurse provides the patient with an opportunity to expand on what could be a significant point. Restating is a useful technique but it needs to be used sparingly or it can hinder effective communication by interrupting the flow of a client's thoughts

Both clarification and restatement can be counterproductive if the listener's tone of voice is accusatory or demanding. However, restating can be used as a positive affirmation of the client. For example, in response to a client who says, *I think I've done quite well with my exercises*, the nurse might restate the fragment . . . *only quite well?* in a warm tone of voice and thus convey to the client a sense of achievement.

To paraphrase is to attempt to put into different words the core elements of another person's message. Paraphrasing a client's thoughts and feelings should always be done tentatively so that the client can correct any misinterpretations or confirm correct understanding. Accurately paraphrasing can mirror the speaker's material but offers the possibility of being clearer and more succinct than the original messages. There is no single correct way of paraphrasing and much will depend on the listener's own choice of words, but if the message has been accurately heard the client is likely to confirm it, for example, *yes, that's right* or *you've got it exactly*.

Using silence

Using silence as an active listening skill offers the patient time to think, and as Arnold and Underman Boggs (2016) note, allows the nurse to step back momentarily and process what they have heard before responding. A natural anxiety on the part of the nurse concerning how to respond or whether the response is appropriate and helpful to the client may lead to filling silences with unnecessary comments. The length of a silence needs to be carefully judged and much will depend on the client's ability to process information and respond to the nurse.

Ending a silence too quickly may not only give the client insufficient time to formulate their thoughts and responses but may convey to the client the nurse's anxiety or discomfort with the topic. Sharing a silence can convey the nurse is willing to 'be with' the client in the sense of attending or presence. Silence may occur for many reasons and might mean that something has touched the client deeply; respecting the client's silence and sitting without breaking the mood can demonstrate an empathic understanding and acceptance of the client's feelings.

Activity 14.7

When you talk with patients be aware of silences as they arise.

- Ask yourself why did the silence occur?
- Look for non-verbal clues that may help you to form an answer.
- Be aware of how silences make you feel.
- Do you try to break a silence as quickly as you can, and if you do, why?
- Is it easier to let the silence continue with some patients and not with others?
- How do you break silences?
- If you cannot break a silence with words (and most of us are often not as articulate as we would like to be) what non-verbal means of communication might be appropriate?

Reflecting feelings

Reflecting feelings can involve paraphrasing but the focus is more on the client's expression of feeling rather than their words. Nelson-Jones (2014) defines the skill of reflection as 'empathising with a client's flow of emotion and communicating this back' (p. 100). Reflection involves the skilled interpretation of verbal and non-verbal clues. Emotions are not always verbalised but may be observed as incongruence between the patient's verbal and non-verbal messages. *I'm fine* might be a verbal response to the question of how the person is feeling but the non-verbal clues of a sad facial expression or tearfulness will undermine the verbal message. Reflection tries to capture the overt and covert messages to reflect them back in an empathetic manner.

Activity 14.8

In the following piece of dialogue a third-year student nurse, Simon, uses reflection in a sensitive and effective way, enabling Clyde, a 17-year-old patient, to express his feelings.

Clyde: I can't bear all the noise in here.
Simon: You are finding the noise upsetting?
Clyde: It's just that there are so many people around all the time. I can't explain it; somehow it makes me feel alone.
Simon: It sounds like you are feeling lonely. Is that how you feel?
Clyde: I guess so. I feel a bit silly really.
Simon: It doesn't sound silly to me at all. Feeling lonely is very upsetting.

Review the skills discussed so far in this chapter and try to identify other elements of therapeutic communication involved in this exchange. You may find this more productive if you undertake this part of the exercise with another student.

Patients may resist revealing their underlying feelings, but gentle and sensitive use of reflection may help the patient to articulate and understand their emotional responses to health-related issues. Egan suggests the following questions may help students to clarify the reflective process at a more advanced level:

- What is this person only half saying?
- What is this person hinting at?
- What is this person saying in a confused way?
- What covert message is behind the explicit message?

(Egan 2014, p. 177)

Listening to self and developing self-awareness

Stickley and Freshwater (2006) assert that before we can listen successfully to others it is important to develop the art of listening to ourselves. This involves becoming conscious of the thoughts, feelings, attitudes, beliefs, prejudices and values likely to affect our interactions with others. Nurses are expected to protect the interests and dignity of patients and clients, and 'avoid making assumptions and recognise diversity' (NMC 2015, p. 4). Arnold and Underman Boggs (2016) indicate that self-awareness helps us to connect emotionally with others. Nurses can learn about themselves through reflecting upon their motives, feelings, responses and behaviours in relation to others. A specific incident, perhaps initially regarded as negative, for example, an unsuccessful confrontation, or an interaction that could be felt to be more positive, such as a warm and caring interpersonal exchange, can be useful in providing a focus for the nurse to reflect critically upon and record both their strengths and the areas in need of further development (see Chapter 17 for more on reflective practice).

Activity 14.9

The five questions below are adapted from Carl Rogers (1958). They are designed to encourage self-awareness in nurse–patient relationships. Think of a client with whom you feel you have a therapeutic relationship. Work through the questions, applying each to your relationship. You might be tempted to simply answer 'yes' and move on but try to think about each question carefully. You could make short notes exploring how you can demonstrate that you are able to answer 'yes'. What areas might still be in need of further development? What steps could you take to start to achieve this?

1 Can I *be* in some way that will be perceived by the other person as trustworthy, dependable, or consistent in some deep sense?
2 Can I let myself experience positive attitudes toward this other person – attitudes of warmth, caring, liking, interest and respect?
3 Can I let myself fully enter into the world of their feelings and personal meanings and see these as they do?
4 Can I accept this person as they are? Can I communicate this attitude?
5 Can I maintain separateness from this person and foster separateness in them?

Burnard (2002) suggests a positive correlation between a nurse's understanding of self and their openness and honesty in interactions with others. By knowing personal prejudices, motivations and current abilities, the nurse can increase their capacity for being empathic with clients.

Setting and maintaining personal boundaries in the therapeutic relationship

One consequence of becoming self-aware is noticing when aspects of the therapeutic relationship serve the nurse's rather than the client's needs. Question 5 above refers to maintaining a sense of separateness from the client. This may seem to contradict the call for 'being with' in attending skills of active listening to build an empathetic understanding of the client. However, a sense of separateness is essential in the therapeutic relationship and maintained through appropriate emotional distancing or emotional boundary keeping.

Therapeutic boundaries are appropriate emotional distances between the nurse and client that help to preserve a sense of separateness and thus allow for safe interactions between the client and the health care professional.

Case 14.3

Jan is a mature student nurse and has formed a close relationship with Georgie, aged 11, who has been a patient on the children's unit for several months. Georgie is aware of his poor prognosis but remains cheerful. From time to time he talks optimistically about his future hopes of being a professional footballer.

Jan has two children, one of whom is the same age as Georgie, and finds it difficult to cope with the knowledge that Georgie is likely to die soon. She feels that she needs to spend as much time with Georgie as she possibly can when she is on duty and is aware that she often thinks about him when she is with her own family. Jan has a strong sense of frustration that little can be done for Georgie. She spends extra time with him before and after each shift. As Georgie becomes increasingly frail Jan finds it almost impossible to hide her distress when he talks about which football club he would like to play for.

Jan's mentor is concerned about the amount of time she is spending with Georgie and has noticed that she seems to resent other nurses being involved in his care. She gently voices her concerns and listens empathically as Jan acknowledges her distress and anxiety about not being able to cope with Georgie's death. She is also able to acknowledge that her emotional involvement with Georgie and his family has led her to think that she has the most important role of all the care team members in being responsible for his care. Her mentor discloses her own similar experience earlier in her career and explains how supportive the care team were in helping each other come to terms with the death of a young patient. Jan and her mentor discuss the nature of empathy and the importance for professional staff of maintaining a sense of separateness or objectivity with a client.

After talking with her mentor Jan was able to relinquish her sense of being solely responsible for Georgie's care and in consequence felt a sense of relief that she was part of a team of professional staff, able to draw on the support and supervision of experienced colleagues.

Therapeutic boundaries are behavioural limits that allow for the safe interaction between client and health care professional (Peterson 1992). According to Malone *et al.* (2004) these limits define and protect the space between a health care professional's power and the client's vulnerability. It is the nurse's responsibility (not the patient's) to set and maintain professional boundaries. The nurse should set clear boundaries when the relationship is first established and must remain consistent in maintaining those boundaries.

A nurse who is emotionally over-involved with the patient is likely to be meeting their own needs rather than the needs of the client. Over-involvement is likely to show itself with the nurse coming to believe that only they are able to fully understand and care for the client, losing the necessary detachment and objectivity needed in accurate assessment and delivery of care. The over-involved nurse may give more time and attention to one particular client, coming to see them in off-duty hours, discounting the efforts of other health care professionals and performing tasks for the client that they could, and probably should, perform for themselves. The over-involved nurse may agree to keep the client's secrets or may not pass on information that should be shared with other members of the health care team. They may also disclose intimate information about themselves and about their experiences in the mistaken belief that they are being empathic or seeking reciprocity with clients.

The NMC requires that nurses maintain appropriate professional boundaries in relationships with patients and clients, ensuring that all aspects of the care focus on the needs of the patient (NMC 2015). However, it may be others, particularly more experienced staff, who first become aware of the over-involvement of the nurse. Dowling (2006) notes that despite a theoretical understanding of the importance of maintaining a therapeutic emotional distance, inexperienced nurses are likely to be less able to maintain an expectation of equal partnership when working with patients, especially patients whose ill-health renders them vulnerable and those who seek dependency upon nursing staff.

Professional boundaries are limits that demarcate the edges of the relationship between the nurse and the client. The parameters of therapeutic boundaries must be embedded in the core conditions of respect, warmth and authentic concern for the client. The development of self-awareness is pivotal in being able to recognise where professional relationship boundaries have become unclear. However, self-monitoring behaviour is an advanced reflective skill that demands honest and unflinching examination of one's motives and behaviours.

Mentor and supervision support is invaluable in helping the nurse discuss and explore the nature of their relationships with clients. Most nurses will be able to recognise the difficulties faced from their own experiences and will be in a position to offer suggestions and support in managing the situation. Hawes (2005) suggests that a culture of nursing colleagues sharing their experiences of the difficulties of managing boundaries needs to be encouraged if junior nursing staff are to feel able to seek advice and support. Gallop (1998) suggests a simple reflective question can help to initiate the process of self-monitoring; for example, *would other nurses or health care professionals think my behaviour with this client appropriate?*

Dowling (2006) suggests that in certain circumstances self-disclosure may be appropriate but requires an acute sense of self-awareness. A parent of a sick child who asks if the nurse has children of their own may be seeking reassurance that someone who understands the needs of both the child and the parent is nursing their child. When a distressed client probes the nurse with a question to ascertain the nurse's personal experiences of coping with stressful events, the nurse needs to measure self-disclosure carefully as the outcome of sharing may have a positive or a negative effect. Before self-disclosure, a useful technique might be to pause and think: in revealing this information, whose need is being met? If the answer appears to favour the nurse's needs then the level of disclosure is likely to be inappropriate.

Relationship boundaries may be tested by patients and might take the form of making unreasonable demands of time and attention, or by indicating that they would like a personal, social or sexual relationship with the nurse. Testing boundaries can also include using behaviours that the patient thinks will provoke a particular response from the nurse, for example, asking for confidential information about fellow patients, making crude sexual innuendoes or telling risqué jokes.

The nurse who deals clearly and directly with boundary testing reasserts the professional parameters of the relationship, allowing both the client and the nurse to refocus on goals that relate to the client's health care. A clear statement from the nurse of what is considered acceptable behaviour, far from damaging the therapeutic relationship, serves to strengthen and underpin future interactions in a constructive and positive manner. Indistinct, ambiguous or violated boundaries undermine the trust necessary for the development of therapeutic relationships.

Barriers to the therapeutic relationship

Factors that can raise difficulties in the nurse–patient relationship, include:

- nurse or patient anxiety;
- specific communication difficulties;
- low emotional intelligence.

Client or nurse anxiety can be a threat to the therapeutic relationship. Common causes of stress for patients are apprehension about their health status or about their current and future treatment options. Anxiety might also relate to uncertainty about future coping and the effects of their ill-health on others, including family members. Nurses may be anxious if they feel under-confident, unsupported by colleagues, inexperienced, or insufficiently competent. Student nurses have the additional pressure of placement assessment.

Anxiety can disrupt and seriously detract from the quality of the therapeutic relationship. Nurse–patient communication is likely to be stilted, superficial and hurried. Concentration is more difficult and active listening and attending are problematic for the anxious nurse. Anxiety will undoubtedly inhibit the degree of warmth and level of genuineness shown to the client.

Patient anxiety may result in a need for repeated reassurance from the nurse. When such reassurance is given but fails to provide the comfort sought, the nurse may feel increasingly unable to meet the client's needs and may begin to avoid further contact.

RESEARCH FOCUS 14.3

Geanellos (2005) found that nurse unfriendliness, characterised by patients as frostiness, officiousness and apathy gave rise to patients feeling unsafe, unwelcome, anxious and unprotected.

In this situation, decreasing patient anxiety is essential if the therapeutic relationship is to flourish, and for patients with severe anxiety, psychiatric and medical interventions may be necessary. Arnold and Underman Boggs (2016) recommend that in mild to moderate levels the nurse can adopt a number of strategies to assist the client. These include:

- active listening to show acceptance;
- honesty – answering all questions at the client's level of understanding;
- clearly explaining procedures, surgery and policies and providing reassurance based on evidence
- acting in a calm, unhurried manner
- speaking clearly and firmly (but not loudly)
- encouraging clients to explore their reasons for anxiety
- using play therapy with dolls, puppets, games and drawing for young clients
- using therapeutic touch, giving warm baths, relaxing music
- teaching breathing and relaxation exercises.

Anxiety levels for the nurse may be reduced by seeking support from mentors, other staff, course and personal tutors, peers and friends. Perhaps the most effective intervention is the one in which the nurse realises that support networks are readily available. Smith (1992) noted that when nurses feel appreciated and supported emotionally by senior staff not only do they have a role model for sensitive and empathic patient care but they also feel able to care for patients in the same way. Chant and colleagues (2002) agree, and suggest that poor support systems and an occupational or ward culture of task-orientated dominance that excludes or diminishes the importance of individualised support for nursing staff has a direct and negative correlation on the quality and standards of care for patients.

Specific communication difficulties can arise with different client groups with different needs and abilities. A detailed exploration of the needs of all client groups cannot be undertaken here but some general comments are offered.

For clients with limited cognitive ability and/or impaired communication the nurse must strive to deliver verbal messages using uncomplicated language in short sentences, containing a single subject or topic in each sentence. Ample time needs to be given and open questions, repeated and rephrased if necessary, will allow the client an opportunity to understand interactions and formulate a response. Frequently checking the client's level of understanding by using clarification through repeating, restating and asking for further explanation, is also likely to be effective.

It may be appropriate for nurses to talk with carers or advocates, particularly if the client's ability to communicate is severely limited; however the individual client should not be ignored or excluded and must be addressed directly during conversation and discussion (Godsell and Scarborough 2006). For clients with sensory impairments, face-to-face communication where the nurse's face can be clearly seen is likely to maximise the client's understanding of what is being said. Increasing the speech volume may be necessary but clear articulation and unhurried speech will be equally or more effective. Para-verbal and non-verbal means of communication can enhance or, if necessary, replace limited verbal exchanges. Touch, body positioning and proximity together with explicit attending skills will help to convey the qualities of genuine interest, warmth and respect for the client.

Pictures, photographs and sign language, known as augmentative and alternative communication systems (AACs), can be used to enhance or supplement verbal communication. Picture boards, simple line drawings or objects can provide easy yet effective methods of communication. Other resources such as leaflets and books with symbols, signs and pictures to explain medical procedures are becoming increasingly available in clinical areas.

Emotional intelligence

Defined as 'a core aptitude related to one's ability and capacity to reason with one's emotions, especially in relation to others' (Freshwater and Stickley 2004, p. 92), **emotional intelligence** plays an important role in effective nurse–patient communication (Cadman and Brewer 2001, McQueen 2004). Being self-aware is part of emotional intelligence, although it encompasses other complex human skills of relationships including empathy, motivation, self-control and adeptness. It is argued that emotional intelligence can be extended and developed through training and that it should be at the heart of education for nursing (Cadman and Brewer 2001, McQueen 2004).

Goleman (1998) suggests it is emotional intelligence that determines an individual's capacity to develop the skills or competencies related to the following five elements of effective communication:

1 *Self-awareness* (emotional awareness, the ability to self-assess with accuracy, high self-esteem).
2 *Self-regulation* (the ability to control emotion and impulse, flexibility in handling change, the ability to innovate).
3 *Motivation* (the need to achieve, need to initiate, optimism).
4 *Empathy* (understanding and developing others, a willingness to meet others' needs, the ability to 'tune into' individuals' or groups' emotional states).
5 *Social skills* (persuasiveness, conflict management, leadership skills).

How does emotional intelligence relate to nursing?

Freshwater and Stickley (2004) claim that emotional intelligence is necessary for effective nursing because nurses work with human emotions such as fear, anxiety, sadness, hope, joy, relief and anger. Cadman and Brewer (2001) hold that the ability to manage one's emotional life while interpreting other people's is a prerequisite skill for any caring professional. In addition to empathy, emotional intelligence includes the ability to manage the emotions we experience as a result of nursing others.

Although it is now acceptable for nurses to show their feelings as they empathise with patients, there is a need to control and manage these emotions if the patient is not to be overwhelmed. Omdahl and O'Donnell (1999) differentiate between acceptable controlled empathic concern and unacceptable overwhelming emotion (or 'emotional contagion'). Thus the type and degree of emotion shown requires self-regulation. This need for self-regulation is particularly important in relation to negative emotional response to, for example, irritation, anger, frustration, or disgust rather than to the many pleasurable emotions associated with nursing practice. A nurse who is unable to exert some control over their negative emotions may damage the therapeutic relationship and the wider professional image of nursing.

Emotional intelligence requires an advanced level of self-awareness; emotional intelligence includes the wider and complex human skills of empathy, motivation, self-control and adeptness in relationships.

Henderson (2001) suggests that emotional involvement is a requirement for nursing excellence, contributing to quality care and the emotional well-being of patients and nurses. However, continuous and intense emotional work can be stressful, demanding and exhausting. Benner and Wrubel (1989) suggest that unrelenting work of this nature can adversely affect the physical and psychological health of the nurse, with the potential to lead to burnout. A balance is needed between providing intimate personal attention to patients and recognising personal limitations. Self-regulation and the adoption of coping techniques such as seeking support and supervision as well as a willingness to accept alternative nurse–patient allocation can be beneficial for both the nurse and the patient.

The complexities of health care provision across hospitals, primary care and the voluntary and independent agencies demand trust, understanding and cooperation. Motivational, social and collaborative working skills are all part of emotional intelligence. The therapeutic relationship is not an isolated entity and directly benefits from the input of all professionals associated with the care of the client. The nurse unable or unwilling to develop and extend their emotional intelligence capabilities threatens to nurse at a mechanistic or task-orientated level and this can be a significant barrier to the richness of the therapeutic relationship.

Disengaging from the therapeutic relationship

By their very nature, therapeutic relationships are time limited; they have a beginning and an end. There are no set time limits for therapeutic relationships; some can last for just a few hours, others may continue for months or even years. Regardless of the length of the therapeutic relationship the same basic principles of disengagement are as follows:

- *Informing*: letting the patient know that the nurse–patient relationship is coming to an end allows an opportunity for the client to acknowledge their feelings on ending the relationship.
- *Maintaining authenticity and boundaries*: it may be necessary for the nurse to restate the professional boundaries required in the nurse–patient relationship, including the need to not make promises to keep in touch or accept invitations for meeting clients once the professional relationship is ended.
- *Acknowledging*: valuing the patient's contribution to meeting their health care goals as well as to the professional development of the nurse.

Some patients develop a close relationship with a particular nurse: when that relationship ends they may experience feelings that lie anywhere in a spectrum ranging from mild disappointment to intense sadness or loss. Arnold and Underman Boggs (2016) draw an analogy between the psychological responses of bereavement and the termination of the therapeutic relationship for both nurse and client. Part of the therapeutic relationship should include the process of preparing the client for ending the relationship by stating when the nurse or patient will need to say goodbye. It may be appropriate from time to time to remind the client of the temporary nature of the relationship, particularly if there is a sense that the patient may have started to become over-reliant on their contact with the nurse. The first principle of disengagement is that the nurse should ensure that patients are made aware of the approaching end of the working relationship and, if appropriate, provide the time and opportunity for the patient to acknowledge their feelings.

Many student nurses will be familiar with the experience of feeling tempted to make promises of keeping in touch with clients once they have finished their clinical secondment, possibly prompted by the patient's responses to saying goodbye. However tempting, making such promises is often unwise. It is likely to be impractical and making a promise to keep in touch would therefore be inauthentic. It is also likely to be contrary to the maintenance of professional relationship boundaries, as it could herald the change from professional to social relationship parameters. The second principle is that, if necessary, nurses must politely but assertively restate that the nature of the professional relationship is such that it must remain focused on the client's health care needs.

It may also be appropriate for the student nurse to express appreciation of having worked closely with the patient and to thank them for their contribution to the nurse's preparation towards becoming a registered nurse. Partnership is a collaborative process, but patients may be unaware of their contribution to the nurse's professional development and unaware of the contribution they have made to meet their own health care goals. It might therefore be appropriate for the nurse to acknowledge how far the goals have been met in the form of a short summary to capture these points. Other resources and future plans for meeting health care needs or the maintenance of health gains can also be discussed, for example, future follow-up care arrangements or referrals to other organisations, agencies and health care teams.

Activity 14.10

Review the basic principles of disengaging from the nurse–patient relationship and write a short response to the scenarios below.

- You have been working with Ian for a number of weeks and feel that you have established a close nurse–patient relationship. He is aware that today is your last working day on the unit. You have come to say goodbye when Ian says, 'I'd really like to keep in touch. Perhaps you could come round for a drink or a meal? I know that my family would love to see you and I'd like to know how you do on your course'.
- Molly has made little eye contact with you and seems distant in her manner since you talked about the transfer of her care to the community team. You open the subject of her future plans but she interrupts with 'I expect you find it hard to remember anyone, you must see so many different patients all the time. This time next week you won't even remember my name'.

CONCLUSION

There is substantial evidence that effective communication plays a pivotal role in successful health outcomes in modern health care provision. At the heart of effective nursing care lies the professional relationship between nurse and patient, a relationship that is founded on the development and practice of the interpersonal and communication skills of each nurse. The therapeutic relationship is vitally important to the effectiveness and quality of care and offers possibilities of deep personal satisfaction and involvement for the nurse in the care of clients.

Reading this chapter has provided the opportunity to explore some of the basic components of communication and interpersonal skills that you can now employ within caring relationships with clients. In acknowledging the importance of communication you can contribute to effective patient care by demonstrating a willingness to enhance your communication and interpersonal skills. Harnessing your skills of listening to the self, developing self-awareness, and enhancing your ability to set and maintain therapeutic boundaries can help you to overcome barriers to effective therapeutic relationships.

SUGGESTED FURTHER READING

Arnold, E. C. and Underman Boggs, K. (2016) *Interpersonal Relationships, Professional Communication Skills for Nurses* (7th edn). St Louis, MO: Elsevier.

Lago, C. (2006) *Race, Culture and Counselling: The ongoing challenge* (2nd edn). Maidenhead: Open University Press.

REFERENCES

Aiyegbusi, A. and Norton, K. (2013) Creating a therapeutic environment in inpatient care and beyond. In *The Art and Science of Mental Health Nursing* (3rd edn), Norman, I. and Ryrie, I. (eds). Maidenhead: Open University Press, pp. 184–284.

Aranda, S. K. and Street, A. F. (1999) Being authentic and being a chameleon: nurse–patient interaction revisited. *Nursing Inquiry* 6 (2), 75–82.

Arnold, E. C. and Underman Boggs, K. (2016) *Interpersonal Relationships, Professional Communication Skills for Nurses* (7th edn), St Louis, MO: Elsevier.

Balzer Riley, J. W. (2012) *Communications in Nursing* (7th edn). St Louis, MO: Elsevier Mosby.

Benner, P. and Wrubel, J. (1989) *The Primacy of Caring*. London: Addison-Wesley.

Burnard, P. (2002) *Learning Human Skills: An experiential and reflective guide for nurses* (4th edn). Oxford: Butterworth-Heinemann.

Burnard, P. (2003) Ordinary chat and therapeutic conversation: phatic communication and mental health nursing. *Journal of Psychiatric and Mental Health Nursing* 10 (6), 678–682.

Cadman, C. and Brewer, J. (2001) Emotional intelligence: a vital prerequisite for recruitment in nursing. *Journal of Nursing Management* 9 (6), 321–324.

Chant, S., Jenkinson, T., Randle, J. and Russell, G. (2002) Communication skills: some problems in nursing education and practice. *Journal of Clinical Nursing* 11 (1), 12–21.

Courtney, R., Ballard, E., Fauver, S., Gariota, M. and Holland, L. (1996) The partnership model: working with individuals, families and communities towards a new vision of health. *Public Health Nursing* 13 (3), 177–186.

Dickson, D. (1999) Barriers to communication. In *Interaction for Practice in Community Nursing*, Long, A. (ed.). Basingstoke: Macmillan, pp. 84–132.

Dowling, M. (2006) The sociology of intimacy in the nurse–patient relationship. *Nursing Standard* 20 (23), 48–54.

Dunn, B. (1991) Communication interaction skills. *Senior Nurse* 11 (4), 4–8.

Egan, G. (2014) *The Skilled Helper: A problem-management and opportunity-development approach to helping* (10th edn). Belmont, CA: Brooks/Cole.

Ekman, P., Friesen, W. V. and Ellsworth, P. (2013) What emotion categories or dimensions can observers judge from facial behaviour. In Ekman, P. (ed.) *Emotion in the Human Face* (2nd edn reprint). Los Altos, CA: Malor Books, pp. 39–55.

Faulkner, A. (1998) *Effective Interaction with Patients* (2nd edn). London: Churchill Livingstone.

Freshwater, D. and Stickley, T. (2004) The heart of the art: emotional intelligence in nurse education. *Nursing Inquiry* **11** (2), 91–98.

Gallant, M. H., Beaulieu, M. C. and Carnevale, F. A. (2002) Partnership: an analysis of the concept within the nurse–client relationship. *Journal of Advanced Nursing* **40** (2), 149–157.

Gallop, R. (1998) Post discharge social contact: a potential area for boundary violation. *American Psychiatric Nurses Association* **4** (4), 105–110.

Gardener, J. (1992) Presence. In *Nursing Interventions: Essential nursing treatments* (2nd edn), Bulechek, G. and McCloskey, J. (eds) Philadelphia, PA: W. B. Saunders, pp. 191–200.

Geanellos, R. (2005) Undermining self-efficacy: the consequences of nurse unfriendliness on client well-being. *Collegian* **12** (4), 9–14.

Godsell, M. and Scarborough, K. (2006) Improving communication for people with learning disabilities. *Nursing Standard* **20** (30), 58–65.

Goleman, D. (1998) *Working with Emotional Intelligence*. London: Bloomsbury.

Gordon, T. (2000) *Parent Effectiveness Training: The proven program for raising responsible children* (30th anniversary edn). New York: Three Rivers Press.

Hall, E. T. (1966) *The Hidden Dimension*. New York: Doubleday.

Hargie, O. (2011) *Skilled Interpersonal Communication: Research, theory and practice* (5th edn). London: Routledge.

Hawes, R. (2005) Therapeutic relationships with children and families. *Paediatric Nursing* **17** (6), 15–18.

Henderson, A. (2001) Emotional labour and nursing: an under-appreciated aspect of caring work. *Nursing Inquiry* **8** (2), 130–138.

Hogg, C. and Holland, K. (2010) *Cultural Awareness in Nursing and Health Care: An introductory text* (2nd edn). Boca Raton, FL: CRC Press.

Knapp, M. L. (1980) *Essentials of Non-verbal Communication*. New York: Holt, Rinehart & Winston.

Lago, C. (2006) *Race, Culture and Counselling: The ongoing challenge* (2nd edn). Milton Keynes: Open University Press.

Liberman, R. P., King, L. W., DeRisi, W. J. and McCann, M. (1975) *Personal Effectiveness: Guiding people to assert themselves and improve their social skills*. Champaign, IL: Research Press.

Macleod Clark, J. (1988) Communication the continuing challenge. *Nursing Times* **84** (23), 24–27.

McQuail, D. and Windahl, S. (1981) *Communication Models for the Study of Mass Communication*. New York: Longman.

McQueen, A. (2004) Emotional intelligence in nursing work. *Journal of Advanced Nursing* **47** (1), 101–108.

Mallett, J. and Dougherty, L. (2000) *Manual of Clinical Procedures* (5th edn). London: Blackwell Science.

Malone, S. B., Reed, M. R., Norbeck, J., Hindsman, R. L. and Knowles, F. E. (2004) Development of a training module on therapeutic boundaries for mental health clinicians and case managers. *Lippincott's Case Management* **9** (4), 197–202.

Nelson-Jones, R. (2014) *Practical Counselling and Helping Skills* (6th edn). London: Sage.

Nichols, K. (1993) *Psychological Care in Physical Illness*. London: Chapman Hall.

NMC (Nursing and Midwifery Council) (2015) *The Code: Professional standards of practice and behaviour for nurses and midwives*. London: NMC.

Omdahl, L. and O'Donnell, C. (1999) Emotional contagion, empathic concern and communicative responsiveness as variables affecting nurses' stress and occupational commitment. *Journal of Advanced Nursing* **29** (6), 1351–1359.

Peplau, H. E. (1991/1952) *Interpersonal Relations in Nursing: A conceptual framework of reference for psychodynamic nursing*. New York: Springer.

Peterson, M. (1992) *At Personal Risk: Boundary violations in professional–client relationships*. New York: W.W. Norton.

Price, B. (2006) Exploring person-centred care. *Nursing Standard* **20** (50), 49–56.

Raeburn, J. and Rootman, I. (1998) *People-Centred Health Promotion*. New York: Wiley.

Victoria Lavender

Rogers, C. R. (1958) The characteristics of the helping relationship. *Personnel and Guidance Journal* **37** (1), 6–16.

Rogers, C. R. (1961) *On Becoming a Person: A therapist's view of psychotherapy*. Boston, MA: Houghton Mifflin.

Sellman, D. (2006) The importance of being trustworthy. *Nursing Ethics* **13** (2), 105–115.

Sellman, D. (2007) Trusting patients, trusting nurses. *Nursing Philosophy* **8** (1), 28–36.

Smith, P. (1992) *The Emotional Labour of Nursing. How nurses care*. Basingstoke: Macmillan.

Stickley, T. and Freshwater, D. (2006) The art of listening in the therapeutic relationship. *Mental Health Practice* **9** (5), 12–18.

Timmins, F. C. (2004) Improving communication in day surgery settings. *Nursing Standard* **19** (7), 37–42.

Wright, S. (2006) The beauty of silence. *Nursing Standard* **20** (50), 49–56.

15

PUBLIC HEALTH

Jane Thomas

LEARNING OUTCOMES

After reading and reflecting on this chapter, you should be able to:

- define public health and health promotion;
- explain the origins of public health, the emergence of the 'new' public health, and their relevance to specialist public health nursing;
- discuss the historical medical dominance of public health in relation to current practice in public health;
- identify the 10 areas of public health practice and reflect on their relevance to your own practice;
- discuss the relevance of public health to nursing with regard to practitioner-level competencies.

INTRODUCTION

Public health is an integral part of nursing practice. The daily work of nurses involves aspects of public health even if this is not always recognised as public health work. This chapter helps to illustrate the myriad ways in which nurses engage with public health work in both specialist and non-specialist environments.

The chapter is divided into three parts. In Part 1, an overview of the range of public health work that goes on in everyday nursing is offered together with a brief explanation of some of the more common public health terms.

In Part 2, an explanation of the importance of public health is offered together with illustrations of how nurses influence the way the public think about health. Awareness of the influence you have in your everyday contact with patients, their families and other members of the public is a starting point for recognising the responsibilities that come with the title of registered nurse. Recognition of this important part of the nursing role

Jane Thomas

Public health
'is the science and art of preventing disease, prolonging life and promoting health through the organised efforts of society' (Acheson 1988, p. 1).

allows you to begin to think more deeply about the influence you have and how you might go about being a positive role model in public health.

In Part 3, some of the history of public health is offered before beginning an exploration of some of the more specialised roles of public health within the overall framework of nursing practice. Some of the barriers to effective public health work are acknowledged and some attention is given to the potential future role of nurses in the public health arena.

PART 1: OUTLINING PUBLIC HEALTH

Case 15.1

Jasmine is a second-year student nurse. On a typical day in practice she washes her hands (often), she encourages healthy eating, she offers reassurance on a variety of health-related topics, she provides advice on lifestyle choices, and she responds to questions about the effects and side effects of drugs or other treatments.

Jasmine is studying to be a mental health nurse, but you cannot tell this merely from the activities listed above. She might just as easily be studying to be a children's nurse, a learning disabilities nurse, or an adult nurse; and she could be working in a hospital or a community setting. Hand washing, encouraging healthy eating, offering reassurance on health-related issues, providing advice on lifestyle choices and answering questions about medications and treatments are all ways in which nurses engage with public health.

These activities are a common aspect of nursing. Of course, the detail will be different within each field, for example:

- A learning disabilities nurse might help residents of a group home to choose their evening meal.
- A children's nurse might help a young child to learn how to brush her teeth.
- An adult nurse might advise on dietary choices for someone recovering from a heart attack.
- A mental health nurse might encourage an individual to practise relaxation techniques.

Nurses do these sorts of things as part of their everyday nursing practice, and each activity contributes in one way or another to the health and well-being of individuals and/or groups. These types of contributions form part of the nature of public health. Thus public health is an essential part of nursing, and this makes public health relevant to all nurses in all fields wherever and whenever nursing takes place. Public health knowledge comes from a number of different subject areas and adds in its own way to the body of professional nursing knowledge. This chapter offers an explanation and exploration of a number of the core concepts of public health that should help you to understand the relevance of public health to your current and future nursing practice.

Public health is difficult to define. It tends to be understood as an umbrella term for a range of activities undertaken by a number of different professionals who come together to study and/or influence health and patterns of disease. Some of the disciplines that contribute to public health are medicine, **epidemiology**, psychology, sociology, health promotion, nursing, social policy, health information, economics and anthropology. From a nursing perspective, public health is wide-ranging and involves nurses in a variety of ways including aspects of lifestyle choices, social change, environmental issues, empowerment and balancing **health intelligence** with lay knowledge. Traditionally, the focus has been on activities related to disease, particularly communicable disease, and priorities are determined by mortality and morbidity information. More recently public health attention has turned towards demographic trends, health improvement and non-communicable disease. There is also a growing awareness of socio-economic and social influences on health status. Public health priorities are identified on account of their impact on health or resources, their suitability for intervention and their public profiles.

Public health or health promotion

The way that the two terms 'public health' and '**health promotion**' are used can be confusing. Naidoo and Wills (2009) suggest combining them and you may see it expressed as 'health promotion/public health' or as 'public health and health promotion'. For this chapter the terminology of new public health has been adopted, where public health is understood as the overarching discipline within which health promotion is recognised as one of the contributing activities.

PART 2: EXPLAINING PUBLIC HEALTH

Why public health is important for nurses

Promoting health has long been recognised as a part of what nurses do and it continues to be the main public health focus for pre-registration nursing students. However, nurses have been involved in broader aspects of public health in one way or another at least since the time Florence Nightingale unpacked her bags at Scutari. Nightingale recognised the harm that could result from patients being nursed too close together and thus illustrated an early awareness of the need to control and prevent the spread of infectious disease. She also kept meticulous records that provided information to show patterns of disease and recovery (an early example of gathering health intelligence). Public health continues to be part of everyday nursing practice. Health visitors, community nurses, school nurses and infection control nurses are among those that have an obvious and clearly defined public health role, but as suggested in Part 1 of this chapter, all nurses have a part to play in public health. Patient education is a key element of how nurses contribute to public health. Hubley and Copeman (2013) offer a useful account of how we have moved from a patient compliance model, where patients are expected to do as asked by health care professionals, to a health empowerment approach. This is important because it moves the focus from the mere transfer of information from health professionals to patients towards a more equal, interactive process of information exchange with clients. This is more appropriate to the current climate in the health service and works well across primary, secondary and tertiary care settings. Keep this in mind as you work through the cases and activities.

Epidemiology involves the study of how, when and how often disease spreads, and of the factors that contribute to health and disease among populations.

Health intelligence is a term used to express the idea of collecting information about health, which can come from a number of sources and in a number of forms.

'**Health promotion** is the process of enabling people to increase control over, and to improve, their health' (WHO 1986).

Jane Thomas

Case 15.2

Linda Wilson is a busy housewife and mother. She has recently been diagnosed with diabetes and is adjusting to her insulin regime. Linda has always been of heavy build and is worried that the more structured eating regime required now will add to her weight. She has been given a lot of information about healthy eating and diabetes but has yet to find time to read it.

Linda enjoys preparing food for the family and often 'finishes off' any food the children leave. She takes an interest in the healthy diet information the children bring home from school but time and cost lead her to stick with what she knows. She is aware that she, her husband and her children are overweight. She worries when she reads about childhood obesity in the newspapers and sees features on TV. She would like to set a good example to the children but worries that the diabetic regime would not suit that. Linda feels that she is 'always on the go' and can't understand why she never loses weight. She has been unable to establish a pattern of exercise beyond walking the children to school.

Linda is the type of client you might meet in a number of different practice settings, such as the diabetic clinic of an outpatient department, an accident and emergency department, a local health centre, or an acute medical or surgical ward. Her situation illustrates many of the issues that currently challenge public health: the steady increase in lifestyle-related health problems such as diabetes; the role of the media and its influence on health behaviour; lifestyle issues such as diet and exercise; the link between poverty and problems such as obesity; the health status of individuals and so on. She benefits from health advice from her general practitioner and practice nurse as well as from the school health service through her children. For Linda, and for any nurse advising her, there are a range of options available if she is to establish a balance in her diabetes and develop a healthier lifestyle. This will inevitably require Linda to make changes in some of her behaviours related to, for example, diet and exercise and it provides the opportunity for the promotion of health through health education.

Activity 15.1

Think about the health care settings you have experienced and try to identify examples of public health activities undertaken by nurses.

As you will probably have identified from Activity 15.1 there are numerous examples of public health activities that take place in everyday nursing practice. For example, during a single working day a nurse might be asked about, among other things, giving up smoking, the effects and side effects of medications, holiday vaccinations, benefit entitlements, children's immunisations and advice on lifestyle, all in addition to the usual role of assessing, planning and delivering nursing care.

Public health embraces a whole range of issues that contribute to health or illness and is concerned with, for example, population and individual issues, lifestyle changes

380

and epidemics and health promotion and health protection, all in relation to both individuals and groups. Nurses have a key role to play in this because of the one-to-one patient contact and because of the unique relationship with patients in primary, secondary and tertiary care. Being in direct contact with the public on issues of public health puts a lot of responsibility on the nurse.

Public health in the UK currently includes diverse professional groups such as nurses, health promoters, **environmental health officers**, epidemiologists, health statisticians, pharmacists, health researchers, therapists, dietitians, doctors and midwives. Within nursing, among those with whom public health nurses work are cardiac rehabilitation nurses, school nurses, occupational health nurses, and respiratory and diabetic specialist nurses. Each of these has a specific profile that relates either wholly or partly to public health work. While each has a contribution to make, interdisciplinary and interprofessional working has become a necessity within the sector as the need to build professional alliances and develop innovative practice is increasingly recognised (for more information on interprofessional working see Chapter 7).

As illustrated above, public health is a broad concept, embracing a range of activities related to nursing and beyond. It includes infection control, disease and accident prevention, health promotion, health protection, health improvement and quality issues in the provision of care and service. It has relevance to the practice of all nurses, whether working with individuals, groups, communities or populations. Many elements of daily nursing practice, such as infection control precautions, notification of infection, statistical reporting and observing policies involve the application of public health practice. Many nurses working in the community have explicit and direct links to public health roles including for example, midwives, school nurses, occupational health nurses, some managers and some educationalists. With such a wide-ranging remit it can be difficult to understand the scope and extent of public health in relation to nursing. It is hoped that by reading this chapter you will be better able to understand public health and to see how it links to your current and future practice.

Environmental health officer is a local government role that has developed considerably in recent years to align with public health. Areas of interest include food hygiene, safe environments and health protection.

Health promotion in nursing practice

Activity 15.2

Sabrina works on a busy cardiac unit in a general hospital. Her role involves caring for patients recovering from acute cardiac episodes and most need to consider lifestyle change as part of their recovery. She has an interest in health promotion, which (as you now know) forms part of public health practice.

Have a go at answering the following questions before reading on:

- What type of lifestyle issues would be relevant for Sabrina to address with patients?
- What methods might she use to promote health?
- Who might her target audience be?
- What approaches might be appropriate?

Jane Thomas

Concordance has replaced the term compliance. Concordance is preferred as it implies patient involvement in agreement to follow the requirements of a treatment regimen.

Lifestyle issues

The lifestyle issues for people who have cardiac problems are well documented and include the need to take regular exercise, eat a healthy diet, reduce or give up smoking, reduce alcohol consumption, avoid substance misuse and try to avoid stressful situations.

Sabrina's methods

Many surviving cardiac patients are keen to make changes in their lifestyle in order to reduce their chance of repeat heart problems (even if in the long term most do not make permanent lifestyle changes). So these types of patients are likely to be receptive, at least in the short term, to advice given to them by health care professionals. Typically, a cardiac unit will be awash with information leaflets on promoting healthy eating, taking regular exercise, giving up smoking and moderating alcohol consumption. So a large part of the 'how' of health promotion here involves health education. Cardiac nurses spend a lot of time with patients re-enforcing the message of the need for permanent lifestyle changes to avoid future heart problems. Sabrina might also be able to refer patients to support groups and rehabilitation programmes where exercise regimens can be tailored to the individual needs of patients.

Sabrina's target audience

Clearly the patient is the primary focus of Sabrina's health promotion activities, and rightly so. However, few individuals can make changes to their lifestyles without it affecting a number of other people. For example, the 48-year-old male who wants to change his diet to eat healthily will need an enormous amount of willpower to make a permanent change if other members of his family continue a regular diet of burgers, chips, chocolate, crisps, doughnuts and other foods high in salt, sugar and saturated fats. This illustrates the point that for health promotion to be successful it needs to do more than merely take aim at individuals.

Sabrina's approaches

These might be thought about in three phases: short, medium and long term. In the short term there are the medical interventions and the immediate changes in behaviour. Sabrina

RESEARCH FOCUS 15.1

An example of the problems of changing lifestyles is found in the work of Lawlor and Hanratty (2001). Their work looked at the effect of advice regarding physical activity in primary care. They found that it was difficult for patients to make long-term changes on the basis of such advice. Studies in other areas of lifestyle have been more successful, for example, Barth, Critchley and Bengel's (2006) work on smoking with coronary heart disease patients. A number of factors play a part in the longevity of lifestyle change and research studies can help us to understand the significance of these for practice.

will need to focus on helping patients to understand the need for **concordance** with treatment. This will include giving information about the effects and side effects of prescribed medications and about when to seek further medical advice or assistance. Sabrina will also work to help patients understand the need to build up their activities gently and to know when to slow down or stop during the initial stages of their cardiac rehabilitation programme.

In the medium term Sabrina will focus on providing information, education and advice about what constitutes a healthy diet, what foods to avoid and the importance of regular exercise. She will also stress the importance of making these sorts of lifestyle changes permanent in order to reduce the likelihood of recurrence of cardiac problems. For obvious reasons, Sabrina will need to ensure the information is accurate and given in a way that the patient can understand. The patients Sabrina has contact with will reflect the profile of individuals within the community so while some will be readers of broadsheet newspapers others will read the tabloids, some may be unable to read (e.g., might have eyesight problems or may never have learnt to read) and some will struggle with English as their second language. If Sabrina is to help each cardiac patient to understand the implications of their medical condition she will need to be able to communicate effectively with all types of people (for more on communication skills see Chapter 14).

Long-term approaches to health promotion require changes in the general environment in which we all live. For example, even in the case of a person who wants to make lifestyle changes, it will not matter how much health education they receive if they cannot get to a shop that sells fresh fruit and vegetables.

It is tempting to think that health promotion is just about giving people accurate information and leaving them to make the right choices. If only it were so easy! Public health in general and health promotion in particular is complicated and there are all sorts of reasons why people do not always behave in ways that contribute to their own health, or to the health of others. Later we will say something about the factors that affect the way people behave in relation to their own health (see Part 3 of this chapter).

Public health with vulnerable groups

Activity 15.3

Sanjay works in a community home supporting clients with learning disabilities. The group is made up of 6 clients – 4 females and 2 males. The youngest client is aged 20 and the oldest is 51. Two residents are in a long-term relationship and one other has a girlfriend living elsewhere. Four of the residents are engaged in sheltered work but two are unable to do so because of health problems.

Have a go at answering the following questions before reading on.

- How might Sanjay achieve health improvement with this client group?
- Using the example of food hygiene, consider Sanjay's contribution to health protection.
- How could Sanjay's preventative practice help his clients?
- What knowledge and skills would Sanjay need to work with these clients?

Health improvement

There are a range of areas that Sanjay might focus on in order to assist the residents to improve their health including: drug concordance, nutrition and diet, alcohol and smoking, and sexual health and contraception.

Health protection

Safe food-handling is an essential component of safe and effective practice for all nurses. It is even more important for Sanjay because the residents of this group home are likely to be vulnerable to poor food hygiene. If only one member of the home has unhygienic habits it can create a danger for all the residents. So Sanjay will be able to contribute to health protection for the group by taking a lead in promoting good practice in food hygiene. This will involve aspects of personal and kitchen hygiene (e.g., effective hand washing); food storage (e.g., keeping raw and cooked meats separate); and thorough cooking (e.g., ensuring frozen food is properly prepared and cooked).

Prevention

Prevention involves some kind of intervention designed to stop something from happening, directly or indirectly. It requires knowledge, skills and attitudes and may encompass health education and protection. Examples include contraception, immunisation, avoiding stress, and anger management.

Knowledge and skills

It should be clear by now that if Sanjay is going to be effective in health improvement and protection he will not only need to be knowledgeable about the things identified as important for his particular area of practice but will also need to be skilled in encouraging and enabling this specific client group to adopt healthy rather than unhealthy behaviour. So Sanjay will need knowledge of, among other things, nutrition, food preparation and hygiene, workplace safety, sexual health and contraception and alcohol and drugs. He will also need to have the skills to communicate effectively with people with different communication abilities and be able to facilitate learning for individuals of varying intellectual capacities (for more about communication skills see Chapter 14; for more about learning and teaching see Chapter 16).

Hospital-based public health

Activity 15.4

Marte is a staff nurse working in a mental health facility. She works on Forsythia Ward, an 18-bed unit where most patients have long-term problems. Some patients spend long periods in supportive care environments, including acute hospital care, and depend on that infrastructure. The ward includes some rotational respite beds so Marte also has a changing group of clients who have home carers and so have different needs and challenges. In this group her care is focused not just on the client but on the carers too.

Have a go at answering the following questions before reading on.

- What contribution might Marte make to public health?
- Identify three priority issues that she could address with this client group.
- What barriers may prevent Marte from working productively with her client group?
- What are the advantages of working in this setting?

Empowerment involves assisting individuals to make independent decisions and so to take control of their lives. In public health terms this relates to enabling people to make autonomous and informed health-related choices.

Contribution

The contribution nurses make to the mental well-being of individuals and groups is often overlooked. Nevertheless, the link between physical and mental health is widely recognised and there is growing understanding of the inter-relationship between physical health and mental health (Naidoo and Wills 2009). There is some recognition of the psychological needs of patients in general health care environments: providing information as a way to reduce anxiety in pre-operative patients is one example of the contribution adult and children's nurses make in this respect (although providing information may increase anxiety in some patients). Mental health nurses make a much more obvious contribution in respect of people with mental health problems as well as to their relatives and carers. Indeed some might say that this is the point of mental health nursing or, to put this another way, mental health nursing can be said to have public health at its very core.

Thus Marte's contribution to public health is both general and particular. The general contribution stems from her everyday work but her particular contribution might involve, among other things, health intelligence (including, for example, the collection of data on inpatient stays and notifiable health problems), health protection (the application of policies to assist in the proactive management of health problems) and health promotion and prevention.

Priority issues

There are a number of priority issues that Marte might focus on depending on the nature of the particular mental health problems of the clients on Forsythia Ward. She might, for example, focus on identifying patients at risk of suicide, following the Suicide Prevention Strategy (DH 2015), or she might focus on **empowerment**, stress management, safety, or lifestyle issues (such as diet, smoking reduction or cessation, alcohol and drug use and abuse, or exercise).

Barriers

Barriers are factors that impede or prevent effective action. For example, institutionalisation, a lack of cooperation from colleagues, and a lack of commitment from colleagues and families can all impede Marte in her public health work with this group of clients.

Advantages

One advantage is that Marte has everyday contact with each client on the ward so they are, so to speak, something of 'a captive audience'. This enables Marte to build relationships over time with the clients as well as with their relatives and carers, which can help Marte to identify priorities for health improvement activities within a supportive environment.

Outbreak of *E. coli*: management of an infectious source

Activity 15.5

Betsan is a practice nurse. Three patients from the practice have been identified as having *E. coli*, a form of food poisoning notifiable under public health regulation. Two of the patients are children attending the local primary school and the third is an 84-year-old lady. There are seven other cases within a 5-mile radius and the public health emergency response team have identified the source of the outbreak as infected meat, sold at the local market.

Have a go at answering the following questions before reading on.

- What role might Betsan have in dealing with patients regarding the *E. coli* issue?
- What issues/topics might she cover?
- Who would she liaise with on this public health problem?
- What information sources could she use?

Role

News of an outbreak of an infectious form of food poisoning (such as the one described here) travels quickly around a community. Local people will soon know about it, it may become a story in the local news media, and it may even make national headlines. As a result Betsan may find she becomes besieged with requests for information and advice, particularly from patients registered with the practice. Thus Betsan will need to act as both health educator and care advisor. She is also likely to have a significant role in relation to the collection and testing of samples of faecal matter in conjunction with the local pathology department.

Topics

Betsan will need to provide information on personal hygiene (particularly the importance of effective hand washing) and food hygiene (including food handling) and she will need to be able to offer advice on care for those suffering from food poisoning.

Liaison

Betsan will need to liaise with a range of different professionals including general practitioners, school nurses, members of the local public health team, pathologists and local government officers (in particular, environmental health officers).

Information services

Betsan will be able to access information from a range of sources (e.g., the health protection agency, NHS Direct, the Internet, leaflets and clients themselves) and work with a range of personnel including specialist colleagues (e.g., environmental health officers and pathologists).

Public health in industrial settings: risk management

Activity 15.6

Kamaria is an occupational health nurse working in a factory where cleaning products are made. Her role involves monitoring the health of the workforce, maintaining health and safety awareness and health promotion.

Several incidents of exposure to noxious substances have attracted attention at the factory in the past 2 years. Two cases involved workers; one a case of accidental spillage when not wearing protective clothing and the second a case of inhalation of fumes caused by the interaction of substances in a storage area. The Health and Safety Inspectorate are investigating both cases.

The third, more recent, case involves a youth who accidentally came into contact with fluids stored securely in the yard area while trespassing at night. Local environmental health officers in collaboration with the police and safety agencies are investigating the incident. The factory owners are cooperating fully and want Kamaria to participate in the public health aspects of maintaining workers' health.

Have a go at answering the following questions before reading on.

- How might Kamaria be involved?
- What are the key aspects?
- What approaches could Kamaria use?
- How might Kamaria organise her intervention?

Involvement

Kamaria is likely to be involved in a number of different ways. In terms of health promotion she will help in educating the factory workforce about the dangers of working with or near noxious chemicals. She may be the first point of contact for employees who are exposed to the chemicals, providing care and ongoing support. She may also become involved with the media, and she will probably contribute to the development of a factory-wide action plan to reduce the likelihood of future incidents of exposure to noxious chemicals.

Key aspects

Kamaria will need to be knowledgeable about the Control of Substances Hazardous to Health (COSHH) regulations, the care and maintenance of safety equipment, good hygiene practice and first aid, particularly in relation to noxious chemical exposure.

Approaches

Kamaria will need to take a number of different approaches if she is to contribute to the way risk is managed in the factory. By providing education she can aim not only to help change the way people behave in relation to noxious chemicals but also to empower individuals to take control of risk management for themselves.

Organising interventions

Kamaria will need to be proactive if she is to make a contribution to the health and well-being of everyone associated with the factory. Given that the factory owners are supportive of her role it should be possible for Kamaria to set out a plan of action on helping manage risk across the organisation. She could engage with labelling products and stored chemicals, and with an information campaign in the local press to remind the public that this workplace houses hazardous materials and is not a place of public access.

She could stage health education sessions for the workforce on:

- safe storage and handling of substances;
- the importance of wearing protective clothing; and
- first aid if accidental exposure occurs.

She might also get involved in spot checks to ensure that protective measures are being taken, which could form part of team-building by praising or rewarding the staff who take the risks seriously and respond accordingly.

Public health and nursing

Each of these examples illustrates ways in which nurses engage with public health. Public health is now understood as reflecting a broad idea of the factors that contribute to the health and well-being of individuals and communities; and it is why nurses are seen as well placed to make a significant contribution.

PART 3: EXPLORING PUBLIC HEALTH

Along with the recognition of public health as an important aspect of nursing comes a responsibility for each nurse to engage with other professionals to enhance and advance the public health agenda (Baggott 2000). Nurses are well placed to make a very real contribution to public health because of their versatility, their wide range of public contact and because of their nursing knowledge, clinical experience and health assessment skills. This potential has been recognised by the Standing Nursing and Midwifery Advisory Committee (SNMAC 1995) and has become increasingly relevant as more and more practitioners, whatever their area of work or specialism, recognise the public health aspects of their daily practice. Craig and Lindsay (2000) have outlined the general nature of the nursing contribution, although they are clear that no one area of nursing can claim the connection exclusively or in isolation. They specifically identify the need for more information and training to equip nurses to fulfil their potential to contribute to public health. This is particularly important as public health is developing quickly with a multidisciplinary focus.

A little bit of history

Public health in the UK began to develop following the 1834 Poor Law Amendment Act and was influenced by the work of Edwin Chadwick, culminating in the first Public Health Act of 1848. Historically, there have been two main thrusts of public health, preventative interventions (including broad improvements in social conditions) and the provision of curative health services (see Figure 15.1).

The social reforms of the nineteenth century provided a series of preventative interventions that laid the foundation for improvements in the general level of health and well-being of the population. During the twentieth century, and particularly after the formation of the National Health Service in 1948, health care provision became increasingly dominated by a focus on curative services for individuals with only minor attention given to preventative interventions. Now, in the early part of the twenty-first century, the recognition of the need to ensure a balance between preventative and curative services is finding a voice in policy statements and in practice. Modern (or new) public health favours a population-based approach in which health promotion, health improvement and health protection lie alongside each other in the attempt to straddle the traditional preventative/curative division (see Figure 15.2).

The development of the UK Public Health Register opened for practitioners in April 2011 and provides the opportunity for nurses and other health care professionals to register as public health practitioners. The skills and knowledge required to register are framed around four areas of practice: professional and ethical practice; technical competencies in public health practice; the application of technical competencies to public health work; and underpinning skills. These are congruent with your nursing registration and work from a similar value base.

Skills for public health

If you have done the activities in Part 2 of this chapter you may have recognised already some of the skills that you will need if you are to engage with public health in ways that

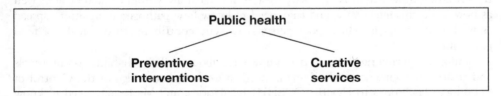

FIGURE 15.1
The two traditional thrusts of public health

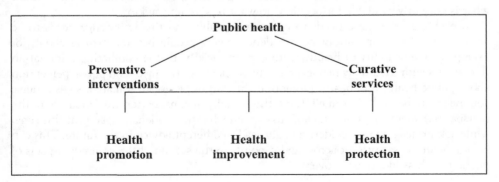

FIGURE 15.2
The new public health

are appropriate to wherever you work as a registered nurse. The good news is that many of these skills are the same skills you need for safe and effective nursing practice, so engaging in public health does not necessarily require you to acquire a new set of special skills. However, if you decide to work in a nursing role that has public health as a primary focus, or if you decide to seek specialist community public health nursing registration, you will need to develop expertise in these skills.

Activity 15.7

Review the information that follows Activities 15.2 to 15.6 inclusive in Part 2 of this chapter. Identify what skills the nurse needs in each case.

The chances are that in doing Activity 15.7 you will have identified some skills that are common across the cases. Perhaps the three most striking common aspects of the public health role are:

1 knowledge
2 communication; and
3 education.

Knowledge

In each scenario the nurse needs to know what they are talking about. If Sanjay and Betsan are to be effective in encouraging good personal and kitchen hygiene among their respective client populations they need to know what good practice in personal and kitchen hygiene actually requires. They need to know about effective hand washing, they need to know why it is necessary to store raw meat away from cooked meat as well as how to do this effectively, and they need to know how pathogenic organisms spread as well as the ways in which poor personal hygiene contributes to outbreaks of food poisoning.

Similarly, Sabrina needs up-to-date knowledge about cardiac rehabilitation protocols and treatment regimens, while Kamaria needs a working knowledge of the Control of Substances Hazardous to Health (COSHH) regulations, and Marte may need to know what is currently available for people who want to give up smoking.

In each case the nurse needs to be knowledgeable and this knowledge needs to be accurate and based on current best evidence. Many people become cynical about, for example, the possibility of healthy eating when faced with the conflicting information that arrives with their daily newspapers. The influence of the media on public perception about public health and health promotion should not be underestimated, so as a nurse you need to be well informed (and this usually means better informed than the newspapers) about the topic and able to explain what the evidence suggests at this time, while acknowledging new evidence might lead to different advice in the future. This can be a difficult message to get across and it points to the second of the common aspects of public health as identified above.

Communication

In each scenario the nurse needs to be able to communicate effectively with a range of different individuals and groups. Sanjay needs to be able to communicate effectively with people who have varying degrees of cognitive and/or physical abilities, Sabrina needs to be able to explain the implications of living with cardiac disease to individuals (and their families) with widely differing understandings of normal and abnormal physiology (in this case how the heart works and what happens when it goes wrong), and Marte will need a range of strategies to ensure she can be heard by those suffering psychotic episodes. Kamaria will be communicating with factory workers and managers as well as with officials (police, safety officers and environmental health officers) and perhaps members of the public. Similarly, Betsan will be communicating with a range of individuals including patients registered with the practice, school children, local government officials and members of the general public. In addition, Kamaria and Betsan may find themselves fielding and responding to media enquiries.

The media plays a significant part in public health in terms of attitude formation and is an important source of health information. Media interest is functional so the portrayal of health issues may be negative or sensational, and may play on the natural fear people feel regarding health, illness, and the health service. That said, staff involved in public health work spend time and effort working to lessen these fears and to provide realistic and accurate information and advice. Harrabin and colleagues (2003) suggest the need for an informed exchange between the media and health (policy makers, managers, and practitioners) on the grounds that such an arrangement would be of greater benefit to the public in the long term. Of course, the media tends not to have public health as its primary concern so any such arrangement might be difficult to initiate or sustain.

While there are some common key skills of communication (see Chapter 14) there are significant differences in applying these skills in different situations and specific techniques may be needed for particular audiences. For example, getting your message across in media-size 'sound bites' for general consumption requires a very different approach than that needed when confronted with 120 young children in a primary school assembly. So when liaising with officials, Kamaria and Betsan will need to use different terminology to that needed when working with health care colleagues and different terminology again when talking to the general public or the media. While perhaps less dramatic, Marte, Sanjay and Sabrina also need to be able to adapt their language and approach depending on the particular individuals or groups they are trying to communicate with at any given time. The skill needed to adapt the message to the audience should not be underestimated and is a skill that takes on even more importance when one of the aims of communication involves education, the third common aspect of public health as identified above.

Education

There are elements of education in each scenario as in each case the nurse has a role in facilitating learning and, as noted with communication above, the nurse needs to be able to adapt their skills to meet the needs of particular learners. For Sanjay this is further complicated because the residents are acknowledged as having learning difficulties: knowing how each of the residents learns best is crucial if they are to develop and retain good hygiene habits. Knowing how people learn best will be helpful in all cases although it is not always possible (nor necessarily desirable) to individualise learning in all circumstances.

When Kamaria or Betsan provide information via the media they will be attempting to educate the public but will need to concentrate on only one or two key messages. This means that they will need to both identify the most important aspects of the situation and be able to articulate those aspects in ways that are accurate, legitimate and believable. Given the media tendency to sensationalise, this might be a difficult task, especially as the public is known to have a healthy scepticism about official pronouncements on health scares.

Facilitating learning is a fundamental aspect of nursing practice. By way of example, nurses help people to learn how to manage their medications, how to care for their indwelling catheters, how to live with long-term conditions (e.g., diabetes, chronic pain), and how to recognise when they need to seek further medical, or non-medical, advice. Nurses also help families to adapt to living with the changing health-related circumstances of one or more of their members, as well as supporting a variety of different learners (nursing and/or other health and social care students, new members of staff, unqualified staff undertaking national vocational qualifications and so on). Nurses also facilitate their own learning in respect of what they need to know in order to remain a safe and effective practitioner beyond the point of qualification.

As Sabrina recognised (see Activity 15.2), merely supplying information does not necessarily mean that the person will learn something. For learning to take place, the learner (in this case the patient and their family) must understand the information in a way that makes sense to them in their particular situation. It is the facilitation of this process of understanding that nurses engage with when they attempt to enable individuals to, for example, learn to live with their newly diagnosed diabetes.

The skills involved in being knowledgeable, communicating and facilitating learning are many and varied and you will find some information about these skills elsewhere in the book (see Chapters 14 and 16). For now the main point is to recognise that public health is a core part of nursing practice, and the skills and knowledge necessary for safe and effective nursing practice are the same skills that enable nurses to make an effective contribution to public health.

Public health nursing as a specialism

Public health nursing is a distinct specialism, and since 2004 in the UK, nurses who are able to demonstrate the necessary competencies can register with the NMC as 'specialist community public health nurses'. Thus the NMC Register has three parts: one for nurses; one for midwives; and one for specialist community public health nurses. For many this registration on what is referred to as the 'Third Part of the Register' follows a period of graduate or postgraduate study leading to an NMC-recognised qualification in public health nursing. Nurses working in public health who do not hold an NMC-recognised public health qualification can apply for specialist community public health nursing registration through the development of a portfolio of evidence demonstrating achievement of the NMC Standards of Proficiency for Specialist Community Public Health Nurses (NMC 2004; see Box 15.1).

New public health

'New public health' is characterised by understandings of the relationship between health and lifestyle, the need to invest resources, policy, programmes and services in healthier

---

BOX 15.1 NMC standards of proficiency for specialist community public health nursing (SCPHN) (NMC 2004)

Four domains:

- search for health needs;
- stimulation and awareness of health needs;
- influence on policies affecting health;
- facilitation of health-enhancing activities.

Specialist community public health nursing (SCPHN) programmes are practice-centred and take account that:

- evidence should inform practice through the integration of relevant knowledge;
- students are actively involved in the delivery of community public health under supervision;
- the NMC code applies to all practice interventions;
- skills and knowledge are transferable;
- research underpins practice;
- lifelong learning and continuing professional development are important.

The **World Health Organization** (WHO) is a global institution, structured on a continental basis. The UK is part of WHO Euro – the European section.

The **Acheson Report** (1988) is the 1988 report produced by Lord Acheson that led to the establishment of annual reporting on the state of the public health and the role of the Director of Public Health in all areas of the UK.

ways of living and better environments. Craig and Lindsay (2000) proposed that nursing and public health come together through the notion of the 'new public health' movement. They concur with Ashton and Seymour's (1988) view of the new public health movement as one in which health is viewed as a function of lifestyle and environment (influenced by biology and care provision) and the social aspects of health. This is important because it governs the way in which we respond to those influences. Approaching the 'problem', if one is identified, may be best from a policy or strategy perspective or it may require a 'grassroots' approach, working from the basics. Current approaches are characterised by terms such as bottom-up (referring to the emphasis of action originating from practice or the population) or top-down (referring to strategists, policy makers and authority) or as upstream or downstream (see Box 15.2).

In this analogy being downstream rescuing drowning people represents a health intervention that reacts to the unfortunate and obvious outcomes of a deeper, more fundamental problem (so it is a reactive approach), whereas in the attempt to be 'upstream' new public health aims to repair the broken bridges of health by taking a preventive and more proactive approach.

The development of public health in the UK and beyond

Major public health development has occurred in recent years on a global scale orchestrated by the **World Health Organization** (WHO), which works to improve health across continents and countries by involving local populations and by providing supporting expertise. In the UK the **Acheson Report** (Acheson 1988) specifically sought to use the term 'public health medicine' rather than 'community health', reflecting the medical dominance and disease focus of the time.

Jane Thomas

BOX 15.2 **Upstream versus downstream**

Imagine you come across a person drowning in a river. You jump in and pull them to safety only to find a second drowning person coming down the same river. You save the second person only to find a third in need of rescue, then a fourth and fifth and so on. Such a process demands a great deal of your time and energy and if it continues, no matter how hard you try you will never be able to save everyone. You might enlist a passer-by to help but even as you take turns in saving the poor souls floating down the river, and even as you get further offers of help, you have a never-ending situation with several people constantly occupied in responding to an ongoing problem.

However, if you make the time to think about it you might start to wonder what is causing so many people to fall into the river in the first place. Assuming you can organise a rota with enough people to continue rescuing drowning individuals, you might venture 'upstream' to try to find out what is going on. Imagine you find people trying to cross a partly submerged bridge only to be swept away by the current. Now that you have identified the root cause of the problem you can try to do something about it. In this case you might work with the local people to raise the bridge above the waterline to make it safe to cross. With few, if any, people now falling into the river the effects downstream will be dramatic and might result in a need only for the strategic placing of an emergency lifebelt.

Lucas and Lloyd (2005) have explored the long-standing medical dominance in public health and the differential between the effects in the UK and America. They have identified the American educational approach as more multidisciplinary and note that the pace of change away from medical dominance in the UK has been slow. The development of public health has been a gradual process following the publication of the Acheson Report for a number of reasons to do with structure and funding. There has been an increased interest since the emergence of the 'new' public health that emanated from work in the UK by Ashton and Seymour (1988) and the **Ottawa Charter** (WHO 1986). This increased interest has been fuelled by theoretical debate, resource pressures and policy drivers and has had the effect of accelerating the development of public health. Changes in public perceptions and media pressure have also had an effect in identifying shortcomings and unmet needs and thereby stimulated public awareness. These factors have combined to create the momentum for change currently evident in public health.

Baggott (2000) recognised the pattern of variation in the dominance (or otherwise) of public health within health care and in the approaches taken to it over time, while Bunton and MacDonald (2002) identify the shift from a social towards an environmental focus as part of the new public health of the late twentieth century. The concerted development of public health on a more international basis in line with Health for All (WHO 1985) has been helped by initiatives such as **Healthy Cities**. This work was based on WHO principles of reorienting health services towards primary care, promoting public participation and partnerships and improving the health of those most in need.

This combined with environmental developments has drawn local authorities into more integrated planning on environmental issues, and helped to establish a more positive and interactive context for health improvement. In considering how best to work with communities in developing all aspects of their health, it is worth considering the key components of space, interests, relationships, shared needs and concerns.

The gradual progression of the public health movement across Europe suggests a higher future profile and the potential for more unified health strategies in the long term. The important thing about strategy is that it provides guidance to enable the operational delivery of better health and a framework for action.

The public health context

Public health focuses on individuals and populations, seeking to protect and improve health through surveillance, notification, regulation and jurisdiction. Public health is described by **Skills for Health** as:

- taking a population perspective;
- mobilising the organised efforts of society and acting as an advocate for the public's health;
- enabling people and communities to take control over their own health and well-being;
- acting on the social, economic, environmental and biological determinants of health and well-being;
- protecting from and minimising the impact of health risks to the population;
- ensuring that preventive, treatment and care services are of high quality, based on evidence and are of best value.

(Skills for Health 2004, p. 6)

This description includes many of the aspects of care and public health with which you have become familiar in nursing. Parts of it may also remind you of the WHO (1986) definition of health promotion in the Ottawa Charter and the Acheson Report.

Activity 15.8

Think about your experience of being a student nurse. Try to identify some of the things you have been told are important considerations in delivering a service to patients and clients in the twenty-first century.

There is a good chance that reflecting on your experiences will lead you to recognise issues such as evidence-based practice, advocacy, interprofessional working, quality assurance and personal responsibility for health. All these issues, in various ways, contribute directly to the purposes of public health. Most are addressed elsewhere in this book so here the focus is on personal responsibility for health.

Personal responsibility for health

There is an often unarticulated and sometimes unacknowledged set of beliefs and values that lie behind the idea that we are all responsible for our own health. The idea is so

Skills for Health is a UK organisation established in 2002 working to integrate skills development in the health sector across the four home nations. Current priorities include the development of competence-based development in public health practice.

powerful and so pervasive that it can be difficult for nurses (as well as other health and social care professionals, policy makers, government spokespersons and so on) to understand why individuals fail to adopt healthy lifestyles. As pointed out in Chapter 3 of this book, this view can lead us to blame some people for their illnesses and might lead us to think that they should wait longer for treatment (or even that they should be denied treatment altogether) on the NHS. For example, in a busy accident and emergency department, the drunk teenager whose fractured fingers resulted from punching a wall on the way home from the pub might not seem to the staff to be as deserving of their attention as the innocent victim of a stabbing. Similarly we might agree with the idea that a person who refuses to give up smoking should not take precedence over the non-smoker on the waiting list for heart bypass surgery (we might even think that they should not be offered surgery at all unless they stop smoking). The basis of this discriminatory view comes from a particular perspective about personal responsibility for health that goes something like this:

- There is a lot of easily available health information.
- A great deal of this information is uncontroversial (for example, few people seriously doubt that smoking, eating a diet high in saturated fats, or drinking excessive amounts of alcohol will have a detrimental effect on the health of an individual).
- Any reasonable person will choose to follow a healthy lifestyle.
- Anyone who does not is to blame for their own ill health.

Some of the limitations of this view include:

1 It takes little account of individual genetic make-up or inherited features

While we all share a common physiology there remain differences in individual physiological responses to threats to health. Not everyone who smokes will develop a life-threatening smoking-related illness (most people claim to know of someone who smoked 20 cigarettes a day for a lifetime without ill effect). Not everyone who comes into contact with a pathogenic organism will contract the disease, and even while those that do will exhibit some common symptoms (that is, after all one of the bases for disease classification) each infected person will suffer some symptoms worse than others. Also, not every cardiac patient who returns to an unhealthy lifestyle will do as badly as we might expect.

2 It takes little account of the social situation of individuals

As pointed out earlier, the person who lives in an environment where healthy lifestyle choices are difficult to make is less likely to make permanent (or even temporary) changes. Those without ready access to fresh fruit and vegetables will find it harder to change their diet; those whose social life consists of '12 pints-a-night and a takeaway on the way home' may find unpalatable the choice between on the one hand eating healthily but losing any form of social life and on the other continuing the unhealthy eating but retaining friends. Put this way, it is not so hard to understand why some people decide against adopting a healthier lifestyle. To assume that individuals will want to extract themselves from their social situation just to follow the health promotion advice of health care professionals is to fail to understand that not everybody values their health equally.

3 It assumes a specific (professional-oriented) view of 'reasonableness'

When health care professionals talk about people being reasonable (or unreasonable), what they often mean is reasonable as defined from a professional perspective steeped in a particular set of values and beliefs about health. Health advice comes from what might be described as an educated and well-informed section of society that does not reflect the diversity of the general population. Arguably, being 'reasonable' in the sense that a reasonable person does not take unnecessary risks with their health can be paternalistic, for it is rather like being told what to do by those who think they know best. Yet health care professionals themselves are often guilty of taking risks with their health. Skiing, bungee jumping, playing rugby, horse riding and driving might seem more respectable pastimes than smoking, drinking or recreational drug use but they all contain elements of risk to the health of participants. The cost to the health service of sporting injuries is significant and yet headlines suggesting skiers should not receive treatment because their injuries are self-inflicted, or that rugby-playing injuries are an unjustified drain on limited health care resources, are noticeable by their absence.

4 It takes little account of people's individual goals or priorities

Similarly, the idea that health has a specific value or that it should be a high-priority 'good' reflects a normative belief (a belief about how things ought to be) rather than an empirical fact (how things really are). Not everyone places their own health above other considerations in their lives. Parents may place the health and well-being of their children over and above their own. Many individuals simply do not believe they will suffer ill effects from unhealthy lifestyle choices, and some (particularly young) people believe themselves to be invulnerable or invincible, or that ill health is something that happens only to other people. Others still may merely think that if they are to suffer ill health it will happen so far in the future as to not be worth worrying about just now. Indeed, health care workers are not immune from this: how else can we explain the fact that some health care workers smoke, drink to excess and eat diets high in salt, sugar or saturated fats?

5 It takes little account of wider considerations

No one would argue with claims about the positive health effects of good sanitation, clean air and clean drinking water. Neither would many argue with the benefits of public health policies such as the compulsory wearing of seat belts or crash helmets. Yet when we advise individuals about ways they might make healthier lifestyle choices we often ignore the powerful influence of factors individuals can do little, if anything, about. The food industry remains a powerful influence and even if our local supermarket offers us choice it is not always easy to understand which products constitute healthy options. Low fat, low salt or low sugar products might not necessarily be healthy options (it all depends on what else they contain).

6 It assumes a common view about risk-taking

Each of us views risk differently. For some the idea of climbing Everest is a complete non-starter because it is just too risky, for others it is the risk itself that makes the idea attractive.

The point is that we each have a different view not only about what constitutes risk but also about how much risk we are prepared to take. For our mountaineer, the risk of not rock climbing may be a life bereft of meaning or a risk of 'death by boredom', and this would compromise her or his well-being. For some, the risk of future ill health is insufficient motivation for changing current behaviour, particularly if that behaviour is pleasurable.

This is a brief overview of some of the difficulties of a simplistic view of health promotion. For a more detailed discussion see, for example, Naidoo and Wills (2009).

Reflection and public health

Reflection can be useful in enabling nurses to assess their beliefs, values and approaches to practice in general and to public health in particular. Reflection is an intrinsic part of nursing practice but has only recently been recognised as an important element of health promotion. Fleming (2006) has explored the value of reflection in relation to his preventive work on managing aggression in occupational settings. While this is a highly specialised area of intervention, he emphasises the way in which reflection can improve practice. To enable health promotion practitioners to engage in reflection in a planned and coherent manner, Fleming (2006) has developed a typology for reflective practice (see Figure 15.3), which focuses on three domains of practice, the role of self (individuals and teams), the influence of the planning context (socio-economic and other environmental and political factors) and issues related to the process of planning/delivery of programmes. Other domains of public health practice could be replaced or inserted, linking your understanding of reflection in general to the specifics of public health. Reflection is a transferable skill and nurses can use it in their daily practice, in health promotion and to help others to understand public health.

The purpose of public health

Skills for Health state that the purpose of public health is to:

- improve the health and well-being of the population;
- prevent disease and minimise its consequences;
- prolong valued life; and
- reduce inequalities in health.

(Skills for Health 2004, p. 6)

Thus the range of activities that fall within the remit of public health practice has extended from the traditional medical model based on epidemiology and disease prevention to more integrated and proactive models combining health statistics and projection, health education, health improvement, harm reduction and health protection. The development of the National Occupational Standards for the Practise of Public Health (Skills for Health 2004) identified the 10 areas of public health practice as:

1 Surveillance and assessment of the population's health and well-being.
2 Promoting and protecting the population's health and well-being.
3 Developing quality and risk management within an evaluative culture.
4 Collaborative working for health and well-being.

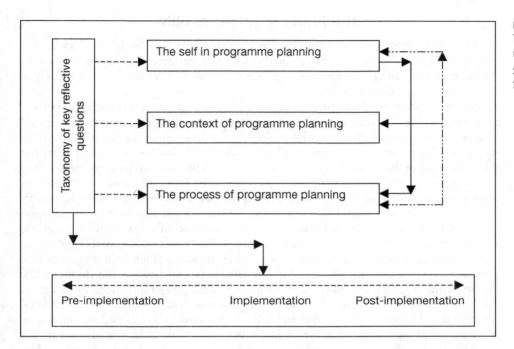

FIGURE 15.3
Typology for
reflective practice

Source: after Fleming
2006.

5 Developing health programmes and services and reducing inequalities.
6 Policy and strategy development and implementation to improve health and well-being.
7 Working with and for communities to improve health and well-being.
8 Strategic leadership for health and well-being.
9 Research and development to improve health and well-being.
10 Ethically managing self, people and resources to improve health and well-being.

(Skills for Health 2004, p. 6)

As you can see these 10 areas of public health are consistent with the general aims of nursing, and most nurses will be contributing to one or more of these ten areas of public health whenever they are engaged in nursing practice.

There are differences in public health provision across the UK. The ways in which health care provision broadly and public health in particular have developed are different and this can be challenging when moving from one area to another. Each of the four UK nations has developed a strategic framework for public health focusing on health improvement with particular emphasis on improving the health of those most disadvantaged. Each nation has devised targets using disease reduction and prevention approaches with a key focus on reducing social exclusion. While the details of the individual strategies and the means for their delivery differ, they share the common aim of seeking to reduce inequalities through health improvement. Devolution has had an effect on policy development and implementation so difference at the strategic and operational level is to be expected and is likely to continue.

The future of public health

Healthy Lives, Healthy People (2011) currently drives the UK health strategy and is supported by the separate initiatives of the four UK nations. The report emphasises the need for core disciplines working in public health to take an integrated approach in improving the health and well-being of the UK population.

The registration of Specialists in Public Health for those practitioners who have attained 'specialist' status as a means of monitoring and supporting excellence and continuing professional development at the highest level in public health practice is subject to change in the near future. This UK Public Health Register differs from the NMC Register in that it has been constructed around a professional grouping rather than by statute and practitioner registration is now in place. There are similarities insofar as both set entry criteria and confer enhanced professional status, but the UK Public Health Register does not have statutory status or mechanisms for the regulation of registration (e.g., regular renewal or the authority to withdraw registration). The NMC Register has one section specifically for specialist community public health nurses, enabling them to register their professional qualification. A specialist community public health nurse cannot practise without such registration but does not need to be registered on the voluntary UK Public Health Register, although they can apply at some other time. Since its inception the Public Health Register has been developed and now contains categories for Defined Specialists and Generalist Specialists and this has attracted medically and non-medically trained practitioners working at senior levels in public health. As specialist status has developed so has the debate around how to support and classify others working in public health, resulting in discussions around the development of 'practitioner' status. As part of the wider group of public health staff, public health nurses, alongside therapists, pharmacists, environment health officers and others can now seek practitioner status in the specialism, developing their careers around the public health career framework.

CONCLUSION

Public health is an important aspect of nursing practice. Wherever and whenever nursing takes place it is likely that it involves some form of public health. Some nursing activity and some nurses will have an obvious and well-developed public health role while others will choose to make public health the focus of their professional careers. However, because the general aims of public health and the general aims of nursing are so closely aligned, most nurses will be making a contribution in one way or another to public health. There is now widespread recognition across the NMC and the public that public health is part of nursing practice as reflected in NMC documentation and the practitioner standards. The opportunity for nurses, in addition to their NMC registration, to seek recognition of their public health practitioner status (UKPHR 2015) is testament to the strength of that relationship and its permanence.

The Code (NMC 2015) outlines the professional standards of practice in terms of prioritising people, practising effectively, preserving safety and promoting professionalism and trust. These values carry effectively into public health practice with their emphasis on accountability and raising concerns and help us to understand public health within nursing practice more effectively.

The dynamic specialism of public health is likely to continue to develop in response to perceived public health needs. The growing prominence of public health and the emerging recognition of its relevance to everyday practice will bring more and more opportunities for nurses to develop their own roles within it. If you now have a clearer understanding of the fundamentals of public health then the aims of this chapter have been met. It is hoped that this understanding will inform your nursing practice and may provide a focus for a stronger interest in the future. However, you should remember that this chapter merely offers an introduction to the complex nature of public health. Should you wish to find out more, one or more of the books on the suggested further reading list will be a valuable resource.

SUGGESTED FURTHER READING

Evans, D., Coutsaftiki, D. and Fathers, C. P. (2014) *Health Promotion and Public Health for Nursing Students*. London: Sage.

Linsley, P., Kane, R. and Owen, S. (2011) *Nursing for Public Health: Promotion, principles and practice*. Oxford: Oxford University Press.

Nutland, W. and Cragg, L. (eds) (2015) *Health Promotion Practice* (2nd edn). Maidenhead: McGraw Hill Education/Open University Press.

REFERENCES

Acheson, D. (1988) *Public Health in England: The report of the committee of inquiry into the future development of the public health function*, CM 289. London: HMSO.

Ashton, J. and Seymour, H. (1988) *The New Public Health: The Liverpool Experience*. Milton Keynes: Open University Press.

Baggott, R. (2000) *Public Health: Policy and politics*. Basingstoke: Macmillan.

Barth, J., Critchley, J. and Bengel, J. (2006). Efficacy of psychosocial interventions for smoking cessation in patients with coronary heart disease: a systematic review and meta-analysis. *Annals of Behavioural Medicine*, **32** (1), 10–20.

Bunton, R. and MacDonald, G. (2002) *Health Promotion: Disciplines, diversity and development*. London: Routledge.

Craig, P. M. and Lindsay, G. M. (eds) (2000) *Nursing for Public Health: Population-based care*. London: Churchill Livingstone.

DH (Department of Health) (2015) *National Suicide Prevention Strategy for England*. London: DH.

Fleming, P. (2006) *Reflection: A neglected art in health promotion*. Oxford: Health Education Research, Oxford University Press.

Harrabin, R., Coote, A. and Allen, J. (2003) *Health in the News: Risk, reporting and media influence*. London: King's Fund.

Healthy Lives, Healthy People (2011) www.rsph.org.uk/en/about-us/latest-news/press-releases/press-release1.cfm/pid/BCB962DB-ADB3–42F3–8D1D1190FDC67E90 (accessed 21 January 2016).

Hubley, J. and Copeman, J. (with Woodall, J.) (2013) *Practical Health Promotion* (2nd edn). Cambridge: Polity Press

Lawlor, D. A. and Hanratty, B. (2001) The effect of physical activity advice given in routine primary care consultations: a systematic review. *Journal of Public Health Medicine* **23** (3), 219–226.

Lucas, K. and Lloyd, B. (2005) *Health Promotion: Evidence and experience*. London: Sage.

Naidoo, J. and Wills, J. (2009) *Foundations for Health Promotion (Public Health and Health Promotion)* (3rd edn). Edinburgh: Bailliere Tindall.

NMC (Nursing and Midwifery Council) (2004) *Standards of Proficiency for Specialist Community Public Health Nursing*. London: NMC.

Jane Thomas

NMC (2015) *The Code: Professional standards of practice and behavior for nurses and midwives* www.nmc.org.uk/globalassets/sitedocuments/nmc-publications/revised-new-nmc-code.pdf (accessed 17 July 2015).

Skills for Health (2004) *National Occupational Standards for the Practice of Public Health*. London: Skills for Health.

SNMAC (Standing Nursing and Midwifery Advisory Committee) (1995) *Making it Happen*. London: DH.

UKPHR (UK Public Health Register) (2015) www.ukphr.org/ (accessed 1 June 2015).

WHO (World Health Organization) Regional Office for Europe (1985) *Targets for Health for All: Targets in support of the European Regional Strategy for Health for All*. Copenhagen: WHO.

WHO Regional Office for Europe (1986) *The Ottawa Charter*. Geneva: WHO.

16

LEARNING AND TEACHING

Derek Sellman and Jane Tarr

LEARNING OUTCOMES

After reading and reflecting on this chapter you should be able to:

- recognise that learning and teaching are an integral part of being a registered nurse;
- develop your own learning capabilities to be an effective learner;
- identify different approaches to and opportunities for learning;
- acknowledge the skills, aptitudes and knowledge required to engage in effective learning and teaching;
- outline factors that contribute to a favourable learning environment;
- acknowledge the value of self-assessment and self-reflection in enhancing learning;
- identify barriers to successful learning;
- discuss the components of effective learning and teaching.

INTRODUCTION

For a registered nurse, a willingness to facilitate learning is an integral aspect of competent nursing practice. Wherever and whenever nursing occurs, learning is almost certainly taking place. Thus a basic knowledge and understanding of learning and teaching is an essential prerequisite for safe and effective nursing. This chapter helps to articulate the professional obligation for learning and teaching that is made explicit in various Nursing and Midwifery Council documents based on the recognition that patients are entitled to a high standard of professional care from registered practitioners.

The chapter is divided into three parts. In Part 1, we outline some aspects of the topic of learning and teaching, and emphasise that the differences between learning and teaching are not as distinct as commonly thought.

In Part 2, we begin to explain further some important aspects of learning and teaching including the role of the teacher in establishing an environment conducive to learning. We suggest some things that make a good or poor teacher and how these things impact

Derek Sellman and Jane Tarr

Learning
is a process that we experience throughout our lives although we do not necessarily recognise or understand this. A few moments of reflection can lead us to identify some instances when we learn easily (e.g., recognition of the tune and rhythm of our favourite song) and other instances where learning is difficult (e.g., completing a self-assessment tax form)

Teaching is a process of sharing one's knowledge, skills, insights, perceptions, values and concepts with another. Teaching can take place in both official/formal settings (e.g., in a classroom) or in classic/informal contexts (e.g., during everyday interactions). Teachers themselves will learn from the process of teaching.

students' learning. We explain Race's (2015) competency model as a way of assisting in identifying learning needs.

In Part 3, we introduce the idea of individual learning styles and begin to explore some aspects of what makes an effective learner. We also stress the important relationship between effective learning and safe nursing practice.

PART 1: OUTLINING LEARNING AND TEACHING

Case 16.1

Sarah is a second-year student nurse. On her current placement she notices that many registered nurses do not wash their hands between patients, and of those who do, many use ineffective hand washing techniques. Sarah has also noticed that quite a lot of nursing staff routinely wear wrist watches, rings with stones, and other assorted adornments that she has been told constitute infection and/or health and safety risks. When she asks her mentor, Steve, about this, he shrugs his shoulders and says that he knows they should pay more attention to hand hygiene but the ward is too busy and anyway the infection rate is no higher here than in any other local practice area.

Those who observe, or are recipients of, nursing care learn much from registered practitioners whether or not these nurses intend to facilitate learning, and regardless of whether this comes from positive or negative experiences. One thing that Sarah has learned from this brief informal interaction with her mentor is that some registered nurses believe it acceptable not to wash their hands between patients. While there may be room for discretion about whether or not to wash your hands between patients the mentor (Steve) demonstrates by his response that in general he knows that ward staff should practise effective hand washing.

Both Steve and Sarah might be surprised to find their brief interaction described as educational, but Sarah has learned something from Steve so in this instance we can describe Sarah as a learner and Steve as a teacher. Indeed, Steve has learned something from Sarah (at the very least he has been reminded of the importance of hand washing), and in this respect Sarah has been a catalyst for Steve to reconsider one aspect of practice of nurses in this placement. Both aspects of learning here can be described as informal because learning occurred by chance, and both Steve's and Sarah's teaching can be described as unintentional because neither set out to teach: there were no set learning objectives or outcomes, and no teaching plan. Nevertheless learning and teaching has taken place.

There are, of course, differences between **learning** and **teaching** but these differences are probably harder to describe than you might imagine: the idea that 'teachers teach' and 'learners learn' is a simplistic view. We will say more about this, but for now it is worth noting that there is more that unites than divides learning and teaching. For the purposes of this chapter we take the view that while some roles within educational settings are formal (i.e., student nurses have a formal learning role while mentors, tutors and lecturers have formal teaching roles) learning and teaching is going on all the time in all sorts of situations, most of which would not normally be described as part of the formal

404

educational process. Yet these informal learning and teaching experiences are inevitable and play an important role in learning to become a registered nurse.

While the distinctions are often blurred between learning and teaching, both are central features of nursing practice. To become an effective nurse it is necessary to be an effective learner and an effective teacher, so it is important to develop your capacities for both. This requires you to recognise not only that you have a preferred way of learning but also that others have preferred learning styles (in other words, not everybody learns in the same way). It also requires an open-minded and flexible approach to both your own and others' learning as well as an ability to engage in a range of different modes of learning and teaching. This is particularly important as you move from the highly structured pre-registration education programme to the often less structured and usually self-directed learning needed for safe and effective practice beyond initial registration.

Learning in practice

Becoming a registered nurse involves spending time in a variety of different practice settings in the company of a number of different professionals. As a student you will find it easier to adapt (i.e., to learn) in some more than other practice environments. Sacks argues that human beings engage in the process of adaptation to such an extent that it may be necessary to:

> redefine the very concepts of 'health' and 'disease', to see these in terms of the ability of the organism to create a new organisation and order, one that fits its special, altered disposition and needs, rather than in the terms of a rigidly defined 'norm'.
>
> (Sacks 1995, p. xvi)

Adaptation in this sense is the ability to learn to respond to changing environments, and just as patients are generally expected to adapt to their situation and learn to take (at least some) responsibility for their own care and treatment, so students of nursing need to adapt to each new situation and learn to take (at least some) responsibility for their own learning.

When do learning and teaching occur?

Pre-registration nurse education involves a structured programme of learning leading to qualification. Learning and teaching take place all the time in informal as well as formal settings. However, learning and teaching do not cease at qualification. Rather registered nurses are expected to engage in both processes in order to remain safe and effective practitioners because the knowledge base from which nursing draws continues to develop. Despite starting as a novice, the student nurse will make a contribution to this development, for example, by asking questions of established and routine practice. The significance on knowledge development of asking questions should not be underestimated: it is through attempts to provide satisfactory answers that insights about what is known and what is not known become apparent.

In this first part of the chapter we have outlined some aspects of the scope of learning and teaching as a topic and we have made the point that the boundary between learning and teaching is not fixed. While the lecturer is required to teach, there are times when the teacher will learn from you (and if they are learning from you, then you are in some sense teaching). The role of the practice mentor may be to facilitate your learning (which might not be the same thing as teaching) but this facilitation of learning applies equally to others, for example, to patients and their families, to other health care workers, to students of other disciplines and so on. You will also recognise that during your practice placements you sometimes help others to learn, for example, you are engaged in facilitating learning each time you help a patient to manage their take-home medication or whenever you explain your placement assessment paperwork to your mentor.

All this illustrates the point that during your nursing course you will learn all sorts of things in all sorts of ways and in all sorts of situations. Only some of these things will be related directly to the learning outcomes of your programme and only some of this learning will take place in formal settings. You will also be involved in teaching and only sometimes will you be intending to teach (often others learn from you without you intending to teach them anything). Thus you are constantly surrounded by learning and teaching. Once you recognise this you can use the knowledge and skills you have to facilitate both your own and others' learning to influence the quality of the provision of patient and client care. In other words a basic understanding of learning and teaching is an essential feature of effective nursing practice. In the remainder of this chapter we will explain and then explore some of these ideas within the context of nursing practice.

PART 2: EXPLAINING LEARNING AND TEACHING

Case 16.2

Mark is a third-year student nurse on his final placement. He is disappointed when his mentor (Khim) tells him that she wants to work alongside him for the first few days. Mark feels that Khim should recognise his seniority and allow him to get on with his work without being constantly supervised. Mark feels constant supervision might be appropriate for a first-year student but is unnecessary for an experienced and competent third-year student.

For her part Khim knows that third-year students ought to be able to work on their own but she feels it important to observe for herself what Mark can do and what he cannot yet do, as this will help her to find out what he knows and what he does not yet know. She tries to explain this to Mark, but she senses he thinks she is demanding an unnecessary level of monitoring.

The role of mentor may be relatively easy to articulate but many qualified nurses find it a demanding addition to what they consider their primary role of providing safe and effective nursing care. In fact facilitation of learning is an integral part of being a registered nurse (NMC 2015).

General everyday (i.e., non-nursing) understandings of mentorship recognise a mentor as someone who encourages, guides and possibly befriends within a relationship that need not be formal or even face-to-face. Writers, artists, musicians, academics and so on sometimes speak of inspirational others as mentors even when they have never met. In this everyday use of the term, a mentor is not allocated but chosen and usually by mutual consent. In nursing the placement mentor role is formalised and is often associated with an assessment function, so much so that many students anticipate being assessed by their mentor (in some places the role is described as the mentor/assessor role).

In the situation described (Case 16.2) both Mark and Khim have expectations of what the mentor relationship entails. Mark thinks he should be allowed to get on with his work; Khim thinks she needs to find out what he can do and what he knows before he is let loose on patients. This is perhaps not the best start to their educational relationship. While Mark may be competent in a wide range of nursing tasks, Khim has a professional responsibility to ensure Mark provides safe and effective care while working under her supervision. This is part of what it means to be a registered and accountable practitioner (see Chapter 2). It is because of this that Khim wishes to be sure that Mark can safely do those things that he says he can do and the only way she can do this is to assess his level of skill and knowledge. Making an assessment of his competencies will help Khim to devise a planned programme of learning related to Mark's individual learning needs. Merely accepting Mark's word that he can or cannot do something would not provide a secure basis for a programme of learning.

Hence Khim wants to work alongside Mark as much as possible during his first few days because she believes this to be the best way to find out what he knows, how he approaches his work, and how he might best learn during the placement. For his part, Mark is interested in learning and believes he knows exactly what it is he needs to learn. He feels that he does not need to waste time demonstrating (yet again) all the things he knows he can do well. He likes to be left alone to get on with his learning in his own way; that is, doing the things he knows he can do and seeking help when he comes across something new. He finds it difficult to understand why he is to be watched so much during his first few days on placement when he has been 'signed off' in earlier placements as competent in many everyday nursing activities. Even if Mark is correct in his claims of competence, Khim has no way of knowing this when they first meet. So unless Khim is ready to accept Mark's word for it, she needs to make an assessment of his competencies. In other words, Khim is asking Mark to provide evidence to support his claims of competence.

Formal and informal learning

There is a tendency to think of learning and teaching as something that happens in formal settings and in relation to specific subjects or for specific purposes. Attending a lecture on infection control or enrolling on a pre-registration nursing course are two examples of what most people would understand as formal education. Yet a few minutes' thought about, for example, how you learned to take a patient's temperature should help you to recognise that this learning came about from a combination of:

- being told how to do it (instruction);
- watching others do it (observation);
- trying to do it (practice).

Of course, learning rarely flows smoothly from the first to the last of these phases. More often a learner will weave in and out of different phases in no particular order, sometimes only being exposed to one phase long after the others. Often one or more of these phases will have been experienced prior to any involvement in **formal learning**. For example, if previously you worked as a health care assistant you probably observed other people taking

Formal learning is intentional and takes place occasionally; it is often hard work and is time limited. It is frequently an individual intellectual activity based upon effort; and often reliant upon rewards and tests related to learning outcomes or objectives.

407

patients' temperatures, you may have had some practice and you may even have had some formal instruction. In fact, you might have arrived as a student fully competent in temperature measurement. Whatever the case, your previous formal or informal learning will have been different to everyone else's. Yet everyone on the course will have learned something in the new formal learning situation, even if only to confirm existing competence.

Smith (1998) identifies 'two visions of learning: an "official" theory that learning is work and a "classic" view that we learn effortlessly every moment of our waking lives' (Smith 1998, p. vii). The classic view of learning (**informal learning**) suggests that learning is based on self-image and is a social activity that takes place continuously, often at the unconscious level.

In the attempt to improve the educational experience of students there has been a move away from concentrating on the development of different teaching strategies towards a focus on understanding the learning process. Claxton's (2002) concept of 'building learning power' seems well suited to pre-registration nursing programmes because of the emphasis on encouraging students to take control of their own learning by **learning-to-learn**.

Approaches to teaching

If learning takes place in different settings and is reliant upon individuals' self-awareness and self-image, then teachers should cultivate the 'necessary circumstances and frame of mind for desired learning' (Smith 1998, p. 5). This can be difficult for teachers (as facilitators of learning) because it requires paying attention to creating an environment in which learning can take place. In the formal learning environment of a classroom, the knowledgeable teacher encourages in students the development of academic skills (e.g., analysis, synthesis and evaluation). In the formal learning environment of the workplace, the skilled teacher encourages students to apply their knowledge to practical situations. In both settings, part of the role of the teacher is to help the student identify appropriate learning opportunities.

Approaches in **formal learning environments** that encourage discussion and dialogue (e.g., seminars and work-based learning days) are designed to help students build their learning power within a social context. According to Vygotsky (1978), learning is a social process where interaction with peers (especially with more able peers) enables each learner to learn more than they would alone and places emphasis on the **social aspect of learning**. Nursing is a social process so social learning can be readily transferred into practice settings where the sharing of knowledge between novice and expert can benefit both. The relationships between, for example, tutor and student, mentor and student, student and patient, and registered nurse and patient can all provide opportunities to learn.

Experiential work-based learning

Learning and teaching occur in the workplace both formally and informally. The more formal aspect of learning in the workplace might be thought of as coaching or mentoring. In a practice setting, a student nurse is normally allocated a **mentor**. Ideally a mentor will be an experienced practitioner who can enable a student to build their learning power as well as a sense of professional identity. The relationship between the novice and the mentor will change over time and each will learn from the other. The student's level of engagement with the social environment that is the work placement will influence their capacity to learn from that experience. As Dewey explains:

> The social environment . . . is truly educative in its effects in the degree in which an individual shares or participates in some conjunct activity. By doing his share in the associated activity, the individual appropriates the purpose which actuates it, becomes familiar with its methods and subject matters, acquires needed skill and is saturated with its emotional spirit.
>
> (Dewey 1916, p. 26)

Thus responsibility for learning is shared between student and mentor in the practice setting, but is affected by the social environment of the workplace, which helps to form part of a **learning community** in which everyone's capacity to learn is enhanced. The existence of special interest groups (SIGs) reflects this idea of learning communities in which professionals demonstrate an understanding of the need to continue to learn from the opportunities that emerge from their work with clients. Wenger (2000) describes such groupings as 'communities of practice' that form the basis of social learning. Members of a community of practice come together through pursuit of a joint enterprise, through mutual engagement and through the development of a shared repertoire of professional aspirations. It is suggested that learning is enhanced within such a social community because it generates credibility and energy, members within the group learn about each other in a positive manner and this encourages self-reflection. Such an approach is thought to be useful in developing professional identity and in enhancing the learning of all participants, whether novice or expert.

> Communities of practice grow out of a convergent interplay of competence and experience that involves mutual engagement. They offer an opportunity to negotiate competence through an experience of direct participation. As a consequence they remain important social units of learning even in the context of much larger systems.
>
> (Wenger 2000, p. 229)

Becoming a nurse in the twenty-first century requires each student to demonstrate their learning by meeting a set of predetermined learning outcomes attached to the different modules that together make up the pre-registration nursing programme of learning. Meeting the learning outcomes of the course requires you to undertake a range of assessments designed to measure your achievement against each of the learning outcomes; hence success on the programme requires success in those assessments. It should be no surprise then that students tend to become **'assessment-driven'**. To focus on educational assessment in this way is not necessarily a bad thing, and the effective teacher can design assessment strategies to capitalise on students' concerns with assessments. So here we offer a few words on the nature of educational assessment.

Most individuals think about assessment as part of the latter stages of an educational experience but, without disputing the value of the end-point assessment, we take the view that it is helpful for both learners and teachers to think about assessment as a process that can be used constructively to enhance the learning experience.

A **mentor** is an experienced practitioner in the workplace who supports trainees in understanding the workplace setting, organises their learning in context and holds overall responsibility for the assessment of their professional practice.

A **learning community** is one where all persons involved engage in developing and enhancing their understanding and insight into the common experience they share.

Assessment-driven is how educationalists describe those students who focus primarily on finding out what it is they need to do to pass assignments.

Derek Sellman and Jane Tarr

Approaches to educational assessment

Educational assessment involves the gathering of a range of forms of evidence of a learner's knowledge, skills, conceptual understanding and values: such evidence is used for different purposes. Formative assessment provides the evidence one requires to be able to teach learners at the right level. Summative assessment summarises the achievement of learners, usually at the end of a period of time. Ipsative assessment is about self-awareness of one's own achievements. Peer assessment is what others perceive one to know.

It would be unusual to join a programme of learning without experiencing **educational assessment**. Even those who undertake a course for which there is no formal assessment will engage in some form of informal self-assessment regarding what they have or have not learned. As a student nurse you will experience a variety of types of educational assessment ranging from the formal written essay or examination to practice-based competency assessment with other less or more formal tests of your knowledge, understanding and skills. One significant feature of this variety of assessment is that different forms of learning will be less or more effective for particular types of assessment. In other words, to be a successful learner requires that you take a learning approach appropriate to whatever assessment type is set for a given unit of learning. For example, if you are required to write an essay then learning how to present information in an academic style (including how to use and present references) becomes an important skill; and if you are required to produce a portfolio then you need to learn how to demonstrate what you have learned from the material you have accumulated. A portfolio is after all a collection of evidence of learning. This skill of working out which approach to learning best suits a specific assessment is an important part of the development of your capacity for self-assessment that in turn is important preparation for assessing your own learning needs as they relate to the needs of patients and clients.

What makes a good teacher?

There are a number of conditions that make effective learning more likely. Most people know something about these conditions simply because everybody has experience of learning. The following activities are designed to help you recognise that you already know quite a lot about learning and teaching.

Activity 16.1

Make a list of the things you think make a good teacher. When you have completed your list, identify the five most important things on your list. Now compare your list with the one we have compiled from nursing students who have undertaken this activity over the years (List 16.1).

We all know a good teacher when we meet one. Most of us will remember the teacher whose classes we most enjoyed. We recognise that we learned more from some teachers than others and if we know this it should only require a little thought to identify some of the things that make a good teacher. Some teachers are inspiring; others boring. Some make learning enjoyable or at least help us to recognise the relevance of whatever material they are trying to teach us. We look forward to the classes of some teachers, the thought of some other classes fills us with dread. In an ideal world we think we would want to anticipate eagerly all scheduled classes, although that might just get to be a little bit too intense. One thing that seems to influence students' experience of higher education is the idea, prevalent in the UK, that it is somehow 'uncool' to want to learn or to be seen to be too enthusiastic about learning.

410

List 16.1 Common responses of nursing students to the question: what makes a good teacher?

We have found that student nurses think good teachers:

- are enthusiastic;
- are knowledgeable;
- are approachable;
- are good communicators;
- have a sense of humour;
- show respect to students;
- respond positively to students' questions;
- are concise;
- are organised;
- interact with students;
- are challenging;
- are flexible with teaching methods;
- are supportive;
- test students' knowledge and abilities.

We suspect that your list will contain similar things.

List 16.2 Common responses of nursing students to the question: what makes a poor teacher?

We have also found that student nurses think poor teachers:

- are too judgemental;
- speak in a monotone;
- are unclear/lack clarity;
- are non-interactive;
- knock one's confidence;
- are aggressive;
- are not open-minded;
- set people up to fail;
- make people feel stupid.

You might be thinking that Khim (Case 16.2) is not the type of mentor you would want in a final-year placement, yet she is displaying several of the features identified by students (List 16.1) as things that make a good teacher. She is keen and enthusiastic. She is interested in Mark's progress, she wants to enable him to have a positive learning experience and she wants to help him make the most of his learning opportunities. Like most teachers and mentors, Khim has expectations (including the expectation that a student will arrive having thought about what they want to learn) and she responds well to students who are interested in learning.

A good teacher is primarily concerned with developing effective learners. Claxton (2002) has identified four ways teachers might talk with learners to help them build learning power, organise learning environments and plan activities. This approach is designed to encourage learners and teachers to develop insight into their own learning processes so as to encourage a learning community. According to Chambers *et al.* (2004) the approach includes:

- *explaining* the learning process to learners by informing, reminding, discussing and training;
- *orchestrating* the resources, environment and activities to support learning to learn through selecting, framing, target-setting and arranging;
- *commentating* on learners' capacities to learn through informal talk and evaluation through nudging, replying, evaluating and tracking;
- *modelling* oneself on being a learner, encouraging collective commitment to learning through learning aloud, reacting, demonstrating and sharing the experience.

This approach seems particularly relevant for the type of practice-based learning experiences of student nurses and particularly suited to work-based learning in which the placement mentor plays such an important part.

Building relationships within the learning environment

To join a pre-registration nursing programme is to join a group of learners. Together the members of the group can offer each other valuable learning resources, and the peer learning that occurs in the group may be more valuable to individual students than the normal interactions between student and tutor. Opportunities for discussion, group work, independent learning and study and so on within the programme provide social learning in which student interactions can play a significant role in the learning of all students.

Vygotsky (1978) describes learning as a social collaborative process in which the group can help each individual to learn to do or understand something and suggests that if you can do something or understand something with help today then you will be able to do it tomorrow without help. He describes this process as the zone of proximal development: the area within which we are able to do new things with assistance. Things that are unknown to us or which we do not understand are outside of this zone. Tharp and Gallimore (1988) have suggested a four-stage process to describe the way learning occurs in the zone of proximal development:

- *Stage 1*: with assistance provided by more capable others, such as peers, tutors, mentors.
- *Stage 2*: assistance is provided by oneself and the capacity is developed.
- *Stage 3*: the capacity becomes internalised and automatic.
- *Stage 4*: one begins to reflect on the capacity and assist others more clearly.

(Tharp and Gallimore 1988, p. 35)

This framework demonstrates the value of being able to mentor others as part of the process of learning to become a nurse, which has become part of the competencies expected of a third-year student nurse. However, it also highlights the importance of interaction in learning as a social process and thus requires the development of effective communication skills (see Chapter 14). Social learning enables peers to exchange stories of their experiences and so develop a narrative about their own learning process.

412

According to Greenhalgh (2006) using such narratives to enhance the quality of health care requires a 'good story' (i.e., one that contributes to the learning of others). A good story is one that meets the following criteria:

- *Aesthetic appeal*: the narrative is pleasing to hear and recount; it contains an internal harmony.
- *Coherence*: the narrative is clear and makes a logical whole; it contains a 'moral order' or sense.
- *Authenticity*: the narrative has credibility, based on the experiences of the listeners/readers.
- *Reportability*: the 'so what' value of what is narrated; its significance.
- *Persuasiveness*: the narrative convinces of the teller's own perspective.

(Greenhalgh 2006, summarised from pp. 9–12)

Work-based learning days seem ideal situations in which stories can provide rich learning opportunities for all or specific learning related to particular contexts. The sharing of stories in this way can be both a learning and a teaching experience for those involved.

While the relationships between students can be varied and educationally important, relationships developed within the placement can be equally valuable. As a student you will work alongside and interact with a wide range of individuals, as such you will engage in dialogue and conversation with more experienced colleagues. These relationships may be structured and formal (as existing between mentor and mentee) or unstructured and informal. The discussion between Sarah and Steve (Case 16.1) in relation to hand washing is an example of an informal conversation that resulted in learning. This type of informal learning is not restricted to the formal type of relationship between mentee and mentor as it is likely that students will learn just as much (if not more) from, for example, health care assistants than from those with formal qualifications and knowledge. Learning conversations are a recognised process of professional development, enabling practitioners to discuss their learning while supporting each other in improving their practice. While Alexander's (2004) exploration of this kind of learning (dialogic teaching) focuses on children, the concept has resonance for adult learning. Dialogic teaching includes the following characteristics:

- *Collective*: teacher and learner address tasks together as a group/whole cohort.
- *Reciprocal*: teacher and learner listen to each other, share ideas, consider alternative viewpoints.
- *Supportive*: learners articulate their ideas freely and help each other to reach common understandings.
- *Cumulative*: teachers and learners build on their own and each other's ideas and chain them into coherent lines of thinking and enquiry.
- *Purposeful*: teachers plan and steer talk with specific educational goals in mind.

(summarised from Alexander 2004, p. 27)

This interactive approach to learning and teaching might be found, for example, in a seminar session in higher education or within a learning community in a health care setting.

Race's competence model

Using uncomplicated language, Race (2015) suggests competence can be understood simply as 'can do': to say that someone has competence in a particular task is to say they can do that task. The simple model of competence Race develops from this essential point provides a basis from which to explore the consequences of either knowing or not knowing what it is that one can or cannot do. This is less complicated than it sounds. The following diagrams and explanations should help to clarify.

Race places competence on a north–south axis with consciousness on an east–west axis (Figure 16.1) providing four quadrants in which to locate competency in relation to awareness.

The competence/uncompetence line (the north–south axis)

Note that Race uses the term *un*competence rather than *in*competence in order to avoid the negative connotations of the latter.

Race notes there are degrees of competence, which means that for any task it is possible to say how well someone can do that task (this is the equivalent of making an assessment about that person's level of competence). So if you think you are highly competent at communicating, you would place yourself somewhere in the top half of the competence/uncompetence line. The exact point will depend on how highly you rate your competence in communicating. Of course, communication is a complex set of skills so it might be better to be more specific. If you are good at finding ways to explain things to patients in words they can understand then you would place yourself near the competence end of the continuum (e.g., at point X in Figure 16.2). However, if you are not very good at active listening then for this skill you would need to locate yourself near the uncompetence end of the continuum (e.g., point Y in Figure 16.2). Thus, it is possible to place yourself on the competence/uncompetence line for any and every task that you might undertake.

The same principle applies to the unconscious/conscious line, only this time with reference to how far you are aware of what you can or cannot do. Of course, everything said so far about the competence/uncompetence line relates to the conscious side (to the right of the line) because you must already know (be conscious of, or aware of) what you can or cannot do in order to locate it on the competence/uncompetence line. You might find this a little confusing but we hope to clarify.

The four quadrants

You should now be able to locate your competence in any specified task in one of the four quadrants (Figure 16.3) as follows:

- *The top right-hand quadrant* = conscious competence (knowing what you can do).
- *The bottom right-hand quadrant* = conscious uncompetence (knowing what you cannot do).
- *The top left-hand quadrant* = unconscious competence (not knowing what you can do).
- *The bottom left-hand quadrant* = unconscious uncompetence (not knowing what you cannot do).

We explain each in turn.

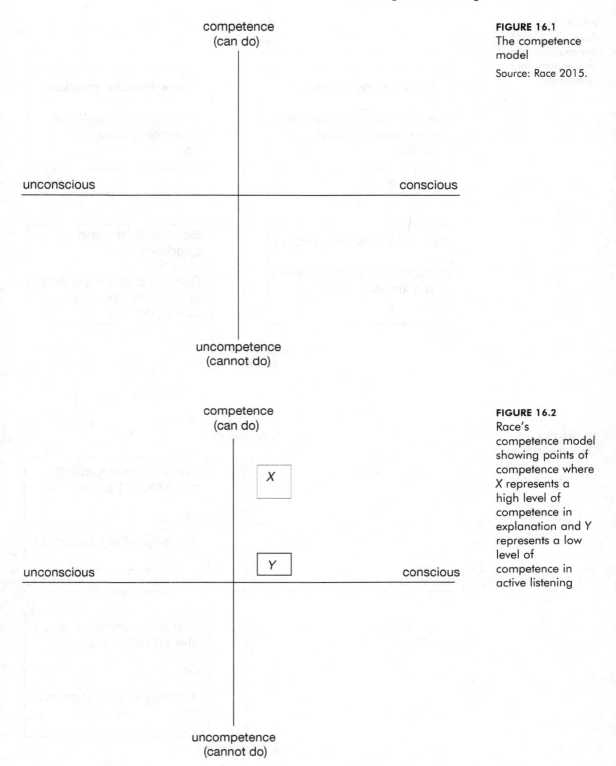

FIGURE 16.1
The competence model
Source: Race 2015.

FIGURE 16.2
Race's competence model showing points of competence where X represents a high level of competence in explanation and Y represents a low level of competence in active listening

FIGURE 16.3
Race's
competence model
showing the four
quadrants

competence
(can do)

Top left-hand quadrant

Unconscious competence
or not knowing what you
can do

Top right-hand quadrant

Conscious competence
or knowing what you can
do

unconscious   conscious

Bottom left-hand quadrant

Unconscious uncompetence
or not knowing what you
cannot do

**Bottom right-hand
quadrant**

Conscious uncompetence
or knowing what you
cannot do

uncompetence
(cannot do)

FIGURE 16.3
Race's
competence model
showing the four
quadrants

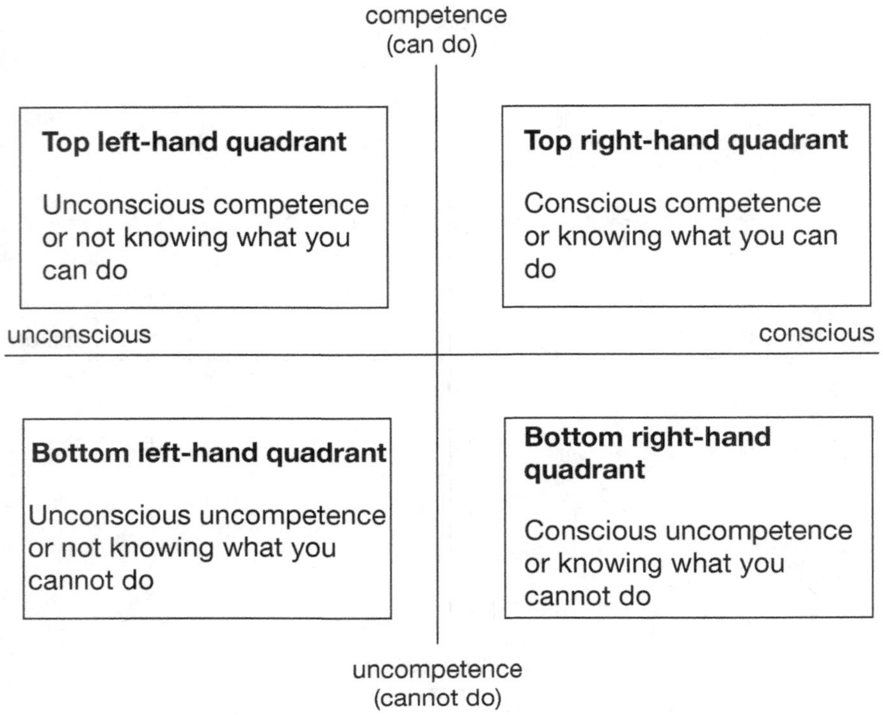

FIGURE 16.4
The conscious side
of Race's
competence model

competence

Conscious competence
(the **TARGET** box)

Or

Knowing what you can do

unconscious   conscious

Conscious uncompetence
(the **TRANSIT** box)

Or

*Knowing what you cannot
do*

uncompetence

416

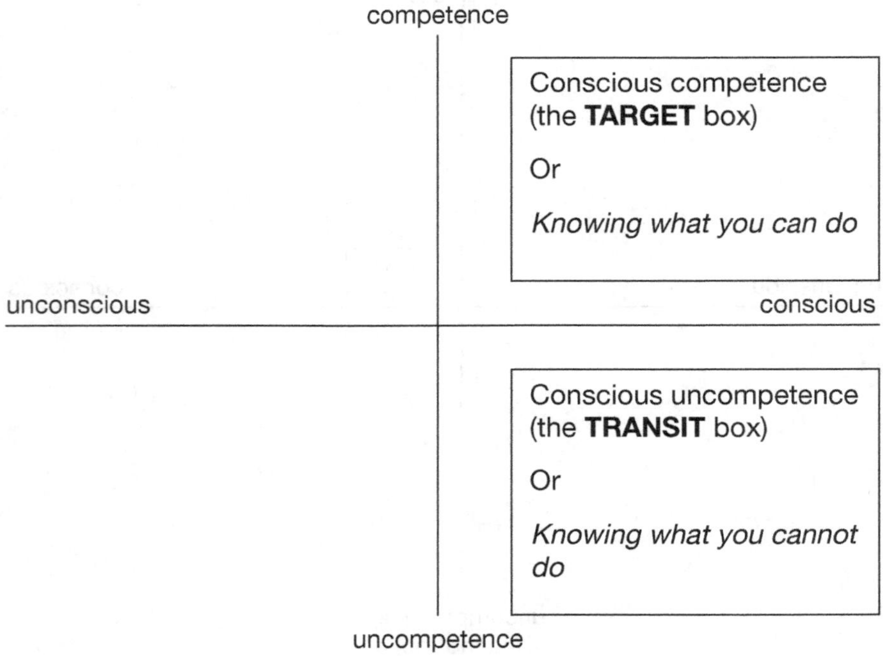

The conscious side of competence

The conscious side of competence includes the two quadrants of 'conscious competence' (*knowing* what you *can do*) and 'conscious uncompetence' (*knowing* what you *cannot do*) (Figure 16.4).

Conscious competence (the target box)

In this quadrant go things you know you can do. Those things you can do very well go somewhere near the top of the box, while those things you can only just about do go near the base. Race calls this the target box because the aim will be to move all the things that you want to be able to do into this box.

Conscious uncompetence (the transit box)

In this quadrant go things that you know you cannot do. Some of the things in this box will be things you neither want nor need to do and these can be safely left in this box. You may not be able to ride a horse but if you have no desire to ride a horse then there is no problem about this 'cannot do' thing being left here. But if you need or want to ride a horse then this will be one of the things you would aim to move into the target box. Because of this potential for movement Race calls this the transit box.

The unconscious side of competence

The unconscious side of competence includes the two quadrants of 'unconscious competence' (*not knowing* what you *can do*) and 'unconscious uncompetence' (*not knowing* what you *cannot do*) (Figure 16.5). Everything on the unconscious side of your competence is invisible to you because as soon as you identify anything you were previously unaware

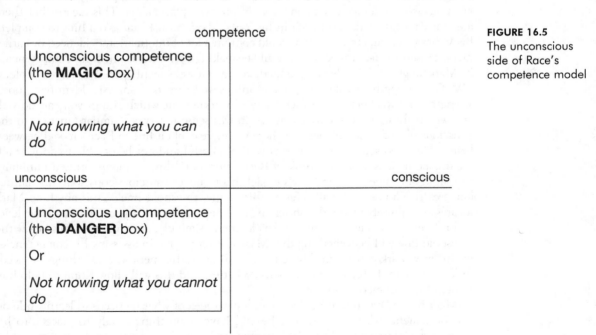

FIGURE 16.5
The unconscious side of Race's competence model

of, it becomes conscious. The implications of this are profound for nursing in general and for learning and teaching in nursing in particular.

Unconscious competence (the magic box)

In this quadrant go things you do not know you can do. Once you become aware that you can do any of the things in this box they are no longer invisible to you and so belong in the conscious competence quadrant (the target box). This means that from your perspective your magic box is always empty. It is empty because by definition you cannot know what is in there. However, many things in your magic box are visible to others, just as the contents of other people's magic boxes are visible to you. Race calls this the magic box because in it are all those things you are good at but do not recognise as anything special or significant.

Unconscious uncompetence (the danger box)

In this quadrant go things that you do not know you cannot do. As with items in the magic box, once you become aware of the things you cannot do they are no longer invisible to you and so belong in the conscious uncompetence quadrant (the transit box). Again, this means that from your perspective your danger box is empty. However, things in your danger box are visible to others, just as the contents of other people's danger boxes are visible to you. Race calls this the danger box because someone who thinks they can do something well but actually does that thing poorly has the potential to be a danger to self and others (the driver who does not recognise how bad their driving is, for example).

If we apply Race's model to Mark and Khim (Case 16.2) we can see how it might benefit their educational relationship.

You will recall that on this new placement Mark wants to be left to get on with the things he knows he can do well. He knows he can do these things well because he has been assessed as competent by mentors in previous placements. This means that there are many things Mark can locate in his 'target' box. So if Khim asked him to complete his 'conscious competence' box it would contain a lot of information evidenced by earlier mentor assessments; in effect Mark would be making a self-assessment of his competencies.

Mark might previously have undertaken a self-assessment by using, for example, a SWOT – strengths, weaknesses, opportunities and threats – analysis. Identifying one's strengths and weaknesses is a useful way of working out which things you can do well and which things need improvement, so in this sense it serves a similar function to the conscious side of Race's model. Yet there is a more explicit line in Race's model between being able to do something (however well or poorly) and not being able to do it at all. At this point it is useful to think of Race's horizontal line as representing a minimum threshold of competence: in Race's model this is the 'unconscious/conscious' line but for our present purposes we will refer to this as the 'threshold line'. Thus anything Mark locates at or just above the threshold line is something he can do but only at a basic level and is likely to benefit from further development; similarly, anything that falls below the threshold line will be something that Mark cannot yet do. In assessing his competencies in this way Mark can see for himself, and indicate to his mentor, those things he needs to learn how to do (or to learn how to do better) and this will allow Khim to help him to plan his placement learning.

Mark has indicated that he does have a clear idea of what he needs to learn while on this placement, which means that he will have some things ready to place into his 'conscious uncompetence' box (things that he knows he cannot yet do, but knows he needs to be able to do). He may even have identified these things as learning objectives or outcomes for the placement. This reflects Mark's strong sense of what he knows and of what he believes he can do well and it is useful for him to focus in this way. However, if he has not taken account of the unconscious side of the competence model his assessment of his learning needs will remain incomplete. Such unrecognised learning needs can lead to poor or even dangerous practice. The following example illustrates the point.

Case 16.2 (continued)

Mark feels slightly aggrieved when Khim asks him if he knows what he is doing when he measures patients' blood pressures. He is surprised to be asked this as he was assessed as competent in this task as a first-year student; and he has been left to get on with doing it without the need for supervision in subsequent placements. In terms of Race's model, Mark would assess himself as scoring high on his level of competence and high on his level of awareness. This means that *he thinks it is something that he knows he can do well*. Because of this Mark resents any implication to the contrary and thinks his mentor is wasting time even asking the question.

However, Khim is a skilled mentor and asks Mark to imagine that she is a first-year student who knows very little about blood pressure measurement. In this way Khim can begin to assess his skill as a facilitator of learning as well as his knowledge of blood pressure measurement and monitoring. Her experience suggests that individuals rarely know how much or how little they really understand about something until they try to share that knowledge. As Mark begins to explain the procedure, Khim plays her part by asking seemingly innocent questions such as:

- Is it best to use the right or left arm of the patient?
- What do you do if the patient is wearing a dressing gown or thick cardigan?

Mark is able to answer Khim's initial questions with ease and begins to warm to his task. He starts to think teaching is not such a big deal and that it should not be too difficult to meet the placement outcomes for learning and teaching. However, as Khim gently increases the probing nature of her questions, Mark begins to flounder and he starts to have trouble answering some parts of her questions.

For example, when Khim asks: 'what do the numbers displayed against MAP mean?', Mark finds himself at a loss. He resorts to telling her what he was told when he first learned about using the machine: that those numbers represent 'mean arterial pressure' and are unimportant. 'If they are unimportant, why are they there?' is Khim's immediate follow-up question, at which point Mark has to admit that he does not know. Similarly, when Khim asks him to demonstrate and explain the use of a manual sphygmomanometer, Mark finds himself on unfamiliar ground. 'I have not been asked to use one of these on a real patient before' he says. Khim then goes on to ask him if he knows when it might be appropriate to use an old-fashioned sphygmomanometer with a stethoscope and about the relationship between Korotkoff's sounds and *systolic* and *diastolic* blood pressure. Mark finds he does not really have satisfactory answers to these questions and finally concedes that his knowledge of blood pressure measurement is less complete than he had previously believed.

419

Khim might have asked other probing questions about the recommended length and width of the inflatable bladder held within the cuff; or about the consequences of using an insufficiently long or wide inflatable bladder, but she decides to stop once Mark admits to not knowing as much as he thought he knew. In this brief interlude, Khim has offered Mark a glimpse into his unconscious uncompetencies; in other words, she has demonstrated to Mark that there are *things he does not know he does not know* and further that *some of these are things he will need to know* (or at least be aware of) if he is to be a safe and effective practitioner. She has also illustrated to Mark the value of receiving feedback from others when undertaking a self-assessment so that one's unconscious competencies and uncompetencies are not ignored.

This is all a bit of a revelation to Mark, who recognises that he does indeed have more to learn than he had realised. As a result of Khim's gently probing questions, Mark has come to realise that his earlier self-assessment was incomplete because he had little input from other, more knowledgeable or more experienced, individuals. Now that Mark has acknowledged this he can, with the help of his mentor, begin to identify a wider spread of learning needs and take more control of his learning.

The value of the unconscious side of Race's model then lies not in filling the quadrants but in acknowledging their existence. The recognition that there are things that you do not know you cannot do is important because it allows you to remain open to the possibility that there are things you need to learn even if you do not yet know what these things are. This may help you to accept that you will not always see the relevance of some of the things other people think you need to learn. In other words, when you struggle to understand what any particular thing you are being asked to learn has got to do with nursing, it may be that you just do not yet know or understand its relevance in relation to the safe and effective care of patients and clients.

PART 3: EXPLORING LEARNING AND TEACHING

In Part 2 of this chapter we outlined some of the things that go to make a good teacher and from this we identified the important role the teacher has in establishing an environment in which learning can take place. As Part 3 progresses we hope you will begin to recognise the limits of the teacher's part in the educational process and start to acknowledge the way in which learners influence the quality of learning and teaching situations. We start here with a brief review of the things identified as making a good teacher.

Activity 16.2

Compare the items in List 16.1 with the items in List 16.2.
  Why do you think the things in one list are not merely the opposite of the things in the other?

As you might suspect, lists of the things that make a poor teacher generally identify things that are the opposite of the features that appear on lists of what makes a good teacher. Yet List 16.2 does not merely list the opposites of features in List 16.1. This suggests that there are some things that students particularly dislike in their teachers, the absence of which does not necessarily make a good teacher and vice versa. So while teacher enthusiasm is something students appreciate, a lack of enthusiasm may not necessarily make a poor teacher; similarly, it may be that a modicum of open-mindedness is sufficient whereas its absence may be a significant obstacle to learning.

Thus far we have contrasted the 'good' with the 'poor' teacher. While these are words that many students use to describe their teachers, the terms have only limited descriptive value. The words good and poor can mean different things to different people, so in the remainder of this chapter we will refer to 'effective' and 'ineffective' rather than 'good' and 'poor' respectively. So we will now be talking about effectiveness in learning and teaching. The effective teacher, then, is the one who provides the environment in which learning is most likely to take place. This is not merely the physical environment of a classroom or a placement but includes a range of factors, some of which have been identified in List 16.1 and List 16.2. However, the importance of the physical environment should not be underestimated. It is, after all, difficult to learn in a cold classroom. Similarly, it may be hard to engage in learning when faced with a heavy workload on placement: if you are worrying that there is not time to get everything done before the end of your shift you are unlikely to give your full attention to the mentor's explanation about, for example, hyper- and hypoglycaemia.

Many factors contribute to the learning environment and other people (mentors and other staff in placement settings; other students and teachers in the classroom and so on) have an important role in determining the effectiveness of any given learning situation. Wenger's (2000) concept of 'communities of practice' is an attempt to describe this social aspect of learning as an essential and necessary feature of a learning environment if an individual is to negotiate the development of competencies. Learning in practice is an important element of becoming a nurse and the practice environment impacts upon a student's capacity to learn. According to Wenger there are a set of specific dimensions necessary for a community of practice if it is to maintain the capacity to develop and support the learning of everyone within it:

- *Enterprise*: the level of learning energy describes the enthusiasm that a community demonstrates for maintaining learning at the centre of its action, a spirit of enquiry and a desire to find out.
- *Mutuality*: the depth of social capital describes the level of trust between people to ensure they feel comfortable addressing problems together; this can often take time.
- *Repertoire*: the degree of self-awareness describes how the concepts, language and tools of the community embody its perspective and own state of development.

(summarised from Wenger 2000, p. 230)

Activity 16.3

Write a short account of a recent or significant learning experience (it can be an effective or ineffective learning experience). Have a go at seeing how far any of the three dimensions described above were present in the setting in which this learning experience took place.

Derek Sellman and Jane Tarr

We anticipate that the more these dimensions were present in the learning situation you describe, the more you learned. You might have described a placement or a classroom learning experience, as these dimensions are relevant across the range of learning situations. For example, seminar groups provide the type of environment where students can learn with and from each other in a way that supports those who at any point may be struggling to learn. In the placement environment the attitudes of the qualified staff can be a significant factor in a student's capacity to learn. It seems that trust has an important part to play if effective learning is to take place. Case 16.3 illustrates a community of practice in which effective learning is occurring:

Case 16.3

Ann, the manager of a unit in a local hospital, understands the value of providing an environment in which learning is encouraged. She contributes sessions to students of nursing at the local university and has appointed an education facilitator to work with staff. Ann encourages all staff to reflect on their practice and to discuss aspects of their reflections with others to help improve practice. The education facilitator contributes to these discussions whenever possible and organises formal study events and training sessions on topics or issues highlighted during the discussions. Over time this has helped the staff to recognise the value of learning in this way and the culture of the unit has developed as a learning community.

In a learning community such as this, everyone is involved and learning takes place both formally and informally, which helps individuals to build their capacity for learning.

Activity 16.4

- Look again at the items in List 16.1 and List 16.2.
- Identify the things in List 16.1 that you think are most likely to aid effective learning.
- Identify the things in List 16.2 that you think are most likely to inhibit effective learning.
- Now swap your new lists with another student, and talk about what you notice.

We think that the things you identify as most likely to aid and inhibit learning will not be exactly the same as those identified by other students. This suggests that individuals learn in different ways. In fact, the idea that not everybody learns in the same way is a well-documented phenomenon referred to as **individual learning style**.

RESEARCH FOCUS 16.1

In a comprehensive review, Coffield *et al.* (2004) found that the literature on learning styles falls into three distinct areas: (1) theoretical, (2) pedagogical and (3) commercial. The review identified 71 models of learning styles. Some discuss the workings of the brain, others explore personality traits, some emphasise the importance of previous experience and environmental factors, and some emphasise the importance of understanding one's own learning biography.

The impact of theoretical frameworks on the teaching and learning process is clear. However, different disciplines have interpreted learning theory in discipline-specific ways: thus learning theory is understood differently in psychology, sociology, management, education, nursing and so on. As a consequence the impact of learning theory varies in the practice of teaching and learning across different disciplines.

The contrast between nursing and teaching is of interest. Teaching began as an academic process and has gradually moved towards an emphasis on classroom practice, whereas nurse education emerged from clinical practice and has developed into an academic discipline. Despite these different antecedents the learning contexts for those learning to become teachers are broadly similar to those learning to become nurses.

Learning styles

There are many ways to categorise how different individuals learn. Common in the different descriptions of learning styles is the idea that people will not simply fit into one category of learner. Rather, most people can be categorised (or will categorise themselves) as having a preferred learning style even if they do not always use that style in all learning situations. This insight is important for several reasons that we will explore shortly. First though we will outline one popular and commonly used learning style; one that has its roots in the psychology of personality.

Honey and Mumford (1992) describe learners as predominately falling into one of four categories: activists, reflectors, theorists, and pragmatists:

- *Activists* like to participate and try things out for themselves. Activists tend to be keen to get involved whenever the opportunity arises.
- *Reflectors* like to think about things first. Reflectors may be content to watch others try things out before getting involved.
- *Theorists* like to use models and theories to understand things. Theorists may try to avoid being swayed by emotions or first impressions.
- *Pragmatists* like to experiment. Pragmatists prefer practical to abstract ideas and like to see how things work in the real world.

Most people find they can identify themselves as fitting one (or more) of these categories and you may already have recognised yourself as primarily a pragmatist, a theorist, a reflector, or an activist. There is no evaluative undercurrent here; this is to say that, in general terms, no one learning style is necessarily better or more effective than another, although there are some situations in which one style is more likely to result in effective learning. For example, students who prefer an activist learning style

Derek Sellman and Jane Tarr

Instrumental understandings of education. Some students (and some teachers) see education purely (or primarily) as a means to a particular end. So the student nurse who thinks classroom teaching is largely irrelevant to the 'real world' of practice might be described as using the classroom primarily as a way of achieving their desired end of becoming a registered nurse. For such a student education is the instrument of getting to where they want to get.

are likely to be most comfortable getting involved in learning the practical skills of things such as cardiopulmonary resuscitation, where theorists might struggle. Nevertheless, the theorist who can adopt an activist approach when faced with learning a practical skill will be an effective learner in that situation. This is important because it suggests that effective learners are those who can adapt their learning style to suit the requirements of learning particular topics in particular situations. Conversely, the student who is reluctant to adopt a different learning style to the one they most prefer is likely to struggle to learn in those situations that benefit most from alternative learning style approaches. The fact that individual students have preferred learning styles also has significant implications for the teacher when designing, planning and implementing programmes of learning.

Activity 16.5 is designed to help you begin to understand some of the ways in which learners influence the learning environment and the quality of learning.

Activity 16.5

Make a list of the things you think make an effective learner. When you have completed your list, identify the five most important things on your list. Now read on and compare your list with the one we have compiled from the responses of nursing students who have undertaken this activity over the years (List 16.3).

One of the implications of individual learning styles is that those students who are able to adapt their learning style to meet demands of particular learning situations are more likely to be effective learners across a wide range of learning opportunities. In addition, teachers think that few learners recognise the role they (the learners) play in influencing the quality of their own educational experiences. Teachers generally understand learning as an active process, whereas (teachers believe) most students think of education as more of a product; this may be in terms of being 'assessment-driven' (see explanation of this point in Part 1 of this chapter) or in terms of education being **instrumental**. If this is true then the learner who takes an active role in the educational process is more likely to benefit from a given learning and teaching situation. In other words: the more active the learner is, the more effective their learning is likely to be.

List 16.3 Common responses of nursing students to the question: what makes an effective learner?

We have found that student nurses think effective learners:

- are committed;
- take a questioning approach to learning;
- are enthusiastic;
- pay attention;
- are keen to learn;
- are motivated;
- have goals/objectives.

424

Just as with the lists for the 'what makes a good teacher' activity in Part 2 of this chapter (List 16.1 and List 16.2) we suspect that your list will contain similar things to the list compiled here. This indicates that you know quite a lot about effective learning and teaching.

List 16.4 Common responses of nursing students to the question: what makes an ineffective learner?

We have found that student nurses think that ineffective learners may:

- not listen;
- be uninterested;
- lack enthusiasm;
- be unmotivated;
- be distracted;
- think they know it all.

One important point here is that there are common aspects of approaching learning that will influence the effectiveness of learning regardless of individual learning styles. The person who thinks they 'already know it all' is likely to be less receptive to new ideas than the person who knows they have things to learn. To return to Race's competence model: the student nurse or practitioner who thinks they 'know it all' is either unaware of their own uncompetencies (i.e., does not know what they do not know or cannot do) or has chosen to ignore their uncompetencies (i.e., knows what they do not know but is unwilling to do anything about it). In either case, such a person is likely to become an unsafe practitioner without recognising this as a danger to their practice and to the patients in their care.

Developing aptitudes to learning

While the characteristics and approach of the teachers will have a significant influence on the learning experience of each student, the role of the learner in creating an effective learning situation should not be underestimated. The teaching style of the teacher will often depend on the nature of the topic being taught but the fine detail of the session will reflect the teacher's own views about how people learn. This alone does not determine the learning that takes place. While the primary responsibility for setting the environment in which learning can take place may lie with the teacher, it is the learner who is ultimately responsible for their own learning. If this is true then it should be clear that each learner needs to build their learning capacity so as to make best use of the available learning resources and opportunities. In other words, what and how much a student learns will be influenced not only by what it is that is to be learned but also by the way in which the learner approaches learning. We will now explore briefly some of the aptitudes that have the potential to enhance students' learning.

Self-awareness

Successful engagement with the learning process requires you as a learner to develop an understanding of how best you learn. This will necessarily require that you engage with some form of self-evaluation in order to gain insight into your particular learning potential and to understand what conditions offer you the best chance of maximising your learning. As mentioned earlier, Claxton (2002) encourages learners to build their learning power through engagement in self-evaluation and through exploration of a variety of approaches to learning in a range of settings.

Claxton suggests that there are four different learning dispositions, which need to be developed and extended in order to build learning capacity. He categorises these as:

- *Resilience*: being ready, willing and able to lock on to learning.
- *Resourcefulness*: being ready, willing and able to learn in different ways.
- *Reflectiveness*: being ready, willing and able to become more strategic about learning.
- *Reciprocity*: being ready, willing and able to learn alone and with others.

(Claxton 2002, p. 4)

These dispositions can be developed in order to understand one's own approach to learning and may involve trial and error by, for example, exploring the best environment for writing essays or by trying to find the most useful person in the workplace with whom to discuss a topic. Both examples require the dispositions described above together with a level of self-confidence in one's own capacities. It may be the case that in professional practice a student nurse is not always aware of all aspects of their learning but that through

> simply interact(ing) with the situation in a 'mindless' but observant manner, they come to master it, at an intuitive level – they do the right thing without knowing why – faster than those who keep struggling for conscious comprehension.
>
> (Atkinson and Claxton 2000, p. 36)

Self-awareness of the learning process is a valuable commodity, particularly in the workplace where formal learning opportunities are not always made explicit. This capacity together with an emergent awareness of learning power can enable a student to recognise informal and formal learning opportunities in the workplace and beyond.

Open-mindedness and flexibility

We have noted that each individual has a preferred learning style and we have suggested that those learners who are able to adopt a style of learning other than their preferred style are likely to increase their learning power. This is important in nursing because learning opportunities occur in various forms (both formal and informal) and learning to be flexible in choosing a learning style to match a specific task will enhance learning, which in turn will help develop and improve practice. For some individuals becoming flexible will require effort but can be assisted by cultivating open-mindedness. Open-mindedness requires a person to remain open to the possibility of being wrong and open to the possibility of a need to change behaviour: including learning behaviour. These are demanding requirements but the alternative is to be either closed-minded or credulous (Sellman 2003), and either of these will reduce learning opportunities available to students and registered practitioners alike.

Reflection

Reflection provides individuals with an opportunity to identify what they know, what they do not know and what they need to do in order to fill gaps in their knowledge, understanding and skills. Reflection is a major theme in Chapter 17 so here we will confine ourselves to a few brief comments. Reflection has become an important aspect of many practical occupations (including nursing and teaching) as a method by which individual practitioners can develop their practice. Schön (1987) presents three levels of reflection: knowing-in-action; reflection-in-action; and reflection-on-action.

Knowing–in-action implies that thinking is embedded in actions, that it is implicit. The student nurse in the workplace would demonstrate their knowledge through their actions. Those students or registered nurses who are unable to enact their knowledge (i.e., unable to use their knowledge to inform their practice) will struggle to be safe and effective practitioners. For Schön, knowing-in-action is demonstrated when, for example, a student successfully gives an injection or accurately assesses the nursing care needs of a patient.

This is distinct from reflection-in-action, which involves a conscious standing back to think critically and to question whether merely continuing with existing knowledge-in-action is appropriate in a particular situation. Reflection-in-action may be momentary and might result in a change of knowledge-in-action and thus a more suitable action in what may be a novel situation. In this respect, reflection-in-action can enable the transfer of skills from familiar to unfamiliar contexts.

Reflection-on-action requires a retrospective review of actions taken and has a more structured purpose in assisting a practitioner or student to evaluate and learn from performance. Many nursing students will be encouraged to reflect-on-action as a way of providing evidence of learning.

CONCLUSION

Wherever and whenever nursing occurs, learning and teaching are almost certainly taking place. Student and registered nurses invariably learn things from and about patients and relatives, while at the same time patients and relatives learn things from and about students and registered nurses. This learning might be incidental or deliberate, and it may be related or unrelated to patient care. When you observe a patient's reaction to a painful procedure you learn something about them and the receptive nurse will make use of that learning to inform future pain management strategies. At the same time the patient will learn something about you: they may learn whether or not you are compassionate and/or trustworthy; they may learn that you care about or are indifferent to their pain and this may affect the way they subsequently behave in your presence. This type of learning may be informal and incidental but as we have indicated, when one person learns something from another then that other is in some sense teaching. When you explain anything to another person, be it how to engage in discussion with a depressed patient, how to manage a long-term urinary catheter, how to measure and monitor blood pressure or how to give advice on healthy eating, you are engaged in a form of teaching because you are trying to get that other person to learn something.

Thus teaching is directly related to nursing practice in myriad ways and it follows that some knowledge and understanding of learning and teaching is an essential aspect of safe and effective nursing practice. As a student nurse, and subsequently as a registered nurse, other people (patients, relatives and carers, students, health care assistants and so on) will learn from you whether or not you intend this to happen. Your choice, then, is to either ignore the influence you have on what it is that others learn from you, or take steps to encourage particular sorts of learning in those around you.

The Nursing and Midwifery Council states that 'you must ... support students' and colleagues' learning to help them develop their professional competence' (2015, pp. 8–9), which makes clear that in addition to the professional requirement to continue to learn, each registered nurse has a professional obligation to facilitate learning for others. This means that as far as the regulatory body for nursing is concerned you do not have a choice. In other words, not only must you be aware of your responsibilities in relation to learning and teaching, but you must also be proactive in assisting in the development of an environment that encourages the development of the learning power of each individual in the environment.

While achieving the minimum threshold level of competence consistent with safe and effective practice is necessary in order to register as a nurse, the importance of developing a positive approach and attitude towards learning for self and others remains the cornerstone of the maintenance of professional nursing practice.

SUGGESTED FURTHER READING

Quinn, F. M. (2007) *Principles and Practice of Nurse Education* (5th edn). Cheltenham, UK: Nelson Thornes.
Race, P. (2015) *The Lecturer's Toolkit: A practical guide to assessment, learning and teaching* (4th edn). London: Routledge.

REFERENCES

Alexander, R. (2004) *Towards Dialogic Teaching: Rethinking classroom talk*. Cambridge: Dialogos.
Atkinson, T. and Claxton, G. (2000) *The Intuitive Practitioner: On the value of not always knowing what one is doing*. Buckingham, UK: Open University Press.
Chambers, M., Powell, G. and Claxton, G. (2004) *Building 101 Ways to Learning Power*. Bristol: TLO.
Claxton, G. (2002) *Building Learning Power: Helping young people to become better learners*. Bristol: TLO.
Coffield, F., Moseley. D., Hall, E. and Ecclestone, K. (2004) *Learning Styles and Pedagogy in Post-16 Learning: A systematic and critical review*. London: Learning Skills Research Centre.
Dewey, J. (1916) *Democracy and Education: An introduction to the philosophy of education*. New York: Macmillan.
Greenhalgh, T. (2006) *How to Read a Paper: The basics of evidence-based medicine*. Oxford: Blackwell.
Honey, P. and Mumford, A. (1992) *The Manual of Learning Styles*. Maidenhead: Honey & Mumford.
NMC (Nursing and Midwifery Council) (2015) *The Code: Professional standards of practice and behaviour for nurses and midwives*. NMC: London.
Race, P. (2015) *The Lecturer's Toolkit: A practical guide to assessment, learning and teaching* (4th edn). London: Routledge.
Sacks, O. (1995) *An Anthropologist on Mars*. London: Picador.
Schön, D. A. (1987) *Educating the Reflective Practitioner: Towards a new design for teaching and learning in the professions*. San Francisco, CA: Jossey-Bass.

Sellman, D. (2003) Open-mindedness: a virtue for professional practice. *Nursing Philosophy* **4** (1), 17–24.

Smith, F. (1998) *The Book of Learning and Forgetting*. New York: Teachers College Press.

Tharp, R. G. and Gallimore, R. (1988) *Rousing Minds to Life*. Cambridge: Cambridge University Press.

Vygotsky, L. S. (1978) *Mind and Society: The development of higher psychological processes*. Cambridge, MA: Harvard University Press.

Wenger, E. (2000) Communities of practice and social learning systems. *Organisation* **7** (2), 225–246.

17

PERSONAL AND PROFESSIONAL DEVELOPMENT THROUGH REFLECTIVE PRACTICE

Clare Hopkinson

LEARNING OUTCOMES

After reading and reflecting on this chapter, you should be able to:

- outline the nature of reflection, critical reflection and reflexivity;
- identify a range of methods for reflecting effectively;
- explain different ways of knowing in nursing;
- begin to develop a professional portfolio and private personal diary;
- raise questions about your own practice;
- recognise the emotional impact of caring for others;
- discuss the importance of continuing professional development.

INTRODUCTION

Personal and professional development is an important part of becoming and remaining a registered nurse. Reflection is recognised as an important aspect of that development for leadership, accountability and service improvement. Nurses need to continue to develop because of the changing nature of what is known, the dynamic nature of practice and the need to constantly improve one's skills to ensure safe and effective evidence-based care. In this chapter I hope to convince you of the value of critical reflection as a systematic and thoughtful way to develop your personal and professional practice either by yourself or with others.

The chapter is divided into three parts. In Part 1, I show the importance of personal and professional development, its relationship with reflection as a way of analysing nursing practice and thus, as a means of quality improvement (Shaw *et al.* 2012).

In Part 2, I outline the nature of reflection offering some definitions while noting that universal agreement about the nature of reflection is not forthcoming. This is unsurprising given that reflection can take a variety of forms and can be undertaken in different ways

A brief discussion about models of reflection is provided together with a short overview regarding their effectiveness.

In Part 3, I explore the explore the framework of ways of knowing developed by Belenky *et al.* (1986), emphasising how this links to the reflective process and how it can help you think about ways to develop your practice. I conclude the chapter with some ideas that may help you to reflect creatively either alone or with others, together with some practical suggestions about keeping and maintaining a reflective portfolio for personal reflection.

PART 1: OUTLINING PERSONAL AND PROFESSIONAL DEVELOPMENT THROUGH REFLECTIVE PRACTICE

Case 17.1

Julia is a third-year student nurse who has been involved in a drug administration error. She has been asked by her mentor (Tariq) to write a reflective piece about the incident. Tariq knows that Julia is not a natural reflector so he has asked her to structure her writing using Johns' model of reflection. For her part Julia is reluctant to put pen to paper, as she knows she will be required to endure a three-way discussion (with her university tutor and her mentor, Tariq) and thinks that this meeting should be the end of it. She finds it difficult to understand why Tariq thinks she should spend time writing about the incident when she already knows what happened and what now needs to be done. In short, she thinks it a bit of a waste of time, furthermore, she thinks Johns' model is repetitive and demands too much detail. However, Julia also knows that Tariq will be responsible for assessing her competencies and she does not want to mess up her chances of getting a good report or reference. She realises that she will need to spend some of her precious spare time tonight before going out writing her reflection in order to have it ready for Tariq in the morning.

As a student nurse you should find it easy to complete the sentence: 'my course would be so much better if only . . . ' This is because most students will have at least one idea of how their programme could be improved. Similarly many students will be able to identify easily what a particular lecturer or mentor needs to do in order to be better at their job. We all engage in the kinds of conversations in which the shortcomings of systems, organisations or other people are identified and where simple solutions for making things better are suggested. Unfortunately, the same cannot always be said in relation to ourselves: indeed, we may not engage in conversations that identify our own shortcomings, let alone provide solutions for improving our performance as nurses. If nothing else, critical reflection provides an opportunity to review the effects and consequences of our behaviour and actions. Tariq has asked Julia to use a structured form of reflection so she can identify her role in the incident because he believes this will enable her to understand how the incident might have been avoided. From this Tariq hopes Julia will agree to construct a plan of action to assist her personal and professional development.

To develop is to improve. Development occurs when things can be said to have improved. Development is intimately bound with thinking; thinking about the way things are now and thinking about the way things might be improved: and to engage in thinking about things in this way is to engage in reflection. Thus reflection is an essential feature of development, and as suggested above, most of us engage in this type of activity on an everyday basis. We might not normally call this 'reflection' but when we think about how things are and how they might be improved we are reflecting on what is and what might be.

Personal development is personal improvement, while professional development involves improving experiences of health and nursing care for patients; in other words, professional development implies service improvement. So in a professional sense, engaging with reflection (i.e., thinking about how things are and thinking about how they might be improved for patients) must be accompanied by action (i.e., actually doing something in an attempt to make things better for patients). Thus reflection is an integral part of personal and professional development and is triggered by our experiences, our

BOX 17.1

A manual handling incident by Clare Hopkinson (2005)

Let's move this patient
From the trolley to the bed
How are we going to do this?
The health care assistant said
All hands to the deck are needed
We could really do with six
Better still, use the slide sheet
Cos we've definitely judged the risk
But the slide sheet can't be found
It's not readily at hand
Oh let's move her anyway then
But be careful how you stand
Fill in the incident form, later
That'll do the trick
But how safe is it to whistle blow?
Cos mud will often stick
Hurry up, time to go home now
The stupid form can wait
We're really fed up of staying behind
So today we won't be late
You need lots of incident forms anyway
Before managers will ever act
What's the point of even trying
There's no money and that's a fact
Staff shortages and cutting corners
Are now part of the working day
Leaving the workforce feeling, what?
Unwilling to have their say?

feelings and our uncertainties (Bradbury-Jones *et al.* 2009). In addition, reflection is now an expectation for registered nursing practice (NMC 2015).

In this chapter the focus is on reflection as a method of pursuing personal and professional development as a way of helping you learn from and about your practice. I hope that reading this chapter will encourage you to have a go at reflection and find out its value for yourself in your development as a professional nurse. In this way you can learn to become a reflective practitioner and begin to use your personal and professional experience as a means for continuing your development.

> **Reflective practice** involves noticing, imagining, challenging, inquiring, reframing, meaningful conscious actions and using different ways of knowing the world of practice to become a more effective practitioner.

Activity 17.1

Consider the feelings evoked by the poem in Box 17.1.

- What questions does it raise?
- What are the assumptions in it?
- What are the tensions and possible contradictions in the poem?
- How does this relate to your own experiences of moving patients?
- Could a poem like this help to change practice for the better?
- What do you imagine might be some of the difficulties in attempting to change practice?
- How effective is the poem for helping to reflect on practice?

I wrote the poem in Box 17.1 following a difficult experience when returning to nursing after a gap of 10 years. In the poem I wanted to capture the reality that practice does not always follow the theory propagated in college (but I am sure you already know this!). I offer this poem not because it is particularly well crafted but because it shows the value of exploring everyday experiences and questioning nursing practices. It illustrates one reflective method for inquiring into some of the difficulties of practising effectively when working with others. Personally I was struck by the power of the group dynamics to silence my objections about moving the patient without a slide sheet and by the general lack of will to feedback to the organisation issues that were affecting practice. Through this poem perhaps you can recognise similar issues and experiences in your own practice.

Reflective practice can be a powerful process for learning from such less than perfect and difficult (although not uncommon) situations. These kinds of experiences are often called critical incidents: not life-threatening, but critical in the sense of questioning taken-for-granted practice norms. In this way, reflective practice can challenge, and help to change for the better, knowledge, attitudes and behaviours, which in turn can lead to improvements in the quality of nursing care as experienced by patients and clients.

Nursing is predominately an oral profession: it seems easier to talk about nursing than to write about it. A feature of this oral tradition is that many nurses find it difficult to articulate the taken-for-granted aspects of nursing knowledge; in particular, the embodied knowledge that guides action because this tacit and intuitive knowledge is difficult to express. Here, I suggest that while there is value in writing reflectively using models of reflection there are other creative ways to reflect that also enable intuitive knowledge to be expressed. For example, I found by using my experiences of practice as poems I could reflect honestly and question my caregiving, values and assumptions. I also suggest that there is value in finding a critically reflexive friend or mentor who can support and challenge your development in a safe environment as you talk about your stories of practice (Clarke 2014, Hopkinson 2009, Taylor 2010). This person must not merely agree with you or take your side, rather they must help you explore your experiences in ways that allow you to see those experiences differently. In other words the critical friend is someone who can help to challenge your assumptions about your practice, to signpost to you potential new knowledge, and to help you integrate learning from your reflections so that you have new actions or ideas with which to improve your practice.

The overall aim of this chapter is to present a realistic picture of the process of reflection and to show that at times reflecting is not an easy process. It takes curiosity, courage, tenacity, commitment, resilience, assertiveness, empathy, a sense of humour and an openness to learn from everyday experiences (Hopkinson 2009). I regard reflection as something of a mystery tour: I think I know where I am going so I tend to jump to conclusions about where I will end up. However, if I do this, I rush to the end too soon and miss both the positive and negative experiences of the journey. In allowing the journey to unfold, the sense of adventure and anticipation of not knowing quite where one will end up allows the learning and the development to take place in sometimes surprising ways. Sometimes this is pleasant, sometimes unpleasant, but either can stimulate strong emotion. A significant proportion of my most important learning has been from the unpleasant experiences.

Despite being in her third year and close to qualification (and registration) and despite being required to incorporate reflection in various assignments throughout her course, Julia has managed to avoid the level of reflection that Tariq is expecting. She thinks she will need only a few minutes to get something written down, just as she has done for those reflective assignments she has completed during her course. She will then be free to enjoy her evening with friends. Sadly for Julia (although she does not know it yet), Tariq will be unimpressed by her half-hearted attempt at reflection and ultimately Julia will find herself slightly embarrassed by her efforts. This chapter follows Julia as she comes to realise that not only is becoming a nurse a more serious business than she has previously taken it to be but also that there may be some value in this thing called reflection after all.

PART 2: EXPLAINING PERSONAL AND PROFESSIONAL DEVELOPMENT THROUGH REFLECTIVE PRACTICE

Case 17.1 (continued)

Tariq is a staff nurse and a mentor to Julia (our third-year student nurse). One of the things Tariq has found so surprising since becoming a staff nurse is the way that so many nurses just keep on doing the same old thing day after day despite being full of complaints about the way things are and full of statements about how much better things would be if only . . .

Tariq knows how busy and pressurised nursing work can be and he is beginning to suspect that the majority of nurses are just too tired and too overwhelmed by the sheer volume of demands on their time to do anything about their complaints or their ideas for improvement. He hears lots of nurses complaining about the way things are but he sees few nurses doing anything to change their situations. Because he has only been qualified a relatively short time and because he feels many of the nurses in his practice area have fallen into the 'this is the way we do it here' trap, he feels he should put his efforts into encouraging students. Thus when the drug administration error occurs he seizes the opportunity to engage Julia with ideas about personal and professional development.

Personal and professional development requires effort and a willingness to continue to learn. Many of the skills and attitudes required for effective learning are explored in Chapter 16, so the focus in this chapter is less on the building blocks of learning and teaching and more on the nature of reflection as a process with which to enable personal and professional development. Reflection is a way of identifying what and how things might be improved. Therefore capturing that learning as well as your contribution to the development of professional practice in a form to be included in a portfolio is one way of demonstrating your personal development. These need not be large-scale efforts in order to improve the service, as often it is the little changes that enhance the patient experience (Francis 2013).

Personal and professional development also requires a willingness to move on from merely complaining about a current unsatisfactory state of affairs; it requires taking action in an attempt to make things better. Nevertheless, arguably, the act of complaining does at least demonstrate a minimum form of reflection (i.e., thinking that things could be better than they are) but without some form of action, complaining tends to become an end in itself and leads to stagnation rather than development. Thus development requires reflection plus action: the term reflective practice captures this requirement for action and is therefore often used as the preferred term in practice-based professional occupations such as nursing.

The language associated with reflection can be difficult to understand. The most common terms in the literature are: 'reflection', 'critical reflection', 'reflective practice' and 'reflexivity'. These terms are sometimes used interchangeably although each has been the subject of a particular definition by different authors; nevertheless it is generally accepted that reflection without some form of development is a sterile activity. Indeed, the majority of the literature on reflection focuses on the personal reflective stories of individuals' experiences as a way of creating, modifying, developing and thus improving practice (e.g., Bolton 2005, Ghaye and Lillyman 2006, Johns 2010, Kim 1999, Moon 2004, Taylor 2010).

Reflection has many definitions. It is variously understood as ranging from casual ways of thinking about practice at one extreme to structured processes based on the philosophical underpinnings of, for example, Dewey, Habermas, Gadamer (Johns 2010, Kember *et al.* 2001, Taylor 2010) at the other. Different levels of reflection are proposed by different authors. For example Mezirow (1990) identified seven levels with each level demanding more intellectual skill while van Manen (1977) described anticipatory reflection through action planning before an event takes place. In the social sciences research literature, the preferred term for looking back and examining the influence and impact of the researcher's experience and values throughout the research process is called reflexivity and is associated with action research, critical pedagogy, critical theory, critical social theory and several qualitative research methodologies such as feminism, heuristic research and ethnography.

According to the *Oxford English Dictionary*, reflection is 'to throw back, reconsider, go back in thought, serious thought or consideration' (OED 2006, p. 1208). This OED definition offers only a simplistic view that corresponds with the 'casual thinking about practice' end of the continuum. The value of this form of reflection tends to remain in the intellectual rather than practical domain and, in common with many other definitions, suggests reflection as a solitary pursuit. Given that nursing is a practical and (more often than not) collective activity, the developmental value of isolated individual reflection may be limited.

> Reflective learning is the process of internally examining and exploring an issue of concern, triggered by an experience which creates and clarifies meaning in terms of self, and which results in a changed conceptual perspective.
>
> (Boyd and Fales 1983, p. 100)

> A process of consciously examining what has occurred in terms of thoughts, feelings and actions against underlying beliefs, assumptions and knowledge as well as against the backdrop (i.e., the context or the stage) in which specific practice has occurred.
>
> (Kim 1999, p. 1209)

The definitions offered by Boyd and Fales (1983) and Kim (1999) recognise reflection as a process for improving practice through increased self-understanding and inquiry into the context and structures that support practice. Kim's notion of 'consciously examining' practice (and this includes examining the context in which care is delivered) implies a depth missing from the OED definition. Johns (2000) described reflexivity as: 'looking back and seeing self as a changed person is the essential feature of reflexivity. It is not an endpoint but is always open to and anticipatory of future experiences' (p. 61). The term 'reflexivity' tends to be used in association with research far more than either reflection or critical reflection. Sometimes there is a distinction between content reflection (what is reflected upon) and process reflection (what happens in a group during group reflection).

Reflection as an effective process has been criticised on the grounds of timing (affecting recall), interference from stress and emotions, particularly anxiety (Ixer 1999, Mackintosh 1998, Newell 1992), self-distortions (Dunning 2005) and lack of universal definition (Mackintosh 1998). This last assumes that a single definition is necessary for understanding a complex phenomenon and that there is only one way of knowing. However, one purpose of reflective practice is to transform and widen one's perspective (Mezirow 1990, Taylor 2010) as well as to appreciate and accommodate alternative perspectives. This makes it unsurprising that numerous definitions exist. I will address additional criticisms that have been levelled at the use of structured reflective models (Coward 2011) later in the chapter.

Using the experience illustrated in the poem in Box 17.1, I would want to explore at least:

- the reason(s) for slide sheets being unavailable in the unit;
- the cost of getting slide sheets;
- why staff are reluctant to use the slide sheets and fill in the risk assessment forms; and
- who would it be necessary to tell to effect a change in practice?

Critical reflection involves reflecting at a deeper level because it focuses on making changes or transforming perspectives (Mezirow 1990). In being reflexive I would be asking myself 'why had I not been my usual assertive self?' and 'what was it that stopped me from completing an adverse incident form?' I might ask myself specific questions such as:

- Did my need to be liked and accepted by the team get in the way of my responsibilities to the patient?
- Could I have exerted a positive influence on those other members of the team who consider form-filling a waste of time?
- Have I learned anything about my own assertiveness in the face of opposition?
- Is there knowledge that would support me to act differently next time I find myself in a similar situation?

This focus on asking questions, on analysis, on evaluation and on possible solutions is central to critical reflection, but more than this, critical reflection also implies an emotional and political awareness that change is needed and what might prevent it from happening. It requires an understanding of power, responsibility, authority and influence. This understanding is important if nurses are to make use of their influence to effect change for the better. A commitment to development then is a commitment to not only acknowledge that one has some influence over the way things are but also to demonstrate leadership in one's role regardless of the level of that role. In other words, a commitment to personal professional development is a commitment to act so as to make a positive difference to practice.

Of course, effecting change is easier said than done. In part this is because we often lack sufficient insight into our own shortcomings (Dunning 2005), and it can be difficult to receive useful and honest feedback about those shortcomings; just as it can be challenging to alert others to their shortcomings. Add to this the unequal power relationship between individual practitioner and institution (hospital system, community provision and so on) then the challenge of effecting change can seem overwhelming.

Activity 17.2

Think of a story from practice that you recently shared with a friend.

- With whom would you share this story?
- What kinds of stories would you not want to share with a consultant? A ward manager? Your mentor? Your personal tutor?
- Why would you tell some people but not others?
- What sort of power relationships might silence your stories?
- Is your reluctance based on fear or anxiety of what might happen to you?
- Is it possible that this fear/anxiety might be more imagined than real?
- To what extent can you realistically influence practice in the area where you work?
- What would stop you trying?
- What would encourage you to give honest feedback to those with whom you work?
- Consider how you might limit your learning by not sharing some stories from practice.

Clare Hopkinson

The literature is further complicated by the various ways in which reflection is categorised. One distinction is between **reflection-in-action** and **reflection-on-action**. In addition, a bewildering array of reflective models can be found (e.g., Boud *et al.* 1985, Bradbury-Jones *et al.* 2009, Gibbs 1988, Johns 2010, Taylor 2010).

Most of the health care literature focuses on reflective practice as a solitary pursuit (Hopkinson 2009) while there is some growing recognition of the value of reflecting in groups through action learning sets (Clarke 2014, Platzer *et al.* 2000, Shaw *et al.* 2012). During my research about whether nurses reflected in a hospital ward while caregiving I saw reflection as three interlinked inquiry processes: that is, first-, second- and third-person inquiry (Hopkinson 2009, 2015, Torbert 2001). Nurses did not connect with these terms so I renamed them respectively: personal reflection (where the nurse reflects on her own); relational reflection (where the nurse reflects as part of a group or in a one-to-one relationship with another person); and organisational reflection (where the nurse contributes to the way the organisation learns and changes its practices as a consequence of reflective activities) – sometimes referred to as organisational learning; an essential part of service improvement (Hopkinson 2015).

Personal reflection

I observe myself and so I come to know others.

Lao-Tze

Personal reflection refers to self-study or self-reflective inquiry (Marshall 1999, 2004). The assumption is that by understanding one's behaviours, communications, intentions, attitudes, values, beliefs, emotions and thoughts this self-awareness enables more effective working relationships and practices. Personal reflection gives the person an opportunity to identify strengths and weaknesses (e.g., contradictions, distortions, defended behaviours, blind spots) as well as values, hopes, intentions, dreams and achievements. It helps in processing emotional aspects of nursing work by removing obstructive negative feelings and by encouraging a reframing to positive feelings thereby facilitating learning (Boud *et al.* 1985). A nurse can imagine how others may be experiencing the event, thereby developing empathy, which can lead to 'checking out' assumptions made about those others or the situation.

Relational reflection

Relational reflection involves other people either in a one-to-one relationship or as part of a group process and can be formal or informal. Torbert (2001) described second-person inquiry as 'speaking-and-listening-with-others' (p. 253) and argued it occurs in dialogue with others where there is 'public testing of our interpretations' (p. 255). Relational reflection often takes place in groups in educational settings such as, an action learning set or a formal clinical supervision process. Process reflection can take place where there is a focus on what happens during a group reflection as well as the content of a story of practice. Relational reflection might take place in, for example, nursing handovers, work-based learning days, multidisciplinary (or nursing) team meetings, over coffee or in everyday conversations. Relational reflection requires the use of appropriate communication skills (see Chapter 14); especially the ability to challenge effectively and supportively while avoiding demonising or blaming specific individuals, so that poor or unsatisfactory practice can be questioned and confronted.

Organisational reflection

Do you continually curtail your effort till there be nothing of it left? . . . By non-action there is nothing which cannot be effected.

Lao-Tze

Organisational reflection takes place at a wider level in an organisation or system, where individual or collaborative efforts of nurses influence or lead to the development of new and effective ways of working. This level of reflection and development can be difficult, but not impossible, to achieve. For example, a change of policy may occur in the workplace as a consequence of the reflection. An example might relate to Julia where she may wear a tabard that signifies she is not to be disturbed during drug administration. Indeed, it may be that the developmental potential of personal and/or relational reflection is restricted unless accompanied by some sense of organisational reflection that leads to change in organisational working. This means reflective practice becomes embedded within the organisation and is not just a deconstruction of practice. For example, this can be achieved through protocols, risk assessments and specific practice developments such as documentation changes.

Reflection-on-action and reflection-in-action

Schön (1983), one of the most influential writers on reflection, suggested practice is messy and complex. He argued the context of practice needs to be explored and understood as a source of knowledge and learning in its own right. He used the term 'theories in use' to describe knowledge situated in practice, which, with Argyris (Argyris and Schön 1978), he found to be different from the theories that practitioners claim to use as a basis for practice (espoused theories).

In the poem in Box 17.1, the use of a slide sheet is the espoused theory, while the 'theory in use' is moving the patient using six people. In other words, we do not always do what we say we do or know we 'should' do. For Schön, practical knowledge arises from what people do and not from what they say they do; and this may be (at least in part) because of the failure of theory to translate into action (i.e., the theory–practice gap, or the need for classroom theory to be adapted before it can be used in practice), or because practice has not been understood sufficiently in its specific context. Schön noted that professionals often find it difficult to articulate their 'theories in use'. It is possible that nurses are drawn to Schön's ideas because of the emphasis on values, the 'difficult to articulate' aspects of nursing work so often devalued by the emphasis on scientific knowledge (Mantzoukas and Jasper 2004).

While difficult to verify, reflection-in-action means nurses in the midst of the action must question whether or not what they are doing is effective and try out alternative actions. This on-the-spot experimentation is something that many nurses claim to do all the time, yet we have all come across nurses who adopt an uncritical and largely uniformed *we-have-always-done-it-this-way* approach to practice. For reflection-in-action

439

to be effective, nurses must know why they are doing what they are doing when they are doing it so that there are fewer habitual practices.

I experienced habitual practice when incontinent following hip replacement surgery. I refused catheterisation whereas the lady opposite in a similar predicament had a catheter *in situ* until her bowels were opened (4 days in her case). She developed a urinary tract infection that delayed her mobilisation programme and her discharge from hospital. When asked about the evidence for the practice of waiting for a bowel movement before catheter removal, the response from the nurses was: 'we do it this way because sister insists upon it'. This story illustrates a singular failure to develop practice precisely because of a reluctance to engage with reflection at either the personal or relational level. It also highlights the power one individual can exert on inhibiting professional development and service improvement among a group of staff.

Activity 17.3

Write a description of your next placement at the end of your first day there. Try to include as much specific detail as possible. The following questions might help in this task.

- What did it look like?
- What did it smell like?
- What kinds of noises did you become aware of?
- How were you welcomed?
- What were you feeling like?
- What nursing did you carry out?
- How well would you judge your nursing ability?
- What helped or hindered your learning that day?
- How do you feel about it now you are looking back on that day?
- How might that day set the tone for your learning experience?

The detail you note on the first day in placement will not be so easy to identify subsequently. If you repeat this exercise a month later you will find it difficult to give such a detailed account. This is because many things you notice now will become routine and taken-for-granted. This means that you will have become part of the culture of that practice environment and consequently will find it harder to identify the need for change and development.

Models of reflection

There are a growing number of models and frameworks for developing reflective skills. Their purpose is to aid the critical reflection on experience and practice and identification of learning needs. Some include a series of prompt questions (e.g., Cook 1999, Driscoll 1994, Gibbs 1988, Holm and Stephenson 1994, Johns 2010). Nurses who find reflecting difficult may find these models helpful. Other models provide a less structured framework for analysing and re-evaluating experiences and when using these nurses can generate their own practice questions (e.g., Atkins and Murphy 1993, Boud *et al.* 1985, Bradbury-Jones *et al.* 2009, Goodman 1984, Kim 1999, Taylor 2010). In addition, there are several models derived from research studies (e.g., Bradbury-Jones *et al.* 2009, Johns 2010, Kim 1999, Taylor 2010). Latterly there has been some criticism about the restrictive nature of models of reflection. Indeed Schön's (1983) work did not suggest a structured approach to reflecting since he was opposed to the technical rationality that constricted creative thinking during practice. Coward (2011) has argued that compulsory and overuse of models for student assessment in nurse education has restricted critical thinking as well as learning from practice and created reflection fatigue. Along the same lines, I find the exposure that comes with reflective writing often results in students reflecting on 'safe' situations or on situations that confirm practice outcomes rather than indicate a need for changes in practice. A brief overview of some models of reflection is given below; however you should note that there are many other models available.

Boud, Keogh and Walker (1985)

Boud, Keogh and Walker's approach is more of a process than a model. This can be a bit daunting for a novice reflector, as it requires a self-generated set of questions and making links between existing and new knowledge. It is designed to enable reflection on new experiences in a cyclical manner and to enable a reframing of negative feelings, although this may be difficult without the help of a critical friend. The process is staged under the following headings.

1 *Experience*:
   - behaviour, ideas and feelings.
2 *The reflective process*:
   - returning to the experience;
   - utilising positive feelings and attitudes;
   - removing negative feelings by reframing and processing them;
   - re-evaluating the experience.
3 *Outcomes/actions*:
   - new understandings and appreciations;
   - new knowledge and perspectives;
   - change in behaviour, attitudes or skills;
   - readiness to put knowledge into practice.

Gibbs (1988)

The simple cyclical structure of Gibbs' model makes it easy to use and popular among nurses, indeed it is the model Julia has previously used for assignment purposes. It is useful because it emphasises the link between reflection and action (and this can assist in setting a personal development plan). However, it neither encourages consideration of other people in (or affected by) the event nor does it require examination of motives, values, knowledge, or congruence between thoughts and actions. While action-based and thus relevant for professional development it may not encourage deeper reflection of self and thus may be limited in terms of personal development (see Figure 17.1).

441

Clare Hopkinson

FIGURE 17.1
Gibbs' reflective
model (1988)

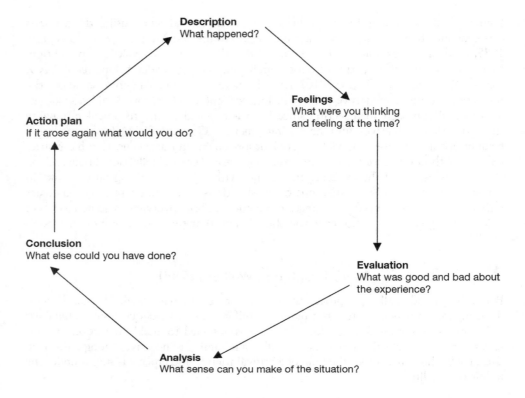

Johns – 'Fifteen A' – (2010)

Since 1990 Johns has frequently updated his reflective model, which was developed through his research study. Some of his earlier versions (e.g., 1995) include Carper's (1978) ways of knowing (aesthetic, personal, ethical and empirical knowing) and add a further section he called reflexivity. This made the model's structure more complex for students. His latest model removes these sections and offers a level of detail that arguably is helpful for those who struggle with reflection. However, in my experience students find the model repetitive and as Coward (2011) argues this model is often perceived as interrogating and complex. It makes direct links between past experiences and values on the one hand and experience on the other. It attempts to develop empathy by asking nurses about the consequences of their actions as well as the feelings of other people associated with the event; which, unless the nurse has asked those others how they feel, can only ever be a best guess assumption. As the point of critical reflection is to move away from assumptions this seems somewhat contradictory. However, the nurse is asked to consider the knowledge base (or ways of knowing) utilised in the event and to identify any gaps in knowledge. It is for these reasons that Tariq has asked Julia to use this model to structure her reflection on the drug administration error.

Johns first asks the nurse 'to bring the mind home'. By this he means become grounded or set aside thoughts of the past or future in order to focus fully on the present. Clearly, this is difficult to do as the past influences the present. However, by focusing on your body and clearing your mind of the chattering thoughts that are often present it is possible to become more attentive and contemplative. Johns' model asks the nurse to describe a significant experience and answer a set of reflective cue questions. His final question asks about insights into the self-realisation of the nurse. Self-realisation is a psychology term and means fulfilling one's potential. In other words it means a self that is honest and true without distortions and delusions and is an ideal to strive towards.

1   Bring the mind home.
2   Write a description of an experience that seems significant in some way.
3   What issues seem significant to pay attention to?
4   How were others feeling and what made them feel that way?
5   How was I feeling and what made me feel that way?
6   What was I trying to achieve and did I respond effectively?
8   What were the consequences of my actions on the patient, others and myself?
9   What factors influence the way I was feeling, thinking or responding?
10 What knowledge did or should have informed me?
11 To what extent did I act for the best and in tune with my beliefs?
12 How does this experience connect with previous experiences?
13 How might I reframe the situation and respond more effectively given this situation again?
14 What would be the consequences of alternative actions for the patient, others, and myself
15 What factors might constrain me from responding differently?
16 How do I NOW feel about this experience?
17 Am I now more able to support myself and others as a consequence?
18 What insights do I draw towards self-realisation?

Holm and Stephenson (1994)

This model was developed by two students who claimed it could be used to structure or act as a checklist for many written assignments. Not all questions will be appropriate in every situation and they suggest it may be helpful to repeat some of the questions at different points during your reflection.
After describing the event ask yourself:

1   What was my role in the situation?
2   Did I feel comfortable or uncomfortable? Why?
3   What actions did I take?
4   Was it appropriate?
5   How could I have improved the situation for myself, the patient, my mentor?
6   What can I change in future?
7   Do I feel as if I have learnt anything new about myself?
8   Did I expect anything different to happen? What and why?
9   Has it changed my way of thinking in any way?
10 What knowledge from theory and research can I apply to this situation?
11 What broader issues, for example, ethical, political, social, arise from this situation?
12 What do I think about these broader issues?

Rolfe, Jasper and Freshwater (2011) and Driscoll (1994)

Both Rolfe *et al.* (2011) and Driscoll (1994) used Borton's 1970 simplistic learning cycle that asks three questions: *What?*, *So what?*, and *Now what?* Driscoll has subsequent questions under each heading. A description of the situation is given, followed by an analysis of that situation, followed by recommendations and conclusions drawn from the analysis for improving future practice. In this way the nurse focuses on developing new knowledge from the experience. This easy to remember framework can also be used for structuring essays.

Taylor (2010)

Taylor based her model on the work of the German philosopher Jürgen Habermas. She identified three types of reflection (technical, practical and emancipatory), each of equal importance. She suggested the nurse could choose the type of reflection based on the nature of the situation and the type of change envisioned.

Technical reflection focuses on the nature and effects of work practices and how they may be changed through technical reflection. It examines empirical knowledge, that is, knowledge obtained from the senses, scientific knowledge and evidence-based practice. This type of reflection allows for prediction when subsequently meeting a similar experience.

Practical reflection relates to the communicative aspects of nursing work and to interpersonal relationships. It is based on personal experience, being subjective and examining the inner self. Practical reflection also examines intersubjectivity, that is, how the nurse relates to others in the social world or her dialogue with others.

Emancipatory reflection requires a more critical view of practice and is linked to transformative action. It involves freedom, choice and empowerment. It challenges power, political aspects of care, and inhibiting cultural and social effects. The nurse is required to be influential and to raise awareness of issues that are often taken-for-granted practices or assumptions.

Bradbury-Jones, Hughes, Murphy, Parry and Sutton (2009)

Rather than focus on one incident Bradbury-Jones *et al.* (2009) developed a different reflective writing approach based on subjective thoughts and feelings, which they have termed the Peshkin Approach. Peshkin (1988) cited in Bradbury-Jones *et al.* (2009) analysed his own subjectivity in his diary writing during his research. Bradbury-Jones *et al.* suggest three prompts for diary entries:

1   Today I have been feeling . . .
2   Today I have been thinking . . .
3   The consequences of thinking and feeling are . . .

Subsequently, diary entries are re-read and analysed to create themes that become the nurse's subjective 'I's; for example, the Angry 'I', the Assertive 'I' and so on. They claim sharing the subjective 'I's in group discussion influences self-awareness and learning in clinical practice.

The benefits of reflective practice

Reflective practice enables nurses to evaluate what they do and the effect they have on other people (patients, relatives, other staff and so on). Reflective practice helps to explore the complexities of practice and practice contexts. It offers a route to critical examination of effective as well as poor, habitual and routine practice (Kim 1999): it is not merely about dramatic events or critical incidents. It offers scope for exploring emotional and ethical dilemmas faced by nurses and a way of encouraging professional and personal development in support of therapeutic relationships with patients, their family and loved

RESEARCH FOCUS 17.1

Mann *et al.* (2009) conducted an extensive literature review and identified more than 600 papers, commentaries and reviews in the literature. Only 29 of those were empirical research studies with the largest percentage of papers from the United Kingdom (25 per cent) and the majority of studies used qualitative approaches. They found no conclusive evidence to prove that reflective practice improves patient care. In addition, they found that not all health care professionals engage and that reflection does not occur in all situations. In fact, they suggest that reflection appeared to decrease both with increasing years in practice and in settings where reflection was not reinforced through mentoring or supervision. However, reflective practice helps in complex situations for meaning-making and extrapolating learning and there are many papers about reflective practice that support its value (e.g., Atkins and Murphy 1993, Clarke 2014, Cook 1999, Freshwater, 2004, Horton-Deutsch and Sherwood 2008, Platzer *et al.* 2000, Rich and Parker 1995). Some qualitative studies have made use of journals and interviews (e.g., Duke and Appleton 2000, Durgahee 1996, Glaze 2001, 2002, Hallet 1997, Smith 1998, Teekman 2000, Wong *et al.* 1995). Teekman (2000) identified three levels of reflection: reflective thinking-for-action (what to do in the here and now); thinking-for-evaluation (integrating different multiple viewpoints) and thinking-for-critical-inquiry (considerations of contexts), which was not demonstrated by any of the participants. Two studies examined perceptions of reflective practice, one by adopting a qualitative design (Burnard 1995), and the other a small sample size quantitative questionnaire approach (Cadman *et al.* 2003).

Even fewer research studies have been carried out in a clinical setting (Hopkinson 2009, Mantzoukas and Jasper 2004, Powell 1989). What remains under-explored is what enables or inhibits interaction with reflection as a learning process. Powell (1989) used a non-participant observation strategy in a small-scale study to inquire into the complex concept of reflection-in-action. Mantzoukas and Jasper (2004) used an interpretive ethnographic approach with unstructured observation, semi-structured interviews and content analysis on written structured reflective writing to examine organisational culture and reflective practices. They found reflection was belittled in the ward setting and that the hierarchical structures and power struggles between the different staff inhibited reflective processes. Where nurses were able to reflect, they did so in their personal time.

There are a growing number of studies using retrospective reflection away from the bedside (e.g., Bradbury-Jones *et al.* 2009, Clarke 2014, Glaze 2001, 2002, Gustafsson and Fagerberg 2004, Johns 1997, Kim 1999). Focusing entirely on personal reflection, Johns (1997, 2000) used a qualitative design to interview practitioners following the introduction of clinical supervision in a primary care nursing unit. He suggests that practitioners could become reflective practitioners by being more available to patients, responding to the person, and knowing and managing the self within caring relationships.

445

ones (Hopkinson 2015). Horton-Deutsch and Sherwood (2008) claim that in developing the skills of reflection nurses can develop as emotionally competent nurse leaders. Reflective practice encourages articulation of the knowledge gained in and from practice as well as of the theoretical knowledge that supports practice. It emphasises the process of learning, not just an outcome to be translated into nursing action. It generates a questioning approach to practice that helps to prevent nurses from becoming complacent about their work.

When Tariq reads Julia's reflection he is not surprised by what he reads. In her writing she provides a full description of the events leading up to the error in drug administration and this part of her reflection is comprehensive. However, the remainder of Julia's reflection is brief and non-committal. She is vague about what she was trying to achieve, why she responded in the way she did, and the consequences for the patient, herself and others. She mentions that she feels 'a bit guilty' but says nothing about her internal state at the time; she is particularly vague about the relationship between her actions and her beliefs and about the knowledge she might have used to inform what she did, although she does mention the NMC *Standards for Medicine Management*. She writes nothing about how this incident relates to previous experience and suggests how she might do things better next time only in abstract terms.

Tariq tries not to show his disappointment as he asks Julia how she went about writing the reflection and if she found the exercise useful. Julia eventually confesses to spending very little time on it and admits that her responses to the cue questions are perfunctory at best. During the discussion with Tariq she does begin to demonstrate greater insight into the issues raised by the error and reluctantly acknowledges that she has learned something about herself in the process. She agrees to revise her reflection in the light of their discussion and to try to give more thoughtful responses to the cue questions. They agree to meet again in a couple of days to review her revised reflective account.

PART 3: EXPLORING PERSONAL AND PROFESSIONAL DEVELOPMENT THROUGH REFLECTIVE PRACTICE

Development is underpinned by knowledge: before you can know what needs to change it is necessary to know how things are. Whether or not there is such a discrete thing as nursing knowledge is the subject of a vigorous debate that will not be discussed here. However, because reflection (as a means to development) requires coming to know something that was previously unknown or at least unacknowledged it cannot be ignored altogether. Many nurses subscribe to the idea that practical knowledge differs from theoretical knowledge, or as Polanyi (1967) describes it: 'knowing how' and 'knowing that' respectively. Reflective practice can be seen as an attempt to bring these two forms of knowledge together so that a nurse may learn in and from practice in the pursuit of development. In this sense, practice can generate knowledge as much as, if not more than, knowledge can inform practice. Some understand this relationship as helping to minimise the so-called 'theory–practice gap' (e.g., Atkins and Murphy 1993, Durgahee 1996, Hallett 1997, Rolfe *et al.* 2011).

The important point here about this distinction between practical knowledge ('know how'/tacit knowledge) on the one hand and theoretical knowledge ('know that'/propositional knowledge) on the other is that while the latter is relatively easy to articulate, the former is not. Propositional knowledge is the kind of knowledge you use

446

when you answer an examination question about, for example, how to catheterise a patient. Tacit knowledge is the type of knowledge demonstrated when you successfully perform a catheterisation.

When composing her reflection on the drug administration error Julia found it easy to write a description of events because it was based on 'know that' type of knowledge. However, she struggled to respond to the cue questions in Johns' model and this can be explained in part by the idea that she needed to draw upon different forms of knowledge. She had always assumed knowledge to be uncontroversial; at school she always turned up for lessons and now at university she attends all scheduled classes, pays attention and does her best to learn and use that learning in her assignments. She does work hard on her assignments but often struggles to know what is required and rarely gets marks above 50 per cent. The idea that there may be different forms of knowledge is new to her and she has agreed to read something about different ways of knowing before revising her reflective piece about the drug administration error. She is not really looking forward to this because she thinks it is going to be difficult.

What knowledge informs nursing practice?

Real knowledge is to know the extent of one's ignorance.

Confucius

Activity 17.4

Spend 10 minutes writing an account of what you do on a typical day working as a nurse. Imagine you are writing this for a friend who knows nothing about nursing. When you have finished writing, think about the following questions:

- Does what you have written capture the essence of nursing?
- From reading what you have written, would your friend have a clear grasp of what being a nurse involves?

If you have done Activity 17.4, then you will have been doing some reflection, but the main purpose of the exercise is to illustrate how difficult it is to articulate the nature of nursing. Like Julia's description of events, the chances are that your description of a typical working day focuses on particular tasks (e.g., washing patients, giving out medications, doing the observations, and so on) because these things are relatively easy to describe: they also tend to fall into the category of 'knowing that'. The other parts of nursing (e.g., the caring, the responding to human suffering, the allaying of fears, the explaining of what is going on) are much more difficult to write down and yet for most nurses, these 'difficult to articulate' things are what make nursing the special occupation that it is. Reflection is one way in which the knowledge that underpins these difficult to articulate aspects of nursing can be expressed.

The implication here should be clear. A large part of what nurses do remains obscure because the emphasis on easily describable knowledge focuses attention on tasks, client group, or speciality: hence the standard categorisations of, for example, mental health

447

Clare Hopkinson

nursing, care of the older person, emergency care and so on. Nursing is more than this: it is a complex social practice requiring a wide and varied knowledge base to support the choices made in caring for the well-being of others. Two different approaches to ways of knowing are explored briefly below.

Ways of knowing 1 (women's ways of knowing)

Silence

The first perspective identified by Belenky and colleagues is silence. The silent women, while few in number in the study, were among the youngest and most socially, economically and educationally deprived. They had no voice and saw words as weapons to be used against them. The silent women described themselves as 'deaf and dumb' in terms of their abilities and found it almost impossible to describe any aspects of themselves as individuals. They used the word dumb to reflect both their feelings of stupidity and their lack of conversation with others. They saw themselves as passive in relation to powerful external authority figures. These women had little sense of their own worth and became uncomfortable when asked to reflect on anything they did. Silent women will only begin to reflect when encouraged within a highly supportive environment because reflection will unlock their silence and attention is drawn to them.

Received knowledge: listening to the voices of others

She never did and never could put words together, out of her own head.

George Eliot, *Middlemarch*

RESEARCH FOCUS 17.2

Belenky *et al.* (1986) researched women in higher education and were interested in their development. In their work they described five different perspectives they called 'women's ways of knowing' and they claim that the self-concepts of women are interwoven with their ways of knowing. They further suggest women struggle to claim the power of their minds because of the stereotypical view of women as emotional and intuitive as opposed to the purported logic and rationality of men. Belenky *et al.* argue that while gender-related, the five identified characteristics (silence, received knowledge, subjective knowledge, procedural knowledge and constructed knowledge) are not gender-specific and may be found in some men. They claim that, unlike male-dominated ways of knowing, women's ways of knowing do not exist as a hierarchy; it is possible to move in and out of these positions depending on the context the women found themselves in.

Belenky and colleagues (1986) identified five characteristics (silence, received knowledge, subjective knowledge, procedural knowledge and constructed knowledge) that they claim typify women's ways of knowing. They suggest these ways of knowing are not hierarchical, which may be important as it leaves the way clear for nurses to draw upon whichever knowledge base best fits a particular practice situation. These different ways of knowing link directly to the reflective process and suggest reasons why some nurses favour a structured rather than a free-form expressive approach to reflection. Additionally, it may be that different levels of structured reflective models are appropriate for different types of experiences.

448

The women in this category learned by listening to others and perceived listening as a way of knowing. They polarised ideas as right or wrong, true or false, good or bad, black or white and so on. They assumed only one answer was correct for a given question and consequently saw alternative answers as just plain wrong. Belenky and colleagues note:

> [W]hile received knowers can be very open to take in what others have to offer they have little confidence in their own ability to speak. Believing the truth comes from others, they still their own voices to hear the voices of others.
>
> (1986, p. 37)

Received knowers have little confidence in their ability to speak out; they tend to perceive authority figures as the source of knowledge. Learning tends to be understood as the regurgitation of facts and they struggle with the idea of being original because they have not learned to trust or value their own opinions; as a result they find course-work challenging when it requires independent creative thought. Belenky and colleagues suggest this type of learner may be successful in courses 'that do not demand a reflective relativistic stance' (1986, p. 42). Received knowers tend to consider the judgements, ideas and opinions of others as more important than their own. They often channel increasing awareness of self into empowering and caring for others through listening and responding, which in certain circumstances may lead to a devaluing of their own judgements, ideas and opinions. While reluctant reflectors, structured models of reflection may assist received knowers to begin at the descriptive level of reflection. Given the appropriate form of encouragement (role models who will encourage the received knower to value their own judgements, ideas and opinions) the received knower may begin to listen to their own inner voice.

Subjective knowledge: the inner voice and the quest for self

Women in this category saw truth and knowledge as subjective, intuitive, personal and private. They relied on gut instinct and refused to accept answers from other people. They tended to mistrust learning from books but valued learning from direct experience or personal involvement, and from their feelings or senses. They preferred to work things out for themselves and because they did not possess a solid sense of self found it difficult to talk about themselves or to ask for help. Nevertheless, they retained a basic commitment and responsiveness to others' needs. Belenky *et al.* suggest this growing reliance on intuitive processes is an important step in the process of women becoming assertive, self-protecting and self-determining; and thus moving towards reflective and critical thought. However, the subjective knower is reticent about sharing personal thoughts in public although they may share them with friends. This makes them reluctant reflectors (despite valuing experience) although structured reflective models may help them to connect with both their own feelings and the feelings of others. Imagining how others might be experiencing a situation can assist subjective knowers to develop reflective skills, which can result in recognising the value of alternative sources of knowledge from which to base decisions and actions (Bolton 2005). This can help the subjective knower to move beyond entrenched positions common among this group.

Procedural knowledge: separate and connected knowing

Men develop their sense of morality from a separateness that emphasises objectivity, evaluation and justice, while women's moral sensitivity arises from a connected, relational

449

Clare Hopkinson

and caring ethic (Belenky *et al.* 1986). Women operating from procedural knowledge invest in learning, which can be either separate, in the sense of being apart from others, or connected (with others). The connected knowing values relations with others, caring, empathy, subjectivity, acceptance and appreciation of others' points of view.

Connected knowers value reflection and find identifying the affective (feeling) component of experience easier than recognising the underpinning knowledge. Hence a structured reflective model could encourage them to identify the gaps in their knowledge base and thus a deeper level of reflection. Connected knowers tend to value conversations with critical friends (Taylor 2010) who will challenge and support their reflections. They may be willing to keep a diary or learning journal.

Separate knowers have difficulty with the ideology of reflection because it challenges the objectivity of separateness. Nurses operating from this perspective prefer a structured reflective model although they tend to have difficulty identifying their feelings and would tend to write themselves out of events. They prefer to focus their analysis on others' experiences because this allows them to be more objective. However, a comprehensive reflective model that encourages consideration of self as well as others, such as Johns' (2010) model, could help separate knowers to move towards deeper reflection.

Constructed knowledge: integrating the voices

Belenky and colleagues describe constructed knowers as articulate and reflective individuals aware of their own thoughts, judgements, desires and moods. They draw knowledge from reason, intuition and others' expertise. They view knowledge as contextual and they notice and care about the lives of other people. They want to make a difference through their actions and are committed to action. Constructed knowers are critical reflectors and probably do not need the security of structured models of reflection as they have an embodied reflexivity that allows them to ask appropriate and probing questions of their practice.

Activity 17.5

Review the five characteristic ways of women's knowing offered by Belenky *et al.* and consider the following questions:

* Do you recognise in yourself one of these ways of knowing?
* Can you identify each of these ways of knowing among others with whom you work in practice?
* If you and your mentor have different ways of knowing, how might this impact on your development as a nurse?

Ways of knowing 2 (Carper 1978)

Carper's (1978) claim of four fundamental patterns of knowing (empirical, aesthetic, ethical and personal) has been influential in nursing. For Carper, each pattern of knowing is of equal value and each has a contribution to make to practice, dependent on the particularities of a given set of circumstances. Carper's work forms the basis for Johns' reflective model (1995).

450

Empirical knowing is gained from the senses and is based on observation, systematic investigation and testing. It can be regarded as the science of nursing; an example would be evidence-based practice. This knowledge is embedded in the positivist or quantitative paradigm.

Aesthetic knowing refers to the action of nursing as it involves perception, understanding and empathy. It is described as the art of nursing in which the value of everyday experience is acknowledged. It is associated with the interpretive, qualitative paradigm and phenomenology. Berragan (1998) links aesthetics to intuitive actions.

Ethical knowing relates to moral issues and value judgements, and enables nurses to engage with difficult philosophical questions about good in relation to health and nursing practice.

Personal knowing recognises that each nurse brings a unique contribution to practice precisely because of a personal history of experience and emotional responses to situations. Carper describes personal knowing as knowing oneself. Personal knowing is a central concept for reflective practice.

Having read this short review of some different ways of knowing you might be getting a sense of where Julia might be located against these different categories. It may not come as a surprise to you to find that Julia is part subjective knower and part separate knower. If you return to these sections you will see that subjective knowers find it difficult to talk about themselves or to ask for help but retain a basic commitment and responsiveness to others' needs and are reticent about sharing personal thoughts in public. Separate knowers tend to have difficulty identifying their feelings and tend to write themselves out of an event. If we were able to point these things out to Julia we can be pretty sure that she would recognise herself in this depiction. It certainly fits with Tariq's impression of Julia and this explains why he was so keen for her to use Johns' model of reflection.

Activity 17.6

Re-read your written account of your typical working day (Activity 17.4).

Try to add some more detail to your description of what it is you do every day, paying particular attention to those 'difficult to articulate' aspects of everyday nursing.

- Make a list of the different types of knowledge needed to complete all the things you describe as the work of nurses.
- Add some brief notes against each type of knowledge you identify explaining where (and when) you obtained that particular type of knowledge (i.e., where and when did you learn to do that particular activity).

Hopefully, this activity has helped you to realise that nursing practice draws on a wide and varied knowledge base. This recognition is important for effective personal and professional development. As suggested earlier, in order to know what needs to be improved (or developed) it is necessary to know what is already known; and this applies to all the different types of knowing that contribute to the knowledge base of nursing. Reflection thus contributes to development by enabling nurses to acknowledge their existing knowledge base and to identify what further knowledge they need in order to be effective in the role of registered nurse.

Of course, knowledge (or more precisely, what is known) changes over time. So nurses will need to review and add to their knowledge if their practice is to remain informed by what is currently known. However, this is complicated by three related factors: (i) what is currently known is often contested; (ii) some types of knowledge receive greater legitimacy than others; and (iii) the type of knowledge valued in the university is not always the same as that valued by practice-based staff.

In order to become a registered nurse, it is necessary to learn both in a practical and an academic setting, integrating rather than separating and then applying all forms of knowledge. As a registered nurse you will need some way of working out which type of knowledge provides the best guide for action in any specific situation. Reflection is one means of achieving this.

Inevitably conflicts of ideas, contradictions and tensions will arise between practitioners who value different aspects of nursing knowledge. This could be seen as an opportunity for development as practitioners engage in critical discussion (in the form of relational reflection) of 'the what' and 'the how' of best practice. Unfortunately, many nurses seem locked into polarised views of practice in which simplistic right or wrong assumptions abound. Reflection as an ongoing process of continuing professional development can assist in more subtle and nuanced thinking about nursing work and I believe this can ultimately benefit patient care.

Activity 17.7

Spend 10 minutes writing about a significant event in your life. Try not to take your hand off the page. Don't worry about sentence construction, punctuation or paragraphs, just let the words flow.

- What did the exercise feel like?
- Is there anything that surprises you as you read over what you have written?

Keeping a reflective diary

How can I know what I think till I see what I say?

E. M. Forster

It is possible to achieve a deeper understanding of ourselves through writing regularly and reflective models are one way of achieving this. Written reflection is a common theme in the literature as a way of reflecting-on-action but it is strewn with confusing language. There are learning logs, journals, portfolios, structured accounts, reflective models, reflective reviews and personal diaries. Some reflective writing is public (e.g., a portfolio for an assignment) while other writing is private (e.g., a diary). Through writing, nurses can be encouraged to reflect on critical incidents from practice (I prefer the term 'stories of experience'). These stories are usually prompted by some emotional or ethical discomfort (Bolton 2005, Ghaye and Lillyman 2006, Glaze 2002, Johns 2010, Moon 2004, Taylor 2010). Stories can focus on positive or negative experiences and allow you the chance to view events from a distance, considering:

- what happened, paying attention to the context and detail of the story;
- what you did and why you did it;
- what you felt about the experience and how this may connect with past experiences;
- what you have learned about yourself, others, your practice;
- what were the gaps in your knowledge, attitudes and skills;
- what could be done differently;
- how your practice has changed now you have read about or considered a different way of working.

The stories help you to identify areas of knowledge and skills for development and help you to explore the context in which you practise. And as the previous discussion on models identified, there are many questions that you can ask yourself to develop your learning. This can form part of your informal diary writing or more formal writing for a public portfolio document. As you get more practised at writing and move through the different ways of knowing you will develop your own ability to ask questions in order to develop your practice insight.

However, writing does not come easily to everyone and some individuals may need regular practice if patterns are to emerge or if deeper learning from experience is to take place. When you first start, it can be useful to share your writing with others: a tutor or a friend, perhaps, who can help you to question your practice. Depending on your preferred way of knowing you may find it more or less challenging. Do not be put off writing just because it is difficult. Try experimenting with different ways of writing, either with different models or just putting your thoughts down in no particular order, just as they come (free-fall writing) and your ability to analyse your experiences will begin to develop. Getting in the habit of writing regularly may also help in your coursework.

My preference is to use an A5-size notebook and write two or three times each week. Like many people, I find it easier to write about negative (rather than positive) experiences. However, this tends to remind me of my weaknesses rather than my strengths and this can undermine my self-esteem. Sometimes I go weeks without writing; other times I write in short bursts of 10 minutes most days.

Writing two or three times a week allows me to process the emotional component of work and re-reading old diaries provides me with insights into my patterns of thinking and behaviour, allowing me to make changes. Several of my diary entries involve pre-planning and these sometimes become 'to do' lists (these help me to clarify my need to act). I have evolved my own method of keeping a diary, which often is just free-fall writing. When I do structure my writing I tend to use the following:

- *I notice*: this tells the story of what happened.
- *I feel*: this notices how I felt and how I feel after writing.
- *I imagine*: this involves me thinking about others involved in my experience. If I am critical of others what is this saying about myself? What might be some of the consequences of this for myself and others?
- *I want*: this often turns into a 'to do' list of actions as it is not always easy to decide what I want. Sometimes I decide what I do not want first!

RESEARCH FOCUS 17.3

Several research studies have analysed nurses' use of diaries/journals during programmes of learning (Richardson and Maltby 1995, Wong et al. 1995) and some have analysed assignments (Duke and Appleton 2000, Jasper 1999, Maclellan 2004, Mountford and Rogers 1996, Watson 2002). As Taylor (2010) notes, few nurses sustain diaries/journals beyond the end of a course and she suggests there is relatively little guidance on how to do reflection in a practical and sustained way. Even portfolios may not be the key factor in promoting reflective learning instead the mentoring or supervision relationship may be more effective (Mann et al. 2009, Gustafsson and Fagerberg 2004, Teekman 2000).

However, Jasper (1999), Smith (1998) and Durgahee (1996) found nurses valued learning about themselves through writing diaries/journals and found emotions from work were released through the process of writing. Nevertheless, Jasper (1999) noted the voyage of self-discovery can be threatening, dangerous and even risky. She advocates developing techniques for 'damage limitation' by, for example, keeping a balance between a focus on strengths and achievements on the one hand and a focus on weaknesses on the other.

- *What have I learned or achieved?*: even if the experience has been difficult this helps to reframe it and allows me to let go of the emotional component.

Keeping a personal diary for professional development raises questions such as:

- For whose benefit am I reflecting?
- If I know others will read my reflections will this have an effect on what I write?
- If I am expected to show my reflections as part of my portfolio, how do I know what is safe to show and what I should keep personal?

Guidelines for starting a reflective diary

Keeping a diary can be time-consuming and I have found it to be a creative and valuable process. You should choose a format that works for you and something that can be carried around easily will allow you to make entries wherever and whenever the need arises. You may find the following considerations helpful.

1. Try a loose-leaf folder (A4). Some people prefer keeping an A5 note book, others prefer to make entries directly onto a computer through an e-portfolio or blog.
2. Writing on one side of the paper or half of the page allows you space to add to your reflections later on (using a second colour for later additions can be useful).
3. Try using different models of reflection until you find your preferred structure. You might find it useful to see what happens when you explore the same incident using different models.
4. Try to write soon after an incident and try not to censor the experiences or forget important contextual information.
5. Let your thoughts flow – do not worry about punctuation, spelling, etc. Doodles and dreams can also be a useful key to your subconscious thoughts.

6. Keep a balance between negative and positive experiences. Writing about successful incidents can help you acknowledge your strengths, develop your self-awareness and unravel your tacit knowledge.
7. Once you get into the habit of reflective writing have a go at free-fall writing – this can be particularly helpful in developing self-awareness and understanding your responses to events.
8. Try to write at least two or three times a week. You may find this requires a bit of effort at first but you should soon find some value in the exercise. Just set aside 10 minutes and see what happens.
9. Experiment with other forms of reflection such as doodling, pictures, painting, or poetry.
10. After you have read an article or book, try jotting down your thoughts about these readings and their impact on your practice.
11. Think of your diary as a friend (rather than an enemy) and make it work for you, not anybody else!
12. Think about converting some of your informal writings into formal portfolio entries.
13. Usually one or two key experiences per placement will build enough evidence for your portfolio but be guided by your place of study.

(Adapted from Bolton 2005 and Boud et al. 1985)

Julia has now spent quite a lot of time trying to write longer and more thoughtful responses to the cue questions in her reflection on the drug incident. Re-reading her work Julia is surprised by what she has begun to reveal about herself. She is fascinated, because she has never really thought about how her behaviour affects other people. Now that she has this insight she is keen to discover more about herself so that she can modify her own behaviour to reduce any negative impact she may have on other people, be they patients, relatives, or other staff. She might benefit from using the Johari window as a way of learning more about herself.

Guidelines for maintaining a reflective portfolio

All nurses, midwives and health visitors on the professional register are required to keep and maintain a profile or portfolio to maintain their registration. A portfolio is a vehicle for encouraging personal and professional development and your portfolio can provide evidence of your learning, which may or may not be related to specific learning outcomes (Timms and Duffy 2011). What you keep in your portfolio really is up to you but as a rule of thumb it might usefully contain your curriculum vitae (CV), evidence of qualifications, evidence of specific study and training and how this applies to your job, and a public section on your learning and reflections. Use dividers for different sections.

Portfolio evidence can be anything that demonstrates your learning and development and might include, for example:

- verification of achievement of specific competencies;
- your job description;
- learning contracts;
- stories from your practice;
- reflective accounts of events;
- learning from your days in college;
- evidence of how your own behaviour has changed during a course;

Clare Hopkinson

- the impact of reading and learning about new subjects and how this has changed your practice;
- accounts of what you have learned from visiting specific agencies or departments;
- summaries of your learning from each placement or job.

This list is neither exhaustive nor definitive. The main thing to remember is that the portfolio captures your development and should be useful for you. Of course, it will be up to you to decide if there are entries that you do not wish to make public and you might keep these in a separate removable section especially if attending interviews where you might be asked to show your portfolio.

Understanding self through using the Johari window

One way of starting a diary is to begin by using a tool such as the Johari window, named after the first names of its inventors (Jo Luft and Harry Ingram). This model helps to describe the process of human interaction and has been used as a way of developing self-understanding. The four-panelled 'window' divides the self into four quadrants: the open, blind, hidden and unknown areas. Luft (1955) argued it is possible to learn about yourself either as you disclose more of yourself to others or as you receive feedback about yourself from others (Table 17.1).

The open area is that part known to ourselves and to others. It contains the information we share with others and is not private.

The blind area is the part of ourselves known to others but not ourselves. It contains our blind spots that we can only become aware of when others tell us.

The hidden area is the part that holds our private information. We know what is in here but generally keep it hidden; although we may allow selected others access to some parts of it.

The unknown area is the part that holds information unknown to ourselves or others. It relates to unconscious processes and can be revealed in dreams, art, writing or, in my case, through writing poetry.

TABLE 17.1 The Johari window

	Known to self	*Not known to self*
Known to others	Open area	Blind area
Not known to others	Hidden area	Unknown area

Source: Luft 1955.

Activity 17.8

Divide a large sheet of paper into four quadrants. Number them as: 1 the open area; 2 the blind area; 3 the hidden area; 4 the unknown area. Make notes in each quadrant using the following guidance.

1   *The open area:*
- Things about myself that I have no difficulty telling others.
- Things about myself that I have some difficulty telling others.

2   *The blind area:*
  •   How do the following people see you?
      −   your best friend;
      −   one of your patients/clients;
      −   a specific person who dislikes you;
      −   a colleague on your course;
      −   someone you have worked with recently.
3   *The hidden area:*
  •   Write some notes about the sorts of things about yourself that you would not disclose to others.
4   *The unknown area:*
  •   This is obviously a difficult part of yourself to write about but try to 'switch off' your logical thinking brain and consider what you are really like underneath the layers of self you present to both yourself and others.
  •   What might you find surprising?
  •   What would surprise others?
  •   Try keeping a dream diary for a week and see if this tells you anything about what is going on in your life at present.

When you have finished each section, reflect on what you have written and consider:

  •   What would happen if you allowed more people to know more about you?
  •   How could you find out more about what others think about you?
  •   What surprises did you find by doing this exercise?
  •   To what extent do you self-disclose to others?

Creativity and models of reflection

As noted earlier, some authors suggest that models of reflection can stifle critical thinking and thus creativity. Arguably one of the difficulties of using reflective models is that they divorce practice from the real context of care and produce formulaic responses. Thus it is possible for reflection to become ritualistic. This would be a shame, because one of the purposes of reflection is to enable a move away from the ritual and routinisation of nursing practice. It is also possible that a nurse may forget what else was happening at the time of the experience and depending on her level of self-esteem, either use the process to berate herself for her shortcomings, or use the model to justify rather than challenge her practice (Hopkinson and Clarke 2002). In this case there would be no evidence of learning or changed perspectives and hence a failure of the purpose of reflection. Sometimes a nurse can become overly descriptive in an attempt to fit answers to the specific questions within a model and in so doing lose sight of the analytical process and the purpose of learning from reflecting (Hopkinson and Clarke 2002). There is some evidence to suggest that successful reflection results from: a protected time to reflect, a facilitated context and a safe environment with peer support and group discussion (Gustaffsson and Fagerberg, 2004, Mann *et al.* 2009). However, in beginning to develop a reflective approach to caregiving, models can be invaluable in getting the nurse to go deeper and look at practice from different angles. Frequently, the nurse will absorb the questioning reflective approach before moving on to develop her own reflective method, which she refers to during (as well as after) caregiving as she becomes more experienced in reflecting (Hopkinson and Clarke 2002).

Creative ways of reflecting

One of the advantages of written reflection is that the nurse can trace her progress and development over time. Yet it is not the only way to reflect. Seekers (2003) linked different ways of reflecting to Gardner's theory of multiple intelligences, suggesting that everyone has a particular preferred way of reflecting (see Table 17.2). However, in order to gain from the process of reflection and particularly from reviewing patterns and development over a longer time frame, there does need to be some form of record keeping. For example, if you only reflect while walking the dog and do not commit anything to paper, those reflections will become more difficult to access as time passes, which can prevent you from identifying patterns in your reflections and reduce your ability to learn about yourself and your practice.

TABLE 17.2 Creative ways of reflecting

Multiple intelligence	Narrative description	Recommended methods for recording reflections
Verbal/linguistic	Preference for using language and reading, writing and speaking to process thoughts	Journals, diaries, written stories, poetry
Logical/ mathematical	Preference for using numbers, maths and logic to find and understand the patterns of everyday life. Often think in conceptual abstract relationships and linkages	Mind-maps, flow charts, pie charts, formulae, tables
Visual/spatial	Preference for shapes, images, patterns, designs and textures	Paint a picture, collage, sculpting, representational construction, photos, artefacts, dreams, images and metaphor
Bodily/ kinaesthetic	Preference for learning by doing and movement Feeling knowledge through the senses is important	Taking a walk, walking the dog, dancing, gardening, cooking, driving, swimming
Musical/ rhythmic	Preference for sound and vibration as a means of gaining understanding	Music which evokes the way you felt/thought acted Repetitive sound can aid reflection e.g roar of the sea
Naturalist	Preference for being outdoors, engaging with eco-systems, plants, animals in order to gain understanding The elements are important aspects of everyday existence	Go on retreat, camping, walk in the rain, lie on the beach, horse riding, stroking and talking to animals

Source: adapted from Seekers (2003).

CONCLUSION

By the time Julia had presented her revised account of the drug incident using Johns' model to Tariq she had become convinced of the value of reflection. Julia was quite surprised to find that in taking reflection seriously, she was able to identify both her strengths and her weaknesses. She has realised that her previous attempts to reflect had all been half-hearted and only done because they were required for assignments or other things unrelated (or so she previously thought) to nursing work. Her motivation to continue to learn about herself and the effect her actions had on others (especially patients) had been gently encouraged by the support from her mentor, Tariq. He had remained non-judgemental throughout, allowing her to arrive at her own conclusions and her own plans for development. Her acceptance of the value of reflective practice as a way of continuing to develop both personally and professionally means that she wants to continue to improve her skills in order to make a positive difference to the patients in her care. In effect, Julia can now relate to and understand the NMC requirement for nurses to reflect on their practice (NMC 2015).

Julia now cannot wait to become a registered nurse and start to inspire the next generation of student nurses to become more reflective as a way of improving the experiences of patients within her sphere of influence.

SUGGESTED FURTHER READING

Bradbury, H., Frost, N., Kilminster, S. and Zukas, M. (2010) *Beyond Reflective Practice: New approaches to professional lifelong learning.* Abingdon, Oxon: Routledge.

Bulman, C. and Schulz, S. (2013) *Reflective Practice in Nursing* (5th edn). Oxford: Wiley Blackwell.

Ghaye, T. (2005) *Developing the Reflective Team.* Oxford: Blackwell.

Rolfe, G., Jasper, M. and Freshwater, D. (2011) *Critical Reflection in Practice* (2nd edn). London: Palgrave.

Taylor, B. (2010) *Reflective Practice: A guide for nurses and midwives* (3rd edn). Buckingham, UK: Open University Press.

Timms, F. and Duffy, A. (2011) *Writing Your Nursing Portfolio: A step by step guide.* Buckingham, UK: Open University Press.

REFERENCES

Argyris, C. and Schön, D. A. (1978) *Organisational Learning: A theory of action perspective.* Wokingham, UK: Addison-Wesley.

Atkins, S. and Murphy, K. (1993) Reflection: a review of the literature. *Journal of Advanced Nursing* **18** (8), 1188–1192.

Belenky, M. F., Clinchy, B. M., Goldberger, N. R. and Tarule, J. M. (1986) *Women's Ways of Knowing: The development of self, voice and mind.* New York: Basic Books.

Berragan, L. (1998) Nursing practice draws upon several different ways of knowing. *Journal of Clinical Nursing* **7** (3), 209–217.

Bolton, G. (2005) *Reflective Practice: Writing and professional development* (2nd edn). London: Paul Chapman, Sage.

Boud, D., Keogh, R. and Walker, D. (1985) *Reflection: Turning experience into learning.* London: Kogan Page.

Clare Hopkinson

Boyd, E. M. and Fales, A. W. (1983) Reflective learning: key to learning from experience. *Journal of Humanistic Psychology* **23** (2), 99–117.

Bradbury-Jones, C., Hughes, S. M., Murphy, W., Parry, L. and Sutton, J. (2009) A new way of reflecting in nursing: the Peshkin Approach. *Journal of Advanced Nursing* **65** (11), 2485–2493.

Burnard, P. (1995) Nurse educators' perceptions of reflection and reflective practice: a report of a descriptive survey. *Journal of Advanced Nursing* **21** (6), 1167–1174.

Cadman, K., Clack, E., Lethbridge, Z., Morris, J. and Redwood, R. (2003) Reflection: a casualty of modularisation? Enquiry-based reflection research group. *Nurse Education Today* **23** (1), 11–18.

Carper, B. (1978) Fundamental patterns of knowing in nursing. *Advances in Nursing Science* **1** (1), 13–23.

Clarke, N. (2014) A person-centred enquiry into the teaching and learning experiences of reflection and reflective practice – part one. *Nurse Education Today* **34** (9), 1219–1224.

Cook, B. (1999) Reflect on the past and plan your future. *Practice Nurse* **17** (2), 98–100.

Coward, M. (2011) Does the use of reflective models restrict critical thinking and therefore learning in nurse education? What have we done? *Nurse Education Today* **31** (8), 883–886.

Driscoll, J. (1994) Reflective practice for practise. *Senior Nurse* **14** (1), 47–50.

Duke, S. and Appleton, J. (2000) The use of reflection in a palliative care programme: a quantitative study of the development of reflective skills over an academic year. *Journal of Advanced Nursing* **32** (6), 1557–1568.

Dunning, D. (2005) *Self Insight: Roadblocks and detours on the path to knowing thyself*. New York: Psychology Press.

Durgahee, T. (1996) Promoting reflection in post-graduate nursing: a theoretical model. *Nurse Education Today* **16** (6), 419–426.

Francis, R. (2013) *Report of the Mid-Staffordshire NHS Foundation Trust Public Inquiry*. London: The Stationery Office.

Freshwater, D. (2004) Analysing interpretation and reinterpreting analysis: exploring the logic of critical reflection. *Nursing Philosophy* **5** (1), 4–11.

Ghaye, T. and Lillymann, S. (2006) *Learning Journals and Critical Incidents: Reflective practice for health care professionals* (2nd edn). Salisbury: Quay Publications.

Gibbs, G. (1988) *Learning by Doing: A guide to teaching and learning methods*. Oxford: Oxford Polytechnic Further Education Unit.

Glaze, J. E. (2001) Reflection as a transforming process: student advanced nurse practitioners' experience of developing reflective skills as part of an MSc programme. *Journal of Advanced Nursing* **34** (5), 639–647.

Glaze, J. E. (2002) Stages in coming to terms with reflection. *Journal of Advanced Nursing* **37** (3), 265–272.

Goodman, J. (1984) Reflection and teacher education: a case study and theoretical analysis. *Interchange* **15** (3), 9–26.

Gustafsson, C. and Fagerberg, I. (2004) Reflection, the way to professional development? *Journal of Clinical Nursing* **13** (3), 271–280.

Hallett, C. E. (1997) Learning through reflection in the community: the relevance of Schön's theories of coaching to nurse education. *International Journal of Nursing Studies* **34** (2), 103–110.

Holm, D. and Stephenson, S. (1994) Reflection a student's perspective. In *Reflective Practice in Nursing: The growth of the professional practitioner*, Palmer, A., Burns, S. and Bulman, C. (eds). Oxford: Blackwell Science, pp. 53–62.

Hopkinson, C. (2009) *More than a Good Gossip? An inquiry into nurses' reflecting in the ward*. University of the West of England, Bristol, unpublished PhD thesis.

Hopkinson, C. (2015) Using poetry in a critically reflexive action research co-inquiry with nurses. *Action Research* **13** (1), 30–47.

Hopkinson, C. and Clarke, B. (2002) Reflection in practice: the level of critical thinking. Presentation at the International Reflective Practice Conference Netherlands 6–8 June.

460

Horton-Deutsch, S. and Sherwood, G. (2008) Reflection: an educational strategy to develop emotionally competent nurse leaders. *Journal of Nursing Management* **16** (8), 946–954.

Ixer, G. (1999) There's no such thing as reflection. *British Journal of Social Work* **29** (4), 513–527.

Jasper, M. (1999) Nurses' perceptions of the value of written reflection. *Nurse Education Today* **19** (6), 452–463.

Johns, C. (1995) Promoting learning through reflection with Carper's fundamental ways of knowing in nursing. *Journal of Advanced Nursing* **22** (2), 226–234.

Johns, C. (1997) *Becoming a Reflective Practitioner*. Open University, Milton Keynes, unpublished PhD thesis.

Johns, C. (2000) *Becoming a Reflective Practitioner: A reflective and holistic approach to clinical nursing, practice development and clinical supervision.* Oxford: Blackwell Science.

Johns, C. (2010) *Guided Reflection: A narrative approach for advancing professional practice* West Sussex: John Wiley.

Kember, D., Wong, F. K. Y. and Young, E. (2001) The nature of reflection. In *Reflective Teaching and Learning in the Health Professions*, Kember, D. (ed.). Oxford: Blackwell Science, pp. 3–28.

Kim, S. H. (1999) Critical reflective inquiry for knowledge development in nursing practice. *Journal of Advanced Nursing* **29** (5), 1205–1212.

Luft, J. (1955) *Of Human Interaction.* San Francisco, CA: National Press Books.

Mackintosh, C. (1998) Reflection: a flawed strategy for the nursing profession. *Nurse Education Today* **18** (7), 553–557.

Maclellan, E. (2004) How reflective is the academic essay? *Studies in Higher Education* **29** (1), 75–89.

Mann, K., Gordon, J. and Macleod, A. (2009) Reflection and reflective practice in health professions education: a systematic review. *Advances in Health Science Education* **14** (4), 595–621

Mantzoukas, S. and Jasper, M. A. (2004) Reflective practice and daily ward reality: a covert power game. *Journal of Clinical Nursing* **13** (8), 925–933.

Marshall, J. (1999) Living life as inquiry. *Systematic Practice and Action Research* **12** (2), 155–171.

Marshall, J. (2004) Living systemic thinking: exploring quality in first person action research. *Action Research* **2** (3), 305–325.

Mezirow, J. (1990) *Fostering Critical Reflection in Adulthood: A guide to transformative and emancipatory learning.* San Francisco, CA: Jossey-Bass.

Moon, J. (2004) *A Handbook of Reflective and Experiential Learning: Theory and practice.* London: Routledge Falmer.

Mountford, B. and Rogers, L. (1996) Using individual and group learning in and on assessment as a tool for effective learning. *Journal of Advanced Nursing* **24** (6), 1127–1134.

Newell, R. (1992) Anxiety, accuracy and reflection: the limits of professional development. *Journal of Advanced Nursing* **17** (11), 1326–1333.

NMC (Nursing and Midwifery Council). (2015) *The Code: Professional standards of practice and behaviour for nurses and midwives.* London: NMC.

OED (2006) *Concise Oxford English Dictionary* (11th edn). Oxford: Oxford University Press.

Platzer, H., Blake, D. and Ashford, D. (2000) Barriers to learning from reflection: a study of the use of group work with post-registration nurses. *Journal of Advanced Nursing* **31** (5), 1001–1008.

Polanyi, N. (1967) *The Tacit Dimension.* New York: Doubleday.

Powell, J. (1989) The reflective practitioner in nursing. *Journal of Advanced Nursing* **14** (11), 824–832.

Rich, A. and Parker, D. L. (1995) Reflection and critical incident analysis: ethical and moral implications of their use within nursing and midwifery education. *Journal of Advanced Nursing* **22** (6), 1050–1057.

Richardson, G. and Maltby, H. (1995) Reflection-on-practice: enhancing student learning. *Journal of Advanced Nursing* **22** (2), 235–242.

Rolfe, G., Jasper, M., Freshwater, D. (2011) *Critical Reflection in Practice: Generating knowledge for care.* Basingstoke: Palgrave Macmillan

Schön, D. (1983) *The Reflective Practitioner*. New York: Basic Books.

Seekers, D. (2003) A journey into reflective space . . . with apologies to Star Trek. *Action Learning and Action Research Journal* **8** (1), 50–58.

Shaw, E. K, Howard, J., Etz, R. S., Hudson, S. V. and Crabtree, B. F. (2012) How team-based reflection affects quality improvement implementation: a qualitative study. *Quality Management in Healthcare* **21** (2), 104–113.

Smith, A. (1998) Learning about reflection. *Journal of Advanced Nursing* **24** (4), 891–898.

Taylor, B. (2010) *Reflective Practice: A guide for nurses and midwives* (3rd edn). Buckingham: Open University Press.

Teekman, B. (2000) Exploring reflective thinking in nursing practice. *Journal of Advanced Nursing* **31** (5), 1125–1135.

Timms, F. and Duffy, A. (2011) *Writing Your Nursing Portfolio: A step by step guide*. Buckingham: Open University Press.

Torbert, W. R. (2001) The practice of action inquiry. In *The Handbook of Action Research*, Reason, P. and Bradbury, H. (eds). London: Sage, pp. 250–260.

van Manen, M. (1977) Linking ways of knowing with ways of being practical. *Curriculum Inquiry* **6**, 205–228.

Watson, S. (2002) The use of reflection as an assessment of practice: can you mark learning contracts? *Nurse Education in Practice* **2** (3), 150–159.

Wong, F. K. Y., Kember, D., Chung, L. Y. F. and Yan, L. (1995) Assessing the level of student reflection from reflective journals. *Journal of Advanced Nursing* **22** (1), 48–57.

18

MEDICINES MANAGEMENT

Claire Fullbrook-Scanlon

LEARNING OUTCOMES

After reading and reflecting on this chapter, you should be able to:

* identify the organisations involved in medicines management;
* discuss the Nursing and Midwifery Council *Standards for Medicines Management*;
* describe current legislation relating to controlled drugs;
* discuss non-medical prescribing;
* describe antimicrobial stewardship;
* discuss the management of medication errors.

INTRODUCTION

Medicines management is an important and growing area of nursing practice, evolving as the demands of modern health care result in the practice of nursing changing to meet patients' needs. Newly qualified nurses are required to know a considerable amount about the medicines that they administer and manage, and at the other end of the spectrum, experienced nurses are able to undertake further training to be able to prescribe from a full range of medicinal products.

The chapter is divided into three parts. In Part 1, the student's role in medicines management is outlined, and some key terms and organisations involved in medicines management are introduced.

In Part 2, the standards for medicines management are explained in more detail and discussed in relation to some case studies.

In Part 3, non-medical prescribing and the avoidance and management of medication errors is explored in more depth and antimicrobial issues are highlighted and discussed.

PART 1: OUTLINING MEDICINES MANAGEMENT

Case 18.1

Josephine is a third-year student who has just started a placement on a rehabilitation ward. During the ward drug round she notices that her mentor doesn't check the name band of all the patients, especially those who have been on the ward for some time, and she doesn't ask patients to confirm their identity. She just hands patients a pot containing their medicines and asks them to take them. Sometimes patients say that they will take the tablets later and put the pot on the locker, where occasionally they remain until the next drug round. Josephine asks why this is done and her mentor replies that the ward is very busy, and there isn't enough time to do things 'by the book'. If that was done the drug round would take all morning. Josephine accepts that the ward is busy, and that managing the medication of 12 patients is a great responsibility as well as a time-consuming one. There haven't been any incidents yet, but surely it's only a matter of time?

Medicines and medicines management

Safe medicines management is integral to the duties of all registered nurses including those working in primary care, in hospitals and in the independent sector. According to the Health and Social Care Information Centre (HSCIC 2014) there were 1.1 billion prescription items dispensed in the community in 2014. The estimated cost of medicines to the NHS for 2013–2014 is £14.4 billion with just over 40 per cent of that cost attributed to hospital use of medicines (HSCIC 2014). As the profession has developed, the responsibilities of the nurse in this area have increased. Not so many years ago, nurses obediently followed doctors' prescriptions and were expected to do no more. Now nurses must have detailed knowledge of the medicines they administer, and make independent judgements about medicines management for those in their care. This shift is recognised in professional language. Where once we discussed the nurse's role in administering medicines, now the emphasis is on medicines *management*, encompassing administration and much more. The term medicine optimisation is often referred to meaning 'optimise', 'to make the best of'. To achieve medicine optimisation for patients requires input from all health and social care practitioners as well as involving a greater patient engagement focus. Many nurses have completed independent prescribing courses and are able to prescribe from a full range of medicines. This is the domain of experienced nurses, but from the first day of their registration all nurses are required to practise according to *The Code* (NMC 2015), and be guided by other Nursing and Midwifery Council (NMC) publications, requiring a considerable amount of knowledge as well as the exercise of professional accountability.

There is a bewildering array of products available, which claim health-giving properties. They may be obviously medicines, or food additives, cosmetics, vitamins or herbs. The Medicines and Healthcare Products Regulatory Agency (MHRA 2012) publishes *A Guide to What is a Medicinal Product*, which uses the definition of 2001/83/EC directive to define a medicinal product as:

Any substance or combination of substances presented as having properties for treating or preventing disease in human beings; any substance or combination of substances which may be used in or administered to human beings either with a view to restoring, correcting or modifying physiological functions by exerting a pharmacological, immunological or metabolic action, or to making a medical diagnosis.

(MHRA 2012, p. 8)

The NMC *Standards for Medicines Management* (NMC 2007) uses a similar definition from an earlier directive. In this and other documents several words are used interchangeably. The standards define 'medicinal products' and then use the words 'medication' and 'medicine'. In this chapter the term 'medicines' is preferred but other terms are used in direct quotations. Occasionally the word 'drug' is used where it is preferred in general usage, for example in 'drug chart' or 'drug trolley'. Medicines management has been described as:

the process of managing the way in which medicines are chosen, bought, delivered, prescribed, administered and reviewed, including appropriate safe, agreed withdrawal, in order to make the most of the contribution medicines can make to improving care and treatment.

(DH 2008, p. 1)

Nurses are generally not involved in the process of choosing, buying and delivering medicines and so these aspects of medicines management will not be discussed in this chapter. However, some nurses are able to prescribe and this role will be examined and explained in Part 3.

The National Institute of Health and Care Excellence (NICE) published guidance on medicines optimistaion in 2015 (NICE 2015a), building on the guide produced by the Royal Pharmaceutical Society: *Medicines Optimisation: Helping people make the most of medicines* (RPS 2013). It has been defined as

a person-centred approach to safe and effective medicines use, to ensure people obtain the best possible outcomes from their medicines. Medicines optimization applies to people who may or may not take their medicines effectively. Shared decision making is an essential part of evidence-based medicine, seeking to use the best available evidence to guide decisions about the care of the individual patient, taking into account their needs, preferences and values.

(NICE 2015a, p. 5)

Nurses are expected safely to administer prescribed medicines and will undoubtedly be involved in reviewing medicines as part of the multidisciplinary team. In some specialties, nurses will also be involved in safe agreed withdrawal of medications. Medicine optimisation requires the nurse to aim to understand the patient experience as well as ensure that medicine use is as safe as possible.

Medicines management is the process of managing the way in which medicines are chosen, bought, delivered, prescribed, administered and reviewed, including appropriate safe, agreed withdrawal, in order to make the most of the contribution medicines can make to improving care and treatment. (DH 2008, p. 1)

Claire Fullbrook-Scanlon

Activity 18.1

This chapter discusses the NMC *Standards for Medicine Management* in some detail. Before you go any further ask yourself these questions.

- Have you heard of the standards?
- Have you read them?
- Were you able to access the standards on your last placement?
- Do you know how the standards relate to student nurses?
- Do you know what is in them in relation to what knowledge is required to administer medicines?

Key Nursing and Midwifery Council documents

The Code (NMC 2015) includes a specific standard regarding medicines. Standard 18 says you 'Advise on, prescribe, supply, dispense or administer within the limits of your training and competence, the law, our guidance and other relevant policies, guidance and regulations' (NMC 2015). This standard and its associated clauses tells nurses that not only must we have knowledge of our patients' health needs, we need to ensure that whatever medication we dispense or administer must be compatible with any other care or treatment they are receiving. This further emphasises the increased safety agenda and nurses' roles and responsibilities within health care.

For nurses the most important publication concerning medicines management is the NMC's *Standards for Medicines Management* (NMC 2007). This document comprehensively sets out what is expected of registrants. It must be considered required reading and is available free to download via the NMC website. If you are using this document online, links to other resources embedded within the text can be used. There are some excellent and free resources available and NMC endorsement validates their use. In 2014 the NMC made it clear in their 'Standards and Guidance Review Cycle' that they expected to publish new guidance on medicines management in the first quarter of 2015 (NMC 2014). However at the time of writing (February 2016) there has been no announcement as whether new standards or guidance will be published. You will need to check on the NMC website and make yourself aware of any new standards while you read this chapter.

Currently there are 26 standards organised in 10 sections, and 8 further annexes,which contain useful further information and guidance. Like *The Code*, the standards are written in clear language often using the imperative 'must', though there are also standards that tell a nurse what she 'may' do. In the standards, a short section of explanatory guidance follows each standard and here the language is more discursive; the word '*should*' replaces the word '*must*'. However, the summary of the standards states that 'it is essential that you read the full guidance and you must follow the advice' (NMC 2007, p. 3). The document is clear that these are *minimum* standards, providing the benchmark by which practice is measured.

In Part 2 of this chapter the standards will be discussed in turn, except for the only one that specifically refers to students, Standard 18, which along with its accompanying guidance is set out in full in Box 18.1. When the term 'standards' is used in this chapter, it refers to the NMC *Standards for Medicines Management*.

BOX 18.1 Standard 18

Students must never administer/supply medicinal products without direct supervision.

Guidance

In order to achieve the outcomes and standards required for registration, students must be given opportunities to participate in the administration of medication but this must always be under direct supervision. Where this is done, both the student and registrant must sign the patient's/woman's medication chart or document in the notes. The registrant is responsible for delegating to a student and where it is considered the student is not yet ready to undertake administration in whatever form this should be delayed until such time that the student is ready. Equally a student may decline to undertake a task if they do not feel confident enough to do so. The relationship between the registrant and the student is a partnership and the registrant should support the student in gaining competence in order to prepare for registration. As students progress through their training their supervision may become increasingly indirect to reflect their competence level.

(NMC 2007, p. 31)

Throughout their programme, students need to gain experience of the duties they will be required to undertake as registrants, and as administration of medicines is integral to the nurse's role, students need continual guidance so that they are fit for practice upon registration. The essential skills cluster concerning medicines management within the standards for pre-registration proficiency (NMC 2010a) provides guidance on how student nurses can progress through their training and demonstrate competence in medicines management as a student and upon entry to the register. For example, the second-year progression point again reinforces that the student nurse: 'Administers and, where necessary, prepares medication safely under direct supervision, including orally and by injection' (NMC 2010a, p. 139).

The Code is clear that registered nurses have a duty to help students to develop their competence and confidence (NMC 2015). Students gain experience and become competent by observing and undertaking tasks in the clinical area. When a student nurse accompanies her mentor on a medicine round it is the mentor who remains accountable for ensuring that medicines are dispensed correctly. As the student becomes more proficient in their role the amount of delegation can be increased but students must be supervised until they become registered. A difficulty for both the mentor and the student is understanding what, exactly, is meant by the term 'direct supervision'.

The guidance accompanying Standard 18 from the NMC appears to contradict itself regarding the question of direct or indirect supervision. The standard clearly states that a student nurse must *never* administer or supply a medicinal product without *direct* supervision, and this apparently unambiguous statement is reiterated in the first line of the guidance that follows. However, later in the guidance it is suggested that as student nurses become more experienced, 'indirect' supervision may be sufficient. It seems clear that the level of supervision required for a student on their first ward does not need to be the same when they are on their final ward. The level of supervision required is a matter for the accountable registered nurse to decide upon, based on a growing knowledge of each individual student's capabilities, though the student must (the standard says 'may') decline tasks they do not feel competent to undertake.

Case 18.2

> Mona is a third-year student on a busy surgical ward. Mr Bellchambers is two days post-surgery and requests analgesia. Mona is able to read and interpret the Medication Administration Record correctly and the patient is prescribed 1 gram of paracetamol orally. Mona approaches the mentor who gives her the keys to the drug trolley and asks her to dispense the medication. Mona hesitates, unsure of whether she should do as she has been asked.
>
> A number of complex issues are presented in this apparently simple scenario. Does Mona know what the standards say about student nurses? Does she feel competent to give the tablets? Is she aware of what she needs to know about the patient, the medicine and how it must be administered? What does local policy say about student nurses having custody of the drug trolley keys, for however short a period? The guidance says that supervision can become more 'indirect' as the student progresses through their training, and Mona is near the end of her programme. The mentor seems to be taking a very slack view of supervision. She has not checked the chart, asked about Mr Bellchambers' pain, checked the medicine or watched it being administered, and could be held to account for these omissions. Perhaps Mona feels capable of doing what is asked, but her mentor will find it difficult to defend supervision such as this.

Activity 18.2

What do you think the difference between 'direct supervision' and 'indirect supervision' is? The NMC does not give any further detail, so there is not a right answer, but thinking about this might help to guide discussions with mentors in practice.

This chapter does not cover aspects of pharmacology. There are several good textbooks that cover this ground, some of which are recommended at the end of the chapter. However, in order to make the standards clear, some terms relating to medicines need to be understood. Medicines fall into a number of categories, and different legal instruments govern the prescription and supply of each category (Downie *et al.* 2008). The categories are shown in Table 18.1.

Loperamide was reclassified from POM to P at the request of the manufacturer in 1983. Since then many more medicines have been reclassified (RPS 2008). It has been claimed that the UK leads the world in allowing patients to purchase medicines over the counter (Gauld *et al.* 2014). These medicines can be prescribed, but they do not have to be. Many prescriptions for medication on the General Sales List (GSL) are issued, allowing prescribers to be aware of the full range of medications taken, as well as being cheaper for many patients.

TABLE 18.1 Types of medicines

Type	Stands for	Explanation	Example
CD	Controlled drug	Addictive drugs which produce dependence. Special controls under the Misuse of Drugs Act 1971	Diamorphine (Heroin)
POM	Prescription only medicine	Medicines that can only be obtained with a prescription from a doctor, dentist, or independent or supplementary prescriber	Most antibiotics
P	Pharmacy	Medicine that can only be purchased from a registered pharmacy under the control of a pharmacist. A prescription is not necessary	Simvastatin, movicol sachets, canestan cream
GSL	General sales list	Medicines that can be bought from any shop (Some can only be bought from a pharmacy but direct supervision from the pharmacist is not required)	Paracetamol, ibuprofen, Paracetamol is limited to a maximum of 32 tablets per sale from a non-pharmaceutical sale due to the risk of permanent liver damage in over-dosage

Organisations involved in medicines management and information

In addition to the NMC there are a number of important organisations involved in medicines management and regulation, and these are excellent sources of information and guidance. Perhaps the most important for students is the NHS Trust or other organisation where they are placed, and their policies of medicines management. Though there are national frameworks and guidance, these are not all implemented in the same way. Not all NHS Trusts use the same prescription charts, for example. Being aware of and being guided by local policy is central to safe medicines management. Many NHS Trusts have an electronic version of their policy available via their website, and if this is the case you should consider downloading it and saving it for reference. An Internet search reveals many examples.

Before medicines are available to the public they have had to go through a licensing procedure. In the UK all medicines and medical devices are regulated and licensed by the Medicines and Healthcare Products Regulatory Agency (MHRA). The MHRA is the government agency responsible for ensuring that medicines are acceptably safe. The MHRA only considers safety and does not take financial considerations into account when granting licences. Their website also contains information about drug safety.

The National Institute for Health and Care Excellence (NICE) is the organisation responsible for providing national guidance in relation to promoting good health and in the prevention and treatment of ill health. In terms of medicines management, NICE is concerned with the costs and benefits relating to medicines available to NHS patients. For example, a new cancer drug would be licensed by the MHRA as safe for use. However, new cancer drugs are notoriously expensive and NICE will undertake a cost appraisal and

Claire Fullbrook-Scanlon

make recommendations as to whether the drug can be used on the NHS and under what circumstances (see Chapter 3). Patients who have been denied drug treatment on the NHS are often discussed in the local and national media.

The National Patient Safety Agency (NPSA) was an arm of the NHS, responsible for promoting patient safety. The NPSA worked with other health care agencies and organisations in identifying risks and helping to promote and develop good practice, including publishing national safety alerts. In relation to medicines management the NPSA has analysed medication incidents reported to the agency and identified areas of risk regarding safety in medications. Some of these findings will be discussed in Part 3. The NPSA ceased to exist in 2012 and its functions were transferred to the NHS Commissioning Board Special Health Authority. This change was to ensure that patient safety is clearly embedded within the NHS, but you will still see the name in important documents.

The National Prescribing Centre (NPC) was formed in 1996 by the Department of Health. The NPC was primarily concerned with information about medicines and their use, education and development, and disseminating good practice. It also provided support to non-medical prescribers, MeRec publications, and new medicine schemes. The National Prescribing Centre integrated with NICE in 2012. The NICE website includes a Medicines and Prescribing Centre. This resource provides information on new medicines, good practice guidance on medications and any alerts regarding medicines or prescribing.

TABLE 18.2 Some organisations involved in medicines regulation and information

Initial	Title	Role	Website
NMC	Nursing and Midwifery Council	Sets standards for practice for nurses and midwives	www.nmc-uk.org
MHRA	Medicines and Healthcare Products Regulatory Agency	Ensures the safety of medicines	www.mhra.gov.uk
NICE	National Institute for Health and Care Excellence	Produces guidance about which medicines should be used	www.nice.org.uk
NPSA	National Patient Safety Authority (now part of NHS Commissioning Board)	Responsible for identifying risk and promoting good practice	www.nrls.npsa.nhs.uk/
NPC	National Prescribing Centre (now part of NICE)	Supports quality and cost-effectiveness in prescribing practice	www.nice.org.uk/about/communities/nice-medicines-and-prescribing
UKMI	United Kingdom Medicines Information	Produces evidence-based information and advice	www.ukmi.nhs.uk
RCN	Royal College of Nursing	Produces some guidelines for practice	www.rcn.org.uk
BNF	British National Formulary	Contains prescribing information	www.bnf.org/

Perhaps the best known resource is the British National Formulary, the brightly coloured paperback that can be found in every drug trolley, but that can now also be found online. A children's BNF and a Nurse Prescribers' Formulary are also published. The BNF is jointly owned by the British Medical Association and the Royal Pharmaceutical Society, professional bodies for doctors and pharmacists. BNF publications reflect current best practice as well as legal and professional guidelines relating to the uses of medicines. Though the BNF gives a great deal of information about indications, contraindications, doses and side effects, it does not give any detail about how drugs work because it is written for prescribers. It is not a textbook or a teaching resource, and so further sources, especially pharmacology textbooks, are needed to increase knowledge and understanding of drugs and the way that they work.

UK Medicines Information (UKMI) is an NHS pharmacy-based service. Its aim is to support the safe, effective and efficient use of medicines by the provision of evidence-based information and up-to-date advice on their therapeutic use. UKMI provides resources through the National electronic Library for Medicines (NeLM), which is the largest medicines information portal for health care professionals in the NHS. The Royal College of Nursing (RCN) also produces a number of influential guidelines. Table 18.2 summarises the organisations and their roles.

A **patient-specific direction** is a written instruction from a qualified and registered prescriber.

PART 2: EXPLAINING MEDICINES MANAGEMENT

This part of the chapter is based on the *Standards for Medicines Management* (NMC 2007). Apart from Standard 18, which was introduced in Part 1, each standard is quoted in at least as much detail as in the summary section and discussed further. Not all clauses are cited. But it should be clear that this chapter serves as a general discussion about medicines management; it cannot replace full reading of the standards, guidance and annexes and local policies. Sections directly quoted from the standards are italicised. A summary of the standards is given in Table 18.3. You need to ensure that you are referring to the latest version of the standards by checking the NMC website.

Standards for Medicines Management

Standard 1: Methods (NMC 2007, p. 13)

Registrants must only supply and administer medicinal products in accordance with one or more of the following processes:

 1.1 *Patient-specific directions (PSD);*
 1.2 *Patient medicines administration chart (may be called a medicines administration record [MAR]);*
 1.3 *Patient group direction (PGD);*
 1.4 *Medicines Act exemption (where they apply to nurses);*
 1.5 *Standing order;*
 1.6 *Homely remedy protocol;*
 1.7 *Prescription forms.*

A **patient-specific direction** (PSD) is the formal name for a written prescription. The prescription is written for a named person. It may be in the form of an instruction, for

Claire Fullbrook-Scanlon

TABLE 18.3 NMC *Standards for Medicines Management*

Section	Section title	Standard number	Subject
1	Methods of supplying and/or	1	Methods
		2	Checking
		3	Transcribing
2	Dispensing	4	Prescription medicines
		5	Patient's own medicines
3	Storage and transportation	6	Storage
		7	Transportation
4	Standards for practice of administration of medicines	8	Administration
		9	Assessment
		10	Self-administration – children and young people
		11	Remote prescription or direction to administer
		12	Text messaging
		13	Titration
		14	Preparing medication in advance
		15	Medication acquired over the internet
		16	Aids to support compliance
5	Delegation	17	Delegation
		18	Nursing and midwifery students
		19	Unregistered practitioners
		20	Intravenous medication
6	Disposal of medical products	21	Disposal
7	Unlicensed medicines	22	Unlicensed medicines
8	Complementary and alternative therapies	23	Complementary and alternative therapies
9	Management of adverse events (errors or incidents) in the administration of medicines	24	Management of adverse events
		25	Reporting adverse reactions
10	Controlled drugs	26	Controlled drugs

Annex 1 Legislation
Annex 2 Guidance on labelling/over-labelling of medicines
Annex 3 Suitability of patient's own medicinal products for use
Annex 4 Exclusion criteria for self-administering medicines
Annex 5 Administering medicinal products in research clinical trial
Annex 6 Information and advice
Annex 7 Glossary
Annex 8 Contributors

472

example, in patients' notes, or in a hospital setting on a patient's medicines administration chart. The prescription may have been written by a doctor or a dentist, or by nurses, pharmacists and some allied health professionals who have qualified as independent or supplementary prescribers (see Part 3).

Patient medicines administration chart (MAR) refers to the patient's own 'drug chart', commonly used in secondary care. Strictly speaking, it is not a prescription but a direction to administer medicine.

Patient group directions (PGDs) are written instructions allowing the supply and administration of prescription-only medications in pre-identified clinical situations without the need for individual prescription. Patients are not pre-identified prior to the treatment, the direction applying to patient groups rather than specific patients. Some GP surgeries operate flu vaccine clinics where the patient will not see the GP but the practice nurse, who can administer vaccination under the direction. It is important to realise that a PGD does not simply allow anyone in that area to administer the medication; the PGD is written for specific indications, and can be operated only by named individuals. Student nurses are not permitted to administer medications under PGDs even if delegated to do so by a registered professional (NICE 2013).

Medications Act exemption. Generally under medicines legislation drugs that are pharmacy-only (P) or prescription-only medication (POM) can only be supplied or sold by a registered pharmacy. However, in certain circumstances some health care professionals, for example occupational health nurses or podiatrists, are able to sell, supply and administer some medicines directly to their patients or clients.

Standing orders. These have in the past been used by maternity services and occupational health departments under local guidelines, to supplement legislation pertaining to medicinal products that midwives or occupational health nurses may supply and/or administer (NMC 2007). Local guidelines are not required under any legislation and indeed 'standing orders' do not exist in current medicines legislation.

Homely remedy protocol. This refers to medicines that are not prescription-only (POM) or pharmacy-only (P) but to medicines from the General Sales List (GSL), for example paracetamol. Homely remedy protocols are usually used in care settings such as nursing or residential homes. If a registered nurse supplies a homely remedy she should ensure that there is written guidance as to the conditions in which she is able to administer the product and that she is competent.

Prescription forms. These are generally used in GP surgeries, hospital outpatients, dental surgeries and by nurse independent prescribers. They are numbered serially and contain anti-forgery and anti-counterfeiting features to reduce the incidence of illegal usage. There are a range of different prescription forms and they are classified as secure stationery, meaning that they have to be kept locked away when not in use.

Standard 2: Checking (NMC 2007, p. 18)

1 *Registrants (1st and 2nd level) must check any direction to administer a medicinal product.*

2 *As a registrant you are accountable for your actions and omissions. In administering any medication, or assisting or overseeing any self-administration of medication, you must exercise your professional judgement and apply your knowledge and skill in the given situation. As a registrant, before you administer a medicinal product you must always check that the prescription or other direction to administer is:*

> A **patient medicines administration chart** refers to the patient's own drug chart.
>
> **Patient group directions** (PGDs) are written instructions allowing the supply and administration of prescription-only medications in pre-identified clinical situations without the need for individual prescription. They must be operated only by named individuals.

Transcribing medication is when a written instruction for a medicine is copied from one place to another.

2.1 *not for a substance to which the patient is known to be allergic or otherwise unable to tolerate;*

2.2 *based, whenever possible, on the patient's informed consent and awareness of the purpose of the treatment;*

2.3 *clearly written, typed or computer-generated and indelible;*

2.4 *specifies the substance to be administered, using its generic or brand name where appropriate and its stated form, together with the strength, dosage, timing, frequency of administration, start and finish dates, and route of administration;*

2.5 *is signed and dated by the authorised prescriber;*

2.6 *in the case of controlled drugs, specifies the dosage and the number of dosage units or total course; and is signed and dated by the prescriber using relevant documentation as introduced, for example, patient drug record cards.*

3 *And that you have:*

3.1 *clearly identified the patient for whom the medication is intended;*

3.2 *recorded the weight of the patient on the prescription sheet for all children, and where the dosage of medication is related to weight or surface area (for example, cytotoxics) or where clinical condition dictates recording the patient's weight.*

This is the minimum required and begins to tell the nurse what must be done in administering medicines. There is some overlap between Standard 2 and Standard 8, in emphasising that the patient must be correctly identified. This is the only standard which has no accompanying guidance.

Activity 18.3

Look at the section of the drug chart shown in Figure 18.1. How many errors can you spot? (Answers are given near the end of the chapter, in Figure 18.2)

Standard 3: Transcribing (NMC 2007, p. 18)

As a registrant you may transcribe medication from one 'direction to supply or administer' to another form of 'direction to supply or administer'.

Transcribing medication is when written prescriptions are copied from one place to another, for example, a direction from a patient's hospital medicines administration record to a new hospital medicines administration record. A nurse transcribing the directions is accountable for the transcription or any omissions in the transcribing process. Any transcribed medications must be signed off by a registered prescriber. It is suggested that this should be undertaken only in 'exceptional circumstances', though many nurses will be familiar with circumstances where the space in a medicines administration record has all been used and the responsible prescriber has not yet completed a new chart to replace it. Local policy is very important here. The *Standards* allow transcription, but some local policies may not. Though the NMC regards transcription as acceptable, nurses are under no obligation to undertake it, and there is the potential that writing new records in this way becomes part of normal practice.

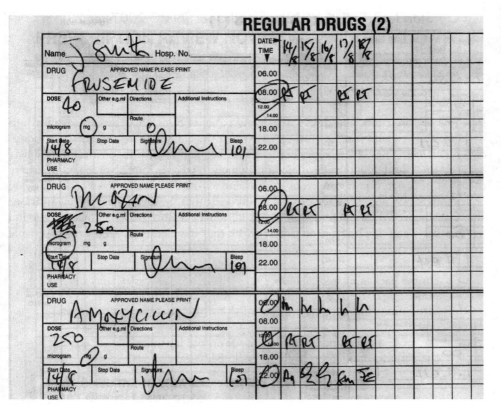

FIGURE 18.1
Drug chart with errors

Standard 4: Prescription medicines (NMC 2007, p. 20)

Registrants may in exceptional circumstances label from stock and supply a clinically appropriate medicine to a patient, against a written prescription (not PGD), for self-administration or administration by another professional, and to advise on its safe and effective use.

The NMC (2007) defines dispensing as 'to label from stock and supply a clinically appropriate medicine to a patient/client/carer, usually against a written prescription, for self-administration or administration by another professional and to advise on safe and effective use' (p. 20). This is different from merely administering a medicine. For example, dispensing a course of antibiotics may involve putting tablets in a box or bottle, and labelling with the patient's name, the dosage and other directions, a process normally undertaken by a pharmacist. Nurses may be called to undertake such activities in dispensing doctors' surgeries. This would be seen as an extension to a nurse's usual professional practice and therefore should be covered by a standard operating procedure. While there is no legal barrier to this practice, the patient can expect to have the dispensing carried out to the same standard that would be given from a dispensing pharmacist (NMC 2007).

Standard 5: Patients' own medicines (NMC 2007, p. 20)

1   *Registrants may use patients' own medicines in accordance with the guidance in this booklet Standards for medicines management.*
2   *The NMC welcomes and supports the self-administration of medicinal products and the administration of medication by carers wherever it is appropriate.*

In a practice welcomed by the NMC, many patients bring their own medicines into hospital, and of course nurses visiting patients in the community normally use patients' own medicines. These may be previously prescribed and current medicines or they may be over the counter purchases including homely remedies, herbal or complementary therapies. It is potentially dangerous if a patient self-medicates unknown to health care professionals, and nurses are responsible for ensuring that they have seen the medications and have checked their suitability for use. Additional guidance on labelling can be found in Annexes 3 and 4. The registrant must check that the medicinal products are suitable for use by ensuring:

- correct packaging and labelling;
- dispensing date;
- instructions for use;
- dose;
- the medicinal product matches what is on the label;
- the patient information leaflet is enclosed;
- correct patient name/ownership.

(NMC 2007, p. 52)

Discussion with the patient is very important. The nurse must explain to the patient the rationale for using or not using them and it must be acknowledged that these medications, including CDs, remain the property of the patient. They must not be removed from the patient unless they have permission and must not be used for other patients (NMC 2007). In accordance with *The Code* (NMC 2015), clear and accurate records of the discussions with patients must be kept especially if a patient refuses consent to use their own medication, disposal of their own medications no longer required or unsuitable for use, or if a patient refuses to allow their medications to be sent home with a relative or carer. Patients' own medications must be stored appropriately and safely if they are to be used or kept while the patient is in a secondary care environment. Additional guidance can be found in Annexe 3.

Standard 6: Storage (NMC 2007, p. 22)

Registrants must ensure all medicinal products are stored in accordance with the patient information leaflet, summary of product characteristics document found in dispensed UK licensed medication, and in accordance with any instruction on the label.

Each NHS Trust should have policies in place to ensure that all medications are stored and kept at the correct temperature according to the licensing guidelines. Examples of these are insulin and antibiotic liquid solutions – which must be kept in a locked refrigerator.

Standard 7: Transportation (NMC 2007, p. 23)

Registrants may transport medication to patients including controlled drugs (CDs), where patients, their carers or reresentatives are unable to collect them, provided the registrant is conveying the medication to a patient for whom the medicine has been prescribed (for example from a pharmacy to the patient's own home).

Although this is permissible it is not considered good practice if it is undertaken routinely. This is more likely to affect nurses working in the community or specialist nurses who perform outreach duties. Medicines must be kept out of sight during transportation and not left in cars or at risk of theft. Where CDs are collected from a pharmacy the nurse will be asked to provide some form of identity, which will usually be identification concerning professional practice, for example a PIN card or identity badge from a current employer. The nurse will also be asked to sign a receipt of CDs at the pharmacy.

Standard 8: Administration (NMC 2007, pp. 24–25)

2   *As a registrant, in exercising your professional accountability in the best interests of your patients:*

    2.1 You must be certain of the identity of the patient to whom the medicine is to be administered.

    2.2 You must check that the patient is not allergic to the medicine before administering it.

    2.3 You must know the therapeutic uses of the medicine to be administered, its normal dosage, side effects, precautions and contra-indications.

    2.4 You must be aware of the patient's plan of care (care plan or pathway).

    2.5 You must check that the prescription or the label on medicine dispensed is clearly written and unambiguous

    2.6 You must check the expiry date (where it exists) of the medicine to be administered.

    2.7 You must have considered the dosage, weight where appropriate, method of administration, route and timing.

    2.8 You must administer or withhold in the context of the patient's condition (for example, Digoxin not usually to be given if pulse below 60) and co-existing therapies, for example, physiotherapy.

    2.9 You must contact the prescriber or another authorised prescriber without delay where contra-indications to the prescribed medicine are discovered, where the patient develops a reaction to the medicine, or where assessment of the patient indicates that the medicine is no longer suitable (see Standard 25).

    2.10 You must make a clear, accurate and immediate record of all medicine administered, intentionally withheld or refused by the patient, ensuring the signature is clear and legible; it is also your responsibility to ensure that a record is made when delegating the task of administering medicine.

In addition:

3   *Where medication is not given, the reason for not doing so must be recorded.*

4   *You may administer with a single signature any prescription only medicine, general sales list or pharmacy medication.*

In respect of controlled drugs:

5   *These should be administered in line with relevant legislation and local standard operating procedures.*

6   *It is recommended that for the administration of controlled drugs, a secondary signatory is required within secondary care and similar health care settings.*

7   *In a patient's home, where a registrant is administering a controlled drug that has already been prescribed and dispensed to that patient, obtaining a secondary signatory should be based on local risk assessment.*

8   *Although normally the second signatory should be another registered health care professional (for example doctor, pharmacist, dentist) or student nurse or midwife, in the interest of patient care, where this is not possible a second suitable person who has been assessed as competent may sign. It is good practice that the second signatory witnesses the whole administration process. For guidance, go to www.dh.gov.uk and search for 'Safer management of controlled drugs: guidance on standard operating procedures'.*

9   *In cases of direct patient administration of oral medication, for example, from stock in a substance misuse clinic, it must be a registered nurse who administers, signed by a second signatory (assessed as competent), who is then supervised by the registrant as the patient receives and consumes the medication.*

10 *You must clearly countersign the signature of the student when supervising a student in the administration of medicines.*

11 *These standards apply to all medicinal products.*

This standard clearly sets out not only what must be checked when administering medications to patients, but also the level of knowledge about each individual medicine, and patient. Practices such as undertaking a medicine round or administering intravenous medicines on other clinical areas present problems as the nurse may not be aware of care plans for the patients.

Clearly a substantial level of knowledge of both drugs and patients is required to comply with this standard, and medicine administration will take some time. It can be difficult to concentrate on a medicine round when the ward is busy, and numerous demands are placed on the nurse. It is imperative that nurses ensure that medicine rounds are given the necessary time for providing a safe environment. This has been recognised in the NHS Institute of Innovation and Improvement with their 'Productive Ward' initiative, which emphasises getting everything ready and ensuring that medicine rounds do not clash with other ward activities. For example, keeping the trolley tidy so that medicines can be found easily will prevent delays. In order to comply with Standard 8 of medicines management it is suggested that nurses develop a structured system of administration that adheres to both Standard 8 and individual Trust policy. The medicine administration records used varies between trusts but many are designed to facilitate checking. A suggested routine is set out in Box 18.2.

This may seem a long-winded method of administering medicines, particularly when the ward is busy and the patients are familiar, but given that medicine administration errors in hospital are between 3 and 5 per cent of total medication errors (Kelly and Wright 2011), nurses must maintain the standard to ensure patients are not harmed.

BOX 18.2 Suggested checking routine

- Check patient's name on the front of the chart and on the inside if double-paged. Confirm the name with the patient.
- Check for allergies.
- Check to see if there are any once-only medicines outstanding.
- Read the chart from left to right by checking the date of the prescription, which medicine, what time should it be administered, has it been signed by a prescriber? Are there any special instructions, for example, before or after meal? What is the duration of prescription and what time was it last given?
- Does the patient's condition give cause for concern based on your knowledge of the medicines and the individual patient? Ask how the patient is. Many side effects are symptoms rather than signs. Symptoms (nausea, dizziness) are felt by the patient. Signs (high or low BP) can be observed or measured. Check the observation chart. Open and closed questions can be used.
- Then find the medicine, check the correct dosage and expiry date. Place medicine in a pot and return the box or bottle to the correct place.
- Check the patient's name band against the patient details on the medication record chart to ensure it is the correct patient, remembering also to ask the patient, if they are able, to confirm their identity. Be prepared to answer any questions.
- Administer the medication, check it has been taken and sign the chart.

How much do nurses need to know?

This is perhaps a more difficult question than might be expected. There are a number of NMC documents that relate to this including the standards, which as indicated, demand a high level of knowledge and understanding of the drugs and how they work in the context of individual patients. As explained in Chapter 1, universities are required to ensure that their programme prepares students for practice and the details are contained in a document entitled *Standards for Pre-Registration Nursing* (NMC 2010a). These standards also apply to registered nurses as *Standards for Competence* (NMC 2010b). In relation to medicines management it simply states that:

> All nurses must practise safely by being aware of the correct use, limitations and hazards of common interventions, including nursing activities, treatments, the calculation and administration of medicines, and the use of medical devices and equipment.
>
> (NMC 2010a, p. 45)

The Essential Skills Clusters that detail what skills must be demonstrated to complete the programme are added to the document as an annex. These are incorporated into courses in different ways, and you may see them explicitly stated as a practice assessment. There are 42 statements of patient/client expectation, of which 10 are concerned with medicines management, and these, unlike the others, also have indicative content. Within

Claire Fullbrook-Scanlon

these statements there are 23 skills relating to medicines management to be met prior to registration including that the student:

35(iv) questions, critically appraises and uses evidence to support an argument in determining when medicines may or may not be an appropriate choice of treatment.

36(ii) applies knowledge of basic pharmacology, how medicines act and interact in the systems of the body, and their therapeutic action related to Branch practice.

(NMC 2010a, pp. 136–137).

It is worth spending a little time to look at the Essential Skills Clusters in conjunction with the *Standards for Medicines Management* and this will tell you that a good knowledge about how drugs work is essential to managing their use safely. However, it is not stated exactly how much needs to be known. The example that the NMC gives about digoxin in Standard 8 illustrates the point. Digoxin acts by slowing heart rate, and contra-indications given in the BNF include heart blocks, which may result in bradycardia. Heart block is also a side effect of digoxin. However, neither the BNF nor the drug information leaflet offers the advice that digoxin should not be given if the pulse is below 60. Nurses must exercise clinical judgement and accountability in viewing the pulse rate in the individual patient and clinical context.

Case 18.3

Martha, a second-year student nurse is asked to second check a controlled drug for Mrs Blackmoor, a 77-year-old woman admitted for pain control following a diagnosis of brain and bone metastases. Mrs Blackmoor is usually orientated in time and place and has not displayed any signs of memory loss or cognitive impairment. Morphine sulphate tablets (MST) 30mg is prescribed for 0800. It is now 0830 and Martha is assisting her patients with washing and dressing, but she agrees to be the second checker. She arrives at Mrs Blackmoor's bedside with the other nurse having already checked the prescription and CD record book in line with hospital policy. Mrs Blackmoor is sitting on the commode by the bedside. The Sister in charge, with whom Martha is checking, tells Martha that she will give the MST to Mrs Blackmoor and she can just sign the CD record book and medicines administration chart and return to her patients. Martha knows the patient on the commode is definitely Mrs Blackmoor, and she has been working with the Sister in charge for several shifts and thinks that she is trustworthy.

This scenario will be familiar to many nurses who may be impatient at having to spend so much time waiting when there is so much to do. Mrs Blackmoor may be some time on the commode (especially if the MST has made her constipated), and she may feel uneasy knowing that the nurses are waiting for her. There are a number of options. The tablet could be returned to the cupboard and signed back in, but this would itself be time-consuming. The tablet could be administered to Mrs Blackmoor while she is on the commode, but this seems undignified and unhygienic, though not completely out of the question depending on the circumstances and the relationship with Mrs Blackmoor; perhaps she has asked for this? What of the suggestion proposed by the ward manager that Martha signs the book and leaves the MST with the Sister? The standards (NMC

480

2007) states that 'it is good practice that the second signatory witnesses the whole administration process' (p. 25).

So it is clear that good practice is that Martha should not do as the Sister asks. However, these documents detail good practice rather than legal requirements, and these must be interpreted in the light of the circumstances. As a student Martha is acting under the accountability of the ward sister who may decide that the situation on the rest of the ward allows her not to follow good practice in this case. However, it is clear that the Sister's proposal should not be followed unless there are compelling reasons. If Martha was a registered nurse, she would be accountable for her actions, and would have to make the decision herself. If she did as the Sister asked she would be unable to sign the medicines administration record as she did not witness the tablet being taken. This is a good example of a decision where being an accountable professional requires more than just following instructions from the NMC or anyone else. It is also a good reason why Martha should know what is in the NMC standards, as they are not presented in a way that readily allows reference at the time a decision is needed. She should also be aware of other relevant documents like those from the Department of Health. These can be referred to when Martha reflects on the experience later.

Standard 9: Assessment (NMC 2007, pp. 26–27)

1   *As a registrant you are responsible for the initial and continued assessment of patients who are self-administering, and have continuing responsibility for recognising and acting upon changes in a patient's condition with regards to safety of the patient and others.*
2   *The NMC welcomes and supports the self-administration of medicinal products and the administration of medication by carers wherever it is appropriate. Registrants may assess the patients as suitable to self-administer medicinal products both in the hospital and primary care settings.*

Patients are encouraged wherever possible to take responsibility for their health. This is increasingly so in relation to self-administration of medicines, supported by many patients and patients' groups. See for example the Parkinson's Disease Society (PDS) 'Get it On Time' campaign (PDS undated), which has resources including an excellent short video. There is much more to self-medication than simply allowing and expecting patients to get on with it unsupported. The nurse retains a duty of care. Patients need to be assessed as to their ability to be able to undertake self-medicating safely. The NMC recommends that patients are assessed at three levels:

Level 1. *The registrant is responsible for the safe storage of the medicinal products and the supervision of the administration process ensuring the patient understands the medicinal product being administered.*
Level 2. *The registrant is responsible for the safe storage of the medicinal products. At administration time the patient will ask the registrant to open the cabinet/ locker. The patient will then self-administer the medication under the supervision of the registrant.*
Level 3. *The patient accepts full responsibility for the storage and administration of the medicinal products. The registrant checks the patient's suitability and compliance verbally.*

> *The level should be documented in the patient's notes.*
>
> (NMC 2007, pp. 26–27)

When patients are self-medicating the nurse is not liable in the case of an error providing the risk assessment was completed and documented in accordance with local policy. There is further guidance about exclusion criteria in Annex 4.

Adherence with medication is an important aspect of medicines management, but not directly addressed in the standards. It is known that there are low levels of adherence across a range of long-term conditions (Bowskill and Garner 2012). Like the NMC standard above, some studies (Carter *et al.* 2005) used the term 'compliance', but this has been criticised as it reinforces the image of a power relationship with the patient complying with the health care professional's instructions. The need for a partnership approach to medicines management is emphasised and NICE has produced guidelines regarding patients achieving adherence with their medications (NICE 2009). The aim of the guidance was to encourage health care professionals actively to involve their patients in the decision-making process by adopting a patient-centred approach, encouraging informed adherence and identifying any perceived or practical barriers the patient may have to taking the medication.

Standard 10: Self-administration – children and young people (NMC 2007, p. 28)

In the case of children, when arrangements have been made for parents, carers or patients to administer their own medicines prior to discharge or rehabilitation, the registrant should ascertain that the medicinal products have been taken as prescribed.

It is recommended that this is performed by direct observation but if appropriate this could be done by questioning the patient, parent or carer. When the nurse has not been involved directly in the administration of the medication the medicines administration record should be initialled and the term 'patient self-administration' documented. Nurses must be aware that while parents or carers should be encouraged to administer medicines to their children caution should be applied as doses may be omitted in error.

Standard 11: Remote prescription or direction to administer (NMC 2007, p. 28)

In exceptional circumstances, where medication (not including Controlled Drugs) has been previously prescribed and the prescriber is unable to issue a new prescription, but where changes to the dose are considered necessary, the use of information technology (such as fax, text message or e-mail) may be used but must confirm any change to the original prescription.

The guidance suggests that a verbal order is not acceptable on its own. There should be an accompanying fax or e-mail confirming any new direction and it is recommended that students refer to local policy.

Standard 12: Text messaging (NMC 2007, p. 30)

As a registrant, you must ensure that there are protocols in place to ensure patient confidentiality and documentation of any text received include: complete text message, telephone number (it was sent from), the time sent, any response given, and the signature and date received by the registrant.

With increasing use of mobile phones and advancing technology it is possible to concede that texts may be used in exceptional circumstances to confirm medication directions. If this does happen it is good practice to ensure that a second nurse observes the text and the subsequent documentation, for example, the medicines administration record, to confirm the text message. In line with maintaining confidentiality all text messages of this nature should be deleted from the phone as soon as possible to comply with information governance directives.

Standard 13: Titration (NMC 2007, p. 30)

Where medication has been prescribed within a range of dosages it is acceptable for registrants to titrate dosages according to patient response and symptom control and to administer within the prescribed range.

This refers to medication regimes such as sliding scales of insulin where the amount of insulin to be infused depends on the blood glucose levels at the time of administration. The nurse must ensure that she is competent to interpret test results such as blood glucose levels prior to administration of the medicinal product. She will also need to be competent in using the specific pump or other medical equipment.

Standard 14: Preparing medication in advance (NMC 2007, p. 30)

Registrants must not prepare substances for injection in advance of their immediate use or administer medication drawn into a syringe or container by another practitioner when not in their presence.

The language in this standard is clear and unambiguous. Practices such as drawing up all the IV drugs in advance are not allowed. There are some exceptions, for example, where an infusion is already running, or where medication has been prepared in the pharmacy.

Case 18.4

Dilip is a staff nurse on a surgical ward. Hannah, one of his colleagues, is finishing her morning drug round and is in the process of drawing up IV medication. Suddenly the emergency call button is activated from one of her patients. Hannah asks Dilip to give the medication telling him that it is the last vial on the ward. She tells him that the medication has been checked by another registered nurse but that the vial has been discarded.

The NMC standard here is unambiguous. Despite an understandable wish to assist his colleague and more importantly ensure that the patient receives timely medication, Dilip should not give the medication, as he has no way of checking the medication against the prescription. Local policy may not require two people to check intravenous injections, though Dilip is aware that Standard 20 states that two registrants should check IV medication wherever possible. He wonders whether this would be considered 'an exceptional circumstance where this is not possible'. Dilip considers putting a sterile cap on the syringe and storing it appropriately in line with the drug information leaflet. However, Standard 14 unambiguously states that substances must not be prepared in advance of their *immediate* use. As in all decisions made by accountable professionals, the details are important; there would be a difference between a minute's delay and an hour's delay. Dilip and Hannah are aware of the importance of ensuring that the patient receives the medicine, and there will be a considerable delay if additional stock has to be ordered and delivered. Perhaps Dilip can assist at the emergency so that Hannah can give the injection. Standard 14 makes it clear that Dilip should not give the medicine, and Hannah may be required to account for her decision if she gives it after a delay.

Standard 15: Medication acquired over the Internet (NMC 2007, p. 31)

Registrants should never administer any medication that has not been prescribed, or that has been acquired over the internet without a valid prescription.

Many medications are available for purchase over the Internet. Increasingly medicines are bought to save patients time or embarrassment or because a request may have been refused by a prescriber. Examples are slimming pills or phosphodiesterase type-5 inhibitors (e.g., Viagra) for erectile dysfunction. The standard uses the word 'never', but the guidance following the standard goes on to give some circumstances when registrants can give medication purchased abroad without a UK product licence.

In a life-threatening situation or where the patient refuses to take anything but the 'unlicensed product' and they are unable to administer themselves the registrant may administer the medication in conjunction with locally agreed policies. In all circumstances a clear, accurate and contemporaneous record of all communication and administration of medication should be maintained.

Standard 16: Aids to support compliance (NMC 2007, p. 32)

1. *Registrants must assess the patient's suitability and understanding of how to use an appropriate compliance aid safely.*

4. *The mechanics of crushing medicines may alter their therapeutic properties rendering them ineffective and are not covered by their product licence. Medicinal products should not routinely be crushed unless a pharmacist advises that the medication is not compromised by crushing, and crushing has been determined to be within the patient's best interest (see Standard 22).*

5. *As a general principle, by disguising medication in food or drink, the patient or client is being led to believe they are not receiving medication, when in fact they are. The NMC would not consider this to be good practice. The registrant would need to be sure what they are doing is in the best interests of the patient, and that they are accountable for this decision. (See chapter 3)*

Standard 17: Delegation (NMC 2007, p. 32)

A registrant is responsible for the delegation of any aspects of the administration of medicinal products and they are accountable to ensure that the patient, carer or assistant is competent to carry out the task.

The guidance following this standard states that this will require education, training and assessment of the patient or carer/care assistant. Records of training received and outcomes should be kept.

Case 18.5

Naomi is a registered nurse working on a medical ward. It is the early shift and she is undertaking the drug round. Mrs Pilot is a 48-year-old lady who has motor neurone disease and is receiving palliative care. Her daughter Jean aged 18 wishes to be involved in her care as much as possible and has been in hospital for the last few days helping with washing, toileting and feeding. Mrs Pilot has some difficulty swallowing her medication and Jean offers to assist her mother.

Mrs Pilot's views about her daughter are very important; she needs to be willing for her daughter to undertake this role in hospital and at home. As the accountable nurse Naomi needs to be sure that Jean is competent to administer the medication. Naomi should arrange to supervise Jean giving the medicine to her mother and this will involve arranging sufficient time to be able to explain how and when to give the medicine. If there are swallowing difficulties, referral to another practitioner may be required. With Mrs Pilot's permission and co-operation, Jean will also need to know what the medicine is for and what to do if there is a problem in giving it. Naomi must ensure that all discussions with Jean are fully documented.

Standard 19: Unregistered practitioners (NMC 2007, p. 33)

In delegating the administration of medicinal products to unregistered practitioners, it is the registrant who must apply the principles of administration of medicinal products as listed above. They may then delegate an unregistered practitioner to assist the patient in the ingestion or application of the medicinal product.

Delegating aspects of medicines management to unregistered practitioners is similar to delegating any other task. Clause 11 of the *The Code* (NMC 2015) requires that nurses be accountable for decisions to delegate tasks and duties to other people. You must:

- only delegate tasks and duties that are within the other person's scope of competence, making sure that they fully understand your instructions;
- make sure that everyone you delegate tasks to is adequately supervised and supported so they can provide safe and compassionate care;
- confirm that the outcome of any task delegated to someone else meets the required standard;
- have in place an indemnity arrangement that provides appropriate cover for any practice you take on as a nurse or midwife in the United Kingdom.

The delegating registered nurse remains accountable to ensure that medicines are correctly administered, and will need to decide if the unregistered practitioner is competent to assist the patient in taking the medicines. For some tasks, there may be local policy detailing required training and assessment of competence, and personal experience of a fellow team member may help the nurse to decide how trustworthy the unregistered practitioner is, whether for example she is likely to forget to give the medicine. It should be remembered that unregistered practitioners are unlikely to know what the medicine is for and may not be able to prioritise. For CDs, the unregistered practitioner must remain under 'direct supervision'. In an exploratory study in inpatient psychiatric wards, Dickens *et al.* (2008) found that care workers administered 17 per cent of medication, just under half of which was administered out of sight of the accountable nurse.

Standard 20: Intravenous medication (NMC 2007, p. 34)

Wherever possible two registrants should check medication to be administered intravenously, one of whom should also be the registrant who administers the IV medication.

The NPSA suggests that the incidence of errors in prescribing, preparing and administering injectable medicines is higher than any other form of medicine (NPSA 2007a, Taxis and Barber 2003). Guidance following Standard 20 suggests that in exceptional circumstances if a second registrant is not available to check the medication then a second person who has been deemed competent to undertake this task should be approached. This may be another health care professional, a parent/carer or the patient. The guidance refers to three other publications. The guidance states that 'registrants should be aware of the risks identified in the NPSA fourth report from the Patient Safety Observatory' (NMC 2007, p. 34, NPSA 2007b). The report is discussed in more detail in Part 3 of this chapter. The guidance goes on to emphasise the duty to monitor the patient and their response during the administration of IV therapy, and suggests that the standards for the administration of IV therapy from the RCN should be viewed. The link is to the RCN homepage and the document can be found by searching under its correct name, *Standards for Infusion Therapy: Third edition* (RCN 2010). It is 94 pages long but it is a comprehensive resource.

Standard 21: Disposal (NMC 2007, p. 35)

A registrant must dispose of medicinal products in accordance with legislation.

Disposal of unwanted/unused or out-of-date medicines is a complex issue governed by legislation. Medicines from a patient's own home and from residential homes are considered household waste. Medicines and clinical waste from hospitals and nursing homes are considered industrial waste. Disposal of medicines into sinks/waste water should be avoided. Hospital and local pharmacies can give advice regarding the safe disposal of medicines.

Standard 22: Unlicensed medicines (NMC 2007, p. 35)

A registrant may administer an unlicensed medicinal product with the patient's informed consent against a patient-specific direction but NOT against a patient group direction.

Unlicensed medicine is one that has no marketing authorisation. Unlicensed medication may be seen for patients who have agreed to take part in research trials of new drugs that have not yet received their product licence from the MHRA. If it is suspected that there has been an adverse drug reaction or there is reason to think that the patient should not be receiving this medicine, the investigator of the trial should be contacted as soon as possible. The nurse has a responsibility to understand potential side effects and contra-indications of unlicensed medications before administration. For example, if a patient is taking a trial medicine that is purported to be a new anti-platelet medication then they would not be able to give any prescribed licensed anti-platelet such as aspirin in conjunction with the trial medication unless authorised to do so. Details about administering medicines in clinical trials are given in Annexe 5.

Some patients have swallowing difficulties, for example people who have had a stroke or have head and neck cancer. When people are unable to take medicines it can be tempting to 'help' the patients with their medicines by opening capsules onto food or to dissolve in water or by crushing medicines and trying to put them into nasogastric tubes or percutaneous gastrostomy tubes. Nurses must be aware that the opening of capsules/crushing of medication can alter the form of the medication so that it is then used in an 'unlicensed' form. The term 'modified release' informs us that the drug is manufactured to allow the medicine to be released over a period of time, and abbreviations in drug names can indicate that their mode of action is modified release (M/R LA, CR, XL, SR, f/c s/c). Words such as slow, continuous or retard in the title also indicate modified release. Opening the capsule for the patient will result in the patient receiving the full dose quicker than intended. Enteric coating (EC) allows the drug to pass through the stomach before being released, so crushing an enteric-coated tablet negates this.

If a drug that is being used outside of its product licence causes harm, manufacturers will not accept liability. It is poor practice to crush a tablet prior to administration unless written authorisation from the prescriber has been obtained. It is also worth noting that even when written permission has been given by a prescriber to use the product unlicensed the administering nurse may still remain partially liable should the patient come to any harm (Wright 2002, 2006).

Standard 23: Complementary and alternative therapies (NMC 2007, p. 36)

Registrants must have successfully undertaken training and be competent to practise the administration of complementary and alternative therapies.

Many members of the public purchase treatments such as plant remedies or undertake therapies such as massage or reiki. These treatments can be taken alone or combined with more traditional medicine. Increasingly, nurses choose to undertake alternative and complementary practices in their career. However, the NMC regulates the practice of nursing and midwifery and is not responsible for overseeing other types of training and education. Therefore nurses must take responsibility in deciding whether they have sufficient qualifications and education to offer such therapies to people in their care. Furthermore, they must ensure that they have sufficient insurance and/or vicarious liability in the therapy they intend to practise within their existing employment. In relation to administration of alternative remedies, nurses must be aware that it is being administered and its possible effects, for example, St John's wort may interact with orthodox medicines.

Standard 24: Management of adverse events (NMC 2007, p. 37)

As a registrant, if you make an error you must take any action to prevent any potential harm to the patient and report as soon as possible the prescriber, your line manager or employer (according to local policy) and document your actions. Midwives should also inform their named Supervisor of Midwives.

According to the NPSA (2007a) 59.3 per cent of medication incidents reported between January 2005 and June 2006 were related to administration errors. The majority of these incidents were related to the patient being given the wrong dose, strength or frequency, the wrong medicine or the dose was omitted. Drug errors are discussed in more detail in Part 3 of this chapter. Be mindful that *The Code* (NMC 2015, p. 9) states that you must 'Be open and candid with all service users about all aspects of care and treatment, including when any mistakes or harm have taken place.' The duty of candour is discussed in Chapter 1.

Standard 25: Reporting adverse reactions (NMC 2007, p. 38)

As a registrant, if a patient experiences an adverse drug reaction to a medication you must take any action to remedy harm caused by the reaction. You must record this in the patient's notes, notify the prescriber (if you did not prescribe the drug) and notify via the Yellow Card Scheme immediately.

Any drug has the potential of causing an adverse drug reaction and causing an unintended harmful effect. Nurses should be aware of potential side effects of all drugs they are administering (see Standard 8), and these are stated in the BNF and in information leaflets. This is important as nurses should understand the difference between possible disease progression and potential side effects. Reporting adverse drug reaction is an easy process. Yellow cards can be found in the BNF and reporting can also be undertaken online at http://yellowcard.mhra.gov.uk/.

Standard 26: Controlled drugs (NMC 2007, p. 38)

Registrants should ensure that patients prescribed controlled drugs are administered these in a timely fashion in line with the standards for administering medication to patients. Registrants should comply with and follow the legal requirements and approved local Standard Operating Procedures for controlled drugs that are appropriate for their area of work.

The use of CDs in England, Wales and Scotland is governed by the Misuse of Drugs Act (1971), and the Misuse of Drugs Regulations 2001. The Act provides the statutory framework for the control and regulation of CDs (DH 2007a), which are addictive and produce dependence (Downie *et al.* 2008). CDs are permitted for use in medicine by the Misuse of Drugs Regulations (MDR) and are classified according to the potential harm they can cause if abused, and there was much debate in the media concerning the reclassification of cannabis from class B to class C and back again (Nutt 2012). Unlawful possession of CDs is a criminal offence and carries stiff penalties, more so on conviction of dealing. Penalties for possession and dealing in CDs are given in Table 18.4.

Procedures relating to CDs were strengthened after the murders committed by Dr Harold Shipman (DH 2004a). Government guidelines relating to CDs were published in 2007 (DH 2007b) and were amended and incorporated into the Controlled Drugs (Supervision of management and use) Regulations (DH 2013a). All NHS Trusts, Foundation Trusts and other independent health care organisations such as nursing homes are accountable for all aspects of monitoring the usage and disposal of CDs. They are required to identify an accountable officer for this specific role. In England these are called NHS England controlled drugs accountable officers (CDAOs) (CQC 2015a). CDAOs

TABLE 18.4 Penalties for unlawful possession of controlled drugs

Class	Examples	Penalties for . . .	
		Possession	Dealing
A	Crack cocaine, cocaine, ecstasy (MDMA), heroin, LSD, magic mushrooms, methadone, methamphetamine (crystal meth)	Up to 7 years in prison or an unlimited fine or both	Up to life in prison or an unlimited fine or both
B	Amphetamines, barbiturates, cannabis, codeine, ketamine, methylphenidate (Ritalin), synthetic cannabinoids, synthetic cathinones (e.g. mephedrone, methoxetamine)	Up to 5 years in prison or an unlimited fine or both	Up to 14 years in prison or an unlimited fine or both
C	Anabolic steroids, benzodiazepines (diazepam), gamma hydroxybutyrate (GHB), gamma-butyrolactone (GBL), piperazines (BZP), khat	Up to 2 years in prison or an unlimited fine or both (except anabolic steroids – it's not an offence to possess them for personal use)	Up to 14 years in prison or an unlimited fine or both
Temporary class drugs (awaiting classification)	Some methylphenidate substances (ethylphenidate, 3,4-dichloromethylphenidate (3,4-DCMP), methylnaphthidate (HDMP-28), isopropylphenidate (IPP or IPPD), 4-methylmethyl-phenidate, ethylnaphthidate, propylphenidate) and their simple derivatives	None, but police can take away a suspected temporary class drug	Up to 14 years in prison, an unlimited fine or both

Source: www.gov.uk/penalties-drug-possession-dealing.

Claire Fullbrook-Scanlon

are responsible for the management of controlled drugs including safe storage, usage, auditing and the investigation of any concerns or untoward incidents involving controlled drugs. They are also responsible for ensuring that relevant staff within their organisation have received information and education appropriate to their needs in order to comply with the regulations. The CDAO should be a senior executive who is not routinely involved in the prescribing, supply, administration or disposal of controlled drugs. This could be a director of nursing, chief pharmacist or medical director. The Care Quality Commission maintains a register of all CDAOs.

Although each organisation has a CDAO, each registered nurse in charge of a ward or department is responsible for the safety and management of the controlled drugs in their clinical area/department. As a registered nurse you can allow access to the CDs by another registered health care practitioner, but the legal responsibility for the CDs remains with you at all times throughout your shift (DH 2007a). Nurses are strongly advised to familiarise themselves with their local policies before undertaking this responsibility.

The guidance that follows Standard 26 is comprehensive, detailing specific arrangements for ordering, transporting and administering CDs. Some Trusts exceed the minimum legal requirements by, for example, extending the arrangements to other medicines. Guidance about administering CDs is contained in Standard 8.

Access to the standards

In some ways the *Standards for Medicines Management* is a frustrating document, posing as many questions as it answers. However, a feature of professional practice is that professionals must be accountable for the decisions that they make, and this precludes a list of actions that must always be followed. Even where wording is apparently unambiguous, cases can be constructed to cast doubt on such certainty. The standards are those against which registrants will be compared in justifying decisions and, if for this reason alone, all students should have access to them. Unfortunately paper copies are not available, but the document and a summary version can be downloaded from the NMC website. As students progress through their programmes, they will be required to take on a greater role in medicines management, and discussions with their mentors must refer to the standards.

PART 3: EXPLORING MEDICINES MANAGEMENT

Non-medical prescribing

Non-medical prescribing is a relatively new area of prescribing. The concept originates from the Cumberledge Report (DHSS 1986), which examined the care given to people in their own homes by district and community nurses. The report found that a lot of time was wasted by nurses in requesting prescriptions from the GP for their patients. The report concluded with recommendations for community nurses to be able to prescribe. In 1989 Dr June Crown was asked to chair an advisory group to investigate the possibility of nurse prescribing (DH 1989). This report made several recommendations suggesting items and situations in which suitably qualified nurses could prescribe. The primary legislation, the Medicinal Products: Prescribing by Nurses Act (1992) allowed nurses to prescribe from a limited formulary for specific conditions. A further Crown Report (DH 1999)

490

recommended that prescribing authority should be made available to other non-medical professionals with appropriate training and expertise.

Supplementary prescribing is a voluntary prescribing partnership between the independent prescriber (doctor or dentist) and a supplementary prescriber, to implement an agreed patient-specific clinical management plan (CMP) with the patient's permission (DH 2006). Supplementary prescribers amend dosages within set limits set by independent prescribers. **Independent prescribing** allows nurse prescribers to prescribe any medication, including CDs, for any medical condition that she is competent to treat.

In order to be able to undertake a training programme enabling nurses to prescribe, eligibility criteria, set by the NMC must be satisfied (NMC 2006). These standards are being reviewed and should be replaced in 2017. There are different qualifications that can lead to nurses being able to prescribe from the Nurse Prescribers' Formulary, (which includes, for example, nicotine replacement therapy and elastic hosiery), or to become supplementary or independent prescribers.

The educational programme for independent prescribers must be approved by the NMC and the face-to-face course must be of a minimum duration of 26 days plus 12 additional days of supervised learning in practice. There are also standards concerning assessment for the programme, including an examination and a numerical assessment for which the pass mark is 100 per cent.

Registered nurses and students working in primary, secondary or tertiary care, will need to be aware of the limitations of the independent prescribers. For instance, a nurse prescriber will not prescribe medication for a patient that the prescriber has not assessed, or that has a condition outside of the prescriber's specialist area. You will also need to be aware of who is a non-medical prescriber so that you are able to refer any issues relating to the medication to the prescriber.

Supplementary prescribing is a voluntary prescribing partnership between the independent prescriber (doctor or dentist) and a supplementary prescriber, to implement an agreed patient-specific clinical management plan (CMP) with the patient's permission

Independent prescribing allows nurses to prescribe any licensed medicine for any medical condition that a nurse prescriber is competent to treat, including some controlled drugs.

Case 18.6

Abdul is a community psychiatric nurse with the early intervention service for adolescents. He has undertaken the independent and supplementary educational training programme and has this qualification recorded on the NMC Register. Among his caseload is William, a 17-year-old with newly diagnosed bipolar disorder. As an independent prescriber Abdul is able to see William regularly in his own home and prescribe valproic acid, a medication licensed for use in manic episodes associated with bipolar disorder. Abdul is able to titrate this medication according to clinical need. By doing this as an independent prescriber, Abdul takes responsibility for clinical assessment and diagnosis of William's presenting condition. He is also accountable for the prescribed clinical management William requires. If Abdul was unable to prescribe then William would need to make frequent visits to the psychiatric hospital to see the medical team. By prescribing independently, Abdul saves William time and also ensures that he gets the right treatment as early as possible.

Antimicrobial stewardship

Antibiotics have been used to treat or prevent bacterial infections since the 1940s following Sir Alexander Fleming's discovery of penicillin. There are many antibiotics available and each antibiotic is used to treat specific types of infection. Antibiotics have

RESEARCH FOCUS 18.1

Tinelli *et al.* (2015) undertook a survey that asked patients about their experiences of being seen by nurses and pharmacists acting as non-medical prescribers. Six sites in the UK were sampled, and the most common clinical conditions were asthma, diabetes and secondary prevention of coronary heart disease. The survey covered a wide range of issues with prescribing practice, but overall, 94.4 per cent of those seen by the nurse prescriber, and 87 per cent of those seen by the pharmacist were satisfied with their consultation. The survey also asked patients to compare the care they received from the independent non-medical prescribers to that they received from doctors. The majority (73.9 per cent) reported no difference with almost the same number (12.7 per cent) reporting better care from the nurse prescriber as reported better care from the doctor (13.4 per cent). Overall the study concluded that independent prescribing by nurses and pharmacists for long-term conditions was well received by patients who reported having established good relationships with their NMP and having confidence in the care provided. Most patients did not express a strong preference for care provided by either their non-medical or medical prescribers with a small subgroup preferring to receive care from their doctor. These findings support the further implementation of non-medical prescribing to support patients with long-term conditions (Tinelli *et al.* 2015, p. 1253).

been used to treat minor infections such as infected toe nails to more serious and life-threatening conditions, for example meningitis. Antimicrobial resistance is a term that refers to the 'loss of effectiveness of any antiinfective medicine, including antiviral, antifungal, antibacterial and antiparasitic' (NICE 2015b, p. 7) and has been cited by the World Health Organization as one of the three greatest threats to human health (WHO 2011, Ness *et al.* 2014). In 2013 the Department of Health set out their Five Year Antimicrobial Resistance Strategy (DH 2013b). The document clearly acknowledges that a case for action is required against antimicrobial resistance. The aim of the strategy is to:

- improve the knowledge and understanding of antimicrobial resistance;
- conserve and steward the effectiveness of existing treatments;
- stimulate the development of new antibiotics, diagnostics and therapies.

(DH 2013b, p. 7)

There are a number of things that nurses can do to support the aims of the antimicrobial resistance strategy. We need to take universal precautions with the prevention and spread of infection. (Please refer to Trust policies for further guidance.) Nurses are well placed to advise patients and the public regarding the appropriateness of antibiotics. McNulty *et al.* (2013) found that patients contacting their general practitioner with respiratory tract infection expected an antibiotic prescription for their symptoms. Nurses can take all opportunities to help educate their patients and the public regarding the misconception that antibiotics are always required for self-limiting illnesses and can help manage patients' expectations. Nurses are also able to explain to patients who are prescribed antibiotics why it is important to complete the whole course and not keep some back for later use. Another way in which nurses can help with antibiotic stewardship is to ensure all antibiotic prescriptions have an end date clearly written. This not only applies to non-medical prescribers who are often required to prescribe antibiotics but also to ward nurses who are reading medicine administration records when undertaking medicines rounds. European Antibiotic Awareness Day occurs on 18 November each year. To help slow the advance of antimicrobial resistance you could visit http://antibioticguardian.com/ and pledge to become an antibiotic guardian.

Managing medication errors

The NPSA (2007a) document *Safety in Doses: Improving the use of medicines in the NHS* reports that between January 2005 and June 2006 NHS staff had reported 59,802 medication safety incidents via the National Reporting and Learning System (NRLS). Approximately 80 per cent of these incidents occurred in acute general and community hospitals: 83 per cent of these errors did not result in any harm, 16.6 per cent caused low and moderate harm and 0.2 per cent resulted in severe harm (54 in total) and there were 38 deaths (NPSA 2007a). The NPSA (2007a) found that the wrong dose, strength or frequency of medication accounted for over a quarter of all medication incidents reported to them (28.7 per cent), indicating that perhaps there are problems in numeracy among nurses. More recently a systematic review covering hospital health care worldwide in the last 28 years by Keers *et al.* (2013) found that medication administration errors are caused by multifactorial systems and processes. The causes identified from the review by Keers *et al.* (2013) included: slips and lapses, that is, misreading of medication charts/drug labels and lack of concentration, calculation errors were commonly reported, nurses feeling fatigued, and sickness as well as stress of the nurses. Inexperienced staff made medication errors as well as nurses who had not received adequate training, and the review highlighted a lack of learning opportunities from previous mistakes. Ofuso and Jarrett (2015) suggested the main causes of medication errors include interruptions and distractions, poor drug calculations skills and inadequate education and compliance. Interestingly Kelly and Wright (2011) found that medication errors were more common in care of the elderly wards rather than general medical or surgical wards.

A common error is giving the wrong medicine, responsible for 11.5 per cent of incidents reported to the NPSA (2007a). This may be attributed to the nurse giving the medication to a patient with a similar name or a similar-sounding medication. It may also be because the nurse was unable to read the writing on the medication administration record. If there is any doubt about a prescription you should *never* administer the medication. If handwriting is illegible the prescriber must be contacted and asked to rewrite the prescription clearly.

Errors can also occur because the incorrect drug formulation is prepared, for example, antibiotics not correctly diluted with water for injection or administered as a bolus injection instead of via an infusion. A drug may be administered via the wrong route, for example, given orally instead of rectally, or may be written intramuscularly but given intravenously by mistake.

Unfortunately nurses and midwives do make medication errors despite the policies, standards and procedures in place to minimise their occurrence. Between 2005 and 2010, 525,186 medication error incidents were reported to the National Reporting and Learning

Claire Fullbrook-Scanlon

FIGURE 18.2
Answers to
exercise in Activity
18.3

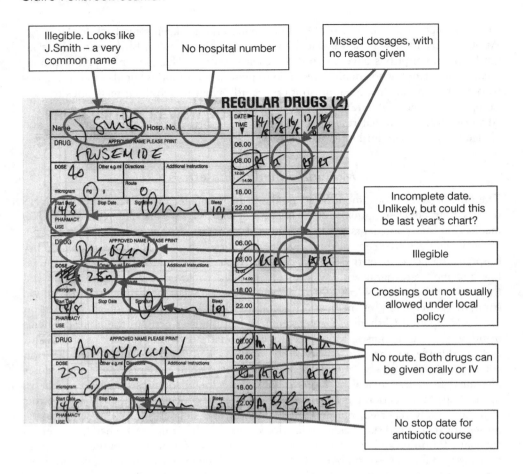

Systems (MHRA 2014). The NPSA (2007b) notes that international research suggests a significant level of under-reporting of errors. Errors can result from genuine mistakes, but failure to report a known error can indicate dishonesty and a breach of *The Code* (NMC 2015), which states that

> you make sure that patient and public safety is protected. You work within the limits of your competence, exercising your professional 'duty of candour' and raising concerns immediately whenever you come across situations that put patients or public safety at risk.

> (NMC 2015, p. 11)

Furthermore, clause 14 states 'You must be open and candid with all service users about all aspects of care and treatment, including when any mistakes or harm have taken place' NMC (2015, p. 11). If you discover a medication error or realise that you have made a medication error you are required to take action to prevent any potential harm to the patient. Below are suggestions as to what you should do in the event of a medication error, but these should be read in conjunction with your local policies.

1   Check that the patient is not in immediate danger, for example, anaphylaxis, respiratory distress. If this occurs start emergency procedures. You must remember to inform the doctors what drug has caused this reaction.
2   A full assessment of the patient must be undertaken, paying particular attention to signs of medication activity. For example, if an antihypertensive drug is given in error to a person who is normally hypotensive, blood pressure will need to be closely monitored.
3   If the patient is not in need of immediate clinical assistance you should inform the nurse in charge of the ward without delay of the error that has occurred.
4   The prescriber/doctor should be informed as soon as possible so that they may take any clinical action necessary. The error and subsequent action should be recorded in the patient's notes.
5   A clinical incident form must be completed. It is a requirement that all serious errors and near misses are reported to the National Reporting and Learning System (NRLS).
6   The error should be discussed with the patient concerned and/or where appropriate with their next of kin. This is following a recommendation of duty of candour to promote a more open culture within the NHS when things go wrong (CQC 2015b).
7   Making a drug error can be very upsetting for the nurse, and you may benefit from discussing it with an experienced colleague, or representative. An investigation may be undertaken, and it is to be hoped that the nurse making the error reflects on the experience and learns from it. Evidence of learning may be required by the employer.

Case 18.7

Jenny is a newly qualified staff nurse working night duty on a medical ward. She is undertaking the medication round at 2300 hours. Mrs Patel is a 45-year-old woman who has recently been admitted with a deep vein thrombosis. She has been treated with Clexane subcutaneously and has now been commenced on a loading dose of warfarin. When Jenny gets to Mrs Patel she discovers that the warfarin due at 1800 has not been signed for on the medication administration chart. Mrs Patel is sleepy and English is not her first language. Due to Mrs Patel's limited understanding, Jenny is unable to ascertain whether Mrs Patel has taken the warfarin. Jenny knows that the nurse on the previous shift has been working for the last 4 days and is due in again the next morning. She is also aware that this nurse is extremely tired and is probably asleep at home. What should she do?

The Code (2015, clause 19) states that you must be aware of and reduce as far as possible any potential for harm associated with your practice. Will Mrs Patel be at risk of potential harm if the warfarin is omitted? The answer here is yes, there is potential harm. Jenny must contact the on-call doctor to ask what action should be taken. Jenny should record all of her actions in the patient's notes and complete a clinical incident form as she has discovered a medication omission that constitutes an error. In an attempt to seek more information, Jenny should also consider ringing the staff nurse on duty the previous evening, depending on the exact circumstances.

Claire Fullbrook-Scanlon

Although it may seem daunting to admit to a medication error, you are bound by the *Code* and your employer to minimise the risk to the patient and to report the incident. It is acknowledged that managers in the NHS historically blame individuals for errors (DH 2000). However, increasingly managers are being urged to look at the numerous complex causes of administration errors (DH 2004b) and use education and retraining as opposed to punitive measures.

CONCLUSION

Administering medicines has been a part of nursing practice for many years. Recently the role of the nurse has extended to management of medicines requiring considerable knowledge and skills. Prescribing medicine is part of practice for more experienced nurses. The growing responsibilities of nurses in the area of medicines management, partly as a result of changes in health policy and technology, have been recognised by the NMC with the publication of a comprehensive set of standards. This chapter has reproduced and discussed these standards in some detail, and they must be considered required reading for all students and nurses.

SUGGESTED FURTHER READING

Websites

A table of organisations and websites is given in Part 1 of this chapter (Table 18.2). All of these have valuable resources.

The NMC *Standards for Medicines Management* are required reading. Available at www.nmc-uk.org

The collection of patient information sheets for drugs is available at www.emc.medicines.org.uk

Textbooks

There are some good pharmacology textbooks for nurses available including:

Barber, P. and Robertson, B. (2015) *Essential Pharmacology for Nurses* (3rd edn). Maidenhead, UK: Open University Press.
Downie, G., Mackenzie, J., Williams, A. and Hind, C. (2008) *Pharmacology and Medicines Management for Nurses* (4th edn). Edinburgh: Churchill Livingstone.
Greenstein, B. and Gould, D. (2009) *Trounce's Clinical Pharmacology for Nurses*, (18th edn). Edinburgh: Churchill Livingstone.

REFERENCES

Bowskill, D. and Garner, L. (2012). Medicines non-adherence: adult literacy and implications for practice. *British Journal of Nursing* **21** (19), 1156–1159.
CQC (Care Quality Commission) (2015a) *The Safer Management of Controlled Drugs: Annual report.* www.cqc.org.uk (accessed 15 February 2016).

Carter, S., Taylor, D. and Levenson, R. (2005) *A Question of Choice: Compliance in medicine taking – A preliminary view*. London: Medicines Partnership.

DH (Department of Health) (1989) *Report on the Advisory Group on Nurse Prescribing* (Crown Report). London: DH.

DH (1999) *Review of Prescribing, Supply and Administration of Medicines* (Crown Report). London: DH.

DH (2000) *An Organisation with a Memory*. London: DH.

DH (2004a) *Safer Management of Controlled Drugs: The Government's response to the Fourth Report of the Shipman Inquiry*. London: DH.

DH (2004b) *Building a Safer NHS for Patients: Improving medication safety*. London: DH.

DH (2006) *Medicines Matter: A guide to the mechanisms for the prescribing, supply and administration of medicines*. London: DH.

DH (2007a) *Safer Management of Controlled Drugs: A guide to good practice in secondary care (England)*. London: DH.

DH (2007b) *Safer Management of Controlled Drugs: Guidance on standard operating procedures for controlled drugs*. London: DH.

DH (2008) *Medicines Management: Everybody's business: A guide for service users, carers, and health and social care practitioners*. London: DH.

DH (2013a) *Controlled Drugs (Supervision of management and use) Regulations* London: DH.

DH (2013b) *UK Five Year Antimicrobial Resistance Strategy 2013–2018*. London: DH.

DHSS (Department of Health and Social Security) (1986) *Neighbourhood Nursing: A focus for care (Cumberledge Report)*. London: DH.

Dickens, G., Stubbs, J. and Haw, H. (2008) Delegation of medication administration: an exploratory study. *Nursing Standard* 22 (22), 35–40.

Downie, G., Mackenzie, J., Williams, A. and Hind, C. (2008) *Pharmacology and Medicines Management for Nurses* (4th edn). Edinburgh: Churchill Livingstone.

Gauld, N. J., Kelly, F. S., Kurosawa, N., Bryant, L. J., Emmerton, L. M. and Buetow, S. A. (2014). Widening consumer access to medicines through switching medicines to non-prescription: a six country comparison. *PloS ONE* 9 (9), e107726.

HSCIC (Health and Social Care Information Centre) (2014) *Hospital Prescribing England 2013–2014* www.hscic.gov.uk/catalogue/PUB15883 (accessed 15 February 2016).

Kelly, J. and Wright, D. (2011) Medicine administration errors and their severity in secondary care older persons ward: a multi-centre observational study. *Journal of Clinical Nursing* 21 (13–14), 1806–1815.

Keers R. N., Williams, S. D., Cooke, J. and Ashcroft, D. M. (2013) Causes of medication administration errors in hospitals: a systematic review of quantitative and qualitative evidence. *Drug Safety* 36, 1045–1067.

McNulty, C. A., Nichols, T., French, D. P., Joshi, P. and Butler, C. C. (2013) Expectations for consultations and antibiotics for respiratory tract infection in primary care: the RTI clinical iceberg. *British Journal of General Practice* 63 (612), e429–e436.

MHRA (Medicines and Healthcare Products Regulatory Agency) (2012) *A Guide to What is a Medicinal Product* London: MHRA.

MHRA (2014) *Patient Safety Alert Stage Three: Directive. Improving medication error incident reporting and learning*. London: MHRA.

Ness, V., Price, L., Currie, K. and Reilly, J. (2014) Antimicrobial resistance and prescribing behaviour. *Nurse Prescribing* 12 (5), 248–253.

NICE (National Institute for Health and Care Excellence) (2009) *Medicines adherence: Involving patients in decisions about prescribed medicines and supporting adherence*. London: NICE.

NICE (2013) *Patient Group Directions*. London: NICE.

NICE (2015a) *Medicine Optimisation: The safe and effective use of medicines to enable the best possible outcomes*. London: NICE.

NICE (2015b) *Antimicrobial Stewardship: Systems and processes for effective antimicrobial medicine use*. London: NICE.

NMC (Nursing and Midwifery Council) (2006) *Standards of Proficiency for Nurse and Midwife Prescribers*. London: NMC.

NMC (2007) *Standards for Medicines Management*. London: NMC.

NMC (2010a) *Standards for Pre-Registration Nursing*. London: NMC.

NMC (2010b) *Standards for Competence*. London: NMC.

NMC (2014) *Standards and Guidance Review Cycle 2014–2017*. London: NMC.

NMC (2015) *The Code: Professional standards of conduct and behaviour for nurses and midwives*. London: NMC.

NPSA (National Patient Safety Authority) (2007a) *Safety in Doses: Improving the use of medicines in the NHS*. London: NPSA.

NPSA (2007b) *Safety in Doses: Medication safety incidents in the NHS. The fourth report from the Patient Safety Observatory*. London: NPSA.

Nutt, D. (2012) *Drugs Without the Hot Air*. Cambridge: UIT Ltd.

Ofuso, R. and Jarrett, P. (2015) Reducing nurse medication administration errors. *Nursing Times* **111** (20), 12–14.

PDS (Parkinson's Disease Society) (undated) *Get it On Time Campaign*. London: Parkinson's Disease Society www.parkinsons.org.uk/content/get-it-time-campaign (accessed 15 February 2016).

RCN (Royal College of Nursing) (2010) *Standards for Infusion Therapy* (3rd edn). London: RCN.

RPS (Royal Pharmaceutical Society of Great Britain) (2008) *RPS e-PIC References on Prescription-Only Medicines Reclassified to Pharmacy-Only Medicines*. London: RPS.

RPS (2013) *Medicines Optimisation: Helping people make the most of medicines*. London: RPS.

Taxis, K. and Barber, N. (2003) Ethnographic study of incidence and severity of intravenous medicine errors. *British Medical Journal* **326**, 684–687.

Tinelli, M., Blenkinsopp, A., Latter, S., Smith, A. and Chapman, S. R. (2015) Survey of patients' experiences and perceptions of care provided by nurse and pharmacist independent prescribers in primary care. *Health Expectations* **18** (5), 1241–1255.

WHO (World Health Organization) (2011) *Antimicrobial Resistance, No Action Today No Cure Tomorrow*. Geneva: WHO.

Wright, D. (2002) Swallowing difficulties protocol: medication administration. *Nursing Standard* **17** (14–15), 43–45.

Wright, D. (2006) Tablet crushing is a widespread practice but it is not safe and may not be legal. *Pharmaceutical Journal* **269** (7208), 132.

19

PRECEPTORSHIP AND TRANSITION

David Cudlip

LEARNING OUTCOMES

After reading and reflecting on this chapter, you should be able to:

*   understand the historical and professional background of preceptorship;
*   understand the contribution preceptorship can make towards your personal and professional development;
*   discuss some of the differing views of preceptorship;
*   recognise the barriers to achieving a successful and satisfying preceptorship experience.

INTRODUCTION

As a student nurse, you will no doubt be anticipating the day you will begin your first job as a registered nurse, perhaps looking forward to operating with greater autonomy and freedom than has so far been the case. Conversely, you may feel some trepidation and are worried about what will be expected of you by both patients and colleagues. Either way, when you start your new job, you will most likely be provided with a period of preceptorship, usually between 4 to 12 months. This chapter aims to explore preceptorship and transition and is divided into three parts.

In Part 1, preceptorship is defined, and its importance is explained. In Part 2, there is some discussion of how and why preceptorship programmes have been developed, and how these differ from mentorship schemes.

In Part 3, current debates about preceptorship are explored. Barriers to successful preceptorship are discussed, and the experiences of newly qualified nurses are used to suggest how such barriers may be overcome.

David Cudlip

PART 1: OUTLINING PRECEPTORSHIP AND TRANSITION

Case 19.1

> Meghan, a student nurse nearing the completion of her course, attends a lecture at her university at which a representative from the local trust describes the preceptorship programme that they run for newly qualified nurses. Meghan has mixed feelings about this; she is pleased that she won't be expected to be the finished article from the start, but was rather looking forward to getting on with just being a nurse. Preceptorship sounds like more study, which she has had enough of. She has heard from some of the nurses that she's worked with on placement that there's a bit of a gap between what you're told will happen when you start, and what actually happens. Also, she wants to work for a different trust anyway, and has no idea whether they do 'preceptorship'. She hopes that all will become clear in time, and decides to worry about this later on.

What is preceptorship?

Preceptorship is defined by the Department of Health (DH) as:

> A period of structured transition for the newly registered practitioner during which he or she will be supported by a preceptor, to develop their confidence as an autonomous professional, refine skills, values and behaviours and to continue on their journey of life-long learning.

(DH 2010, p. 11)

This definition actually contains quite a lot of information in a small space. The style of writing and the expressions used will become familiar to you as you read DH documents and it's worth becoming familiar with what is meant early on, as these ideas will form the basis of how post-registration progress can be measured. There are a number of elements present in this definition:

- structured transition;
- supported by a preceptor;
- to develop . . . confidence as an autonomous professional . . . refine skills, values and behaviours;
- continue on their journey of life-long learning.

Structured transition

This term suggests that you will be in transition but it doesn't say from what to what. The idea referred to here is one developed by Patricia Benner (1984), who developed a model of nursing skill development *from novice to expert*. There are five stages in the model:

1 *Novice practitioners* require a rules-based approach to their work, usually outlined prior to carrying out the required task, and often in a classroom environment. Consider

the structure of your initial clinical skills classes, where you learned factual information such as about anatomy, and applied that knowledge in carrying out straightforward tasks in a controlled, protocol-driven manner. This approach was devised to allow you to complete required tasks safely. Perhaps you can recall the first time you were asked to take a patient's blood pressure, when you followed a set procedure: seeking consent, feeling for the pulse, applying the cuff and so on. This step-by-step approach can be seen on competency assessment sheets.

2   *Advanced beginners* begin to use acquired clinical experience, such as that gained on practice placement, to inform their approach. The focus begins to broaden out from a task-oriented approach such as 'I must take this patient's blood pressure' to a more holistic one, such as 'I must take this patient's blood pressure in such a manner that he feels comfortable, and confident in me'.

3   *Competent practitioners* have a good grasp of the main tasks expected of them in their work, and are able to use their experience as a basis for problem-solving, such as: 'the blood pressure monitor is not working; I'll use the manual sphygmomanometer'.

4   *Proficient practitioners* are able to understand situations that they encounter in their work as part of a broader picture. For example, they will understand the importance of consistent, competent monitoring of patients' vital signs as part of the evidence needed to treat patients appropriately.

5   *Expert practitioners* are able to use their wealth of experience and knowledge to provide leadership in the use of new approaches to their work. They use what Benner calls 'intuition' as a basis for their decisions. You may have encountered this on placement where some staff have a 'feel' for what is going on with their patients that seems unerring, appearing to the novice as verging on the uncanny.

The stages are understood as being a continuum. You are unlikely to go to work one day and realise or think that you have made a step change so that now you are a 'competent practitioner'. It is more likely that as you spend more time with patients, gaining more experience, you will feel a sense of development along similar lines to those described above. There is no clear timetable for how long it takes to move from novice to expert, and the mechanisms by which transition occurs are not entirely clear, although the process of structured reflection is considered pivotal (see Chapter 17). Attempts have been made to identify the number of years required to attain expert status (Benner et al. 1996), and it is possible to draw an interesting parallel with the work of Malcolm Gladwell (2000), an author and philosopher who has suggested that many skill-based tasks (piano playing, for example), take a similar amount of time to master, his golden figure being 10,000 hours. Gladwell's figure equates to about 6 years working, and expert nurses have a much longer gestation. Bear in mind, though, that just as I am never going to be a concert pianist, not all nurses will become expert, some becoming 'stuck' at earlier stages.

There are critiques of Benner's theory. It is, however, still the case that Benner's thinking forms the basis of how nursing progression is understood, and her terminology is explicitly used in the DH Preceptorship Framework (DH 2010), which outlines current guidance on the subject, so it is worth becoming familiar with her work.

I briefly alluded to the problem of *how* we as nurses can progress our understanding, whether you choose to characterise it in Benner's terms or others' (Gobet and Chassy 2008, Paley 1996). This is where the structured part of structured transition comes in.

501

David Cudlip

Preceptorship aims to give you a programme through which you can progress from novice (although not to expert) within the first months of your time as a registered nurse. The exact content of preceptorship programmes is not standardised, but the Preceptorship Framework (DH 2010) gives what it calls an 'indicative content of preceptorship', that is, what the DH currently regards as desirable. It comprises:

- decision-making;
- team working;
- leadership and management development;
- negotiation and conflict resolution;
- equality and diversity;
- manage risk and not being risk averse;
- interpersonal skills;
- advocacy;
- develop an outcome-based approach to continuing professional development;
- reflection and receiving feedback;
- understand policies and procedures;
- integrate prior learning into practice;
- increase knowledge and clinical skills;
- implement the codes of professional values;
- develop confidence and self-awareness;
- confidence in applying evidence-based practice.

Some of these elements will have formed part of your pre-registration course, and so will be familiar to you, others less so. There is a mix of information, skills and attributes but no prescribed method of delivery. The DH states that 'A variety of learning methods should be integrated into preceptorship so that programmes can be personalised to meet the needs of each newly registered practitioner to build their confidence as a practising professional' (2010, p. 18). Although this may at first glance appear to be a lack of leadership at a time when you may feel the need of some nice clear certainties, consider how varied are the workplaces covered by this guidance. How would you apply the same methods to district nursing, with its extended periods of lone working as you would to work in an intensive care unit or an operating theatre? The precise design of your preceptorship course may differ from that of your recently qualified friends in other areas. You should expect learning methods to include:

- action learning sets;
- self-directed learning;
- clinical practice focus days;
- reflective practice;
- shadowing;
- one-to-one support either in person or electronically;
- preceptorship via higher education institutions;
- work-based learning;
- web-based learning;
- attitudinal and behaviour-based learning, perhaps through role-modelling.

(DH 2010, p. 18)

. . . *supported by a preceptor*

Your preceptor should have been assigned to you prior to your first day in post. Being a preceptor is a formal responsibility, yet it requires no specific training. Instead, the attributes and responsibilities of an effective preceptor are outlined by the DH, and include the ability to 'act as an exemplary role model'. This is also reflected in the Nursing and Midwifery Council (NMC) *Code* where clause 20.8 states that you must 'act as a role model of professional behaviour for students and newly qualified nurses and midwives to aspire to' (NMC 2015a). This NMC injunction applies to all nurses (including newly qualified ones) but more realistically, the way your preceptor conducts themself could tell you about what your practice area's manager regards as desirable. There is a suggestion that the qualities required to become an effective preceptor take around two years to acquire post-registration (DH 2010), and it has been claimed that those relatively recently qualified are better able to empathise with new registrants (Cowan and Flint 2012) and support them effectively. This may differ to some extent from your experience in pre-registration, where you may have been mentored by relatively senior staff. The DH offers a list of the skills attributes of an effective preceptor as follows:

- giving constructive feedback;
- setting goals and assessing competency;
- facilitating problem-solving;
- active listening skills;
- understanding, demonstrating and evidencing reflective practice ability in the working environment;
- demonstrating good time management and leadership skills
- prioritising care;
- demonstrating appropriate clinical decision-making and evidence based practice;
- recognising their own limitations and those of others;
- knowing what resources are available and how to refer a newly registered practitioner appropriately if additional support is required, for example, pastoral support or occupational health services;
- being an effective and inspirational role model and demonstrating professional values, attitudes and behaviours;
- demonstrating a clear understanding of the regulatory impact of the care that they deliver and that ability to pass on this knowledge;
- providing a high standard of practice at all times.

(DH 2010, p. 17)

This group of attributes and skills is not written with you, the preceptee, in mind. It is aimed more at those in the position of appointing members of staff to the role of preceptor. That does not mean, however, that you shouldn't consider them as you work with your preceptor. Note the repeated use of certain words within this document, particularly 'demonstrating'. You will have been expected to demonstrate knowledge, skills and attributes in the course of your undergraduate study. How did you do this? You will be in a position to see how your preceptor demonstrates their attributes to their colleagues including you. This may prove to be an instructive exercise in how (or maybe how not) to perform this aspect of nursing work. Finally, remember that it will be important to cultivate a good working relationship with your preceptor. You may not like them – indeed, working well with those we would not seek out as friends is a significant part of success in the workplace – but you should be able in all honesty to state that you work with them in an atmosphere of mutual respect and trust.

. . . confidence as an autonomous professional . . . refine skills, values and behaviours

Preceptorship should help you to grow in confidence, through your experiences of work and reflections on those experiences, the structured learning elements outlined above, and the input and feedback of your preceptor. What, however, do we mean by an 'autonomous professional'? The *Oxford English Dictionary* defines autonomy in the sense it is meant here as 'acting independently or having the freedom to do so', and a profession as 'a vocation or calling, especially one that involves some branch of advanced learning or science' (OUP 2015). Although both are complex ideas, these definitions give a good basic sense of what is intended. You should be able competently and confidently to apply what you have learned in order to carry out your nursing duties without inappropriate levels of supervision or assistance. You'll be expected to have basic levels of these attributes, but will 'develop' and 'refine' them through your preceptorship programme.

. . . continue on their journey of life-long learning

This is the bit that Meghan was concerned about. Although she knew that she would have to develop her knowledge and skills, she was hoping for a bit of time to relax and get used to her new role. However, the NMC *Code* states clearly that you must 'keep your knowledge and skills up to date, taking part in appropriate and regular learning and professional development activities that aim to maintain and develop your competence and improve your performance' (NMC 2015a, clause 22.3). You may be surprised at how seriously this aspect of your career will be taken. You are not just to pay lip service to this as an ideal; it will be expected of you. Although this can be tiring, it is part of what differentiates a profession from a job, and it is best to cultivate a positive attitude towards the situation. Be pleased that your employer wishes to invest in you and your future, and relish where possible the opportunity to show yourself what you are capable of. You will be required to demonstrate learning as part of periodic revalidation.

Why should I worry about this now?

As you approach registration, you will of course have a lot on your mind, perhaps awaiting vital results, arranging interviews and accommodation. Remember that your first job as a registered nurse will have a profound and lasting effect on the rest of your career, for good or ill. Being well prepared for the transition from student to registered nurse will ease some of the anxieties that this time inevitably brings. Preceptorship is designed in part to help you with this process, so the better your understanding, the more you will gain from it. Less time worrying about support and transition will give you more time to think about other things. Because a well-organised preceptorship programme can make such positive impact on the early stages of your career (Morgan *et al.* 2011, Oxtoby 2012), it is wise to enquire at interview or earlier about the arrangements put in place by your prospective employer. There will be a good deal of variation between and within organisations, partly because their requirements and staffing levels are variable. Remember that the NHS is not the only provider of health care, and like it or not, the number of other providers will most likely increase. This will add to the variety of approaches available. Remember also that at present it is not mandatory for organisations to provide a preceptorship programme. My first position after graduation was in a minor injuries unit. Although the preceptorship programme was relatively informal, it was an excellent experience, because all my colleagues were happy to support me. I was surrounded by experienced senior nurses every day. Whitehead *et al.* (2016) found that the idea of a one-to-one relationship was in places replaced by a sort of informal collective preceptorship. It can be seen that my good experience resulted from a combination of a positive working culture and the staffing requirements of the unit; also perhaps a good fit with my preferred learning style. Clearly a more structured approach would be required in an area with a different skill mix, with less access to senior staff. I did enquire about preceptorship provision at interview, but not particularly deeply. With the benefit of hindsight, here are a few questions I would consider asking if I were to repeat the interview today:

- Do you run a preceptorship programme?
- Is it published so that I can look at it? (If you are really canny, you can look on the Internet prior to interview.)
- How long does it last?
- Will I be assigned a single preceptor? Will this be arranged prior to my arrival on the first day?
- Are preceptors adequately supported and given time to carry out their responsibilities towards me?
- Does the preceptorship programme carry academic credit?
- Does your preceptorship programme allow for accelerated pay progression?

NHS terms and conditions (NHS 2005) state that 'Staff joining Band 5 as new entrants will have accelerated progression through the first two points in six monthly steps (that is, they will move up one pay point after 6 months and a further point after 12 months) providing those responsible for the relevant standards in the organisation are satisfied with their standard of practice as outlined in the KSF profile'. Is this the case within your organisation?

The final question is important, because it relates directly to pay. Though accelerated pay progression is part of the NHS pay structure that should be organised for you, you have a direct financial interest in ensuring that progress is maintained and documented. As a final note to this section, I do not expect, and would not advise that you focus solely on preceptorship provision when considering where to work. There will be other considerations, from the type of clinical area you want to work in to the distance of your workplace from home, to consider. I would urge you, however, to give careful consideration to this aspect of any offer made to you by a prospective employer, not least because it offers an insight into the levels of investment they are willing to put into your career development.

If you work for NHS Scotland, you will very likely be offered the opportunity to enrol on the 'Flying Start' program, which is a standardised, mixed-method platform for preceptorship, linking directly to your Knowledge and Skills Framework (KSF) profile, making it simpler to develop a practice portfolio that you can use to evidence your professional development. If you do not work for NHS Scotland, you can still use Flying Start, but you should check with your employer that it will integrate into their preceptorship programme. Have a look at the website at: www.flyingstart.scot.nhs.uk for details.

BOX 19.1 Getting registered and staying registered

At the end of your course your university will forward your documentation to the NMC who will process it and add your name to the register. You'll be able to look yourself up on the online checking system and you will be a registered nurse, entitled to put the initials RN after your name along with your university degree. Unlike some other professional groups there is no reduction in fees for nurses at initial registration, so you will have to pay the full annual fee, which is currently £120, having been increased from £100 in 2015 and £76 in 2012. This may seem a lot of money to pay, but most of the NMC spend is accounted for by fitness to practise hearings (see Chapter 2), for which the process is largely determined by legislation. Part of the fee can be recouped by claiming tax relief, but this is only done by about 30 per cent of nurses (NMC 2014a). When combined with allowances for union fees and laundry expenses, tax relief can be worth up to £177 per year. You can get details from your union, or go to the HMRC website www.gov.uk/government/organisations/hm-revenue-customs and search for 'tax relief for employees'.

When the fees were increased to their current level a consultation exercise was carried out and 96 per cent of just over 4,500 responses opposed the increase. The previous increase in 2012 was also preceded by a consultation, which elicited over 25,000 responses (NMC 2014b). There were 1,649 responses to the consultation about *The Code*, and it will be seen that although the latest consultation about fees was answered by considerably fewer than the last, it is still an issue that provokes strong opinions. The decision to implement the increase in the face of opposition in the consultation may justify some scepticism about the value of responding. For every person completing the online consultation, over 25 signed an e-petition, which when it closed had collected 113,797 signatures (Petitions 2015).

Once you are on the register you need to pay the fee on an annual basis. Reminders are sent out but these can get mislaid and if you forget to register you will be de-registered and won't be able to practise until you have reapplied. Readmittance is not guaranteed. This can have serious implications for your career (and finances), so it is highly recommended that you pay by annual direct debit. You can manage your registration online by registering with NMC online – and this is also highly recommended though not yet compulsory.

Every 3 years you will need to revalidate. This is new process that requires continual engagement. You should be aware of what will be required as soon as you register as you will need to collect information for this when you have your appraisals. There is extensive guidance available at http://revalidation.nmc.org.uk/. For each 3-year period you will need to provide records of:

- 450 hours of practice (900 for jointly registered nurses and midwives – 450 for each);

- 35 hours of continuous professional development of which 20 must be participatory;
- 5 pieces of practice-related feedback;
- 5 written reflective accounts – these must be presented on the form provided by the NMC;
- a reflective discussion with another NMC-registered practitioner;
- a confirmation form signed by your confirmer (who is likely to be your line manager);
- a declaration of good health and character;
- a professional indemnity arrangement.

This process can be co-ordinated with your appraisal and preceptorship activities. It's recommended that you download and read the guidance (NMC 2015b) and keep good records from the start. This may avoid much stress later on!

PART 2: EXPLAINING PRECEPTORSHIP AND TRANSITION

Case 19.2

Following the lecture she attended on preceptorship, Meghan goes into her placement, and on shift she asks the nurses she is working with about their first days and weeks in post. She hears a mixture of stories ranging from the terrifying to the merely worrying. On further discussion, however, some of her colleagues begin to talk about the more positive experiences they had; good days among the bad, supportive staff, particularly moving or happy experiences with patients, and so on. It is almost as though some of her friends take a certain pleasure in frightening her; either that, or they remember bad experiences more clearly than good ones.

Feeling somewhat discomfited by these stories, Meghan heads home at the end of her shift wondering whether the start of her career will inevitably be stressful and possibly unpleasant.

What would you do in Meghan's position?

Having calmed down a little at home, Meghan wonders how to make sense of these stories. She remembers her training; the tools she has been given to make sense of the things that happen. That's right: reflection. She begins to deconstruct these stories in her mind. Who had bad experiences? What, specifically were they? Were there solutions? Did these people have preceptorship, and if so, did it help? If not, why not? Meghan is not satisfied to settle for the surface of the story; she digs a little deeper to get to the sense behind the experience. She resolves not to allow herself to become frightened, because these are not her experiences. Meghan reminds herself through this process that she is in charge of the place she ends up in, and that nothing is inevitable if she takes control of her situation.

Perhaps, like Meghan, you have heard some alarming stories about the early stages of nurses' careers. You may even have spoken to people who decided that nursing wasn't for them, and left the profession. It is entirely natural that you should feel nervous about your first days as a registered nurse, and wonder whether this will turn out to be the start of an illustrious career or a descent into hell. In reality, things are unlikely to be that dramatic, so take heart and know that you are far from the first person to be in this situation.

A brief history of preceptorship

We have seen that the intention behind preceptorship programmes is to provide you with a period during which you'll be supported in practice. This was devised to minimise or even prevent what became known as 'reality shock', a negative response to the differences between nursing students' perceptions of what nursing would be like and the reality of practice on the ground described in a early account as 'the impact of the schism between school-bred values and work-world values.' (Sardis 1974). The term originated from the work of Marlene Kramer in the United States (1974), so you can see that this is not a new phenomenon or a knee-jerk reaction to some of the negative press nursing has received of late. The full title of the book was *Reality Shock: Why nurses leave nursing* indicating the primary concern of the study. Retention rates among nurses were problematic, and Kramer hypothesised that a programme of support and education incorporated into their 3-year training period might be beneficial. She took two year-groups, and gave one the support programme; the other, the control group, did not receive additional support. Having allowed for confounding variables, it appeared that the supported group, broadly speaking, did better than the control. This seminal work has attained broad acceptance within the profession and forms the foundation on which preceptorship has been built. Since that point, the proposed benefits of preceptorship programmes have gone beyond those proposed by Kramer (see lists below). The results of research into preceptorship and will be discussed further in Part 3.

In the UK, nurse training had evolved from its origins in the Nightingale School for Nurses at St Thomas' Hospital in London in 1860, with degree courses being launched at the University of Edinburgh in 1960, followed by the University of Wales in 1972 and the University of Manchester in 1974. Starting with the now confusingly entitled Project 2000 educational review, nursing pre-registration courses gradually moved away from hospitals and into universities and other higher education institutions (Meerabeau 2001). This process of change and development from practical, embodied knowledge to a more academic, theoretical approach has been controversial and you will no doubt have heard the expression 'too posh to wash', which neatly, if not glibly, encapsulates the problems some feel have been caused by these changes. It is easy to imagine that UK nursing education was ready to consider the implications of Kramer's research, with the gradual and broadening introduction of preceptorship programmes of various design from around 1985 onwards, with a desire for some standardisation eventually leading to the publication of the DH Preceptorship Framework (DH 2010), which set out desirable structure, content and implementation of preceptorship pro-grammes in the UK. It is notable, however, that at the time of writing, the provision of preceptorship remains optional.

What does it do?

Kramer's work broadly suggested that her support programme positively affected their abilities to 'operationalize their professional values', increased job satisfaction and success. Subsequent research has examined the impact of preceptorship on meeting newly qualified nurses' needs for support, improving confidence and competence, improving quality of care and reducing sickness and absence while improving staff retention. We can see here that the proposed benefits seem to be multiplying: The DH Preceptorship Framework (2010) offers an extensive list of benefits, both to you and your employer, as follows:

Benefits to you

The benefits of the DH Preceptorship Framework (2010) to you are that it:

- develops confidence;
- offers professional socialisation into working environment;
- gives increased job satisfaction leading to improved patient/client/service user satisfaction;
- makes you feel invested in and enhances future career aspirations;
- makes you feel proud and committed to the organisation's corporate strategy and objectives;
- develops understanding of the commitment to working within the profession and regulatory body requirements;
- encourages personal responsibility for maintaining up-to-date knowledge.

(DH 2010)

Activity 19.1

Take a moment to look closely at this list. If you have the time, reflect on it, perhaps by putting the contents in order of importance to you. This may tell you something about which of these aspects you feel you need support with.

Benefits to your employer

The benefits of the DH Preceptorship Framework (2010) to your employer are:

- enhanced quality of patient care;
- enhanced recruitment and retention;
- reduced sickness and absence;
- enhanced service user experience;
- enhanced staff satisfaction;
- opportunity to 'talent spot' to meet the leadership agenda;
- progression through pay-band gateways for those organisations who implement Agenda for Change;

- registered practitioners who understand the regulatory impact of the care they deliver and develop and outcome/evidence-based approach;
- identify staff that require further/extra support.

(DH 2010)

Again, examine this list. Clearly your interests and those of your employer overlap. Who wouldn't want to be 'talent-spotted', for example? The evidence for these bold claims is discussed in Part 3.

Agenda for Change and the KSF

The Agenda for Change system has been designed in order to bring transparency and fairness to the NHS pay structure. Any given post is ascribed to a set pay band, ranging from 1 to 9 according to the demands of the job in terms of knowledge, responsibility, skills and effort. This is done using a system called the Job Evaluation Scheme. As a newly qualified nurse, you'll be paid at Band 5. At the time of writing (January 2016), annual pay at this scale starts at £21,692 and progresses through seven incremental pay points to £28,180 (NHS 2015). Clinical areas have individual structures, but broadly, Band 6 posts used to be called senior staff nurse or junior sister, Band 7 posts are Senior Sisters, in charge of a larger clinical area, and Band 8 posts are matrons and senior clinical nurse specialists. To progress through the pay points within your band, you must demonstrate development of your knowledge and skills against a benchmark called the Knowledge and Skills Framework, or KSF, which comprises six core dimensions:

- communication;
- personal and people development;
- health, safety and security;
- service improvement;
- quality;
- equality and diversity.

All NHS workers are assessed according to these criteria. There are 24 more specific dimensions, which apply to some jobs but not others and your job description will contain a KSF outline so that you know how your performance and development will be measured. Although your development should be continually assessed by your senior colleagues, you will be involved in an annual formal discussion on this matter, known as an appraisal or personal development review. At this meeting you will be expected to show how you have developed professionally and how you will continue to do so. Training opportunities will be agreed upon, and any support required will be planned. All staff are assessed using the same framework so that fairness is assured as far as possible. As you settle into your role, you may find yourself considering how to progress up the NHS pay structure. You don't have to progress through all Band 5 increments. If you wish, you can apply for a Band 6 post once you feel that you have the required knowledge and skills and one becomes available. It is often the case that employers ask for 2 years' post-registration experience as a minimum for Band 6 posts, but this may be flexible, so if in doubt, ask. There is more detail about the KSF at the nhs employers website www.nhsemployers.org/SimplifiedKSF.

As higher band roles are increasingly specialised, they usually require specific post-graduate qualifications. You may find that your manager has a clear development plan in place for you, which involves the achievement of these. Remember that you can always ask universities whether they will give academic credits for particular pieces of work and some are willing to give credits for completion of a preceptorship course. The downside of this is that universities will charge a fee for this, which may not be paid by your employer. Recent proposed changes to nurse education and post-graduate funding mean that individuals paying for their own education has become more common. This isn't popular, but you should consider paying as an investment in your future career. It is sometimes possible to add up various credits gained through completion of courses and modules to achieve a master's degree, which is a requirement for some roles. A word of caution, however: not all courses can be bolted together to give a master's degree, and not all master's degrees accept credit from elsewhere. It may be that you need to develop a clear idea of where you want to specialise before investing too heavily in this. It is worth keeping in touch with your university after you graduate; they'll be happy to provide information and assistance with this. Also consider attending open days to gain an idea of what's on offer, and don't be wary of ringing for advice or seeking an appointment. Outside of specialist areas, there is considerable competition among universities, which rely on student funding. Flexible delivery of courses including study blocks and e-learning mean that the days of confirmed and recurring contracts between employers and local universities are nearly over. They should be very happy to talk to you as a potential student.

The Shape of Caring Review (Health Education England 2015) undertaken by Lord Willis examined how the education and training needs of the health workforce will be met over the next 10 to 15 years. It is clear from this review that preceptorship programmes are likely to become more formalised, with suggestions that their contribution towards post-graduate credits could become the norm. The value of master's-level educated nurses is also explicitly recognised in the review and it seems that the enormous potential of the nursing workforce is now being recognised. Whether such well-intentioned plans can actually be adequately operationalised remains to be seen, but the NHS will have need of highly qualified, forward-thinking nurses, so any investment you make in this direction is likely to be rewarded in the longer term. Nurses are fortunate in that their noble academic pursuit of knowledge can often be readily translated into improved earnings. Sadly this state of affairs is not universal in our society.

Preceptorship and the Francis Report

Perhaps the most significant claim put forward for preceptorship is that it can improve the quality of care that we provide to patients. There have been numerous accounts over the last few years of nurses both failing to provide adequate care to patients, and even actively seeking to harm and humiliate them. The most widely publicised of these was the inquiry into events at Mid-Staffordshire NHS Trust (Francis 2013). These events have been ascribed to numerous causes, including perceived inadequacies of nurse education overall, with a degree of emphasis on post-qualification support, that is, preceptorship. The reports are lengthy documents, but nursing is largely discussed in a single chapter (chapter 23). I urge you to read it. The following quotation helps to illustrate the importance of the skills that preceptorship aims to develop. A patient describes an incident he witnessed while an inpatient at Mid-Staffordshire Hospital:

David Cudlip

I mean, 10 minutes was nothing, sometimes longer. And it was worse, I thought, for the old lady next to me, who couldn't get out of bed, and she was on a commode at least 15 minutes ringing and ringing, and it went on and on, and she was a very ill lady. I mean, everybody seems old to me because I feel only 50, but she did seem very old. And she was ill, truly ill. And . . . then at last the nurse came. And she said 'Do you want to go back to bed or will you sit in the chair?' And before the lady could answer, the cleaning lady said 'If she can sit on a commode she can sit on a chair. Don't put her back to bed'. So the young nurse didn't, she sat her in a chair.

(Francis 2013, p. 1501)

Activity 19.2

What are the issues from this account that illustrate the importance of preceptorship?

Perhaps the most important issue is the nurse's decision to acquiesce to the 'cleaning lady's' call that she should sit her patient in a chair. I do not seek to apportion blame here, and I have chosen this example in part because I have experienced similar situations myself; when I was a student nurse, support workers often offered their opinions and advice. In some instances, this was entirely valid and at the start of my course especially, experienced health care assistants knew far better than I how to provide basic patient care and I learned a great deal from them. What appears to have happened in the above scenario, though, is that a significant boundary has been crossed. A non-clinical member of staff is advising a registered nurse on how she should care for her patient. What has gone wrong here? How would preceptorship help in this instance?

The cleaner has gone beyond her remit

Clearly the cleaner feels that it is valid, indeed entirely acceptable, that she should offer an opinion regarding the nursing care of a patient. It sounds from the account that this is not the first time this has happened, as the cleaner is intervening in a relatively routine decision, rather than preventing what anyone would be qualified to recognise as an obviously dangerous or malicious act, in which case she would be entirely right to step forward on the patient's behalf. It seems that, for some reason, the cleaner has become so accustomed to the clinical environment, perhaps being exposed to the clinical decision-making process on a daily basis, that she has begun to regard herself as a member of clinical staff; she over-identifies with the nurses' professional role. It is understandable that this phenomenon may occur, but not acceptable that the clinical staff on the ward have either not noticed that this is happening, or have noticed, but have not done anything about it.

The nurse has abdicated responsibility

It might be that the ward nurses may be averse to conflict, not wishing to upset the cleaner by reminding her of her role within the ward team. This suggests a lack of

512

confidence, and a failure properly to understand what it means to be a professional nurse. Nursing is now, and to some extent always has been, a management role. Nurses are responsible for the smooth and safe running of their practice areas, and although in this instance the nurse may not have line-management responsibility for the cleaner (this may be the housekeeping manager's job), she absolutely has the authority to remind the cleaner (in a private area, of course) of her remit, and point out that further attempts to interfere in nursing decisions will not be welcomed. Even though the nurse may have been young and inexperienced, she should act as a leader and here the nurse has not performed well in this role. Perhaps she does not feel confident in her decision. Perhaps she feels that if she were to challenge the cleaner's intervention she would not be supported by her senior nursing colleagues. Either way, perhaps preceptorship could help.

How would preceptorship have helped here?

Nursing is a professional role that requires us to step beyond the limits of established comfort zones on an almost daily basis. What did you struggle with on your first placement? I am a quietly spoken person, so it felt like I was shouting sometimes to make myself heard. I also found it difficult at first to walk up to complete strangers and begin to interact with them in a way that would be considered intimate or invasive in other contexts. Over time, I got used to these things, not least by understanding that an element of theatre is involved. When you put on your uniform (if you are required to wear one) or when you walk into the space occupied by your patient, you take on an identity beyond that which you inhabit outside work. Understanding this is part of becoming a professional. It seems that the nurse in the account above may be experiencing dissonance between her view of herself as a private person (perhaps she is shy, and naturally averse to imposing her views on others) and herself as a professional person, which in this instance requires her to do something she finds difficult or distasteful. It is this kind of situation that preceptorship aims to help with. There is no additional clinical knowledge to be imparted here; the nurse made her decision. What she would benefit from is a senior colleague helping her to understand how to resolve this issue comfortably and professionally.

How is preceptorship different from having a mentor?

You'll be familiar with mentorship from your practice placements. Under this system, a registered professional is tasked with facilitating your learning, and assessing your levels of competence against specific outcomes and skills. In the event of your involvement in an adverse incident, your mentor will bear a significant share of the responsibility for your actions or omissions. This is not the case in preceptorship, as 'From the moment they are registered, practitioners are autonomous and accountable' (DH 2010, p. 10). Though some areas will offer a short period of supernumerary practice (Whitehead et al. 2016), it is important that you understand that you will be regarded as a fully qualified professional, and expected to behave as such. Should these expectations seem vague, carefully read the NMC Code, which details 'the professional standards that registered nurses and mid-wives must uphold' (NMC 2015a, p. 2). Note the use of the word 'must', there is nothing optional or discretionary about this (see Chapter 2). Although your preceptor and indeed the team you work in as a whole should support you throughout your career, it will be up to you to ensure that you practise within your levels of competence, and that you raise concerns promptly should they arise. Remember that everyone will be busy, and that you

David Cudlip

are no longer supernumerary, and nor will there be a set number of hours that your preceptor must work with you. People will help you, but they'll expect you to help yourself and others also.

Should you want to read about preceptorship in the research literature, caution is advised: a significant proportion of the research into this subject comes from North America, where the terms 'mentorship' and 'preceptorship' tend to be used interchangeably (Marks-Maran *et al.* 2013), so your initial database search will offer you papers that are about undergraduate training programmes, which while interesting, will lack the fundamental point that preceptorship programmes are designed for post-registration staff. You could try extending your search by putting the terms 'post-registration' or 'post-graduate' into your search. You will need to maintain your academic skills as your career progresses, as you will be expected to attend numerous career development courses; for example, after a year in post you will be eligible to train as a mentor, and it won't be long before you are trained to be a preceptor yourself. Keeping up your data-searching skills will not only make your life a lot easier, but will be of help to the student nurses for whom you will be responsible. It may sound crazy that you may be expected to teach others so soon, but from experience I can tell you that your first year will fly by, and that you will learn very quickly. You should consider keeping a concise reflective diary of experiences so that you'll be able to look back in a year's time to see how far you have come. There is sound thinking behind this approach: as Sellman and Tarr explain in Chapter 16, it is widely held that teaching is learning. I have experienced this when trying to explain things to my children. If I don't really know what I'm talking about, I cannot clearly explain it. I read up on the subject myself, and then can do a

---

BOX 19.2 Standards of competence for registered nurses

As a student nurse you will have been assessed against some key documents, notably the *Standards of Proficiency for Pre-Registration Nursing* and the Essential Skills Clusters (NMC 2010). These standards direct the content of pre-registration courses at universities and together they represent the nearest that there currently is to a national curriculum. The NMC do not tell universities how to meet the standards, but all students must meet them before they are allowed to register, and they must be maintained to remain on the register. The Francis Report and the *More Care, Less Pathway* report (DH 2013) into the Liverpool Care Pathway, called for information and clarity about what standards can be expected from nurses. *The Code* gives standards for performance and behaviour, but the statements are general and cannot really guide action and do not say in any detail what nurses must be able to do (Snelling 2015). In order to clarify what can be expected by all registered nurses, the NMC reissued the *Standards of Proficiency for Pre-Registration Nursing* as *Standards for Competence for Registered Nurses* (NMC 2010b). The standards contain generic and field-specific statements. Your preceptor will probably be familiar with these as they probably also act as a mentor to student nurses. This is an important document and you would do well to continue your familiarity with it. Like other NMC standards documents, the statements begin with the words 'Registered nurses must . . . ' indicating that they are non-negotiable.

514

better job of teaching them. It has also been suggested that mentors should be of the same generation as students, so that their experiences of training are comparable (Cowan and Flint 2012), so that what you perceive as a weakness may actually be a strength.

In the final section, a brief overview of the research base for preceptorship will be conducted, using it to assess what evidence there is to suggest that preceptorship works.

PART 3: EXPLORING PRECEPTORSHIP AND TRANSITION

What evidence is there for the effectiveness of preceptorship?

Throughout your education programme you will have studied evidence-based practice, which is intended to ensure that professional actions are based on sound evidence rather than tradition or just opinion, and that we change our practice to stay in line with new developments. This section will give a brief survey of the evidence supporting preceptorship, but it should be remembered that research papers are published at a much higher rate than textbooks, so if you want to stay up-to-date, keep an eye on recent research by carrying out regular searches on your database, and by signing up to online table-of-contents (toc) from selected journals. You'll currently have access to papers through your degree provider and once you graduate, you can continue access through the NHS, which will give you an Open Athens account.

The first review of this subject in the UK was published in 1996. Its aims were to 'review the current literature addressing . . . themes of role definition, preceptor selection, preceptor programmes, the preceptorship experience and the limitations of preceptorship in clinical practice' (Bain 1996, p. 104). There is no clear evidence presented regarding the effectiveness or otherwise of preceptorship. Bains states:

> Preceptorship is an important element of the United Kingdom Central Council's post-registration education and practice proposals. Therefore, there is a great need for educationalists and clinical practitioners to explore the issues surrounding preceptorship and to come to informed decisions on how they intend to implement preceptor programmes.
>
> (Bain 1996, p. 104)

In effect this says that preceptorship is important because people say it is important. The problem that it was originally intended to counter, the theory–practice gap identified by Kramer in the USA in the 1970s, is not examined. To some extent this is understandable, because in 1996 the subject was in its infancy, so there was not a great deal of research to draw upon. In a statement echoed in subsequent literature reviews, Bain states that 'The empirical evidence addressing preceptorship programmes is contradictory and inconsistent. Unfortunately much of the literature lacks the essential elements of replication and compatibility for scientific credibility' (Bain 1996, p. 107). She then remarks that: 'However, one need only reflect upon personal experience as a newly qualified practitioner to identify the need for a period of support' (Bain 1996, p. 107). This approach is a challenge to evidence-based practice, as it suggests that individual experience can be a reliable substitute for research. Worryingly, this brief, somewhat exploratory and now dated review was the only research paper in the references section of the DH Preceptorship Framework, which as noted above, forms the basis for all programmes in the UK.

A subsequent literature review was carried out in Canada in 2007 (Billay and Myrick 2007). Clearly over the intervening period more research has been conducted, although the picture is confused by the elision of undergraduate and post-graduate programmes limiting its usefulness. In its opening sentence, the paper states that 'The preceptorship model is as an effective teaching and learning strategy' (Billay and Myrick 2007, p. 258). There is no evidence presented in support of this claim, however. Intended, and by now familiar benefits are mentioned, these being the socialisation into the registered nursing role and a reduction in the assumed theory–practice gap. The quality of the papers reviewed is questioned by the researchers and clearly significant work remained at this point.

In 2009, a scoping review was carried out by the National Nursing Research Unit, commissioned by the DH (Robinson and Griffiths 2009). This report specifically addresses the question of the effectiveness of preceptorship programmes, specifically its effects on:

- providing support to newly qualified nurses (positive);
- bolstering their confidence and competence (positive);
- improving quality of care (no studies found that investigated this);
- increasing staff retention rates while reducing sickness and absence rates (limited evidence that dissatisfaction with a preceptorship programme contributes to leaving a job);
- helping nurses to choose suitable career pathways (no evidence);
- effects on preceptors themselves (preceptors seek tangible benefits to aid commitment);
- impact on organisational resources (no evidence).

Similar to Bain's paper, the report points out that 'most of the evidence relied on self-report, primarily by the preceptee' (Robinson and Griffiths 2009, p. 11). Overall, there are some benefits to the newly qualified nurse, but it is startling that the impact of preceptorship on the quality of nursing care has not been investigated, particularly as improvement in this area is one of the 'benefits to employer' explicitly stated in the DH Preceptorship Framework (DH 2010).

A further review was conducted in 2012 by Currie and Watts. This work set out to discover 'the benefits of, and approaches to, supporting new graduate nurses in post-registration role transition through preceptorship programmes in the UK' (2012, p. 1). Once again it is stated that there is no evidence on the clinical or cost-effectiveness of preceptorship provision in the UK and that studies cited are generally descriptive and based on self-report. 'Although mutual benefits of preceptorship programmes for new qualified nurses, preceptors and organisations are well documented, there is little evaluation of programmes demonstrating effectiveness in terms of quality of care or making recommendations concerning best practice' (Currie and Watts 2012, p. 1). Finally, a comprehensive review of the effectiveness of strategies and interventions to improve the transition from student to newly qualified nurse was published in 2015 (Edwards et al. 2015). This review looked at a number of strategies to support transition but only assessed quantitative studies. The conclusion was that any process was better than none – that the focus on investment is significant rather than leaving newly qualified nurses to acclimatise themselves. 'The findings of this review are based upon weak evidence which concurs with earlier reviews and shows that there has been very little advancement in this area' (Edwards *et al.* 2015, p. 1267).

Overall, then, the effectiveness of preceptorship is not proven. There is limited evidence supporting the idea that a good preceptorship experience will ease your transition

---

RESEARCH FOCUS 19.1

Marks-Maran *et al.* (2013) undertook a mixed-methods study in London, which evaluated an academically accredited preceptorship programme. Ninety preceptees completed the programme but fewer than half (44) completed the questionnaire, which comprised 52 four point Likert style statements. Qualitative data were collected by open-ended questions and self-recorded video diaries. Generally the evaluation was positive, although 82 per cent of respondents were challenged by making time for meetings. The impact of communication, personal development, role development, professional relationships and clinical skills development were all evaluated positively, and 80 per cent of preceptees said that they would recommend the programme to colleagues. Qualitative data supported these findings. For example:

> I now understand the importance of reflection on my experiences to develop my skills and understandings as a professional nurse. My preceptor helped me reflect on things that happened in my practice and as a result I have a clearer understanding of my strengths and where I need to develop. I have a greater understanding now of being a nurse.
>
> . . . there were moments when I felt like leaving the job but my preceptor was always there to encourage me to face my fears and persevere. She always gave me encouragement and advice.
>
> (Marks-Maran *et al.* 2013, p. 1432)

A further parallel study (Muir *et al.* 2013) investigated the experiences of the 90 preceptors. Despite being given the questionnaires in a face-to-face meeting and again by preceptees, only 40 (44 per cent) returned them. Qualitative data were obtained by interviews with a purposive sample of nine preceptors. There were two research questions. First the study aimed to assess the preceptors' views of the impact of the programme, and second, the impact of the programme on their own role development. Generally the Likert responses were similar to the preceptees', with generally positive views for development in the areas identified. There were questions relating to the value of preceptors' own development but these weren't reported, and the qualitative data were only reported to the extent that it claimed that the scheme contributed to the preceptors' development in a number of ways:

- impact on their own knowledge;
- impact on the teaching/staff development role;
- understanding the needs and issues of newly qualified staff;
- impact on their emotional support skills.

Taken together these studies claim that the programme has positive outcomes, but there are acknowledged limitations. There is scant detail of the programme given, the response rate for the questionnaires is poor, and the reporting of data collected in the papers is less than complete. The papers investigate perceptions rather than actual benefit. However, the programme apparently worked for them, so despite the poor quality of the evidence it's difficult not to conclude that there was some benefit.

from student to registered nurse, which is clearly a good thing, but there is currently no evidence to justify the assertion that preceptorship improves standards of patient care. Finally, it should be remembered that the absence of evidence is not the same as evidence of absence; that is, there may be benefits in all the areas outlined by the Preceptorship Framework, and perhaps more besides, but these have not as yet been uncovered by research, for two main reasons. First, historically, nursing research was not of the highest quality, although this is changing rapidly, and a number of the literature reviews cited above make suggestions as to how the evidence base for preceptorship can be improved. Second, the questions raised are difficult to answer; as Currie and Watts state: 'It may not be possible to compare the quality of care delivered by those nurses who had received preceptorship against those who had' (2012, p. 5).

Are there potential problems?

It is claimed that one of the main benefits to you will be an easier socialisation into the profession. The process of internalising the values and *culture* of nursing in general, and your place within it in particular will be more straightforward (Higgins *et al.* 2009). This sounds somewhat abstract, but in practical terms it means that you should be helped to feel more comfortable at work sooner with the help of a preceptor. There has been a lot written and said about the culture of nursing in recent years. 'Culture' is one of those words that can have very different meanings depending upon who is using it. In general terms, it means the complex of attitudes and behaviours that we absorb as members of society, rather than inheriting biologically from our parents. It can, however, be used differently by specialists: in archaeology, for example, a culture is held to mean a particular set of finds (pottery, metalwork and so on), which provide evidence for a defined group of people, so people talk about the 'beaker culture' on the basis of digging up a particular type of pot on a number of sites of the same date. What, then, does culture mean in nursing?

Think about the practice areas where you have been placed, and your first impressions of them. Was it noisy, quiet, welcoming, tidy or untidy? Did it feel chaotic or controlled? Were you made to feel welcome by the staff? Were they neatly dressed? Were there information boards charting how well the ward (or other area) was doing at meeting targets for infection control, pressure sores and patient satisfaction? Did you know who was in charge? Were patients attended to promptly? All of these first impressions are good indicators of how the area is run, and how clearly the staff understand what their purpose is. Over time, you would have noticed deeper signs, such as how handover was conducted, how different professions communicated with each other, whether patients were treated with kindness, and so on. All these factors, both immediate and subtle, influence the feel of the environment and its effectiveness. This complex interaction of people and place gives rise to the 'culture' of a given practice area. Clearly, becoming used to this culture (acculturated) is a highly complex process. You may have a great time on a given ward while one of your friends struggles; the 'cultural fit' is difficult to predict and more so to obtain.

One of the most far-reaching findings of the report into events at Mid-Staffordshire was that standards of nursing had deteriorated to an unacceptable level. Causes of this included 'inadequate staffing, poor leadership, poor recruitment, deficiencies in initial and continuing training, undervaluing of the nursing task and those who perform it, and declining professionalism' (Francis 2013, p. 1498). To counter this, the report suggested

518

that 'Much of what needs to be done does not require additional financial resources, but changes in attitudes, culture, values and behaviour' (Francis 2013, p. 1499). This is a controversial claim, given that low staffing levels caused by poor resourcing may have contributed to the problems noted (Paley 2014). At any rate, there was a high turnover of staff on the wards particularly affected and there must, therefore, have been acculturation taking place. People were starting to work there, and either leaving to find work elsewhere as they could not fit in, or staying and becoming effectively socialised into the negative culture of the wards. What was the difference between those who left and those who stayed? Was it that those who stayed were inherently less caring? If you think that this might be the explanation, here's a cautionary tale.

In 1971 a psychologist at Stanford University called Philip Zimbardo conducted an experiment in which he randomly divided a set of his students into two equal groups (Zimbardo 2008). One group were to be prison guards, and the other prisoners in a mock-up prison built in the basement of the university psychology department. The participants had been screened to check that they were in good mental and physical health and as far as possible it was ensured that there were no differences between them that would affect the outcome. The experiment was set to run for two weeks, but within days the 'guards' began to mistreat the 'prisoners' to such an extent that the experiment was ended. When questioned about their behaviour after the events, the 'guards' were troubled by the ease with which they had acted cruelly to the 'prisoners', although at the time, they were so absorbed in their roles, in the prison environment itself, that they had not stopped to think. Zimbardo concluded from this that the influence of the prison environment, the system, was so strong that it overwhelmed individuals' capacity to resist. In a neat phrase, he described the problem as a 'bad barrel', rather than 'bad apples'.

Think about the implications of this for you as a nurse. You will be given a uniform, a name badge, and authority over people. How will you ensure that you do not take the same road as some of the staff in the troubled wards at Mid-Staffordshire, or the 'Guards' of the Stanford Prison Experiment? Could it be that too successful an acculturation, perhaps through a preceptor, could make you more susceptible to negative acculturation? The answer to this must lie with you. You must accept full responsibility for your acts and omissions, as you would outside work. You must be able to retain a detached ability to judge whether the culture within which you are working is focused on providing the best possible patient care. Although the pressures of our lives can have a powerful influence on how we behave, it is up to us to retain agency:

It matters not how strait the gate,
How charged with punishments the scroll,
I am the master of my fate,
I am the captain of my soul.

(William Henley)

Barriers to successful preceptorship and how to overcome them

There will be times when your preceptorship experience does not proceed smoothly; indeed you may feel that it is not proceeding at all. There may be a number of factors contributing to this unfortunate situation, but broadly speaking they will be assignable to four major sources:

David Cudlip

- you (intrinsic factors);
- your preceptor (extrinsic factors);
- the organisation you work for (organisational factors);
- a combination of the above.

Even if you don't have any difficulties, your friends and colleagues might, and analysing their situations will help you to become the kind of preceptor you want to be when you are asked to take on the role. First, in order to work out where the problem lies, you'll have to reflect (yes, again!) very carefully on what you think and feel is going wrong. A clear-minded and honest review will be needed. This isn't always possible to do alone, because the preceptorship period can be emotionally and psychologically demanding. The strains of the situation can deplete your ability to take an objective view. Also, the intrinsic ability to do this varies between individuals. Therefore, you would do well to find a friend or colleague who knows you well, and whose opinion you trust. This person should be able to give you a full and honest appraisal of the situation, not just reassure you with platitudes or tell you what you want to hear. I have found that nurses tend to be very good at this; just the other day I was talking about a problem I'd had at work with a colleague and the person I was talking to suggested that I go and talk to the colleague about it. This simple solution had occurred to me, but for various reasons I had not done so. Let's use this simple scenario as the basis for what be considered under the 'intrinsic factors' heading, also known as 'What's my problem?'

Intrinsic factors

I am by nature averse to conflict, and have a tendency to leave discussion of problems too late, until I have become irritated or angry. In this way, my reluctance to raise issues early actually leads to a greater likelihood of conflict and I end up in the situation I wish to avoid by mistakenly confusing assertiveness with aggression. I am male, and part of me feels uneasy entering into potentially controversial conversations with female colleagues in case I appear to be overbearing. Here, I am being sexist and I need to realise that my colleagues are capable of defending their views and actions, and that I am able to make my points without being rude.

Before I was a nurse, I was an archaeologist. That line of work has a very different culture from nursing, and it would generally be seen as a bit odd to discuss emotional responses to colleagues' actions in an open and straightforward manner. Such discussions did take place, but usually at Christmas parties, and seldom ended well. I need to readjust to my current situation.

The above list (there's more, believe me) is not meant as a catalogue of excuses for my not taking what appears to be straightforward and obvious action to deal with a problem; rather it is an honest consideration of my reasons for not doing so. Note how irrational they are. Note also that these factors recur in my conduct and I have to guard against them all the time. It is possible that you will also have similar dysfunctional attitudes. There is no magic pill to resolve these, but I would say that being aware of when these issues are coming into play and colouring your perceptions will allow you to combat and hopefully overcome them.

Extrinsic factors

It may be that having reflected as honestly as you can, and perhaps having sought the opinions of a friend or colleague, that the source of your difficulties is your preceptor. The list of what can go wrong here is lengthy as we are dealing with human beings, but perhaps a straightforward way to reduce potential issues down to manageable proportions would be to look at the list of attributes of an effective preceptor drawn up by the DH (2010) and invert them. For example, perhaps your preceptor is not good at giving constructive feedback, either dwelling on the negative or simply saying that everything is okay when you think (or are told by others) that it isn't. Perhaps she does not set clear goals and assess competency adequately and you feel that either goals are unrealistic or too lax; that competency is either assumed or refuted unfairly.

In contrast to intrinsic factors, where a careful internal audit had value, there doesn't appear to be much point in you attempting to discover on a psychological level why your preceptor is not performing as you'd like. In any case, you need to find practical solutions to your challenges. What will help is the part I'm not good at: sit down and talk it through with your preceptor early on. Have a clear, objective list of concerns, and stay away from personal comments or vague, subjective statements. A large part of the art of being happy at work is getting along with those you wouldn't usually spend time with, so don't use personal incompatibility as a basis for these discussions. Following a good, honest and clear conversation, if either or both of you feel that a change is needed, then ensure that you have documented the discussion clearly in a way that satisfies both parties, and then approach your manager. Lack of time has been offered as a barrier to structured preceptorship programmes, and this will be familiar to many student nurses and mentors who struggle to find time to compete what is sometimes called 'paperwork'. There's no easy answer for this, except to give the activity a higher priority among competing demands.

Organisational factors

As we have discussed above, there is great variability in the provision of preceptorship programmes. You should gain a clear idea of what the organisation you intend to work for will offer you in this regard. If you feel that it is not adequate, yet you decide to accept their job offer on the basis of other factors then consider signing up to Flying Start to provide a clear structure and documentation for your portfolio. If on the other hand, your employer isn't providing what they said they would, then you need to be prepared either to move, or to hold them to account. The events at Mid-Staffordshire were as much about leadership as anything else. It may be that their omissions are easy to resolve; perhaps they need to provide a quiet space and time for you and your preceptor to discuss issues. On the other hand it may be that there is a lack of understanding of what they need to provide, in which case consider making a clear case to your manager. Although you may feel worried, consider this: would you want to work for an organisation that doesn't prioritise your professional development, aiming to help you to become the best nurse you can be? Perhaps by presenting your views in a clear and well-informed way, and displaying courage, you'll get yourself noticed in a positive light.

A combination of the above

A good example of this would be that your preceptor does not feel engaged with your development because he or she has been told rather than asked to carry out this role

521

(Kelly 2011). In such a case, it can be seen that two things have gone wrong: the organisation has not respected your preceptor's requirements for autonomy; also your preceptor has failed to take seriously their professional duties. In such a case as with those above, it will be pivotal to gain a clear understanding of what has happened and how people feel about it in order to formulate a plan. Although this sounds like a distraction from your nursing work, it is in fact precisely the process that your nursing assessment training should have provided you with the skills to carry out. Thus, at the end of this discussion it can be seen that the process of negotiating your preceptorship programme will provide you with experiences directly applicable to your clinical nursing work. Good luck!

CONCLUSION

In this chapter we have considered some of the features of transition to registered nurse. Schemes to aid transition are offered by many employers and while these generally are considered worthwhile there is little high quality evidence available to validate their use. When you first register you will lose, at a stroke, your protected status as a student nurse and gain the professional responsibility and autonomy that are the hallmarks of a profession. You will join over half a million other registered nurses in providing care for young and old, rich and poor at home and in hospital. Nursing has had a difficult time so far in this century and there are considerable challenges ahead. But you are joining a worthy profession with an honourable history and an exciting future.

SUGGESTED FURTHER READING

Burton R. and Ormrod, G. (2011) *Nursing: Transition to professional practice (prepare for practice)* Oxford: Oxford University Press.
Richards, A. and Richards S. L. (2012) *A Nurse's Survival Guide to the Ward* (3rd edn). Edinburgh: Churchill Livingstone.

REFERENCES

Bain, L. (1996) Preceptorship: a review of the literature. *Journal of Advanced Nursing* **24** (1), 104–107.
Benner, P. (1984) *From Novice to Expert: Excellence and power in clinical nursing practice*. Menlo Park, CA: Addison-Wesley.
Benner, P.,Tanner, C. and Chesla, C. (1996) *Expertise in Nursing Practice: Caring, clinical judgement and ethics*. New York: Springer.
Billay, D. and Myrick, F. (2007) Preceptorship: an integrative review of the literature. *Nurse Education in Practice* **8** (4), 258–266.
Cowan, F. and Flint, S. (2012) The importance of mentoring for junior doctors. *British Medical Journal* **7886** (345), 1–48.
Currie, L. and Watts, C. (2012) *Preceptorship and Pre-Registration Nurse Education: A rapid review.* London: The Willis Commission.
DH (Department of Health) (2010) *Preceptorship Framework for Newly Registered Nurses, Midwives and Allied Health Professionals.* London: DH.

DH (2013) *More Care, Less Pathway*. London: DH.

Edwards, D., Hawker, C., Carrier, J. and Rees, C. (2015) A systematic review of the effectiveness of strategies and interventions to improve the transition from student to newly qualified nurse. *International Journal of Nursing Studies* **52** (7), 1254–1268.

Francis, R. (2013) *Report of the Mid-Staffordshire NHS Foundation Trust Inquiry*. London: HMSO.

Gladwell, M. (2000) *The Tipping Point: How little things can make a big difference*. New York: Little, Brown.

Gobet, F. and Chassy, P. (2008) Towards an alternative to Benner's theory of expert intuition in nursing: a discussion paper. *International Journal of Nursing Studies* **45** (1), 129–139.

Health Education England (2015) *Raising the Bar: The Shape of Caring Review*. London: Health Education England.

Higgins, G., Spencer, R. and Kane, R. (2009) A systematic review of the experiences and perceptions of the newly qualified nurse in the United Kingdom. *Nurse Education Today* **30** (6), 499–508.

Kelly, M. (2011) Preceptorship in public health nursing. *Journal of Community Nursing* **25** (5), 10–15

Kramer, M. (1974) *Reality Shock: Why Nurses Leave Nursing*. St Louis, MO: Mosby.

Marks-Maran, D., Ooms, A., Tapping, J., Muir, J., Phillips, S. and Burke, L. (2013). A preceptorship programme for newly qualified nurses: a study of preceptees' perceptions. *Nurse Education Today* **33** (11), 1428–1434.

Meerabeau, E. (2001). Back to the bedpans: the debates over preregistration nursing education in England. *Journal of Advanced Nursing* **34** (4), 427–435.

Morgan, A., Mattison, J., Stephens, M. and Medows, S. (2011) Implementing structured preceptorship in an acute hospital. *Nursing Standard* **26** (28), 35–39.

Muir, J., Ooms, A., Tapping, J., Marks-Maran, D., Phillips, S. and Burke, L. (2013). Preceptors' perceptions of a preceptorship programme for newly qualified nurses. *Nurse Education Today* **33** (6), 633–638.

NHS (National Health Service) (2005) *Agenda for Change: NHS terms and conditions of service handbook*. London: NHS.

NHS (2015) *Agenda for Change: NHS pay bands and points 2015*. www.nhsemployers.org (accessed 23 January 2016).

NMC (Nursing and Midwifery Council) (2010) *Standards of Proficiency for Pre-registration Nursing*. London: NMC.

NMC (2014a) 70 per cent of nurses and midwives are missing out on over £170 a year. www.nmc.org.uk/news/news-and-updates/70-percent-of-nurses-and-midwives-are-missing-out-on-over-170-a-year/(accessed 23 January 2016).

NMC (2014b) Decision on the registration fee level. Board paper presented to Council meeting 1 October 2014. Contained in bundle of papers pp. 41–60. www.nmc.org.uk/globalassets/sitedocuments/councilpapersanddocuments/council-2014/october-council-open-papers-october-2014.pdf (accessed 23 January 2016).

NMC (2015a) *The Code: Professional standards for practice and behaviour for nurses and midwives*. London: NMC.

NMC (2015b) Revalidation. London: NMC. www.nmc.org.uk/globalassets/sitedocuments/revalidation/how-to-revalidate-booklet.pdf (accessed 23 January 2016).

OUP (Oxford University Press) (2015) *Oxford English Dictionary*. www.oed.com

Oxtoby, K. (2012) Vital support that pays off. *Nursing Standard* **26** (37), 64.

Paley, J. (1996) Intuition and expertise: comments on the Benner debate. *Journal of Advanced Nursing* **23** (4), 665–671.

Paley, J. (2014). Cognition and the compassion deficit: the social psychology of helping behaviour in nursing. *Nursing Philosophy*, **15** (4), 274–287.

Petitions (2015) No to proposed increases in fees for nurses and midwives. https://petition.parliament.uk/archived/petitions/60164 (accessed 23 January 2016).

David Cudlip

Robinson, S. and Griffiths, P. (2009) *Preceptorship for Newly Qualified Nurses: Impacts, facilitators and constraints*. London: National Nursing Research Unit.

Sardis, N. (1974) A review of *Reality Shock* by Marlene Kramer. *American Journal of Nursing* **75** (5), 691.

Snelling, P. C. (2015) Can the revised UK code direct practice? *Nursing Ethics*. Published online before print November 30, 2015, doi: 10.1177/0969733015610802

Whitehead, B., Owen, P., Henshaw, L., Beddingham, E. and Simmons, M. (2016) Supporting newly qualified nurse transition: a case study in a UK hospital. *Nurse Education Today* **36** (1), 58–63.

Zimbardo, P. (2008) *The Lucifer Effect: How good people turn evil*. London: Rider.

INDEX

Page numbers in *italics* denotes a figure/table